Basic Neurology
Second Edition

PERGAMON TITLES OF RELATED INTEREST

Garcia/DIAGNOSTIC NEUROPATHOLOGY
Hartman/NEUROPSYCHOLOGICAL TOXICOLOGY: Identification and Assessment of Human Neurotoxic Syndromes
Lavine/NEUROPHYSIOLOGY: The Fundamentals
Pansky/REVIEW OF NEUROSCIENCE, Second Edition
Smith/**van der Kooy**/BASIC NEUROANATOMY, Third Edition

RELATED JOURNALS
(Free sample copies available on request.)

Biogenic Amines
Brain Research Bulletin
Current Advances in Neuroscience
International Journal of Developmental Neuroscience
Neural Networks
Neurochemistry International
Neuropharmacology
Neuropsychologia
Neuroscience

Basic Neurology
Second Edition

John Gilroy,
M.D., F.R.C.P. (CAN), F.A.C.P.

Clinical Professor of Neurology, Wayne State University, Detroit, Michigan;
Chairman of Neurology, William Beaumont Hospital, Royal Oak, Michigan;
Former Professor and Chairman, Department of Neurology,
Wayne State University, Detroit, Michigan

PERGAMON PRESS

Member of Maxwell Macmillan Pergamon Publishing Corporation
New York • Oxford • Beijing • Frankfurt
São Paulo • Sydney • Tokyo • Toronto

U.S.A.	Pergamon Press, Inc., Maxwell House, Fairview Park, Elmsford, New York 10523, U.S.A.
U.K.	Pergamon Press plc, Headington Hill Hall, Oxford OX3 OBW, England
PEOPLE'S REPUBLIC OF CHINA	Pergamon Press, 0909 China World Tower, No. 1, Jian Guo Men Wai Avenue, Beijing 100004, People's Republic of China
FEDERAL REPUBLIC OF GERMANY	Pergamon Press GmbH, Hammerweg 6, D-6242 Kronberg, Federal Republic of Germany
BRAZIL	Pergamon Editora Ltda, Rua Eca de Querios, 346, CEP 04011, Paraiso, Sao Paulo, Brazil
AUSTRALIA	Pergamon Press Australia Pty Ltd., P.O. Box 544, Potts Point, N.S.W. 2011, Australia
JAPAN	Pergamon Press, 8th Floor, Matsuoka Central Building, 1-7-1 Nishishinjuku, Shinjuku-ku, Tokyo 160, Japan
CANADA	Pergamon Press Canada Ltd., Suite No. 271, 253 College Street, Toronto, Ontario, Canada M5T 1R5

Copyright © 1990 Pergamon Press, Inc.

All Rights Reserved. No part of this publication may be reproduced in a retrieval system or transmitted in any form or by any means: electronic, electrostatic, magnetic tape, mechanical, photocopying, recording or otherwise, without permission in writing from the publishers.

First Edition 1982
Second Edition 1990

Library of Congress Cataloging in Publication Data

Gilroy, John, 1925-
  Basic neurology/by John Gilroy.—2nd ed.
    p.   cm.
  Includes bibliographical references.
  ISBN 0-08-040297-6:   ISBN 0-08-040301-8 (soft):
  1. Nervous system—Diseases. 2. Neurology. I. Title.
  [DNLM: 1. Nervous System Diseases. WL 100 G486b]
  RC346.G53   1990
  616.8—dc20
  DNLM/DLC
  for Library of Congress   89-26650
                                                                        CIP

Printing: 1 2 3 4 5 6 7 8 9 10   Year: 0 1 2 3 4 5 6 7 8 9

Printed in the United States of America

⊗™ The paper used in this publication meets the minimum requirements of American National Standard for Information Sciences -- Permanence of Paper for Printed Library Materials, ANSI Z39.48-1984

PREFACE

The revision of a textbook is a combination of pleasure and challenge. The author is pleased and grateful that the previous edition has been well received and at the same time challenged to improve the new edition as much as possible. This challenge has been accepted in the preparation of the second edition of Basic Neurology where once again I have relied heavily on the suggestions made by medical students, residents, and fellow physicians in preparing the text.

There have been tremendous advances in neurology in the eight years that have passed since the first edition was published. Consequently, I have had to be selective in choosing new material for inclusion in the second edition. I have tried my best; there are bound to be omissions but I hope that the more important changes are included and the book continues to be well received by students and residents.

There is little to change in the first chapter. The neurologic evaluation remains firmly established as the keystone in neurological practice. It is time honored; a combination of art and science; a logical process which guides one to a diagnosis or differential diagnosis and which leads to a logical selection of the correct diagnostic procedures that are offered to the neurologist in increasing profusion. The exquisite anatomical detail of magnetic resonance imaging does not substitute for the careful sifting of evidence created by the clinical evaluation. Clinical neurology survives and is well.

The second chapter has been extensively revised and rewritten to reflect the increasing participation by neurologists in the emergency center and intensive care units. The remaining chapters contain a great deal of new material and have been brought up to date at the time of completion of the manuscript for the second edition. Chapter 11 has been deleted and completely rewritten as Strokes in Children and Young Adults. This change is more in keeping with a text largely devoted to adult neurology but also reflects the increasing knowledge about stroke in the younger population.

Most of the figures have been replaced with MR scans and up-to-date CT scans. In addition, I have added some excellent photographs of optic nerve and retinal abnormalities in the appropriate section. None of the line drawings have been replaced because the originals were so well produced. Credit should be given to the medical illustrator, Mr. Williams Loecher. Illustrations of the optic nerve and fundus, and the new MR and CT scans were produced by the Department of Medical Photography William Beaumont Hospital, Royal Oak, Michigan.

The revised manuscript was prepared by Karen Richardson, Regina Wierzbicki, and Teresa Maslowski, who were always willing to meet my deadlines often at short notice. I also wish to thank the medical section of Pergamon Press under the direction of Mr. Roger Dunn, who gave me total support and encouragement in the preparation of the second edition. The efficiency of the medical library at William Beaumont Hospital was outstanding and I am particularly grateful to Ellen Carey who obtained innumerable articles for me at short notice.

In addition, I am indebted to several colleagues at William Beaumont Hospital for advice in the preparation of the manuscript and selection of illustrations:

Wayne Burkle, Pharm. D.
Assistant Director of Pharmacy
Clinical Services
William Beaumont Hospital

Edward M. Cohn, M.D.
Chief, Section of Neuro-Ophthalmology
William Beaumont Hospital

Roger B. Fenton, D.O.
Medical Director
Magnetic Resonance Imaging Center of Michigan

Juliette Saad, M.D.
Neurologist
William Beaumont Hospital

Ay Ming Wang, M.D.
Co-Chief of Neuroradiology
William Beaumont Hospital

David Wesolowski, M.D.
Co-Chief of Neuroradiology
William Beaumont Hospital

John Gilroy, M.D.

CONTENTS

CHAPTER 1

THE NEUROLOGIC EVALUATION

The neurologic evaluation (See Table 1–1) should be conducted in a relaxed atmosphere. The examiner should face the patient, who may be accompanied by relatives or close friends, and all should be seated comfortably. Children aged six or older usually feel most secure when seated between parents, while younger children are less apprehensive when seated on the lap of one of the parents.

HISTORY

The history begins with the identification of the chief complaint. The patient may be asked, "Mr. X, why have you come to see me?" If the patient cannot answer the question through apparent failure of comprehension or lack of insight, the query should be addressed to those accompanying the patient. The individual answering can then be asked to supply the remainder of the history.

The chief complaint is the focal point of the history and is the key to the subsequent analysis of information leading to a differential diagnosis. Once the chief complaint has been identified, the examiner should record the history of the present illness in chronological order up to the time of the interview. This provides an excellent opportunity to analyze the information associated with the chief complaint and develop an appropriate differential diagnosis. The examiner must learn to encourage the flow of information and at the same time minimize the interjection of valueless statements made by the patient or relatives. The experienced examiner is polite, firm, and tactful in maintaining control of the interview and keeping the history "on track" so that the·maximum amount of relevant information is obtained. It is important to realize that patients and their relatives are usually incorrect in their interpretation of symptoms. There is a tendency to misconstrue statements made by other physicians and to misinterpret the results of diagnostic studies performed in the past.

It is often possible to obtain additional information by observation of the patient during the interview. The patient may appear to be comfortable, apprehensive, alert, or drowsy. The facial expression is important in assessing appropriate or inappropriate affect. Lack of facial expression may indicate depression, early parkinsonism, or failure of comprehension. Ptosis, involuntary eye movements, tics, myokymia, hemifacial spasm, or facial asymmetry may be observed during the interview. The examiner may see intermittent involuntary movements or tremors affecting the limbs, head, or trunk, or may observe abnormal posture as the interview proceeds. The interplay between the patient and spouse, relatives, or friends is important in determining closeness or conflict in their relationships and is apparent only on continuing observation.

1

History
  Chief complaint
  History of the present illness
  Neurologic review
  Past medical history
  Family history
  Social history

General Physical Examination

Neurologic Examination
  Mental status examination
    Speech, orientation, current events, judgment, insight, abstraction, vocabulary, perception, emotional response, memory, calculation, object recognition, praxis
  Cranial nerve examination
    I. Olfaction
    II. Visual acuity, ophthalmoscopic exam, visual fields
    III,IV,VI. Pupils, eye movements
    V. Corneal reflex; jaw jerk; sensation—face, scalp; motor function—muscles of mastication
    VII. Motor function—facial muscles; taste—anterior ⅔ tongue
    VIII. Hearing, equilibrium
    IX,X. Motor function, palate and pharynx, phonation, taste, posterior third of tongue
    XI. Motor function—sternocleidomastoid and trapezius
    XII. Motor function—tongue
  Motor
    Inspection, posture, tone, and power
  Coordination
    Rapid alternating movements, finger-to-nose and heel-to-shin tests
  Gait and station
    Gait testing, tandem gait, walking on heels and toes, Romberg test
  Sensory
    Touch, pinprick, vibration, position, and temperature senses
  Reflexes
    Stretch reflexes, plantar response, abdominal reflexes, release phenomena

The next step in the history is the neurologic review, which supplies additional information and is a logical extension of the history of the present illness. The neurologic review consists of a series of questions about the presence of common neurologic symptoms (see Table 1–2). If the answer is affirmative, the examiner must decide whether to continue interrogating the patient until the maximum amount of information is obtained or to discontinue questioning if the symptom adds little to the total picture. The decision to

disregard or pursue a positive response to a question is often a matter of experience or may be based on information already obtained from the patient. For example, the question "Do you suffer from headaches?" is likely to receive the answer "Yes" in the majority of cases. However, the examiner will benefit from additional questioning about headache only if the headache is of recent origin or if there has been a recent change in the frequency or severity of chronic headaches. A headache pattern that has been present and unchanged for many years, and is not the primary complaint, is unlikely to be related to the chief neurologic complaint. Conversely, if the examiner decides that the headache is relevant to the neurologic complaint, a series of subsidiary questions must be posed to the patient to obtain the maximum information about the headache. This includes such questions as: "How often does the headache occur? What factors precipitate the headache? When does it occur? Are there any early warning symptoms? Where is the pain? What kind of pain is it? How long does it last? Does anything relieve the pain? Does anything make it worse? Are there any associated symptoms during the headache? How do you feel after the headache has resolved?"

The question regarding visual symptoms is related to sudden dimness or blurring of vision which may occur in neurologic conditions such as transient cerebral ischemia or multiple sclerosis. For example, transient visual loss in one eye (amaurosis fugax) is a feature of internal carotid artery disease. The next series of questions on diplopia, hearing, tinnitus, and vertigo are related to the function of other cranial nerves and their central connections (the third, fourth, and sixth nerves, and the acoustic and vestibular divisions of the eighth nerve). The examiner is advised to avoid the use of the term "dizzy" and to seek clarification of the term if it is used by the patient. "Dizzy" or "dizziness" may be used to describe vertigo, ataxia, lightheadedness, transient impairment of consciousness, or minor seizure activity. These conditions are unrelated pathophysiologically, and the term "dizzy" is meaningless without clear definition.

There are several reasons for ataxia, including weakness, poor coordination, sensory loss, or transient impairment of consciousness. Focal weakness is a condition that alarms patients, and a history of recent focal weakness is usually obtained as one of the ini-

TABLE 1–2. Neurologic Review

Subject	Question
Headache	Do you suffer from headaches?
Visual symptoms	Have you experienced sudden dimness or sudden loss of vision in one or both eyes?
Diplopia	Have you had any double vision?
Hearing	Has there been any change in your hearing?
Tinnitus	Do you get any buzzing or ringing in your ears at any time?
Vertigo	Do you ever get a sensation that objects are moving around you or feel that you are moving or spinning?
Ataxia	Are you unsteady when you walk or are you clumsy when using your hands?
Focal weakness	Have you ever had weakness of an arm, hand, or leg on one side?
Focal numbness	Has there been any numbness or tingling involving an arm, hand, leg or any part of your body at any time?
Sphincter problems	Do you ever get a sensation that you may suddenly lose control of your bladder? Do you have to rush to the bathroom to empty your bladder? Have you ever lost control of your bladder?
Speech	Have you noticed any slurring of speech recently? Do you find that you are unable to understand other people or that you cannot produce the right word in conversation?
Writing	Has your writing changed recently?
Reading	Do you have any difficulty in reading or understanding what you have read?

TABLE 1–2. Continued

Subject	Question
Memory	Have you had any difficulty with memory recently?
Loss of consciousness	Have you ever lost consciousness, fainted, or felt that you were not aware of what was going on around you?

tial complaints. However, transient episodes may not be remembered unless the patient is asked about this symptom. Paradoxically, transient numbness or paresthesias affecting a limb or part of the trunk are often tolerated without seeking medical opinion and frequently forgotten if they resolve. Impairment of bladder function is not unusual with lesions at almost all levels of the central nervous system and in many peripheral neuropathies. Urgency, frequency, and incontinence frequently indicate impairment of neurologic control of the bladder in patients with suspected neurologic disease. However, the symptoms are often misinterpreted by patients and their physicians as bladder infections.

Obvious language problems are readily recognized as the patient communicates with the examiner, but many patients can recognize subtle changes in speech or recent difficulties in communication which may only be revealed by direct questioning. Writing is usually affected by any condition involving the function of the dominant hand. Deterioration in writing may be due to dysgraphia secondary to a lesion in the frontal or parietal lobe in the dominant hemisphere or may indicate weakness, tremor, ataxia, sensory loss, spasticity, or rigidity of the hand and upper limb. Thus, a change in writing is a nonspecific complaint but is often an early indication of impairment of the neuromuscular control of the hand. A problem with reading may occur in patients with visual failure or diplopia, or when there is a failure of comprehension of printed or written material. This latter condition is not uncommon in early dementia but will be uncovered only if the question is posed to the patient. Many patients with failing memory recognize this problem but are reluctant to disclose the symptom unless asked directly by the examiner. Thus, patients with early dementia frequently resort to writing notes to compensate for this situation. These notes are often produced during the interview, and the patient uses them as a guide when giving the history.

The last question in the neurologic review is concerned with impairment or loss of consciousness. The cause is apparent in the great majority of cases if the examiner listens carefully to the description of the syncopal episode and obtains a total picture of the event by direct questioning. The examiner should adopt the same approach to this problem whether the symptom is disclosed as the chief complaint, during the history of the present illness, or in the neurologic review. The patient must describe the attack, or each attack if there seem to be several types of syncopal episodes, from the time there was a sensation of something abnormal to loss of consciousness. If there appears to be some difficulty, the examiner might begin the process by saying: "I want you to describe the last attack for me. Can we go back to the time when you felt perfectly normal? I would like you to describe every event as it occurred until you lost consciousness." Having obtained the preictal history, the examiner should obtain as much information as possible about events after return of consciousness: "How did you feel? Were you confused? Now tell me everything you remember from that moment until you felt absolutely normal." The examiner now has a complete description of the preictal and postictal symptoms. The patient cannot, of course, describe events during loss of consciousness, and this gap should be closed by questioning an observer. However, the observer may augment the information already given by the patient regarding the preictal and postictal states. Therefore, the observer should be asked to describe the state of the patient from the moment that there seemed to be some abnormality up to the loss of consciousness. This is followed by observations during loss of consciousness, and finally a description of events that occurred from the moment the patient recovered consciousness up to the time that the patient appeared to be functioning normally. In the great majority of cases the combined description by the patient and observer should give the examiner a clear history of the attack and provide sufficient information for diagnosis.

The interview now continues with the recording of the past medical history, family history, and social history.

The past medical history should be recorded in chronological order beginning with any unusual diseases during childhood. A history of systemic disease such as diabetes mellitus or hypertension is important.

The family history is important for two reasons. A number of neurologic conditions are inherited, and there will be a strong family history of neurologic problems when the condition is inherited as an autosomal dominant trait. A sex-linked recessive form of inheritance is apparent when only males are affected. Many patients with cerebrovascular disease have a family history of stroke, diabetes, hypertension, and/or ischemic heart disease. The examiner should inquire about the presence of these conditions in family members.

The social history includes questions about the patient's occupation. The physician should learn something about the activities of people in the community and show an interest in the patient's occupation. This helps to form a rapport with the patient and may provide useful information. Questions about smoking, alcohol consumption, and the use of drugs are routine during the social history. Patients should be asked about exposure to any unusual chemical or toxic substances. The examiner should record the marital status of the patient, the number of children, and the health of the children.

Finally, a list of all medications used in the preceding two years, the reason for prescription, and possible side effects to the drugs should be obtained.

GENERAL PHYSICAL EXAMINATION

Many neurologic problems are associated with systemic diseases, and the patient should have a general physical examination either before or following the neurologic examination. During this examination the blood pressure should be measured with the patient lying prone, immediately followed by measuring the blood pressure with the patient standing erect, to detect any tendency toward postural hypotension. This procedure should be routine in all examinations, but it is particularly important to look for postural hypotension in patients with cerebrovascular disease or Parkinson's disease, in patients taking antihypertensive medication, and in all elderly patients.

NEUROLOGIC EXAMINATION

The neurologic examination begins with the assessment of mental status.

MENTAL STATUS EXAMINATION

Speech

Since most of the mental status examination requires verbal communication, the first task in assessing mental status should be an assessment of language functioning. The exchange of information between the patient and the examiner has already given the examiner an opportunity to make an assessment of the patient's ability to communicate and to express ideas. During this period of observation it may be possible to identify the presence of dysarthria, dysphonia, or dysphasia.

Dysarthria may be defined as difficulty in articulation. Dysarthria is due to some abnormality in the neuromuscular control of the articulation process. In practice, this usually means difficulty in movements of the palate, tongue, and/or lips during articulation.

Dysphonia is a difficulty in phonation with alteration in the normal volume and tone of the voice. Dysphonia occurs in the presence of neuromuscular impairment of function involving the vocal cords or palate.

Dysphasia is a difficulty with comprehension or production of language due to disease involving the cerebral hemisphere. Total loss of language function is termed aphasia. There are several types of dysphasia, each producing a pattern of abnormalities that can be recognized in conversation with the patient and by a number of simple tests. Recognition and classification of dysphasia require an understanding of language function, which is an extremely complex subject. A simplified concept of language function is illustrated in Figure 1-1.

All auditory stimuli are transmitted from the periphery through the auditory system to the primary auditory areas in Heschl's gyrus in both temporal lobes. In the dominant hemisphere the information is directed from the primary auditory area directly to the auditory association area in the posterior aspect of the superior temporal lobe. Information from the nondominant hemisphere is transmitted through the corpus callosum to the auditory association area in the dominant hemisphere. This area can be regarded as a word identification center and has long been termed Wernicke's area. Once the sound has been identified as a language symbol, the information is transmitted to a word recognition area which probably lies in the inferior portion of the parietal lobe in the dominant hemisphere. Recognition of the language symbol is based on past experience, and the function of the language recognition area is not only the recognition of language symbols but also the relationship of one symbol to another. When this function has been accomplished, information is transmitted back to or through Wernicke's area to areas of the brain concerned with encoding of or response to language. The generation of language by an individual is probably mediated through the word recognition area, followed by passage of information to the word identification area. Communication is established between the word identification area and a motor encoding area via association fibers, which connect

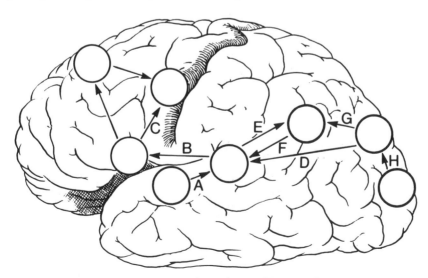

FIGURE 1-1. A simplified concept of language function.

the posterior portion of the superior temporal gyrus to the opercular area of the frontal lobe. The motor encoding area (Broca's area) is responsible for the preliminary conversion of language symbols into motor activity. Information from the motor encoding area is then transmitted to the primary motor area of the dominant hemisphere to be converted into the necessary motor movements, which produce speech. At the same time there is a communication from Broca's area to the supplementary motor area, which lies on the medial aspect of the superior frontal gyrus. There is a further communication from the supplementary motor area to the primary motor area. This reflex loop from Broca's area through the supplementary motor area to the primary motor area seems to be responsible for the smooth conversion of information in the primary motor area into impulses that generate speech.

Visual language symbols are received as visual impulses in the primary visual center in the occipital lobes of both hemispheres. Information is then passed to the visual association areas where object recognition and identification of language symbols occur. There are two main pathways from the visual association areas concerned with language. In the first pathway information from the dominant visual association area passes directly to the word identification area. Information from the nondominant visual association area crosses to the dominant hemisphere via the corpus callosum. Information concerned with object-naming passes from both visual association areas to the word recognition area in the dominant hemisphere. At this time, impulses concerned with object-naming enter the language system and are transmitted forward through Wernicke's area.

It is possible to recognize 13 abnormal conditions in comprehension or production of language. The 13 conditions are outlined in Table 1–3.

Testing Language Function. History-taking provides an opportunity to detect language problems. There is no difficulty in cases with a well-developed dysphasia, but subtle dysphasic states may not be noticed unless the examiner is alert and attuned to the flow of language. Under these circumstances it may be possible to identify:

1. Minor difficulties in expression
2. Occasional failure to comprehend simple statements
3. Occasional failure to name an object
4. A tendency toward circumlocution

Formal testing of language function should include the following:

1. Asking the patient if there is any difficulty in finding the right word during conversation
2. Showing the patient several familiar objects (e.g., watch, ring, pencil, comb, key, etc.) and asking the patient to name each object
3. Asking the patient to repeat a simple phrase
4. A verbal request to perform simple acts (e.g., close your eyes, put out your tongue)
5. A similar request, as in #4, with the instructions written on cards
6. Selecting a passage from a newspaper or magazine and asking the patient to read and then to give an interpretation of the material that has been read
7. Asking the patient to write his name and to write a simple sentence without prompting
8. The patient copies a simple sentence written by the examiner

The remainder of the patient's mental status examination can now be conducted with the examiner making allowances for any deficits in comprehension or communication detected in the patient.

The first task is to ascertain the patient's general cerebral functioning.

Orientation

Orientation to time, place, and person indicates an ability to correlate environmental clues with past experience. The patient should be asked:

1. The day of the week
2. The date
3. The name of the building where the examination is taking place
4. The occupation of the examiner

Current Events

A knowledge of current events requires intact orientation, recent memory, and the ability to think in an abstract fashion. The patient should be asked to give the name of the President of the United States, the governor of the state, and the mayor of the city. This is followed by a request for information on current events anywhere in the world with an interpretation of these events.

TABLE 1–3. Abnormalities in the Comprehension or Production of Language (see Fig. 1–1)

Area Involved	Language Impairment	Language Functions Retained	Synonym
Primary auditory area (bilateral)	Comprehension of spoken language, repetition of spoken language. Patient does not respond to nonlanguage sounds	Spontaneous speech, naming objects, reading comprehension	Cortical deafness, auditory agnosia
Connection A	Comprehension of spoken language, repetition of spoken language	Spontaneous speech, naming objects, reading comprehension	Pure word deafness
Auditory association area (Wernicke's area)	Comprehension of spoken language, repetition of spoken language, naming comprehension of written language, spontaneous speech	None. Spoken language is fluent but impaired (jargon)	Wernicke's aphasia
Connection B	Repetition of spoken language, spontaneous speech, naming, reading aloud, writing	Comprehension, spoken language is fluent but paraphasic	
Motor encoding area (Broca's area)	Spontaneous speech, repetition, reading aloud, naming (but recognizes object), writing	Comprehension of both spoken and written language	Broca's aphasia
Connection C	Spontaneous speech nonfluent, reading aloud, naming (but recognizes objects), writing	Comprehension of both spoken and written language, repetition	Transcortical motor aphasia
Supplementary motor area	Spontaneous speech, flow of speech impaired and irregular	All other language functions retained	Supplementary motor aphasia
Connection D	Comprehension of written language, reading aloud	Normal except for reading	Alexia without agraphia
Connection E	Comprehension of spoken language, comprehension of written language	Repetition, naming objects, reading without comprehension	Transcortical aphasia, naming intact
Word recognition area	Comprehension of spoken and written language, reading aloud, naming objects, writing	Repetition, spoken language, fluent paraphasia and echolalia	Transcortical sensory aphasia
Connection F	Naming objects, spontaneous speech	Repetition, comprehension of both spoken and written language. Spoken language fluent but rambling and vague.	Nominal aphasia (anomic aphasia)
Connection G	Naming objects	All other language functions intact	Associative agnosia without alexia
Connection H	Naming objects, naming colors, reading aloud, comprehension of written language	Comprehension of spoken language	Visual agnosia

7

Judgment

The ability to give a reasonable assessment of the situation or a failure to do so may be apparent from the examiner's contact with the patient up to this point. Judgment may, however, be tested by asking the patient to interpret a simple story requiring judgment.

Example 1. What would you do if you were walking along a street and saw an envelope lying on the sidewalk? The envelope is sealed, addressed, and has an unused stamp in the corner.

Correct Answer. Pick it up and mail it.

Incorrect Answer. Pick it up, open it, and read it or leave it alone.

Example 2. What would you do if you were sitting in the middle of a crowded theater and you were the first person to notice that smoke was pouring out of a ventilator?

Correct Answer. Get up quietly, find an usher or the manager and inform him that this was occurring and request immediate action.

Incorrect Answer. Stand up and shout "Fire."

Insight

Insight may be defined as the awareness of a reason for a given situation. An experienced examiner can usually tell whether insight is intact on obtaining the history from the patient. When there is doubt, the patient may be asked to give an explanation for consulting the examiner.

Abstraction

Abstraction is an intellectual function of high order requiring comprehension, understanding, and judgment. This can usually be tested by asking the patient to interpret proverbs such as:

1. Don't put all of your eggs in one basket.
2. People in glass houses should not throw stones.
3. The grass is always greener on the other side of the fence.

The patient may fail to interpret the proverb, give a concrete interpretation such as "It might break the glass" in response to proverb 2, or make a correct abstract interpretation of the proverb.

Another way of testing abstract thinking is to ask for similarities and differences. Example: "What is similar about a bicycle and an airplane?"

Vocabulary

The examiner is now in a position to assess the patient's vocabulary, which is one of the best methods of assessing the patient's premorbid intellectual capacity. Patients with progressive dementia tend to retain a premorbid vocabulary which often gives a false impression of their intellectual abilities. When dementia is suspected, the patient should be asked to give the definition of words presented at increasing levels of difficulty, for example, dog, winter, assemble, reluctant, tangible, and abstruse.

Perception

Perceptual difficulties are often experienced by patients with neurologic problems. The following may be encountered:

Delusion. A delusion is a false belief.

Illusion. An illusion is a false interpretation of a sensory perception.

Hallucination. An hallucination is a false sensory perception which does not result from an external stimulus.

Déjà Vu Phenomenon. This phenomenon is a sudden feeling by the patient that he or she has experienced an event in the past identical to the event that is occurring at the time of the experience (e.g., the patient suddenly has an intense feeling that he or she has been in the examiner's office in the past, having never done so). The déjà vu phenomenon is not unusual in patients with disease involving the temporal lobes, particularly in partial complex seizures (psychomotor seizures).

Emotional Response

It is not unusual to obtain a history of change in mood when a patient has a neurologic problem. In addition, chronic diseases and ill health often result in depression that may be obvious to the examiner. Nevertheless, it is useful to inquire whether there has been a change of mood and to assess this change in terms of depression, elation, irritability, anger, or anxiety. At the same time an estimate of the patient's affect should also be made. Affect may be defined as an emotional response to a situation. The response may be appropriate or flat. An example of an inappropriate response would be laughter while discussing an obviously sad situation or spontaneous laughter during the interview, suggesting hypomania or euphoria. A patient who fails to show an appropriate emotional response is said to have inappropriate affect. A patient with flat affect has little or no emotional response. Patients with bilateral damage to the cerebral hemispheres lose finer control of emotional response. Their response may be said to be "all or none." Usually this takes the form of crying in a situation that would normally produce only a mild emotional response. Pathologic laughing is less frequently encountered. These types of emotional response are usually associated with pseudobulbar palsy, with bilateral spasticity and rigidity indicating damage to both cerebral hemispheres.

Memory

A number of the tests employed in the mental status examination evaluate a function mediated through a well-recognized anatomic site in the brain. Abnormalities in a specific test may therefore indicate some abnormality in a focal area of the brain.

Both recent and remote memory depend upon the integrity of the hippocampal complex in the temporal lobes. Progressive disease involving the temporal lobes usually results in loss of recent memory with retention of remote memory. Loss of memory for remote events indicates severe involvement of both cerebral hemispheres. The formation of a memory requires the retention of information. The ability to retain information may be tested by asking the patient to remember the names of three objects, two similar and one dissimilar, for a fixed period of time (e.g., three minutes) and then asking the patient to recall the names of those objects. This test should not present any difficulty. If the patient fails to recall the names, an assessment of the deficit of retention and recall can be gauged by presenting the patient with the names of three additional objects, continuing the examination, and then asking the patient to recall the names of the objects after two-and-a-half minutes. The time scale is reduced progressively by 30 seconds when the patient fails to answer correctly, until an assessment of the period of time taken to retain and recall the information is obtained. The most severe failure of retention and recall occurs in acute lesions involving the temporal lobes such as *Herpes simplex* encephalitis or Korsakoff's psychosis.

Calculation

Recognition and intellectual manipulation of mathematical symbols depend upon the integrity of the angular gyrus in the dominant hemisphere. This faculty can be tested by asking the patient to perform simple arithmetic problems such as subtracting seven from 100, then subtracting seven from the result and continuing to do this in serial fashion (reversed serial sevens). If the patient fails to perform serial sevens, the patient should be asked to perform simple addition. Difficulty with subtraction or simple addition is called dyscalculia. Failure to utilize mathematical symbols constitutes acalculia.

Object Recognition

The individual may recognize an object by use of one or more of the primary senses. Agnosia may be defined as a failure to recognize objects in the presence of adequate primary sensation. A number of agnosias recognized in clinical practice include:

Visual Agnosia. Visual agnosia is the failure to recognize an object visually in the presence of adequate vision and suggests that the patient may be suffering from a lesion involving the visual association areas of the brain. In this condition the patient can see the object but cannot recognize or name it. It is possible to exclude nominal aphasia if the patient can name the object by tactile contact. There are a number of subtypes of visual agnosia, including failure to recognize familiar surroundings and failure to maintain orientation in a previously known environment *(visual spatial agnosia)*.

Finger agnosia. Finger agnosia is a condition in which the patient shows inability to identify fingers on request (e.g., "Show me your right index finger; now show me your left thumb"). Finger agnosia is often associated with right-left disorientation *(allochiria)*, agraphia, and acalculia. These symptoms constitute Gerstmann's syndrome and are associated with lesions involving the angular gyrus in the dominant hemisphere.

Autotopagnosia. Autotopagnosia is a failure to recognize a body part. The patient with this affliction may fail to recognize his own hand or arm and may readily accept the examiner's hand or arm as a substitute. This condition occurs in lesions of the nondominant parietal lobe.

Anosognosia. Anosognosia is denial of disease and is a condition in which the patient will deny loss of function of a body part. The loss of function is usually severe and the patient may, for example, deny paralysis in the presence of an obvious hemiplegia. Anosognosia is a feature of disease of the posterior frontal and parietal lobes of the brain and is more often seen when the lesion involves the nondominant hemisphere.

Tactile Agnosia. Tactile agnosia is a condition in which there is failure to recognize an object by palpation in the absence of a primary sensory deficit. The condition is sometimes called *astereognosis* and occurs with lesions involving the nondominant parietal lobe.

Auditory Agnosia. Auditory agnosia is a failure to identify the meaning of sounds in the presence of adequate hearing. Auditory agnosia occurs when there is bilateral damage to the primary auditory cortex.

Praxis

Dyspraxia may be defined as difficulty or absence (apraxia) of ability to perform a planned motor activity in the absence of paralysis of the muscles normally used in the performance of that act.

A number of dyspraxic states are recognized:

Ideational Apraxia. In this condition the patient is unable to formulate a plan of action. The request to perform the act is clearly understood, but the patient is unable to develop a sequence of activities that will result in the movement necessary to complete the requested action. This condition is said to resemble absentmindedness. The patient is asked to pour water from a jug into a glass and then drink the water from the glass. The patient may fail to pour the water into the glass and attempt to lift the empty glass to his lips or may lift the jug and take a drink of water directly from the jug.

Ideomotor Apraxia. This condition occurs when there is failure to transmit the plan of action and convert the plan into motor movement in the frontal lobes of the brain. Patients with ideomotor apraxia may be unable to close the eyes on request, yet are seen to blink spontaneously; they may be unable to protrude the tongue on request yet tongue movements are adequate in conversation. Patients with ideomotor apraxia have great difficulty in performing simple tasks such as dressing, combing the hair, and using eating utensils.

Motor Apraxia. Motor apraxia is an inability to perform finely coordinated skilled movements in the absence of weakness or paralysis of the involved muscles. This presents as a loss of dexterity in handling small objects, particularly in the performance of rapid finger movements.

Constructional Apraxia. Constructional apraxia is an inability to construct simple models or simple designs, although visual perception and object recognition are intact and there is no apparent paralysis of muscles of the hands. Patients with constructional apraxia cannot copy simple designs or copy simple models with wooden blocks. The condition appears to be a failure of revisualization of the task and occurs in the presence of lesions affecting the visual association areas in the posterior portion of the parietal lobe. Constructional apraxia is often considered to be indicative of involvement of the visual association areas in the nondominant hemisphere, but it is probable that the condition is more apparent with nondominant hemisphere involvement because of the preservation of language.

CRANIAL NERVE EXAMINATION

The cranial nerve examination should be carried out in an orderly and efficient manner. Table 1–4 lists the cranial nerves, their components, their function, and the clinical findings with lesions. Figures 1–2 and 1–3 illustrate the sensory and motor cranial nerve nuclei and their approximate location in the brainstem.

The First Nerve (Olfactory Nerve)

Anatomy. The peripheral portion of the olfactory system consists of nerve endings which arise from bipolar cells located in the mucous membrane of the upper portion of the nasal cavity. The central processes of the bipolar cells pass in bundles through the cribriform plate of the ethmoid bone to enter the olfactory bulb on the floor of the anterior cranial fossa. These afferent fibers synapse with the dendrites of the mitral and tufted cells in the olfactory bulb, and the axons of the mitral cells pass through the olfactory bulb and divide into medial and lateral olfactory striae. Fibers in the medial olfactory striae terminate in the paraolfactory area, subcallosal gyrus, and the inferior portion of the cingulate gyrus. Fibers from the lateral olfactory striae enter the gyriform area, which contains the uncus and the anterior portion of the hippocampal gyrus.

The rhinencephalon (olfactory bulbs, olfactory tracts, olfactory striae, and central connections) constitutes one of the phylogenetically oldest portions of the cerebral hemisphere, and olfaction plays a major role in the functional response of many animals. Consequently, there are several anatomic pathways that connect the olfactory areas of the frontal

TABLE 1–4. Components and Functions of Cranial Nerves

Cranial Nerve		Component° and Location	Function	Clinical Findings with Lesion
Olfactory (I)	SVA	Neurosensory cells of sup. nasal concha and upper ⅓ of nasal septum → bipolar cells of olfactory epithelium → olfactory bulb	Smell	Anosmia
Optic (II)	SSA	Bipolar cells of retina → ganglion cell layer of retina → lateral geniculate → visual cortex	Vision	Amaurosis, anopia
Oculomotor (III)	GSE	Oculomotor nucleus → levator palpebrae; medial, sup., inf. recti; inf. oblique	Eye movements	Diplopia, ptosis
	GVE	Edinger-Westphal nucleus → ciliary and episcleral ganglia to sphincter pupillae and ciliary muscle	Pupillary constriction, accommodation	Mydriasis, loss of accommodation
Trochlear (IV)	GSE	Trochlear nucleus → superior oblique	Eye movement	Diplopia
Trigeminal (V)	GSA	Sensory endings of skin of face, mucous membranes, teeth, orbital contents, supratentorial meninges → trigeminal ganglion → spinal trigeminal and chief sensory nucleus	General sensation	Numbness of face
	GSA	Muscles of mastication and ext. ocular muscles → mesencephalic nucleus	Proprioception	———
	SVE	Motor nucleus → masseters, temporalis, pterygoids, mylohyoid, tensor tympani, ant. belly digastric	Mastication	Weakness, wasting
Abducens (VI)	GSE	Abducens nucleus → lateral rectus	Eye movement	Diplopia
Facial (VII)	SVA	Taste buds of ant. ⅔ tongue → chorda tympani → geniculate ganglion → rostral tractus solitarius	Taste	Loss of taste ant. ⅔ tongue
	GVA	Sensory receptors of tonsil, soft palate and middle ear to geniculate ganglion → caudal tractus solitarius	General sensation	———
	GSA	Sensory receptors of ext. auditory meatus and ext. ear → geniculate ganglion → spinal trigeminal nucleus	General sensation	———
	GVE	Sup. salivatory nucleus → greater petrosal n. → pterygopalatine ganglion → maxillary n. → lacrimal gland, nasal and palatal mucosa: chorda tympani to lingual → submandibular post. gang. to submandibular and sublingual glands	Secretion	Dry mouth, loss of lacrimation
	SVE	Motor nucleus → facial muscles, stylohyoid, and post. belly digastric	Facial expression	Paralysis of upper and lower facial muscles

TABLE 1–4.   Continued

Cranial Nerve		Component° and Location	Function	Clinical Findings with Lesion
Vestibulocochlear (VIII)	SSA	Hair cells of organ of Corti → bipolar cells of spiral ganglion → dorsal and ventral cochlear nucleus	Hearing	Deafness, tinnitus
	SSA	Hair cells of crista ampullae, semicircular canals and maculae of saccule and utricle → vestibular nuclei and cerebellum	Equilibrium	Vertigo, dysequilibrium, nystagmus
Glossopharyngeal (IX)	SVA	Taste buds post. ⅓ tongue → inf. petrosal ganglion → rostral tractus solitarius	Taste	Loss taste post. ⅓ tongue
	GVA	Sensory receptors of ant. surface epiglottis, root of tongue, border of soft palate, uvula, tonsil, pharynx, auditory tube, carotid sinus and body → caudal tractus solitarius	General sensation	Anesthesia of pharynx
	GSA	Sensory receptors of middle and external ear → geniculate ganglion → spinal trigeminal nucleus	General sensation	————
	SVE	Nucleus ambiguus → stylopharyngeus	Elevates pharynx	————
	GVE	Inf. salivatory nucleus → tympani nerve to → lesser petrosal nerve → otic ganglion → auriculotemporal n. → parotid gland	Secretion	Partial dry mouth
Vagus (X)	SVA	Taste buds in region of epiglottis → inf. (nodose) ganglion → rostral tractus solitarius	Taste	————
	GVA	Sensory receptors post. surface epiglottis, larynx, trachea, bronchi, esophagus, stomach, small intestine, ascending and transverse colon → inf. (nodose) ganglion → caudal tractus solitarius	General sensation	————
	GSA	Sensory receptors in ext. ear and meatus → sup. (jugular) ganglion → spinal trigeminal nucleus	General sensation	————
	SVE	Nucleus ambiguus → pharyngeal constrictor and intrinsic muscles of larynx, palatal muscles	Delglutition, phonation	Dysphagia, hoarseness, palatal paralysis
	GVE	Dorsal motor nucleus → thoracic and abdominal viscera	Cardiac depress., visceral movement, secretion	————
Spinal accessory (XI)	SVE	Caudal nucleus ambiguus → vagus → muscles of larynx	Phonation	Hoarseness
	GSE	Ant. horn cells C1–5 → sternocleidomastoid and trapezius	Head and shoulder movement	Weakness, wasting
Hypoglossal (XII)	GSE	Hypoglossal nucleus → muscles of tongue	Tongue movements	Weakness, wasting

° GSA—general somatic afferent, GSE—general somatic efferent, GVA—general visceral afferent, GVE—general visceral efferent, SSA—special somatic afferent, SVA—special visceral afferent, SVE—special visceral efferent.

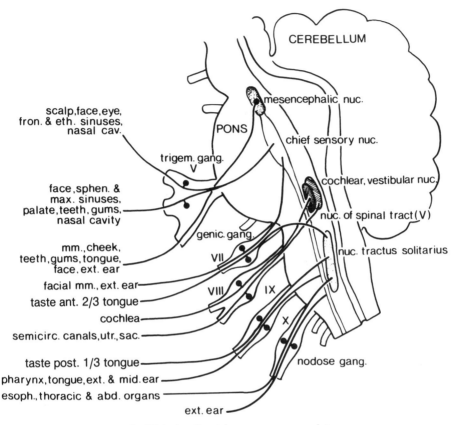

FIGURE 1–2. Cranial nerve sensory nuclei.

and temporal lobe to the hypothalamus, thalamus, and brainstem nuclei. Thus, olfactory stimuli give rise to autonomic responses that are well developed and often critical to survival in lower animals but are less essential in man.

Examination of the Olfactory Nerve. The patient is asked to close the eyes and inhale with one nostril occluded as the examiner brings the test substance close to the nonoccluded side. Test substances, which must be nonirritating, include, freshly ground coffee, tobacco, or volatile oil solutions such as oil of lavender, oil of cloves, or oil of lemon. Each nostril is tested separately, and the examiner notes that inhalation is adequate, then requests the patient to identify the test substance. A consistent loss of sense of smell on one side, unilateral anosmia, is usually more significant than a bilateral loss, unless the patient's chief complaint is of sudden total anosmia. Unilateral anosmia is indicative of a lesion involving the olfactory nerves, olfactory bulb, or olfactory tract. Central lesions in the hemispheres do not produce anosmia because

of the decussation of olfactory fibers in the anterior commissure.

Many neurologists omit tests of olfaction unless the clinical examination is abnormal and indicates that examination for loss of the sense of smell might give a positive result. A unilateral anosmia suggests compression of the olfactory bulb or olfactory tract by a frontal lobe abscess or glioma, olfactory groove meningioma, sphenoid ridge meningioma, and pituitary and parasellar tumors. Tumors may extend posterolaterally to involve the ipsilateral optic nerve causing optic atrophy. The same tumor mass may also cause increased intracranial pressure with papilledema of the opposite optic nerve. The combination of unilateral anosmia with ipsilateral optic atrophy and contralateral papilledema is known as the Foster-Kennedy syndrome.

The Second Nerve (Optic Nerve) and Visual System

Anatomy of the Visual System. Retina. The receptors for visual stimuli are of two types—rods and cones—and are the outer

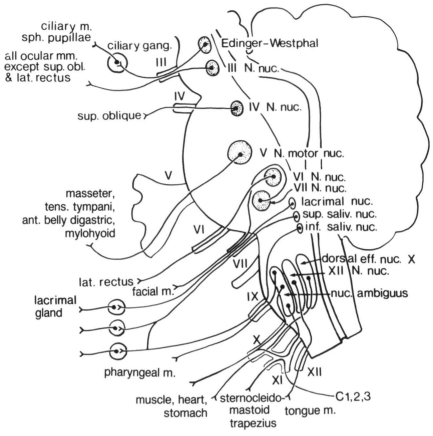

ciliary m.
sph. pupillae
ciliary gang.
Edinger–Westphal
all ocular mm.
except sup. obl.
& lat. rectus
III
III N. nuc.
IV
sup. oblique
IV N. nuc.
V N. motor nuc.
V
VI N. nuc.
VII N. nuc.
masseter,
tens. tympani,
ant. belly digastric,
mylohyoid
lacrimal nuc.
sup. saliv. nuc.
inf. saliv. nuc.
VI
dorsal eff. nuc. X
XII N. nuc.
VII
nuc. ambiguus
lat. rectus
facial m.
IX
lacrimal
gland
X
pharyngeal m.
XI
XII
muscle, heart,
stomach
sternocleido-
mastoid
trapezius
tongue m.
C1,2,3

FIGURE 1–3. Cranial nerve motor nuclei.

segments of the cells in the outer nuclear cell layer. The rods and cones are specialized photosensitive receptors. The cell bodies of the rods and cones are located in the outer nuclear layer of the retina and the afferent processes synapse with dendrites of bipolar cells lying in the bipolar cell layer. The bipolar cells in turn synapse with dendrites of ganglion cells lying in the ganglion cell layer of the retina. The unmyelinated axons of the ganglion cells converge in centripetal fashion in the superficial, nerve fiber layer of the retina and from the optic nerve.

Optic Nerve. The optic nerve is situated slightly to the nasal side of the retina. The fibers that compose the optic nerve become myelinated as they pierce the lamina cribrosa of the sclera. The optic nerve courses caudally and medially, surrounded by a sheath of dura, arachnoid, and pia. It traverses the optic foramen of the orbit accompanied by the ophthalmic artery and is joined by the central artery of the retina. The course within the cranial cavity is short and the optic nerve

is closely related to the olfactory tract, internal carotid, and anterior cerebral arteries as it terminates in the optic chiasm.

Optic Chiasm. The optic chiasm is located superior and slightly anterior to the pituitary fossa, pituitary gland, and infundibulum. The anterior communicating artery lies superior and just anterior to the optic chiasm, and the lamina terminalis and hypothalamus are immediately superior to the chiasm.

Nerve fibers from the nasal half of each retina decussate in the optic chiasm and enter the opposite optic tract. Fibers from the inferior nasal quadrant of the retina loop forward into the opposite optic nerve just before they turn into the optic tract (see Figure 1–4).

Optic Tract. The optic tract receives fibers from the temporal half of the ipsilateral retina and the nasal half of the contralateral retina (see Figure 1–4). The optic tract passes posterolaterally around the cerebral peduncle and terminates in the lateral geniculate body of the thalamus. The infundibulum

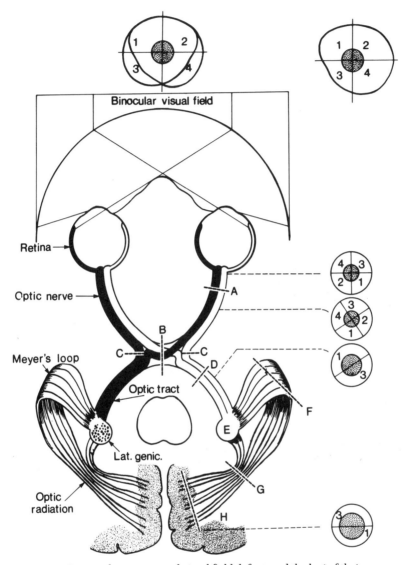

FIGURE 1–4. Commonly encountered visual field defects and the loci of their corresponding lesions.

A. Right anopsia
B. Bitemporal hemianopsia
C. Binasal hemianopsia
D. Left homonymous hemianopsia
E. Left homonymous hemianopsia
F. Left homonymous superior quadrantanopsia
G. Left homonymous inferior or superior hemianopsia
H. Left homonymous hemianopsia

and tuber cinereum of the hypothalamus lie between the two optic tracts anteriorly, and each optic tract is closely related to the posterior communicating and posterior cerebral arteries.

Optic Radiation. The optic radiation arises from the lateral geniculate body and passes laterally in the retrolenticular portion of the internal capsule anterior to the descending portion of the lateral ventricle. Fibers that arise in the medial portion of the lateral geniculate body, which represent the lower visual fields, pass dorsally along the lateral wall of the posterior horn of the lateral ventricle and terminate in the superior lip of the calcarine fissure. Fibers from the lateral portion of the lateral geniculate body, which represent the upper visual fields, pass forward in the roof of the temporal horn of the lateral ventricle. They then loop backward (Meyer's loop) and pass inferiorly into the parietal lobe in the lateral wall of the posterior horn of the lateral ventricle and terminate in the inferior lip of the calcarine fissure.

Examination of the Visual System. Examination and interpretation of abnormalities of the visual system can be performed satisfactorily only if the examiner has an adequate knowledge of the anatomy and physiology of the optic nerve and its peripheral and central connections. The examination is divided into three parts:

1. Visual acuity
2. Ophthalmoscopic examination
3. Plotting of visual fields

Visual Acuity. The examination of visual acuity involves evaluation of distant vision and near vision.

Distant Vision. The subject is seated 20 feet from a well-illuminated Snellen test chart. Each eye is tested separately, followed by testing of binocular vision. Visual acuity is expressed as a fraction. The numerator is the distance between the subject and the chart (i.e., 20 feet). The denominator is obtained by finding the smallest type read without error. The number printed at the side of this type is the maximum distance at which a subject with normal vision can read the type. Normal vision is usually expressed as 20/20 or as a fraction with denominator below 20, i.e., 20/15. Impaired distant vision might be measured as 20/60 when the subject is only able to read material at 20 feet that a normal individual could read at 60 feet.

Near Vision. The reading card published by the American Medical Association is probably the best of the many test cards available for evaluation of near vision acuity. This card is read at 14 inches from the eyes and gives a measure of near vision expressed in fractional form similar to the Snellen type. The patient should always wear his or her glasses or bifocals when near vision is being evaluated. Impaired visual acuity may occur under the following conditions:

1. A structural lesion involving the cornea, lens, or vitreous humor
2. A refractive error in which the object is not projected or "focused" sharply onto the fovea of the retina
3. A structural lesion involving the visual pathways from the retina to the occipital cortex
4. Conversion (hysterical) reaction (hysterical blindness)
5. One amblyopic eye from an old squint or asymmetric refractive error

Determination of the cause of impaired visual acuity requires an adequate ophthalmologic and neurologic examination. A number of findings suggest the presence of a conversion reaction. These include:

1. Good visual acuity is a function of the fovea and is represented by the central five degrees of visual field; a complaint of poor visual acuity without loss of this small central field suggests a conversion reaction.
2. The presence of stereopsis when visual acuity is impaired in one or both eyes suggests a conversion reaction, since stereopsis requires good binocular visual acuity.
3. The presence of optokinetic nystagmus in one eye with greatly reduced visual acuity or blindness in that eye is also a feature of a conversion reaction, since optokinetic nystagmus depends upon appreciation of and accurate pursuit of moving stripes on a rotating drum.
4. The presence of tubular (cylindric) fields in patients who demonstrate no difficulty in ambulation is strongly suggestive of hysteria.

Ophthalmoscopic Examination. The patient is asked to fix the gaze on a distant object at approximately eye level. The examiner focuses the light from the ophthalmoscope onto the cornea using a 10+ lens and examines the cornea for abrasions or opacities. The aqueous humor, iris, lens, vitreous humor, and retina are then examined by interposing lenses of decreasing power between the light source and the patient's eye. When a clear outline of the retina is obtained, the examiner evaluates the optic nerve head, the blood vessels, and the retina.

The optic nerve head or optic disk is a yellowish-white structure situated slightly to the nasal side of the optic axis. The temporal margin of the disk is clearly outlined in the majority of cases but may be blurred in myopic subjects. The nasal margin is often indistinct, but this finding is of no significance. The optic disk contains a smaller, whitish, eccentric depression known as the optic cup, where the central retinal artery enters and the retinal veins leave the optic nerve. Careful examination will reveal venous pulsation in the majority of cases. Venous pulsation is present in about 80 percent of individuals and is indicative of normal intracranial pressure. Conversely, absence of venous pulsation does not invariably indicate increased intracranial pressure. Occasionally the optic cup is enlarged and occupies most of the surface of the optic disk. Since the cup has a whiter appearance, enlargement may lead to a spurious impression of optic atrophy.

Papilledema. Papilledema is defined as edema of the optic disk. The pathogenesis of papilledema is uncertain but is believed to be the result of increased intracranial pressure, venous stasis and/or lymphatic stasis. The rate of development depends upon the degree of increased intracranial pressure or venous stasis and the consistency of elevation. There are two forms of papilledema.

1. Noninflammatory papilledema. In noninflammatory papilledema the patient may report transient 5- to 10-second episodes of grayness or blackouts of vision. Sudden standing or excitement may precipitate these visual difficulties. Chronic papilledema may eventually result in blindness. Symptoms of increased intracranial pressure such as headache, nausea and vomiting, sixth nerve palsies, or alteration of consciousness may be present. Noninflammatory papilledema is characterized on ophthalmologic examination by cylindric elevation of the nerve head, obliteration of the disk margins, hyperemia of the disk, venous distention, absence of venous pulsations, loss of optic cup, and the appearance of concentric ripples of the retina on the temporal side of the disk (Paton's lines). (See Figure 1–5.) Noninflammatory papilledema may be difficult to distinguish in its early stages of development. Hemorrhages associated with papilledema due to increased intracranial pressure are usually located in the peripapillary area, while hemorrhages that occur in papilledema due to hypertension are widespread and accompanied by hypertensive retinopathy. Examination of the visual fields in noninflammatory papilledema usually reveals enlargement of the blind spot and constriction of peripheral visual fields. Noninflammatory papilledema may be seen with mass lesions of the intracranial cavity (e.g., tumor, abscess, or subdural hematoma); in subarachnoid hemorrhage; in various infectious diseases; and in metabolic conditions (e.g., hypertension, anemia, emphysema, and benign intracranial hypertension [pseudotumor cerebri, otitic hydrocephalus]).

2. Inflammatory papilledema (optic neuritis) (see Figure 1–6). Inflammatory papilledema is characterized by sudden unilateral amaurosis, ocular pain, particularly on eye movement, and palpable globe tenderness.

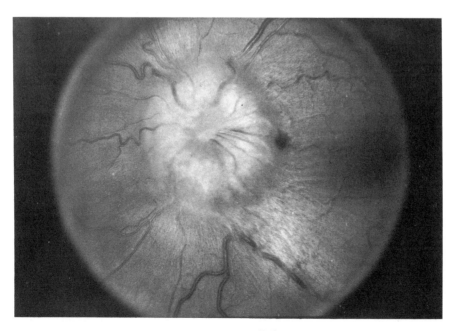

FIGURE 1–5.   Papilledema.

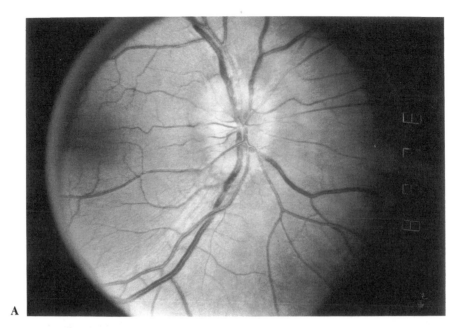

FIGURE 1–6.   **A.** Optic neuritis. There was retrobulbar pain on eye movement. Visual acuity 20/80. **B.** Normal opposite fundus and disc.

Ophthalmologic examination may reveal findings similar to those of noninflammatory papilledema plus inflammatory cells in the vitreous. The elevation of the nerve head may appear more gradual rather than cylindric. Examination of the visual fields may reveal a central, paracentral or cecocentral scotoma of the involved eye. An afferent pupil defect is likely to be present (see p. 21). Optic neuritis is a frequent occurrence in demyelinating diseases, particularly multiple sclerosis. It may also be seen when there is infection involving the nerve (e.g., meningitis, encephalitis); in metabolic diseases (e.g., diabetes mellitus, thyroid dysfunction, vitamin B_1 or B_{12} deficiency); in toxic conditions (e.g., methylalcohol poisoning); and in vascular disorders (e.g., giant cell [temporal] arteritis).

Retrobulbar Neuritis. Retrobulbar neuritis is a form of inflammatory edema of the optic nerve in which the edema remains confined to the retrobulbar portion of the optic nerve and does not extend into the optic nerve head. The clinical features are those of optic neuritis, but the optic disk has a normal ophthalmologic appearance.

Optic Atrophy. Optic atrophy is defined as pallor of the optic disk due to demyelination and axonal degeneration of the optic nerve. Primary optic atrophy occurs without evidence of preceding papilledema. The disk typically appears uniformly white with a clearly outlined margin. Secondary optic atrophy follows papilledema and the disk is white, but the margins are grayish and indistinct.

Optic atrophy may occur in hereditary cerebral degenerations, for example, cerebral lipidoses, metachromatic leukodystrophy, and Leber's optic atrophy. It may follow inflammatory or noninflammatory papilledema, or it may be associated with compressive lesions of the nerve, trauma, glaucoma, vascular disorders, or exposure to toxins.

Examination of the Visual Fields. The method employed in office practice or at the bedside is called confrontation and compares the examiner's field of vision with that of the patient. The patient should be seated facing the examiner at eye level. The patient is instructed to look at the examiner's nose and the examiner looks at the patient's nose. The examiner extends his arms to each side in a position roughly midway between patient and examiner so that the fingers are beyond the periphery of the examiner's visual field. The patient is instructed to indicate when he sees the examiner's finger move, and the examiner begins to rhythmically move his right index finger and at the same time advances it slowly toward the center of his own visual field. The patient with a normal peripheral visual field will indicate that the moving finger is visible at the same time as it appears at the periphery of the examiner's visual field. The process is then repeated with the left index finger. The test should be carried out in the following order: patient's left upper quadrant, right upper quadrant, left lower quadrant, and right lower quadrant. The examiner

then brings his fingers to the periphery of the midfield (equivalent to three o'clock and nine o'clock) and moves both index fingers simultaneously. The movement (bilateral simultaneous stimulation) should be appreciated in the right and left visual fields by the patient. Failure to appreciate movement of one finger in an intact visual field on bilateral simultaneous stimulation is termed visual extinction. This phenomenon occurs in the presence of an early lesion of the opposite parietal lobe that has not developed sufficiently to produce a homonymous visual field defect.

Testing of binocular visual fields should be followed by testing of the visual fields in each eye. This is accomplished by asking the patient to close one eye or cover one eye with a hand. The examiner closes the opposite eye and instructs the patient to gaze into the examiner's open eye. The examiner then maps the periphery of the visual fields for each eye using the method previously described.

The following abnormalities may be observed during the examination of the visual fields:

1. Immediately after the examiner has instructed the patient to look at the examiner's nose and has extended his arms laterally, the patient moves his gaze from the examiner's nose to the hand on one side. This suggests the presence of a homonymous hemianopia on the side opposite to the patient's eye movement.

2. The patient changes his gaze from the examiner's nose to the moving finger on either side despite repeated instructions to continue looking at the examiner's nose. This condition is called impersistence and represents an inability to maintain gaze on a designated object when another stimulus enters the visual field. Impersistence suggests the presence of degenerative disease of the brain.

3. The visual fields appear to be intact by confrontation when binocular testing is performed. However, a partial superior temporal quadrantanopsia is observed on one side only when the eyes are tested individually. This defect would not be apparent unless the eyes were tested individually, since the intact field on one side compensates for the partial loss of the temporal field on the other side. The reason for this partial visual field loss is illustrated in Figure 1–4.

Testing for Scotomata. Patients with inflammatory papilledema, retrobulbar neuritis, or optic atrophy may develop scotomata. These scotomata may be central, involving the central portion of the visual field; paracentral, involving an area near the central field; or cecocentral, involving the central portion of the visual field and extending to the blind spot.

Scotomata are usually detected by using a tangent screen, but it is possible to test for the presence of a scotoma in the office. The patient is instructed to maintain a steady gaze into the pupil of the examiner's eye. The examiner brings a small white object, such as the head of a corsage pin, from the periphery across the visual field, moving steadily from the temporal to the nasal side (see Figure 1–7). Under normal conditions the patient and examiner will observe that the object disappears momentarily in the physiologic blind spot but remains clearly visible in the central area of the field. However, the patient will report that the object disappears again if there is a central or paracentral field defect. The boundaries of the scotoma can be defined by bringing the object from the periphery in vertical diagonal planes. Scotomata are usually larger when measured with colored objects, particularly red objects.

The Third, Fourth, and Sixth Nerves (Oculomotor, Trochlear, and Abducens)

Anatomy. The motor fibers of the third nerve supply extraocular muscles, which control eye movement and instrinsic muscles,

which control accommodation and pupilloconstriction.

The third nerve arises from a compound nucleus located in the midbrain immediately ventral to the cerebral aqueduct. The fibers pass through the tegmentum of the midbrain and emerge as a series of rootlets in the sulcus oculomotorius on the medial aspect of the cerebral peduncle. The rootlets unite to form the oculomotor nerve, which passes between the posterior cerebral artery and the superior cerebellar artery to enter the lateral wall of the cavernous sinus. The oculomotor nerve is situated immediately above the fourth, fifth, and sixth nerves in the lateral wall of the cavernous sinus and emerges anteriorly to enter the orbit through the superior orbital fissure. At this point the nerve divides into a superior branch, which supplies the levator palpebrae and the superior rectus, and an inferior branch, which supplies the medial rectus, inferior rectus, and inferior oblique muscles. The inferior branch also contains the parasympathetic fibers, which have their origin in the most superior portion of the third nerve nucleus (Edinger-Westphal nucleus). These fibers synapse in the ciliary ganglion, and a series of postganglionic fibers pass through several short ciliary nerves to supply the ciliary and sphincter pupillae muscles of the eye.

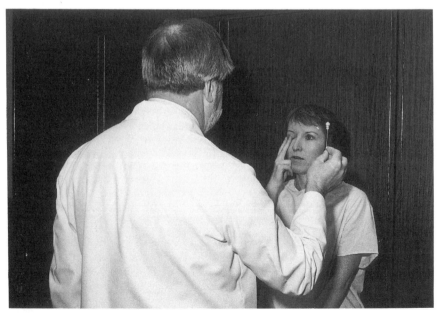

FIGURE 1–7. Testing for scotomata.

The nucleus of the fourth nerve lies ventral to the cerebral aqueduct in the midbrain at the level of the inferior colliculus. Fibers emerging from the nucleus pass dorsally and decussate in the anterior medullary velum immediately below the inferior colliculus on the dorsal surface of the midbrain. The trochlear nerve then passes ventrally around the cerebral peduncle and pierces the dura to enter the lateral wall of the cavernous sinus. The nerve passes through the superior orbital fissure to innervate the superior oblique muscle.

The sixth nerve arises from the abducens nucleus, which lies in the dorsal pons ventral to the floor of the fourth ventricle. The nerve has an anteroventral course through the pons and emerges close to the midline at the junction of the pons and medulla. There is a relatively long course in the posterior fossa where the nerve is in contact with the ventral surface of the pons. The nerve crosses the apex of the petrous temporal bone and enters the lateral wall of the cavernous sinus to lie below and medial to the third and fourth cranial nerves and ophthalmic and maxillary divisions of the fifth cranial nerve and lateral to the internal carotid artery. The sixth nerve then enters the orbit through the superior orbital fissure and supplies the lateral rectus muscle.

Pupillary Reflexes. *Types.* There are three pupillary reflexes: the light reflex, near-vision reflex, and reflex dilatation.

Light Reflex. The afferent pathway for the pupillary light reflex is activated by light which stimulates the rods and cones in the retina. The afferent pathway passes via the optic nerve with partial decussation in the optic chiasm and then continues bilaterally through both optic tracts and the brachium of the superior colliculi to the pretectal region of the midbrain. From the pretectal region the fibers pass forward close to the aqueduct to enter the Edinger-Westphal nucleus on the same side or pass through the posterior commissure to enter the nucleus on the opposite side. The efferent side of the reflex is completed by fibers that pass from the neurons in the Edinger-Westphal nucleus through the oculomotor nerve to the ciliary ganglion, and thereafter by short ciliary nerves to the constrictor muscles of the iris.

Near-Vision Reflex. Afferent impulses for the pupillary constrictor reflex for near-vision are transmitted through the visual pathway to the visual cortex. Impulses then pass from cortical neurons through the corti-cotectal tract to synapse with neurons in the pretectal area of the midbrain. The connections from the pretectal area to the Edinger-Westphal nucleus on either side pass ventrally to the fibers for the pupillary light reflex to reach the Edinger-Westphal nucleus. The remainder of the efferent pathway for the near-vision reflex is similar to that for the pupillary light reflex.

Pupillary Dilatation. Almost any emotional or sensory stimulus (with the exception of light and near-vision) may produce pupillary dilatation in man. One well-known example is the ciliospinal reflex in which there is pupillary dilatation on pinching the skin on the side of the neck. The pupillary dilatation reflex is probably mediated through the posterior hypothalamus with activation of sympathetic fibers, which pass down through the brainstem to the superior cervical ganglion and via the carotid plexus to the radially arranged dilator muscle fibers of the iris. The reflex activity also includes a simultaneous inhibition of the Edinger-Westphal nucleus through hypothalamic connections via the reticular activating system to the Edinger-Westphal nucleus in the midbrain.

Examination of Pupil. In the majority of cases, the pupils will appear to be equal, round, and centrally placed in relation to the cornea. It is not unusual to see some mild inequality of pupils, "anisocoria," and observation will show that this difference in size may fluctuate over a relatively short period of time.

The pupillary light reflex is tested by flashing a bright light into each eye and quickly swinging the light between the two eyes. Under normal conditions there is an immediate constriction of the pupil in the eye stimulated by light and an immediate constriction of the pupil on the other side (consensual response). When the light is swung to the other side, the pupil dilates momentarily and then constricts when the stimulus is perceived. Occasionally there may be a sustained dilatation followed by delayed constriction after the light is directed into the eye. This suggests some delay in the afferent pathway of the light reflex and is commonly seen in optic neuritis, retrobulbar neuritis, and optic atrophy. This delay in pupillary constriction on stimulation, sometimes called the Marcus-Gunn phenomenon, is often present in multiple sclerosis.

It is not unusual to see a brisk pupillary constriction to the light stimulus, followed by rhythmic relaxation and contraction of the iris. This condition, which is called *hippus*, is a normal response and is also said to be more common in multiple sclerosis and in barbiturate poisoning.

Abnormalities of Pupillary Light Reflex. The pupillary reaction to light may be absent or impaired if there is a lesion involving the reflex pathway at any site. These include:

1. Failure of light to reach the retina—local diseases of the eye (e.g., vitreous opacities, as in diabetes)
2. Diseases of the retina—retinitis pigmentosa, macular hemorrhage or scar
3. Diseases of the optic nerve—severe inflammatory papilledema, retrobulbar neuritis, optic atrophy
4. Diseases involving the optic tracts and the connections to the midbrain
5. Diseases of the midbrain
6. Diseases involving the third nerve or ciliary ganglion

Argyll Robertson Pupil. The Argyll Robertson pupil is said to occur when there is impairment or failure of the pupils to react to light but preservation of reaction to near vision. It should be noted that the classical description of the Argyll Robertson pupil, as an irregular miotic pupil that fails to react to light, is only a partial description of this abnormality. In fact, the Argyll Robertson pupil may be present when:

1. The pupil shows absence of response to light with preservation of constriction to near vision.
2. The pupil shows some response to light, but this response is reduced and is much less than the pupillary response to near vision.
3. In early cases the pupil may be normal in size, since the development of miosis is a late feature of the Argyll Robertson pupil.
4. The pupils are often round, and it is only later when they become scarred by synechiae and atrophy from inflammatory iris disease that they appear irregular and unequal.

The Argyll Robertson pupil is the result of a lesion involving fibers that pass from the pretectal area of the midbrain to the Edinger-Westphal nucleus. However, only the rostrally placed fibers subserving the light reflex are involved, while the more caudally located fibers responsible for the near-vision reflex are unaffected. The Argyll Robertson pupil was first described in neurosyphilis, in which neuronal destruction and gliosis occurred in the periaqueductal area of the midbrain with destruction of fibers involved in the light reflex. Consequently, the Argyll Robertson pupil is a feature of tabes dorsalis, general paresis, and meningovascular syphilis. Other causes of the Argyll Robertson pupil are rare and include viral encephalitis, Wernicke's encephalopathy, cerebrovascular disease and infarction of the midbrain, multiple sclerosis with demyelination of the midbrain, and neoplasm involving the rostral midbrain. This pupillary abnormality may also be seen in advanced cases of chronic degenerative diseases involving the central nervous system, including Alzheimer's disease, spinocerebellar degeneration, and chronic hypertrophic interstitial polyneuropathy.

Spastic Miotic Pupil. This condition can be regarded as a variant of the Argyll Robertson pupil. In the spastic miotic pupil the reaction to light and to near vision is poor or absent. This condition indicates the presence of a lesion in the midbrain involving nerve fibers serving both light and near vision.

Lesions of the Third Nerve. Pupillary constrictor fibers form an outer sheath on the third nerve and surround the inner core of nerve fibers which supply the extraocular muscles. Therefore, pressure on the third nerve will produce pupillary dilatation, which may occur before paralysis of extraocular movement. This is commonly seen:

1. When the third nerve is stretched over the free edge of the tentorium cerebelli during herniation of the medial aspect of the temporal lobe
2. When the third nerve is compressed by a mass such as a posterior communicating artery aneurysm

Lesions of the Ciliary Ganglion: The Tonic Pupil (The Holmes-Adie or Adie Syndrome). Injury to the cells of the ciliary ganglion or to the short ciliary nerves may result in denervation of the pupil. The subsequent reinnervation from surviving ganglion cells is such that the majority of regenerating nerve fibers reach the ciliary muscle. This leaves the iris relatively denervated and produces a condition known as the tonic pupil. The condition is usually unilateral. The pupil is large and fails to contract, or shows a very slow, delayed contraction to light and to near vision. In each case the pupil contracts slowly and then remains small for some time before returning to normal size with an equally slow movement. The tonic pupil is exquisitely sensitive to local application of 0.125 percent fresh solution of pilocarpine with prompt constriction. A similar application would not affect a normal pupil.

Disorders of Eye Movement. Eye movements are tested by asking the patient to look to the right, look to the left, look upward, and look downward. The patient is then instructed to follow a moving object, which is moved by the examiner in the same fashion.

Three types of eye movement disorder can be recognized. The patient may have a disturbance of conjugate eye movements, nystagmus, or paralysis of individual extraocular muscles.

Conjugate Eye Movements. Fibers arising in the frontal cortex, the occipital cortex, the vestibular system, and the cerebellum converge in the pons and terminate in the paramedian pontine reticular formation (PPRF). The PPRF is the center for coordinating nerve impulses concerned with conjugate gaze. Fibers from the PPRF pass to the ipsilateral abducens nucleus and terminate on neurons in that nucleus. The abducens nucleus gives rise to fibers that enter the sixth nerve and terminate in the lateral rectus muscle. A second pathway from the abducens nucleus enters the contralateral medial longitudinal fasciculus and terminates in the oculomotor nucleus. Abnormalities of conjugate eye movement include:

1. Conjugate deviation of the eyes at rest. This may be due to:
   a. A destructive lesion involving one hemisphere. This produces conjugate deviation of the eyes toward the side of the destructive lesion. A destructive lesion produces imbalance of cortical activity transmitted to the PPRF, and conjugate movement is influenced only by the intact hemisphere with deviation of the eyes toward the destructive lesion.
   b. An irritative lesion involving one hemisphere. This results in deviation of the eyes away from the side of the irritative lesion. In this case the irritative influence is stronger than the normal activity generated in the opposite hemisphere.
   c. A destructive lesion in the brainstem below the decussation of the corticobulbar fibers. This produces deviation of the eyes away from the side of the lesion.
   d. An irritative lesion of the frontal lobe. This results in conjugate vertical deviation of the eyes. Prolonged tonic deviation of the eyes in an upward direc-

tion, "oculogyric crisis," has been described in postencephalitic parkinsonism.

2. Dysconjugate deviation of the eyes at rest. This may be the result of:
   a. A destructive lesion of one oculomotor nucleus or oculomotor nerve. This results in outward deviation of the eye on the affected side due to unopposed activity of the abducens nerve and the lateral rectus muscle.
   b. Destruction of one abducens nucleus or abducens nerve. This results in inward deviation of the eye on the affected side due to the unopposed activity of the oculomotor nerve and medial rectus muscle.
   c. A destructive lesion involving the tectooculomotor pathway on one side. This produces vertical deviation of the eye on the opposite side.
   d. A destructive lesion involving the medial longitudinal fasciculus on one side in the pons. This lesion results in skew deviation of the eyes with one eye elevated and the other eye depressed.

Voluntary Conjugate Eye Movements. Abnormalities of voluntary conjugate eye movements may be due to:

1. Disease of one frontal lobe. This causes paralysis of voluntary conjugate gaze to one side. There is an inability to direct the gaze away from the side of the lesion on command.
2. Diffuse disease involving both hemispheres. This results in impairment of smooth pursuit conjugate eye movements. These are replaced by coarse, interrupted, conjugate saccadic movements and occur when the patient attempts to follow a moving object in a horizontal plane.
3. Diffuse degenerative processes involving both hemispheres. This may result in ocular impersistence. The patient cannot sustain gaze on an object once movement of it ceases.
4. Bilateral involvement of corticobulbar tracts which enter the brainstem at the level of the midbrain. This can produce loss of gaze in any direction on command, or in following a moving object. Initial impairment is usually in upward gaze.

Reflex conjugate eye movements occur:

1. In response to a moving visual stimulus.
2. In response to tonic neck and vestibular

reflexes in the absence of a visual stimulus.

In reflex conjugate eye movements which depend upon the integrity of the visual cortex afferent stimuli are received in the primary visual cortex, which is located on the upper and lower borders of the calcarine fissure, and are then transmitted to the visual association areas. The visual association areas project to the brainstem via internal corticotectal fibers, which pass to the tectum of the midbrain, and via corticotegmental fibers, which pass through the pons and terminate in the PPRF.

Abnormalities can occur when there are:

1. Lesions involving the internal corticotectal pathway or tectooculomotor connections in the midbrain. This results in impairment of upward gaze. The commonest cause of this phenomenon is compression of the middle of the superior colliculi by a pineal tumor resulting in loss of upward gaze (Parinaud's syndrome).
2. Lesions involving the pons. This produces paralysis of reflex conjugate horizontal gaze. This commonly occurs in multiple sclerosis and in infarction and tumors of the pons which impair the function of the PPRF and its immediate connections.

In the absence of visual stimulation, reflex mechanisms, such as tonic neck reflexes and vestibular reflexes, can produce reflex conjugate eye movements. These movements can be elicited in unconscious patients in the absence of visual stimuli. When the head is turned in one direction reflex conjugate movement of the eyes occurs in the opposite direction. These movements have been termed *doll's eye movements*. Reflex conjugate eye movements are impaired or lost in bilateral destructive lesions of the brain stem, which interrupt the connections between the vestibular nuclei and the third, fourth, and sixth nerve nuclei. Consequently, loss of doll's eye movements is usually an indication of bilateral pontine dysfunction.

Nystagmus. Nystagmus is an involuntary rhythmic movement of the eyes, which may be present at rest or occur with eye movement. In the latter case it persists for an interval after eye movement has ceased. Nystagmus may be bilateral or unilateral, although unilateral nystagmus is rare.

Nystagmus may result from imbalance of coordinated reflex activity involving the labyrinth, vestibular nuclei, cerebellum, medial longitudinal fasciculus, or nuclei of the third, fourth, and sixth nerves. It may also occur from remote influences that affect this reflex system. These include disease of the retina; disease of the third, fourth, and sixth cranial nerves; and disease of the cervical cord, Drugs may also act as a remote influence on the central reflex mechanisms and produce nystagmus. Nystagmus may be horizontal, vertical, oblique, or rotatory (clockwise to the right, counterclockwise to the left) in nature. Nystagmus may be pendular or jerk.

Pendular Nystagmus. This is characterized by a regular to-and-fro movement of the eyes in which both phases are equal in duration. In jerk nystagmus one phase of eye movement is faster than the other. Jerk nystagmus may result from loss of central vision. Pendular nystagmus occurs in:

1. Spasmus nutans. Spasmus nutans is a benign condition which appears in infants between three and eight months of age and lasts months to years. The onset is thought to be related to a viral illness. It is characterized by pendular nystagmus, usually horizontal, occasionally vertical, and often monocular; rhythmic head nodding, usually up and down; and head tilting.

2. Patients with defective vision since birth. Infants with congenital cataracts, central corneal opacities, or chorioretinitis may develop pendular nystagmus, which is coarse, slow, and usually horizontal.

3. Occupational nystagmus. Miners' nystagmus occurs in individuals who work in poorly illuminated surroundings. Rods are required for vision under these conditions, and there are no rods in the macula. Consequently, there is constant movement of the eye in an attempt to project the image on more peripheral parts of the retina.

4. Congenital nystagmus. Congenital nystagmus is inherited as an autosomal dominant or sex-linked recessive trait. It appears at birth, persists throughout life, and is occasionally accompanied by titubation of the head. On deviation of the eyes it may become jerk in nature.

Jerk Nystagmus. This occurs in:

1. Optokinetic nystagmus. Optokinetic nystagmus is a normal physiologic response to a series of objects moving in the same direction across the visual field. The eyes follow one object to the edge of the visual field, then rapidly return to the central fixation point to focus the next object. Optokinetic nystagmus can be produced by rotation of a drum with alternating vertical black and

white stripes before the patient's eyes. There is a slow movement in the direction of the movement of the drum with a quick return in the opposite direction. Testing is usually carried out in a horizontal or vertical plane but can be carried out in any direction of gaze. Optokinetic nystagmus is a reflex phenomenon dependent upon the integrity of the cortical visual pathways. It may be absent or reduced in deep parietal lobe lesions and infrequently in temporal and frontal lobe lesions.

2. Vestibular nystagmus. Vestibular nystagmus is the result of asymmetric impulses from the semicircular canals. It is independent of visual stimuli and is inhibited by fixation. It may be elicited by rotation in a Barany chair, by caloric irrigation of the external auditory canals, or by galvanic stimulation of the labyrinth or vestibular nerve. Abnormal occurrence of vestibular nystagmus may occur when there is disease of the labyrinth, such as labyrinthitis, hemorrhage, or hydrops (Ménière's disease). Peripheral disease is usually associated with spontaneous nystagmus (horizontal and rotary) and is accompanied by vertigo. When the brain stem is involved, the spontaneous nystagmus may be horizontal, rotary, or vertical, and vertigo is not a prominent feature. Rotary nystagmus is characteristic of vestibular nystagmus.

3. Nystagmus of neuromuscular origin. This occurs with:

a. Fatigue. It is not unusual to see irregular jerking movements of the eyes on extreme lateral gaze during fatigue. This is of no significance.
b. Paresis. Contraction of paretic extraocular muscle will produce irregular nystagmoid movements. This condition can occur in myopathies, in myasthenia gravis, and in partial lesions of the oculomotor nerves.

4. Cerebellar nystagmus. Although cerebellar nystagmus can occur with lesions involving the cerebellum, the majority of cases are due to involvement of cerebellar connections in the brain stem including the vestibular nuclei, vestibular cerebellar tracts, cerebellar pathways in the brain stem, and medial longitudinal fasciculus. The nystagmus is horizontal and more pronounced on looking to the side of the lesion.

5. Nystagmus due to lesions of the medial longitudinal fasciculus.

a. The nystagmus of internuclear ophthalmoplegia is described on page 27.

b. Nystagmus occurs with involvement of the medial longitudinal fasciculus in any portion of the brain stem and also occurs with involvement of the medial longitudinal fasciculus in the upper portion of the cervical cord tumors.

6. Miscellaneous forms of nystagmus. These include:

a. Drug-induced nystagmus. Many drugs can cause nystagmus, the commonest being barbiturates and phenytoin. Other causes include alcohol, nonbarbiturate sedatives, and quinine. This is typically a horizontal nystagmus.
b. Seesaw nystagmus. Seesaw nystagmus is a rare condition usually associated with a parasellar lesion such as a craniopharyngioma. It is characterized by a seesaw displacement of the eyes in the horizontal plane with intorsion of the globe on depression and extorsion on elevation.
c. Retraction convergence nystagmus. This is a rare type of nystagmus associated with tectal and pretectal lesions of the midbrain. The eyes jerk back into the orbits with simultaneous adduction of both eyes. The optokinetic drum is an excellent way of eliciting this condition.
d. Vertical nystagmus. Vertical nystagmus that occurs when the eyes are in the primary position is indicative of a lesion involving the anterior vermis of the cerebellum or medulla. Vertical nystagmus that occurs on downward gaze is found with lesions of the cervical medullary junctions such as basilar impression or the Arnold-Chiari malformation.
e. Ocular bobbing. Ocular bobbing consists of brisk, downward conjugate movements of both eyes followed by a slow return to position of rest, and occurs in destructive lesions of the caudal pons and cerebellar hemorrhage.
f. Ocular flutter. Ocular flutter, consisting of rapid, rhythmical eye movements of decreasing amplitude when the eyes fix on an object, is characteristic of cerebellar disease, and is a form of ocular dysmetria.
g. Irregular jerking of one eye in the presence of coma. This can occur in lateral vertical, or rotary form and is indicative of severe destructive lesions involving the pons.
h. Opsoclonus. Opsoclonus consists of totally random clonic conjugate movements of the eyes in any direction and occurs in diffuse bilateral brain stem disease.

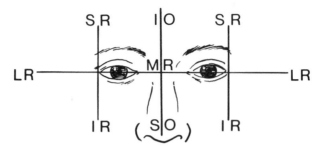

FIGURE 1–8. Clinical actions of the extraocular muscles.

Paralysis of Extraocular Muscles.   Actions of the extraocular muscles are illustrated in Figure 1–8 and outlined in Table 1–5. The eye findings in individual muscle paralysis are listed in Table 1–6. There are several rules for determining the cause of diplopia and determining paralysis of extraocular muscles:

1. Diplopia will be present at rest and there will be an apparent ocular deviation at rest when one or more of the extraocular muscles is paralyzed on one side.
2. Diplopia will increase when gaze is attempted in the direction of pull of the paralyzed muscle.
3. The ocular deviation will increase when the eyes are moved in the direction of action of the paralyzed muscle.
4. When the paretic eye attempts to look at any object in the field of action of the paralyzed muscle, there is overaction or secondary deviation of the sound eye. Central neuronal discharges are enhanced in this situation, and because of reciprocal innervation a stronger impulse is received by the nonparalyzed muscles producing reciprocal movement of the eye. The secondary deviation is always greater than

primary deviation in paralytic squint, whereas the deviation remains the same in all directions of gaze in nonparalytic or concomitant squint.

5. When an attempt is made to fix an object on the macula in the direction of pull of the paralyzed muscle, the image is projected onto the retina outside of the macular area. This produces a false projection of the image, incorrect localization, and past pointing by the patient.
6. If the affected eye is occluded, then the occlusion quickly removed, the eye will have deviated in the direction opposite to the pull of the paretic muscle.
7. If the sound eye is occluded and the affected eye is made to fix on an object in the direction of pull of a paretic muscle, the sound eye will seem to deviate excessively in the same direction (secondary deviation) when the occlusion is removed.

Summary of Disorders of Eye Movement Seen with Pontine Lesions.   These include:

1. Lesion of the sixth nerve in the pons produces internal strabismus at rest due to paralysis of the lateral rectus muscle, dip-

TABLE 1–5.   **Clinical Actions of Extraocular Muscles**

Muscle	Cranial Nerve	Action
Medial rectus	III	Adduction
Superior rectus	III	Elevates when eye abducted
Inferior oblique	III	Elevates when eye adducted
Inferior rectus	III	Depresses when eye abducted
Superior oblique	IV	Depresses when eye adducted
Lateral rectus	VI	Abduction
Levator palpebrae	III	Elevates upper lid
Müller's muscle	Sympathetic	Elevates upper lid
Orbicularis oculi	VII	Closure of eyelids

TABLE 1–6. Eye Findings in Cases of Individual Muscle Paralysis

Paralyzed Muscle	Upper Lid	Eye at Rest	Movements	Images	Head
Superior rectus	Ptosis	Normal position	Limited elevation particularly on abduction	Oblique, false above true—diplopia increases on attempted elevation and abduction	
Inferior oblique	Normal	Normal position	Limited elevation when eye adducted	Oblique, false above and lateral to true—diplopia increases on attempted elevation and adduction	
Medial rectus	Normal	Abducted	Limited adduction	Crossed, parallel, diplopia increasing on attempted adduction	
Inferior rectus	Normal	Normal position	Limited depression particularly on abduction	Oblique, false image below and medial to true image—diplopia increases on attempted depression and abduction	
Superior oblique	Normal	Normal position	Limited depression when eye adducted	Oblique, false image below and lateral to true—diplopia increases on attempted depression and adduction	Head tilted toward sound side
Lateral rectus	Normal	Adducted	Limited abduction	Parallel, uncrossed—diplopia increases on attempted abduction and distance vision	Head turned toward affected side

lopia at rest, and increased diplopia on attempted gaze toward the side of the lesion.

2. Destruction of the sixth nerve nucleus produces all of #1 and in addition is usually associated with seventh nerve paralysis on the same side because of close association of seventh nerve to the sixth nerve nucleus in the pons.

3. Lesion of the medial longitudinal fasciculus in the pons produces double vision or oscillopsia. The patient is unable to adduct the eye on the side of the lesion because of paralysis of the connections to the medial rectus muscle. In addition, there is nystagmus of the abducting eye, which is occasionally accompanied by slight skew deviation. In midbrain lesions there is an additional failure of convergence (anterior internuclear ophthalmoplegia), while in pontine lesions (posterior internuclear ophthalmoplegia) the ability to converge the eyes is maintained. Bilat-

eral internuclear ophthalmoplegia occurs most frequently in multiple sclerosis.

The Fifth Nerve (Trigeminal Nerve)

The trigeminal nerve supplies sensation to the face, the buccal and nasal mucosa, sinuses, contents of the orbit, teeth, gums, and part of the scalp. The motor root supplies the muscles of mastication.

Anatomy. The gasserian ganglion is located on the floor of the middle fossa and contains the unipolar cells subserving touch, pain, and temperature sensation. The peripheral fibers leaving the ganglion enter the three major subdivisions of the trigeminal nerve, the ophthalmic, maxillary, and mandibular nerves. The proximal fibers enter the lateral pons at the junction of the pons and middle cerebellar peduncle. Fibers that carry discriminatory touch information ascend and synapse in the chief sensory nucleus of the trigeminal complex. The mesencephalic nucleus contains the cells of origin subserving proprioception. The peripheral fibers are located in the maxillary division and carry proprioceptive information from the muscles of mastication. Fibers that carry pain, temperature, and crude touch descend and synapse in the nucleus of the spinal tract of the trigeminal nerve, which extends to the upper cervical portion of the spinal cord. The nucleus of the tract is divided into three portions: the oralis, which extends from the midpons to olive; the interpolaris, which extends from the olive to the pyramidal decussation; and the caudalis, which extends from the decussation to the C_2 level. Axons carrying pain information synapse in the caudalis, while axons carrying temperature information synapse in all three portions. Fibers carrying crude touch information synapse in the oralis and interpolaris. Fibers from the mandibular portion of the nerve are most dorsal in the tract, while fibers from the ophthalmic portion are most ventral. The maxillary fibers occupy an intermediate position. The dorsal trigeminothalamic tract arises from the chief sensory nucleus, contains crossed and uncrossed fibers, and ascends to the posteromedial ventral nucleus of the thalamus. Tertiary neurons send fibers through the posterior limb of the internal capsule to the lower one-third to one-half of the postcentral gyrus. Fibers arising in the spinal nucleus decussate and form the ventral trigeminothalamic tract, which ascends in the medial aspect of the medial lemniscus to synapse in the posteromedial ventral nucleus of the thalamus. Pain, temperature, and crude touch sensations are then relayed through the posterior limbs of the internal capsule to the postcentral portion of the parietal lobe.

The motor neurons of the motor nucleus of the trigeminal nerve lie in the midpons, central and slightly medial to the chief sensory nucleus. Axons of the motor neurons pass in the motor portion of the trigeminal nerve to exit from the pons and pass beneath the gasserian ganglion to join the mandibular division.

The three divisions of the trigeminal nerve are distributed as follows;

1. The ophthalmic division passes along the lateral wall of the cavernous sinus, enters the orbit through the superior orbital fissure, and divides into a number of branches which supply the frontal and ethmoid sinuses, the conjunctiva, cornea, upper lid, bridge of nose, forehead, and the scalp posteriorly as far as the vertex of the skull.

2. The maxillary division enters the lateral wall of the cavernous sinus and leaves the middle cranial fossa through the foramen rotundum to enter the sphenomaxillary fossa. The nerve enters the orbit through the inferior orbital fissure, passes through the floor of the orbit in the inferior orbital canal, and emerges below the orbit through the inferior orbital foramen. The maxillary division supplies sensation to the skin of the cheek, the sphenoid and maxillary sinuses, the lateral aspect of the nose, the upper teeth, and the mucous membrane covering the nasal pharynx, hard palate, uvula, and inferior part of the nasal cavity.

3. The mandibular division leaves the middle cranial fossa through the foramen ovale accompanied by the motor branch of the trigeminal nerve. Sensory fibers are distributed to the skin over the chin and lower jaw, extending as far back as the pinna of the ear; the anterior portion of the external auditory meatus; the anterior two-thirds of the tongue; the lower teeth; the gums and floor of the mouth; and the buccal surface of the cheek. The motor fibers supply the muscles of mastication, tensor tympani, anterior belly of the digastric, and mylohyoid.

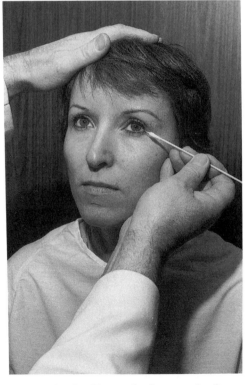

FIGURE 1–9.   Testing for the corneal reflex.

Examination of the Trigeminal Nerve.
Examination of the trigeminal nerve includes evaluation of the corneal reflex, sensation over the face and scalp, motor function, and the jaw jerk.

Corneal Reflex. This reflex is tested by the light application of cotton to the cornea. The examiner takes a cotton applicator and pulls the cotton head into a fine point. The patient is asked to look upward, and the cotton is brought toward the eye from a lateral position and gently applied to the cornea (see Figure 1–9). Application should produce a prompt bilateral reflex closure of the eyelids. The response is compared on the two sides, and the patient is asked whether the sensation appears to be equal on the two sides. The afferent loop of this reflex is via the ophthalmic division of the trigeminal nerve. The efferent side of the reflex is conducted through the facial nerve.

Sensation over the Face and Scalp. The patient is asked to close the eyes and to respond if touched. The cotton is applied to the forehead on one side, followed by application to the forehead in a similar position on the other side, then to the cheeks on the two sides, then to the jaws on the two sides. The patient's responses are monitored, and the patient is asked whether the sensation appears to be equal on the two sides of the face. The same test is then repeated using a sharp pin with gentle application in the ophthalmic, maxillary, and mandibular area, alternating between the two sides.

Motor Function. The examiner places the fingers over the temporalis muscles and asks the patient to clench the teeth or bite. The temporalis muscle will be felt to contract under the examiner's hands on both sides. A similar maneuver is performed with the fingers over the masseter muscles. The pterygoids can be tested by having the patient deviate the jaw to one side against resistance. In unilateral lesions the jaw deviates toward the side of the lesion.

Jaw Jerk. The jaw jerk is tested by lightly tapping the anterior, lower jaw with the reflex hammer (see Figure 1–10). Normally, there is a slight upward movement of the mandible. The jaw jerk is increased in destructive or compressive lesions involving the

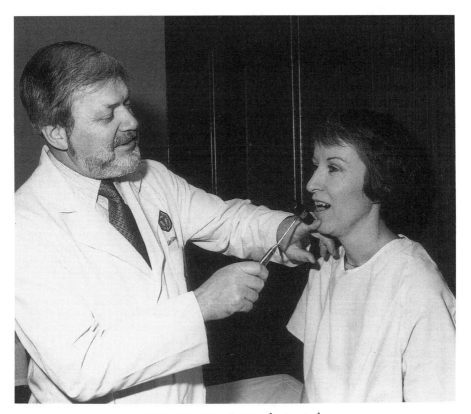

FIGURE 1–10.   Testing the jaw jerk.

corticopontine pathways and is discussed in more detail on page 42.

The Seventh Nerve (Facial Nerve)

The seventh nerve innervates the facial muscles and supplies taste sensation to the anterior two-thirds of the tongue and general sensation to a small portion of the external ear.

Anatomy. The motor neurons of the seventh nerve are located in the facial nucleus in the tegmentum of the pons. The motor fibers pass dorsally and medially from the nucleus, loop around the nucleus of the sixth cranial nerve, and then proceed in a ventrolateral and caudal direction to emerge at the lateral pontomedullary junction. The facial nerve immediately enters the internal auditory meatus in association with the eighth cranial nerve. The seventh nerve leaves the internal auditory canal, enters the facial canal, and passes through the facial canal to emerge through the stylomastoid foramen at the inferior border of the temporal bone. The nerve then penetrates the parotid gland and divides into several branches, which supply the muscles of the face, the stylohyoid, the buccinator, the posterior belly of the digastric muscle, and the platysma. The facial nerve also gives off a branch to the stapedius muscle in the facial canal.

The facial nerve carries parasympathetic motor fibers that arise from the superior salivatory nucleus in the pons. These fibers leave the facial nerve via the greater superficial petrosal nerve and pass to the sphenopalatine ganglion. The postganglionic fibers innervate the glands and mucous membranes of the palate, nasopharynx, and paranasal sinuses. The remaining parasympathetic fibers leave the facial nerve via the chorda tympani and terminate in the submaxillary ganglion. Postganglionic fibers innervate the sublingual and submaxillary salivary glands.

The sensory neurons of the seventh nerve are located in the geniculate ganglion, which is situated in the proximal portion of the facial canal. The peripheral branches of these nerve cells transmit taste sensation from the anterior two-thirds of the tongue and reach the geniculate ganglion via the lingual nerve, chorda tympani, and a short portion of the facial nerve. The central branches pass from the geniculate ganglion, form a separate bundle called the nerve of Wrisberg, enter the pons, and terminate in the nucleus of the tractus solitarius.

The facial nerve has a relatively small general somatic sensory component. These sensory fibers supply sensation to a small portion of the external ear, and the impulses are transmitted to the unipolar cells in the geniculate ganglion and through the facial nerve into the pons.

Examination of the Facial Nerve. The patient is asked to contract the facial muscles and show the teeth. The contraction should be symmetric on the two sides and simultaneously performed. The patient is then asked to close the eyes tightly and the examiner attempts to open the lids (see Figure 1–11). Normally this is not possible even when the examiner uses considerable force. Finally, the patient is asked to wrinkle the forehead in an upward direction. Again, this should be symmetric on the two sides.

Two types of facial weakness may be observed:

1. Upper motor neuron lesions involving the corticobulbar pathways will produce weakness of the lower portion of the face with normal function when the patient is asked to wrinkle the forehead. The lower portion of the face has unilateral innervation from cortical centers, while the forehead is bilaterally innervated from cortical centers.

2. Involvement of the facial nucleus in the pons or the facial nerve will produce total involvement of the facial muscles on the same side, and the lower facial muscles and forehead are equally involved in the process.

There are three forms of taste sensation: sweet, sour, and bitter. The sense of taste is tested by placing a test substance, sugar (sweet), vinegar (sour), or quinine (bitter), on the tongue. The test is best conducted by asking the patient to protrude the tongue, exposing one side. The side of the tongue is then dried and the test substance that has been prepared in solution is gently applied with a cotton applicator. The patient signals when the test substance is identified and can then draw the tongue back into the mouth and verbally identify the solution.

The Eighth Nerve (Acoustic Nerve)

The eighth nerve, or acoustic nerve, is a compound nerve with two divisions: the cochlear, subserving hearing, and the vestibular, subserving motion, balance, and an awareness of position in space.

Anatomy. The Cochlear Nerve. The ganglion cells in the spiral ganglia of the cochlea have short peripheral and long central processes. The peripheral processes terminate around the hair cells of the organ of

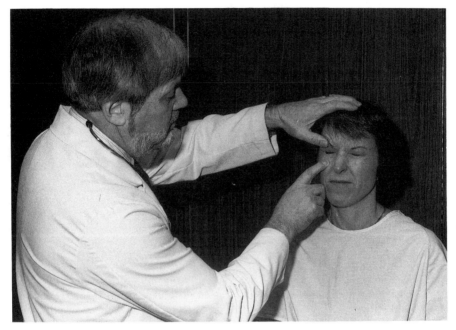

FIGURE 1–11. Testing for weakness of the face.

Corti, while the central processes pass to the cochlear nuclei in the brain stem. The cochlear nerve and the vestibular nerve form a common trunk, the acoustic nerve, which is closely related to the facial nerve in the internal auditory meatus. The two divisions of the acoustic nerve separate, and the cochlear nerve enters the brain stem lateral to the vestibular nerve at the junction of the pons and medulla. On entering the pons, the cochlear nerve divides, and fibers synapse in the dorsal and ventral cochlear nuclei.

Axons from cells in the ventral cochlear nucleus enter the trapezoid body and pass: 1) to the contralateral lateral lemniscus and medial longitudinal fasciculus, and 2) to the ipsilateral superior olivary nucleus and then to the medial longitudinal fasciculus and the nucleus of the sixth cranial nerve.

Axons from neurons in the dorsal cochlear nucleus cross the midline immediately below the fourth ventricle and enter the contralateral lateral lemniscus. The lateral lemniscus is a multisynaptic pathway, and the fibers within the structure may synapse as they pass through the pons and lower midbrain and ascend to the inferior colliculus. There are also several commissural connections which cross between the two lateral lemnisci. The inferior colliculus is a relay station in the auditory

pathway which may also be concerned with the interpretation of sound stimuli. Consequently, the majority of fibers from the lateral lemniscus enter and synapse with cells in the inferior colliculus, while a few fibers bypass the inferior colliculus and enter the brachium of the medial geniculate to terminate in neurons within this latter structure. Fibers arising from neurons in the inferior colliculus also terminate in the medial geniculate body.

The axons of neurons within the medial geniculate body form the auditory radiation, which passes through the sublenticular portion of the posterior limb of the internal capsule to the superior transverse temporal gyri. These structures constitute the primary auditory reception areas of the cerebral cortex and are located on the opercular surface of the superior temporal gyrus.

The Vestibular Nerve. The vestibular ganglion is attached to the vestibular nerve and is situated just within the internal auditory meatus. The ganglion contains bipolar cells with peripheral processes distributed to the maculae of the utricle and saccule and to the ampullae of the superior, lateral, and posterior semicircular canals. The central processes form the vestibular nerve, which accompanies the cochlear nerve and enters the brain stem. The vestibular nerve then passes dorsomedially between the inferior cerebellar peduncle and the spinal tract of the fifth cranial nerve to reach the vestibular nuclei. The vestibular nuclei consist of four separate structures: the medial vestibular nucleus, which extends from mid medulla to the inferior pons forming the vestibular area of the fourth ventricle; the lateral vestibular nucleus, which extends from the medulla, caudally, to the level of the sixth cranial nerve in the pons; the inferior (spinal) vestibular nucleus; located almost entirely within the medulla; and the superior vestibular nucleus, which is situated in the floor of the fourth ventricle and extends through the pons into the lower portion of the midbrain.

Efferent fibers from the vestibular nuclei pass to the medial longitudinal fasciculus, which brings the vestibular system into communication with other cranial nerve nuclei. Other fibers enter the pontine reticular formation or descend into the upper spinal cord to communicate with motor neurons. There are additional connections to the cerebellum and an ascending fiber system, which takes an unknown course and terminates in the temporal cortex in the posterior aspects of the superior temporal gyrus.

Tests of Auditory Function. Testing for hearing at the bedside is inaccurate. Audiograms should be obtained in all cases where there is doubt about the patient's ability to hear properly.

Conduction tests are useful, however, since in the normal state air conduction is much more sensitive than bone conduction. Testing is carried out by placing a tuning fork over the mastoid process and asking the patient to indicate when the sound is no longer audible. At this point the fork is placed at the level of the external auditory meatus and the patient is asked whether the sound is audible. Under normal circumstances this will be so, since air conduction is better than bone conduction. This test, the *Rinné test,* is said to be positive when air conduction is more sensitive than bone conduction. In conditions where bone conduction is more sensitive than air conduction, the Rinné test is negative. This indicates some obstruction of transmission of sound by disease involving the external auditory meatus, such as foreign bodies or wax, some malfunction of the drum, or some malfunction of the middle ear. Diseases of the cochlea or cochlear nerve produce impairment of hearing, and both air and bone conduction are diminished, but the Rinné test remains positive.

The examination continues with the performance of the *Weber test,* in which the tuning fork is placed on the center of the forehead and the patient is asked to indicate the location of the sound. This will usually be heard equally in both ears or appreciated at the site of the tuning fork on the forehead. When there is impairment of air conduction on one side, the Weber lateralizes to that ear. On the other hand, if there is disease of the cochlea or cochlear nerve, the Weber will lateralize to the side opposite the diseased ear.

Test of Vestibular Function. The vestibular system is an extremely sensitive system, and disturbances of function of the vestibular system or the vestibular division of the eighth nerve are accompanied by vertigo. Vertigo is a sensation of movement in which objects seem to be moving in a rotating fashion around the subject, or when the subject has an illusion of rotation. Occasionally vertigo may present with an illusion of tilting of objects in a horizontal or vertical plane without a rotary component. Vertigo is always accompanied by nystagmus because of the connections between the vestibular system and third, fourth, and sixth nerves via the medial longitudinal fasciculus. This anatomic pathway can be tested as follows.

Barany Test. Labyrinthine nystagmus may be induced by rotating the subject in a Barany chair. The patient's eyes are closed and the head is inclined forward 30 degrees to test the lateral semicircular canal, or extended backward 60 degrees to test the anterior canal. Under these circumstances, the canal to be tested is in the horizontal plane. The chair is then rotated 10 times in 20 seconds, which produces stimulation of the cristae in the canal. When the movement of the chair is stopped, the inertia of the endolymph continues to stimulate the cristae, producing a sensation of vertigo in the direction opposite to the previous rotation of the chair. This is accompanied by nystagmus, past pointing, and deviation of the eyes in the direction of the previous rotation. The sensation of vertigo usually lasts about 35 seconds under normal circumstances. Vertigo is reduced in disease of the stimulated canal or vestibular nerve. The vertigo may be increased in certain conditions that produce dysfunction of the vestibular system.

Caloric Testing. Caloric testing can be performed by tilting the head of a supine patient forward 30 degrees and irrigating the external auditory canal of one side with 5 to 10 ml of iced water or warm water for 30 seconds (see p. 51). The effect of caloric stimulation is reduced in disease of the external auditory canal, the vestibular apparatus or the vestibular nerve, and the central connections.

The Ninth Nerve (Glossopharyngeal Nerve)

This nerve supplies (a) motor fibers to the stylopharyngeus muscle; (b) sensation to the pharynx, tonsillar fossa, posterior third of the tongue, ear canal, and tympanic membrane; (c) secretomotor fibers to the parotid gland; and (d) taste sensation to the posterior third of the tongue

Anatomy. Motor fibers to the stylopharyngeus muscle arise from a rostral extension of the nucleus ambiguus in the upper medulla. Secretomotor fibers arise from the inferior salivatory nucleus in the medulla.

Both motor and secretomotor fibers leave the medulla in the groove between the inferior olive and the inferior cerebellar peduncle in a series of rootlets lying rostral to the rootlets of the vagus nerve. The rootlets unite to form the glossopharyngeal nerve, which passes from the skull through the jugular foramen. The nerve descends between the internal jugular vein and the internal carotid artery, crosses the styloid process, enters the pharynx between the middle and inferior constrictors, and is distributed to the pharyngeal structures. The majority of the secretomotor fibers leave the glossopharyngeal nerve as it emerges from the jugular foramen and form the tympanic nerve, which passes into the middle ear to join the tympanic plexus. The lesser superficial petrosal nerve arises from the tympanic plexus and passes to the otic ganglion. Postganglionic fibers from the otic ganglion enter the auricular temporal branch of the fifth cranial nerve and are distributed to the parotid gland.

Fibers that carry sensation from the pharynx, tonsils, and posterior third of the tongue arise from neurons in the petrosal ganglion, which is situated in the jugular foramen. The central fibers enter the brain stem and terminate in the nucleus of the tractus solitarius. Taste sensation from the posterior one-third of the tongue is transmitted by neurons in the petrosal ganglion, which have central fibers terminating in the nucleus of the tractus solitarius in the brain stem.

The glossopharyngeal nerve also carries impulses from the carotid sinus and the carotid body. The fibers arise from ganglion cells in the petrosal ganglion and enter the nucleus solitarius.

Examination of the Glossopharyngeal Nerve. Examination of the glossopharyngeal nerve includes evaluation of:

1. Taste sensation. The taste sensation of the posterior third of the tongue is tested in the same manner as taste over the anterior two-thirds of the tongue (see p. 30).
2. Gag reflex. The glossopharyngeal nerve forms the afferent loop of the gag reflex, which can be tested by stimulation of the pharyngeal wall. The efferent part of this reflex is served by the vagus nerve.

The Tenth Nerve (Vagus Nerve)

The vagus nerve supplies (a) autonomic fibers to viscera of the thorax and abdomen, (b) motor fibers to the pharynx and larynx, (c) sensation to viscera of the thorax and abdomen, and (d) sensation to the external ear and dura of the posterior fossa.

Anatomy. Autonomic (parasympathetic) fibers arise from neurons in the dorsal nucleus of the vagus, which lies immediately beneath the floor of the fourth ventricle in the dorsal medulla. The fibers pass between the nucleus ambiguus and tractus solitarius and emerge in the ventral medulla between the inferior olive and inferior cerebellar peduncle. The emerging fibers form a series of rootlets, which unite to form the vagus nerve, which leaves the skull through the jugular foramen. The vagus nerve then passes between the carotid artery and internal jugular vein to the root of the neck and enters the thorax. The vagus nerves supply branches to the heart, bronchi, and esophagus in the chest and to all of the abdominal viscera.

Motor fibers to the pharynx and larynx arise from neurons in the nucleus ambiguus, which extends through the whole length of the medulla. The fibers form a dorsal loop, then turn ventrally and laterally to join with other fibers of the vagus complex and emerge as a series of rootlets on the ventral surface of the medulla. The motor fibers are distributed to:

1. The pharynx through a series of pharyngeal branches, which supply the muscles of the pharynx and soft palate
2. The inferior constrictor of the pharynx and cricothyroid muscle through the superior laryngeal nerve
3. The intrinsic muscles of the larynx except the cricothyroideus through the recurrent laryngeal nerve. The recurrent laryngeal nerve arises from the vagus nerve at the level of the anterior aspect of the subcla-

vian artery on the right side and at the level of the aortic arch on the left side. Both nerves wind around the vessels and ascend between the esophagus and the trachea to enter the larynx.

Sensory fibers arising in the viscera have cell bodies located in the inferior ganglion. The peripheral processes are distributed with the vagus nerve to thoracic and abdominal viscera. The central processes terminate in the tractus solitarius.

Cutaneous sensation fibers arise from neurons situated in the superior jugular ganglion. The peripheral processes are distributed to the external auditory meatus, the skin on the back of the auricle, and the dura of the posterior fossa. The central processes join the spinal tract of the fifth cranial nerve in the medulla.

Examination of the Vagus. Changes in Speech. Paralysis of the vagus nerve or its branches may give rise to dysphonia or dysarthria.

Dysphonia may be defined as difficulty in phonation and occurs when there is paralysis of the larynx or vocal cords due to a lesion of one or both recurrent laryngeal nerves. The voice is hoarse and the volume reduced. Bilateral recurrent laryngeal paralysis produces stridor due to unrestricted activity of the cricothyroid muscles, causing the partially paralyzed cords to lie close to the midline.

Dysarthria, or difficulty in articulation, has many causes, but unilateral or bilateral vagal paralysis results in weakness of the soft palate and imparts a nasal quality to the voice.

Examination of the Soft Palate. The patient is asked to open the mouth and say "Ah." Under normal circumstances the soft palate elevates symmetrically and the uvula remains in the midline. Unilateral vagal paralysis results in a failure of palatal movement on one side. The palate does not elevate on the affected side, and the uvula is drawn to the opposite side by the contraction and arching of the palate on the nonaffected side.

Dysphagia. Dysphagia, or difficulty in swallowing, occurs when vagal nerve paralysis produces weakness of the pharyngeal muscles. This weakness can be demonstrated during phonation as the pharynx fails to contract.

The Eleventh Nerve (Accessory Nerve)

The accessory nerve is a purely motor nerve supplying the sternocleidomastoid and trapezius muscles.

Anatomy. The motor neurons of the accessory nerve lie in the intermediate column of gray matter in the upper five segments of the cervical cord. Fibers that emerge from these motor neurons pass dorsolaterally and emerge midway between the anterior and posterior roots and unite to form an ascending trunk, which passes through the foramen magnum into the posterior fossa. The spinal portion of the accessory nerve then joins the bulbar accessory nerve, which is the lowest portion of the vagus nerve, and leaves the posterior fossa through the jugular foramen. The bulbar portion then joins the vagus nerve while the spinal portion descends in the neck to terminate in the sternocleidomastoid and trapezius muscles on the same side.

There is evidence that the motor neurons in the upper cervical cord supplying the sternocleidomastoid and trapezius muscles have a segmental distribution, the more rostral cells supplying the sternocleidomastoid while the caudal neurons supply the trapezius.

Examination of the Accessory Nerve. The sternocleidomastoid is examined by asking the patient to turn the head to one side against resistance by the examiner's hand. The belly of the sternocleidomastoid can be felt to contract firmly if the examiner palpates the opposite side of the neck (see Figure 1–12). The trapezius is tested by the examiner placing both hands on the patient's shoulders and palpating the muscle on each side between the thumb and forefinger. The patient is then asked to elevate the shoulders against the examiner's resistance; equal contraction of the trapezius should occur on the two sides.

The Twelfth Nerve (Hypoglossal Nerve)

The hypoglossal nerve is a purely motor nerve that supplies motor fibers to the muscles of the tongue.

Anatomy. The motor neurons are contained in the hypoglossal nucleus, which lies in the dorsal and inferior portion of the medulla immediately below the floor of the lateral ventricle. The nerve passes ventrally through the substance of the medulla to emerge between the medullary pyramid and the inferior olive as a series of rootlets, which unite to form the hypoglossal nerve. The nerve leaves the posterior fossa through the anterior condyloid foramen and traverses the neck to terminate in a series of branches, which supply the ipsilateral muscles of the tongue.

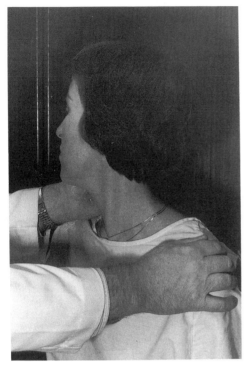

FIGURE 1–12. Examination of the sternocleido-mastoid muscle.

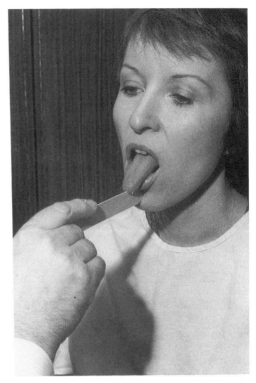

FIGURE 1–13. Testing for deviation of the tongue.

Examination of the Tongue. The tongue should be inspected with the mouth open and the tongue lying quietly on the floor of the mouth. This is the only way to see involuntary movements, particularly fasciculations, since the protruded tongue always has some involuntary movement. The tongue should also be inspected for asymmetry indicating wasting and scarring. The latter condition is not infrequent in a patient with a generalized seizure disorder. The examiner then places a wooden tongue blade edged upward in the midline, immediately below the lower lip, and the patient is asked to protrude the tongue. Under normal circumstances the tongue is protruded and lies symmetrically on the edge of the tongue blade (see Figure 1–13). This method allows the examiner to detect slight deviations of the tongue that otherwise might not be noticeable if the patient is simply allowed to protrude the tongue without a clear indication of the midline. The paralyzed tongue deviates toward the side of a lower motor neuron lesion.

When the tongue is protruded, the examiner should take the opportunity to examine the tongue more closely for the presence of scars and the state of the mucous membrane. Glossitis is not unusual in patients suffering from vitamin deficiency. An atrophic membrane can occur in long-standing pernicious anemia due to vitamin B_{12} deficiency.

The examiner then removes the tongue blade, and the patient is asked to move the tongue back and forth in rhythmic fashion as rapidly as possible. Rapid alternating movements of the tongue should be smoothly performed and rhythmic in character. Slowing or dysrhythmia can occur in the presence of weakness and in cerebellar dysfunction. Cerebellar difficulties can also be recognized by asking the patient to repeat syllables such as "mi-mi-mi" or "la-la-la." Again, this should be performed rhythmically, without any irregularity.

The remainder of the neurologic examination consists of evaluation of the motor system, coordination, gait and station, sensation, and reflexes. In the ambulatory patient it is most convenient to evaluate the upper extremities completely, and then evaluate the gait and station and lower limbs.

EXAMINATION OF MOTOR FUNCTION

The examination of motor function begins by inspection. The examiner stands in front of the patient who is seated and suitably clothed to expose the upper limbs, shoulders, and lower limbs. The contours and muscle development of the two sides should be equal. It is important to observe the limbs from the front and sides and to walk behind the patient and inspect all muscle groups. During this inspection, which is primarily directed toward the detection of muscle wasting, the presence of muscle fasciculations or involuntary movements of the limbs should be noted.

Muscle tone is tested by passively moving the joints and comparing the two sides. The examiner quickly learns to appreciate the smooth sensations of normal tone, and experience permits the detection of even a slight increase in tone when it is present. Palpation of the proximal muscle with one hand during passive movement will detect the presence of cog-wheeling, which is a ratchety jerkiness associated with extrapyramidal disease. In the lower extremities, the examiner should grasp the foot and perform several passive dorsiflexion and plantar flexion movements followed by sudden forced dorsiflexion of the foot. The presence of involuntary rhythmic dorsiflexion/plantar flexion movements is termed ankle clonus and occurs only in the presence of increased tone. Ankle clonus is occasionally present in healthy athletic individuals but is not sustained. The presence of sustained clonus or unilateral clonus with absence on the other side is abnormal.

Strength is tested by asking the patient to contract a muscle group against resistance applied by the examiner. It is important to compare the two sides. As a minimum the examiner should evaluate: abduction, arm at 90 degrees; flexion and extension, forearm; flexion and extension, wrist; grip; flexion and extension, thigh; flexion and extension, leg; dorsi and plantar flexion, foot; inversion and eversion, foot; extension, great toe (see Figure 1–14); flexion, toes. A more detailed evaluation is indicated when the history suggests the presence of a spinal cord or peripheral nerve lesion (see Table 1–7).

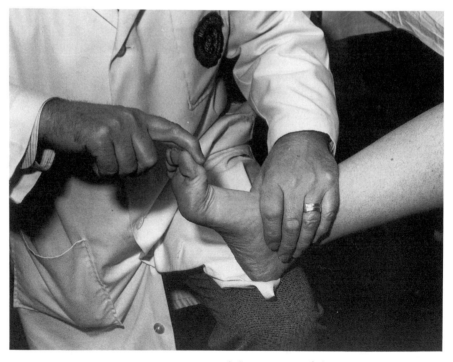

FIGURE 1–14.   Examination of the extensors of the great toe.

TABLE 1–7. **Muscle Innervation—Action**

Muscle	Nerve Root Level	Action
Rhomboids	Dorsal scapular N C_4–C_5	Adduction–scapula
Supraspinatus	Suprascapular N C_4–C_5	Abduction–arm
Infraspinatus	Suprascapular N C_4–C_6	Lateral rotation–arm
Serratus anterior	Long thoracic N C_5–C_7	Draws scapula forward during pushing
Subscapularis	Subscapular N C_5–C_6	Medial rotation–arm
Latissimus dorsi	Thoracodorsal N C_6–C_8	Adduction, medial rotation–arm
Teres major	Lateral subscapular N C_5–C_7	Adduction, extension, medial rotation–arm
Deltoid	Axillary N C_5–C_6	Abduction–arm
Biceps brachii	Musculocutaneous N C_5–C_6	Flexion–forearm Supination–hand
Triceps	Radial N C_6–C_8	Extension–forearm
Brachioradialis	Radial N C_5–C_6	Flexion–forearm
Extensor carpi radialis	Radial N C_5–C_7	Extension, abduction–hand
Supinator	Radial N C_5–C_7	Supination–hand
Extensor digitorum	Radial N C_6–C_8	Extension–wrist, phalanges
Extensor carpi ulnaris	Radial N C_6–C_8	Extension adduction–hand
Abductor pollicis longus	Radial N C_6–C_8	Abduction–thumb
Extensor pollicis longus	Radial N C_6–C_8	Extension–second phalanx thumb
Extensor pollicis brevis	Radial N C_7–T_1	Extension–first phalanx thumb
Pronator teres	Median N C_6–C_7	Pronation–hand
Flexor carpi radialis	Median N C_6–C_7	Flexion, abduction–hand
Flexor digitorum sublimis	Median N C_7–T_1	Flexion–second phalanx–fingers
Flexor digitorum profundus	Median N C_7–T_1	Flexion–terminal phalanx–fingers
Flexor pollicis longus	Median N C_6–C_8	Flexion–second phalanx thumb
Abductor pollicis brevis	Median N C_7–T_1	Abduction–thumb
Opponens pollicis	Median N C_7–T_1	Abduction, flexion–thumb
Flexor pollicis brevis	Median N C_7–T_1	Adduction, flexion–thumb
Flexor carpi ulnaris	Ulnar N C_7–T_1	Flexion, adduction–hand
Abductor digiti quinti brevis	Ulnar N C_8–T_1	Abduction–little finger
Flexor digiti quinti brevis	Ulnar N C_8–T_1	Flexion–little finger
Opponens digiti quinti	Ulnar N C_8–T_1	Abduction, flexion–little finger
Abductor pollicis	Ulnar N C_8–T_1	Adduction–thumb

TABLE 1–7. Continued

Muscle	Nerve Root Level	Action
Interossei	Ulnar N C_8–T_1	Dorsal–abduction fingers from middle finger
Lumbricals	1,2–median 3,4–ulnar C_8–T_1	Palmar–adduction fingers toward middle finger
Neck flexors	C_1–C_6	Flexion–neck
Neck extensors	C_1–T_1	Extension–neck
Diaphragm	Phrenic N C_3–C_5	Diaphragmatic breathing
Abdominal muscles upper lower	T_5–T_9 T_{10}–L_3	
Iliopsoas	Femoral N L_2–L_4	Flexion–thigh at hip
Adductor magnus, longus, brevis	Obturator N L_2–L_4	Adduction–thigh
Gluteus medius minimus	Superior gluteal N L_4–S_1	Abduction, medial rotation–thigh
Gluteus maximus	Inferior gluteal N L_4–S_2	Extension, lateral rotation–thigh
Quadriceps femoris	Femoral N L_4–S_1	Extension–leg at knee
Hamstrings	Sciatic N L_4–S_1	Flexion–leg at knee
Tibialis anterior	Deep peroneal N L_4–L_5	Dorsiflexion, inversion–foot
Extensor hallucis longus	Deep peroneal N L_4–S_1	Extension–great toe dorsiflexion–foot
Extensor dig. longus	Deep peroneal N L_4–S_1	Extension–lat. 4 toes dorsiflexion–foot
Extensor dig. brevis	Deep peroneal N L_4–S_1	Extension–all toes except little toe
Peroneus longus brevis	Sup. peroneal N L_5–S_1	Eversion–foot
Gastrocnemius soleus	Tibial N L_5–S_2	Plantar flexion–foot
Tibialis posterior	Posterior tibial N L_5–S_1	Inversion–foot
Flexor dig. longus	Posterior tibial L_5–S_2	Plantar flexion–toes
Flexor hallucis longus	Posterior tibial L_5–S_2	Plantar flexion–great toe
Foot intrinsics	Posterior tibial L_5–S_2	

The differentiation of lower motor neuron lesions from upper motor neuron lesions is listed in Table 1–8.

Muscle strength can be graded on a scale of 0 to 5, with 5-normal strength, 4-slight weakness, 3-marked weakness, 2-ability to contract against gravity, 1-inability to contract against gravity, and 0-total paralysis.

EXAMINATION OF COORDINATION

The cerebellum located in the posterior cranial fossa, coordinates muscle movement and maintains body equilibrium and muscle tone. The main anatomic divisions of the cerebellum consist of two large lateral hemispheres, an anterior lobe, and a flocculo-nodular lobe. There are connections to the midbrain, pons, and medulla by the superior, middle, and inferior cerebellar peduncles. Disease of the cerebellum produces ataxia, intention tremor, nystagmus, dysmetria (disturbed ability to gauge distances), dysdiadochokinesia (disturbed ability to perform rapid alternating movements), hypotonia, and rebound. See Table 1–9 for correlation of areas of cerebellum involved and symptoms and signs produced.

TABLE 1–8. Differentiation of Upper Motor and Lower Motor Neuron Lesions

	Tone	Muscle Bulk	Reflexes	Fasciculations
Upper motor neuron lesion	Spastic—may be flaccid early	Min. atrophy only after long period of disuse	Increased—may be clonus, plantar extensor	Absent
Lower motor neuron lesion	Flaccid	Decrease in bulk	Decreased or absent, plantar flexor	Present

TABLE 1–9. Signs and Symptoms of Cerebellar Disease°

	Cerebellar Hemisphere (Posterior lobe– neocerebellum)	Rostral Cerebellum (Anterior lobe– paleocerebellum)	Caudal Cerebellum (Flocculonodular lobe–archicerebellum)
Ataxia	+	Truncal ataxia + upper extremity ataxia	Truncal ataxia + lower extremity ataxia
Nystagmus	+	0	±
Intention tremor	+	0	0
Hypotonia	+	+	±
Rebound	+	±	0
Dysmetria / Dysdiadochokinesia / Dysarthria	+	0	0

° It is important to remember that cerebellar lesions tend to produce ipsilateral symptoms and signs.

Testing for abnormalities of coordinated movements of the upper limbs is carried out by asking the patient to extend the arms forward 90 degrees with the forearms and hands supinated. The patient is then asked to close the eyes and maintain the limbs in the extended position without movement. There may be a very slow "drift" of one of the upper limbs. This usually takes the form of very slow pronation of the affected limb and then gradual descent. Drifting may be seen with minimal weakness of the affected limb or sensory (proprioceptive) impairment of the limb. Upward or lateral drifting is seen occasionally in the presence of impaired proprioception or cerebellar disease. Rebound may be tested by depressing one of the extended limbs and releasing it rapidly. The extended arm in the intact individual will immediately reassume the initial position, but the arm of the patient with cerebellar disease will make several oscillations of decreasing amplitude before it assumes the resting position.

The patient is then asked to rapidly pronate and supinate the extended forearms and hands. These rapid alternating movements should be of equal rate and amplitude on the two sides. Slowing may be present on one side in the presence of weakness, increased tone, dyspraxia, disturbed sensation, or cerebellar impairment. Cerebellar ataxia produces slowing and overflinging, which is an increased amplitude of the supination/pronation movement. The patient is next asked to hold one hand in a pronated position and to tap the back of the hand rhythmically with the fingers of the other hand as rapidly as possible. This is normally performed in a rhythmic fashion, but the rhythm is variable and the amplitude inconsistent in cerebellar disease. The patient is then instructed alternately to supinate and pronate one hand on the dorsal surface of the other hand as rapidly as possible. Again, the rate is slowed, the rhythm is abnormal, and there is overflinging in the presence of cerebellar disease. The activity on the two sides is compared in all of these maneuvers.

Testing is continued by asking the patient to perform the finger-to-nose test. The examiner holds his extended index finger at arm's length from the patient. The patient is asked to touch the finger then touch his nose. This should be performed slowly. In many cases a patient will reach out and tap the examiner's finger and then rapidly return his finger to the nose. This will effectively block a mild degree of tremor. Cerebellar disease is characterized by past-pointing, with the patient's index finger repeatedly overshooting the target, and intention tremor, a terminal tremor that increases as the finger approaches the target.

Cerebellar function of the lower limbs is evaluated by the heel-to-shin test, in which the patient slides the heel of one lower extremity down the anterior tibial surface of the other. This should be a smooth movement, and the heel should be a remain on the tibial crest without ataxia. Other tests include the toe tap test, in which the patient taps the patella of one extremity with the toes of the other; and foot tapping test, where the patient stands with one foot placed forward and slightly to the side, rests the heel on the floor, and rapidly taps the floor with the toes.

EXAMINATION OF GAIT AND STATION

The patient is asked to walk across the examining room while the examiner observes the gait. The patient should have normal posture. The feet should be a normal distance apart, and there should be good associated movement of the arms. A loss of associated movement of the arm on one side indicates the early development of either spasticity or rigidity in that limb. Particular attention should be given as the patient turns; this movement is likely to produce slight ataxia or a shuffle indicating early dyspraxia of gait. After the patient has walked back and forth several times, the examiner demonstrates tandem gait and asks the patient to walk toward the examiner, with one foot placed in front of the other, the heel touching the toes at each step. This is normally performed without any undue unsteadiness or sudden lateral placement of one foot to maintain balance, which would indicate the presence of ataxia. The patient is then asked to walk across the examining room on his heels and return on the toes. These maneuvers not only tend to accentuate ataxia but can also disclose unexpected weakness in the lower limbs. The ability to perform heel walking and toe walking indicates good strength in the dorsiflexors and plantar flexors of the feet.

The examiner then requests the patient to stand with the feet together and parallel so that the heels and toes are touching. The examiner stands at the side of the patient and extends one arm in front of and one arm behind the patient at chest height. The patient is now ready to perform the Romberg test and is requested to close the eyes. The examiner maintains the arms in an extended position ready to give support to the patient should the patient fall. The patient should be able to maintain posture without movement of the feet with the eyes closed indefinitely. The Romberg test is then said to be negative. The Romberg test is positive if the patient has to move one or both feet in order to mainain balance. When there is marked loss of proprioception due to peripheral neuropathy or posterior column disease, the patient with a positive Romberg test may fall suddenly on closing the eyes and the examiner must always be prepared to give support to the patient.

EXAMINATION OF SENSORY FUNCTION

Tests of sensory function are concerned with appreciation of primary or cutaneous sensation and evaluation of cortical integration of sensory impulses.

The examination of cutaneous sensation begins with an evaluation of light touch. The examiner takes a wisp of cotton and applies it lightly to the skin. The patient closes the eyes and is instructed to answer yes when the stimulus is appreciated. The examiner alternates between the two sides, examining the homotopic areas. The patient sits with the hands supinated, and the cotton is applied to the skin of the neck beginning in the C_3 dermatome on each side and passing down the neck to the shoulder and the lateral aspect of the arm and forearm to the hand. The fingers are tested individually and the cotton is then applied up the medial aspect of the forearm and upper limb to the chest. Sensation in the lower limbs is examined in a similar fashion with an alternating application of the cotton down the lateral aspect of the thigh, leg, and foot and up the medial aspect of the foot, leg, and thigh.

Pain sensation is tested with a corsage pin or pinwheel. The examiner begins distally on the index finger and progresses to the lateral border of the hand, forearm, upper arm, and across the shoulder to the neck, up to the angle of the jaw. The two sides are compared and the patient is asked whether there is any difference between the two sides and whether there is any change as the pin is moved between the distal and proximal areas. The examiner then applies the pin to the middle finger, progressing to the palm and forearm, which tests sensation in the C_7 dermatome. Again, the two sides are compared. Finally, the pin is applied to the little finger, the medial aspect of the hand, the medial forearm, and the upper arm as high as the axilla. Once more the patient is asked to compare the two sides and to indicate whether there is any change as the pin is moved from distal to proximal areas. In testing pain over the lower limbs, the examiner begins distally at the level of the little toe and moves the pin up the lateral border of the foot and lower limb as high as the inguinal area. The two sides are compared, and the medial aspects of the foot, leg, and thigh are tested in similar fashion. Once again the patient is asked to compare the two sides and to indicate whether there is any change in pin sensation as it is moved from distal to proximal areas. When there is an indication of possible spinal cord lesion, it is important to test pinprick over the abdomen and thorax as high as the neck, again comparing the two sides (see Figure 1–15).

Vibration sense is tested by placing the base of the tuning fork over a bony prominence and instructing the patient to indicate when the sensation of vibration is no longer appreciated. Tests of vibration should be car-

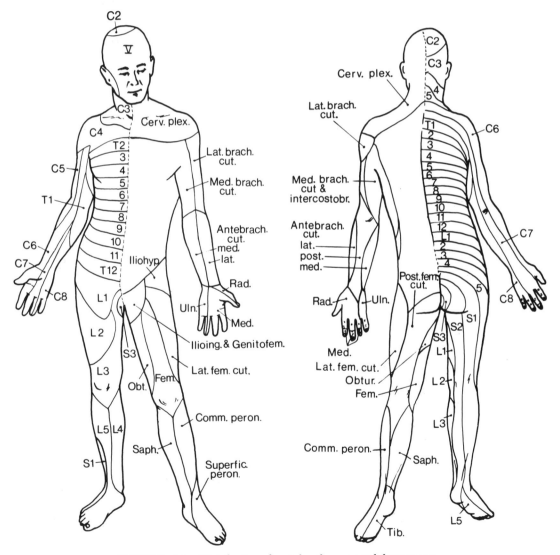

FIGURE 1–15. Distribution of peripheral nerves and dermatomes.

ried out over the terminal phalanx of the index finger bilaterally and over the terminal phalanx of the hallux bilaterally. If vibration is not appreciated at these sites then the examination is conducted more proximally at the level of the wrist and ankle. Under normal circumstances the patient indicates that vibration sense is no longer appreciated at the same time as the examiner loses the sense of vibration from the tuning fork. Vibration is decreased when the examiner appreciates the continuation of vibration that is no longer appreciated by the patient. Vibration sense should be equal on the two sides of the body.

Position sense or proprioception is tested by gently moving a terminal phalanx. The examiner grasps the terminal phalanx at the sides and gently moves it a few degrees in an upward or downward direction while the patient is instructed to close the eyes and indicate whether the digit is moved up or down. It is important that the examiner grasp the digit only on the sides so that the patient does not obtain indication of movement by alteration of pressure from above and below. It is customary to test movement at the terminal phalanx of the index finger and the terminal phalanx of the hallux and compare the two sides. Loss of position sense at these sites is an indication for testing movement of the finger at the metacarpal phalangeal joint and the hallux at the matatarsal phalangeal joint. Position sense will be lost at these joints only when this modality is severely impaired.

Temperature sensation is evaluated by application of glass tubes filled with hot or iced water to the skin. The examiner applies the two tubes in a random fashion and alternates to each side of the body as described under light touch. The patient is asked to identify whether the stimulus is hot or cold.

Discrimination of tactile stimuli is a cortical function sometimes termed cortical sensation, which may be evaluated by testing for tactile localization, extinction, two-point discrimination, graphism, and stereognosis.

Tactile localization is tested by asking the patient to close the eyes and to name the body part that is touched with a piece of cotton. This is a complex sensory task requiring cortical integration. The patient is then touched at an identical site on both sides of the body at the same time. Under normal circumstances the patient will appreciate both stimuli. However, if there is an early lesion involving the parietal lobe, the patient will appreciate only one stimulus and will fail to appreciate the stimulus applied to the side

opposite the parietal lobe lesion. This failure is termed extinction.

Two-point discrimination tests the ability of the patient to differentiate one stimulus from two. The ability to appreciate two stimuli shows great variation; the fingertips have the most sensitivity and are able to differentiate two points 2 mm apart. The test is carried out by asking the patient to close the eyes and applying either one or two points over the fingertips (see Figure 1–16). The patient is asked to indicate whether one or two points were applied. The fingertips over the right and left hand are compared. Two-point discrimination is impaired in parietal lobe lesions.

Stereognosis is an integrative function of parietooccipital location in which the patient attempts to identify familiar objects placed in the palm of the hand when the eyes are closed. Astereognosis, the inability to identify the object, is associated with parietooccipital lobe lesions and is usually easy to identify when the nondominant lobe is involved. Graphism is tested by asking the patient to close the eyes and extend the hand in a supine position. The examiner then constructs numbers in random fashion from zero to nine over the finger pad of the terminal phalanx. The patient is asked to identify each number. The number of incorrect responses can be compared on the two sides. Graphesthesia or impaired graphism is a very sensitive indicator of parietal lobe damage.

EXAMINATION OF REFLEXES

Reflexes are of three types: (a) stretch or tendon reflexes, (b) superficial reflexes, and (c) release reflexes.

The jaw jerk is obtained by placing the examining index finger in the midline on the patient's jaw and asking the patient to open the mouth about 30 degrees and then relax. The examiner then strikes the index finger with the tendon hammer. This produces stretching of the masseter and pterygoid muscles, followed by reflex contraction of these muscles, and the jaw jerks toward a closed position. The jaw jerk is often absent in normal individuals or may be present with minimal movement of the jaw. This movement is exaggerated in corticobulbar tract lesions above the midpons. The jaw jerk is important since it is the highest stretch reflex that can be elicited in the neurologic examination. An increased jaw jerk means that the lesion is above the midpons. A normal jaw jerk with

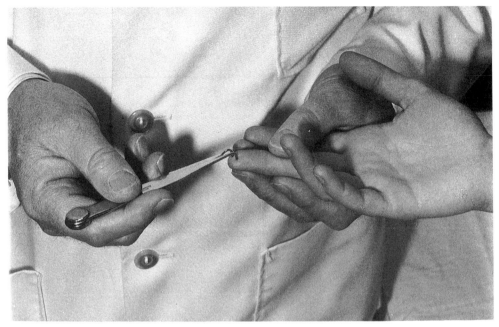

FIGURE 1–16. Testing two-point discrimination.

increase in the tendon reflexes in the upper limbs indicates that the lesion lies below the pons but above C_5.

The stretch or tendon reflexes of the upper limb are tested with the patient seated and the hands in a supine position on the thighs. The patient is instructed to relax. The examiner tests the brachioradialis reflex by percussion of the radius proximal to the wrist joint. The stimulus causes contraction of the brachioradialis (C_5–C_6) with a flexion movement at the elbow. The response on the two sides is compared. The examiner then places his index finger on the patient's biceps tendon and gently strikes the finger with the tendon hammer. This produces contraction of the biceps (C_5–C_6) and flexion at the elbow. The two sides are compared. To test the triceps reflex, the elbow is flexed to 90 degrees and the wrist is supported by the examiner's left arm. The triceps tendon is percussed by the tendon hammer just above the elbow, producing extension of the elbow. The triceps reflex (C_6–C_7) is compared on the two sides. Finally, the finger jerk (C_7–C_8) is tested by flexing the patient's fingers over the examiner's index and middle finger (see Figure 1–17). The examiner then strikes his index and middle fingers with the tendon hammer. This produces flexion of the fingers.

The stretch reflexes in the lower limbs are tested with the patient seated and the legs relaxed and flexed at right angles to the thighs. The examiner then strikes the patellar tendon and notes the response. The patellar reflexes should be symmetric. When these reflexes (L_2–L_4) are depressed, the patient is asked to perform the Jendrassik maneuver by hooking the fingers of the two hands together and attempting to pull the hands apart (see Figure 1–18). This often suffices to accentuate or reinforce the patellar reflexes. In testing the ankle jerks (S_1–S_2) the patient is asked to apply gentle plantar flexion onto the palmar surface of the examiner's hand. The examiner notes the pressure on the hand and using the tendon hammer in his other hand strikes the Achilles tendon. The degree of plantar flexion is noted. The examiner then asks the patient to apply the same pressure on the examiner's hand on the other side and once again strikes the Achilles tendon with the tendon hammer. The response should be symmetric.

Stretch reflexes should be graded as follows: 0, absent; 1+, diminished; 2+, normal; 3+, increased; and 4+, clonic.

Superficial reflexes are elicited by applying gentle pressure to the skin in a specific area. The abdominal reflexes can be elicited by stroking the skin of the abdomen gently with a blunt object such as the wooden end of

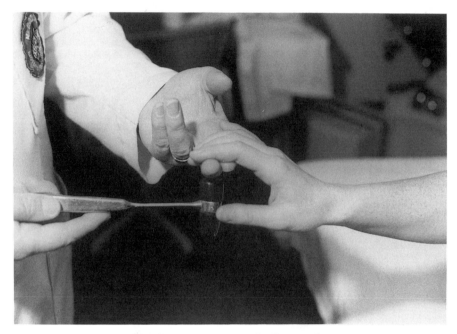

FIGURE 1–17.   Testing the finger jerk.

a cotton applicator. The skin is stroked in a diagonal fashion moving downward lateral to medial toward the midline. The sites stimulated are above the umbilicus, at the level of the umbilicus, and below the umbilicus. The abdominal muscles contract beneath the stimulus under normal circumstances. The abdominal reflexes are absent on the side of the corticospinal tract lesion but also may be absent if the innervation of the stimulated quadrant is interfered with for any reason. It is often difficult to observe abdominal reflexes in obese individuals.

The plantar response is elicited by stimulation of the lateral aspect of the sole of the foot with a blunt object. The movement is carried along the lateral aspect of the sole and then across the head of the metatarsal bones. This gentle stimulus should produce flexion of the hallux, which is a normal plantar flexor response. Any extension movement is abnormal and should be recorded as an extensor plantar response. The Babinski response consists of extension of the hallux and extension of the other toes, which separate in a fanlike fashion (see Figure 1–19).

The cremasteric reflex can be obtained in the male by stroking the anterior medial aspect of the upper thigh with a blunt object. The stimulus results in contraction of the cre-masteric muscle and elevation of the testis on the same side. This reflex is lost in corticospinal tract lesions and in lesions involving the lower segments of the spinal cord. The anal reflex is produced by gently stroking the skin around the anal margin which produces contraction of the anal sphincter. The anal reflex is lost in lesions involving the sacral segments of the spinal cord and cauda equina.

Release reflexes are reflex responses present in the newborn infant. These reflexes disappear with maturation of the central nervous system but can reappear in degenerative diseases associated with loss of inhibitory activity in the brain. The glabellar reflex is elicited by gently tapping the forehead in the midline just above the bridge of the nose. Under normal circumstances this produces rhythmic contraction of the eyelids, which disappears after a few seconds. The abnormal response consists of persistent closure of the eyes and blepharospasm in response to each stimulus which is persistent as long as the stimulus is applied. The glabellar reflex is indicative of degenerative disease of the brain and is frequently seen in Parkinson's disease, Alzheimer's disease, other forms of dementia, frontal lobe infarction, and frontal lobe tumors. The snout reflex cannot be elicited in normal individuals but appears in patients each stimulus. The sucking reflex can be obtained by gently stroking the upper or lower lip from the midline to the lateral border of the mouth with the finger or with a tongue blade. The lips contract in a sucking movement. This reflex, which is normally present in infants, reappears in diffuse disease of the brain and is usually noted in patients with Alzheimer's disease and other dementias. The chewing reflex is an abnormal response obtained by placing a tongue blade in the mouth. The patient begins to make chewing movements, and when the reflex is well developed the jaws may bite down on the tongue blade and make removal difficult. This has been called the bulldog response. The presence of a chewing reflex is indicative of diffuse bilateral lesions involving the cerebral hemispheres.

The grasp reflex is a response obtained by stimulation of the palm of the patient's hand. The examiner grasps the patient's hand as if to shake hands and then strokes the palm of the patient with his fingers. The reflex is positive when the patient's fingers flex and grasp the examiner's fingers. In the early stages of this abnormality the patient can release the examiner's fingers on request. Later, release is not accomplished on request and the grasp is sustained. The release can then be accomplished by gently stroking the dorsal surface of the patient's hand. The extreme form of the grasp reflex is the groping reflex, in which the patient actively seeks objects to grasp in the hand and may be frequently found tightly clenching the bed clothes. The grasp reflex is indicative of diffuse bilateral disease involving the cerebral hemispheres. It is commonly seen in the dementias but can occur in many other diseases producing bilateral cerebral damage.

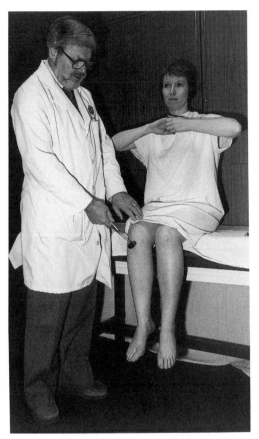

FIGURE 1–18. The Jendrassik maneuver.

with bilateral cerebral damage, often associated with pseudobulbar palsy. The reflex is elicited by tapping the face between the upper lip and the nose gently with the finger. There is a pursing of the lips in response to

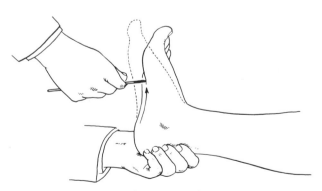

FIGURE 1–19. The extensor plantar response.

FINAL TOUCHES OF EXAMINATION

The examination should be concluded by the performance of several observations which may add to the total picture of the patient's disability.

Examination of Peripheral Pulses

The radial pulses should be of equal volume at the wrist and the dorsalis pedis, and posterior tibial pulses should be palpable in the feet. Peripheral vascular disease often accompanies cerebrovascular disease, and the examiner should auscultate for the presence of bruits over the femoral arteries if the peripheral pulses are absent in the feet.

Auscultation for Bruits

Auscultation should be carried out over the carotid arteries during the general physical examination for the presence of bruits after the heart has been examined. This will help to localize the bruit to the carotid artery and eliminate the possibility of transmission from the heart. The examiner should also auscultate over the eye for the presence of intracranial bruits. This is accomplished by using the bell of the stethoscope, which is placed over the closed eyelid. The patient is then asked to open the opposite eye, which removes the sound of muscle artifact and permits auscultation into the cranial cavity (see Figure 1–20). Intracranial bruits are usually associated with arteriovenous malformations and are occasionally heard in other conditions such as severe stenosis of the carotid artery or persistent trigeminal artery. As already indicated, auscultation should be carried out over the femoral arteries as they enter the thigh in the inguinal region, particularly when the pedal pulses are absent, since this latter condition is often associated with atherosclerotic narrowing of the iliac or femoral arteries.

Nuchal Rigidity

Every patient should be examined for the presence of nuchal rigidity. This can be performed at the end of the cranial nerve examination. The examiner asks the patient to flex the head and place the chin on the chest. The performance of this simple maneuver will lessen the risk of overlooking an early encephalitis, early meningitis, or subarachnoid hemorrhage. The patients who seem to have nuchal rigidity can also be tested for the presence of Brudzinski's sign, which consists of

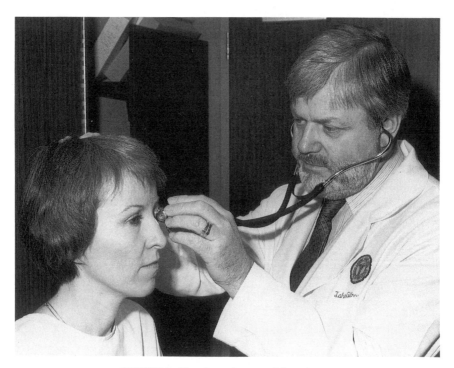

FIGURE 1–20.   Auscultation of the orbit.

flexion of the knees when the head is flexed on the chest, and of Kernig's sign, which is characterized by back pain and sciatic pain on attempting to straighten the leg when the thigh is flexed at the hip.

Examination of the Peripheral Nerves

Palpation of peripheral nerves should be carried out in all cases of suspected peripheral neuropathy. The ulnar nerves are easily palpated in the ulnar groove on the medial aspect of the elbow joint. The common peroneal nerve can be felt as it winds around the head of the fibula. Enlargement of nerves occurs in some cases of chronic peripheral neuropathy.

Examination of the Spine

A short cervical spine with low head line may indicate the presence of some congenital abnormality at the base of the skull, such as platybasia or odontoid compression. The cervical spine may show limitation of movement in the presence of cervical spondylosis. Scoliosis is a feature of a number of neurologic conditions, including the spinocerebellar degenerations. Scoliosis also occurs in patients who have some degree of paralysis of the paraspinal muscles following poliomyelitis and trauma. There is loss of lumbar lordosis in degenerative diseases of the lumbar spine, particularly in herniated lumbar disk. This may be associated with a mild degree of scoliosis and spasm of the erector spinae. There is usually limitation of straight-leg raising (Lasegue's sign) in patients with herniation of lower lumbar disk and sciatic pain.

Pes Cavus

The examination of the gait and the Romberg test give the examiner an opportunity to observe the patient's feet for the presence of pes cavus. This condition is found in a number of chronic neurologic conditions including the familial spinocerebellar degenerations and may be observed in patients who have congenital or long-standing lesions involving the corticospinal tracts dating from infancy or early childhood.

CHAPTER 2

COMA

Definition

Coma is a state of unresponsiveness in which the patient is unable to sense or respond to the environment.

Etiology and Pathology

Coma occurs in response to four conditions:

1. A focal supratentorial lesion, meningeal infection or subarachnoid hemorrhage producing increased intracranial pressure, which is transmitted to the ascending reticular activating system
2. A lesion in the posterior fossa or brain stem directly affecting the ascending reticular activating system
3. Metabolic encephalopathy with diffuse involvement of the cerebral hemispheres
4. Generalized tonic-clonic seizures.

There are many causes of coma, and a systemic approach is required in the examination of comatose patients to avoid overlooking potentially remediable situations. Table 2–1 lists the more common causes of coma.

Examination of the Acutely Comatose Patient

The evaluation of the acutely comatose patient is a common situation encountered in the emergency room. The examination should begin by attempting to obtain information from those who are familiar with or who have had some contact with the patient, including relatives, police, and the emergency services team. A history of hypertension, diabetes, drug abuse, epilepsy, or recent head trauma is invaluable.

Immediate Action. Although the patient may have already been seen by others in the emergency room, the examiner should check to see whether immediate action is necessary. The patient's airway should be clear, and there should be no signs of respiratory obstruction. If there is evidence of respiratory failure, the patient should be intubated and placed on a mechanical respirator. The comatose patient may be hypotensive or become hypotensive at any time. This complication should be immediately treated with fluid challenge, transfusions, or, if necessary, dopamine infusion. Hypotension is rarely caused by intracranial lesions. If the patient is in cardiac arrest or showing severe cardiac arrhythmias the cardiopulmonary resuscitation team should be called immediately.

Stabilization. The neurologic evaluation begins by ensuring that the patient's condition is stable. Two peripheral intravenous lines, one measuring central venous pressure and the other for the administration of intravenous fluids, should be inserted. A Foley catheter should be placed in the bladder, and a nasogastric tube should be passed into the stomach. A cervical collar should be applied until a cervical fracture can be ruled out by x-ray. A blood sample should be drawn and

TABLE 2–1.   Causes of Coma

1. Intracranial
   a. Vascular—infarction, intracerebral
      hemorrhage, venous-sinus thrombosis.
   b. Trauma—penetrating injury; closed head
      injury—concussion, contusion,
      intracerebral hemorrhage, subdural
      hematoma, epidural hematoma.
   c. Infection—encephalitis, meningitis,
      abscess.
   d. Epilepsy—status epilepticus
   e. Neoplasm

2. Metabolic
   a. Electrolyte and acid base disorders—
      increased or decreased sodium, potassium,
      calcium and magnesium levels; acidosis and
      alkalosis.
   b. Endocrine disorders—diabetic coma,
      hypoglycemia, nonketotic hyperglycemic
      hyperosmolar coma, adrenal insufficiency,
      Cushing's disease, myxedema coma,
      thyrotoxicosis, hypo- and
      hyperparathyroidism.
   c. Hepatic coma.
   d. Uremia.
   e. Hypoglycemia.
   f. Anoxia—airway obstruction, pulmonary
      dysfunction, anemia, cardiovascular
      dysfunction.
   g. Vitamin deficiencies—thiamine
      (Wernicke's encephalopathy), niacin,
      vitamin B-12, pyridoxine.
   h. Poisons and intoxications.
   i. Hypothermia, hyperthermia.

sent for electrolytes, glucose, blood urea nitrogen (BUN), serum creatinine, complete blood count, a drug screen, and a blood alcohol level in cases of suspected alcohol intoxication. Arterial blood gases should be drawn if hypoxia is suspected. The patient is attached to a cardiac monitor and an electrocardiogram is obtained to rule out a recent myocardial infarct, detect arrhythmias, or discover evidence of electrolyte imbalance. The urine should be tested for the presence of glucose and blood and sent for urinalysis. The nasogastric tube aspirate may be sent for analysis if poisoning or intoxication is suspected.

Once the patient is stabilized, 50 ml of a 50 percent dextrose and water solution should be administered intravenously. This should be preceded by an intravenous injection of 100 mg of thiamine if there is any suspicion that the patient may be suffering from Wernicke's encephalopathy. In suspected cases of opiate usage 0.4 mg (1 ml) of naloxone (Narcan), a narcotic antagonist, should be administered intravenously. The injection can be repeated at two- or three-minute intervals. If there is no improvement following two or three doses of naloxone, the patient's comatose state is unlikely to be due to opiates.

General Physical Examination. A systematic examination of the patient should be carried out. The patient should first be observed. The dress; age; stigmata of chronic illness, such as gingival hypertrophy in the epileptic patient on phenytoin therapy; pattern of respiration; and position of the body and limbs should be noted. The comatose patient with an acute hemiplegia lies with the affected lower limb externally rotated. The examiner notes the presence of spontaneous movements such as myoclonic jerks or spontaneous decerebration. A general physical examination should be done in an attempt to identify evidence of organ failure or trauma. The odor of the breath should be noted. The examiner may detect the odor of alcohol, the smell of ketones in diabetic coma, of urine in uremia, and fetor hepaticus in liver failure. The scalp should be palpated by running the fingers of both hands through the hair from the frontal area to the occiput in an effort to detect any depressed fractures or lacerations. The external auditory meatus should be examined for the presence of cerebrospinal fluid or hemorrhage indicating fracture of the petrous temporal bone. The mastoid area should be examined for the presence of bruising (Battle's sign) indicating a fracture of the middle cranial fossa. The zygomatic arches should be palpated. The sclera of the eyes should be examined for hemorrhages. A hemorrhage of the lateral aspect of the eye that is not bordered posteriorly by normal sclera is indicative of a fracture of the anterior cranial fossa. The nose should be examined for fractures of the nasal bones and epistaxis. Persistent drainage of a clear, watery fluid suggests the possibility of a fracture of the cribriform plate with drainage of cerebrospinal fluid. The mouth should be examined and any broken or loose teeth removed to prevent aspiration. Lacerations of the tongue are almost always caused by a recent generalized seizure and most commonly occur on the lateral borders of the tongue. The neck should be palpated for the presence of hematomas and abnormalities of the vertebral bodies. The examination continues with palpation of the clavicles and auscultation and observations of the chest to detect absence of breath sounds and paradoxical respirations. The chest should be palpated for rib fractures. The trachea should be in the midline, and the examiner should palpate the left side of the chest for the apex beat and note its position. Auscultation of the heart is carried out and the presence of dysrhythmia or murmurs noted. The abdomen is palpated for the presence of muscle rigidity indicating possible abdominal hemorrhage or infection. The limbs are then examined for the presence of fractures.

Neurologic Examination. Since the comatose patient is unable to respond, the neurologic examination must be modified to obtain responses that are largely reflex and vegetative in nature.

Appreciation of the respiratory pattern and rhythm is important when examining a semicomatosed or comatosed patient (see Table 2–2). Posthyperventilation apnea is present when three minutes of hyperventilation are followed by a period of apnea of more than 30 seconds. This respiratory response is associated with diffuse metabolic or structural forebrain damage. Cheyne-Stokes respiration is characterized by rhythmic waxing and waning of respiration separated by periods of apnea. This type of respiration is frequently associated with early brain stem compression or bilateral deep cerebral hemisphere damage. Central neurogenic hyperventilation is characterized by regular, rapid, deep, machinery-like breathing and is associated with lesions of the midbrain and/or pons. Apneustic breathing is characterized by a pause at the completion of inspiration and is associated with pontine lesions. Ataxic breathing is characterized by an irregular rhythm and depth of respiration and is associated with dysfunction of the medullary respiratory centers.

The pupils should be equal in size and briskly reactive to light. Constricted pupils occur when there is paralysis of sympathetic function or stimulation of parasympathetic connections. This occurs in severe bilateral hemorrhage, or following ingestion of narcotics. Dilated pupils indicate paralysis of parasympathetic function or stimulation of sympathetic connections, which occurs following overdosage with hallucinogens, central ner-

TABLE 2–2. Signs of Rostral-Caudal Deterioration and Level of Dysfunction*

Level of Dysfunction	Pupil Size and Pupillary Light Reflex	Oculocephalic Reflexes ("Doll's eye movements") Caloric Testing	Respiratory Pattern	Response to Painful Stimuli
Normal	Normal Briskly reactive	Calorics; normal nystagmus present	Normal	Appropriate
Hemispheres	Small Reactive	Doll's eyes present Calorics; eyes may be tonically deviated	Cheyne-Stokes or posthyperventilation apnea	Decorticate posturing
Diencephalic	Small 1–3 cm Reacting	Doll's eyes present Calorics; brisk may be tonic deviation	Normal	Decorticate
Midbrain	Midposition 3–5 cm fixed	Doll's eyes present Calorics; poor response, may be internuclear ophthalmoplegia	Central neurogenic hyperventilation	Decerebrate posturing
Pons	Midposition	± present	Central neurogenic hyperventilation or apneustic	Decerebrate or flaccid
Medulla	Midposition and fixed Terminally dilated and fixed	Absent	Ataxic or absent	Flaccid

* From Plum, F.; Posnov, J. *Diagnosis of Stupor and Coma.* Philadelphia: F. A. Davis Co.; 1980.

vous system stimulants, or anticholinergic drugs (see p. 326). A unilateral fixed and dilated pupil is indicative of a third nerve paralysis in a comatose patient, providing a mydriatic agent was not applied in an effort to obtain a better view of the fundus, a procedure that should never be performed in an emergency room. Pressure on the third nerve results in pupillary dilatation, which precedes paralysis of extraocular muscles because the fibers subserving the light reflex surround an inner core of fibers that innervate the extraocular muscles. Dilatation of the pupil may indicate herniation of the medial aspect of the temporal lobe over the free edge of the tentorium cerebelli (uncal herniation). This ominous size indicates the need for immediate treatment of increased intracranial pressure. A metabolic abnormality should be suspected when the patient is nonresponsive with absent corneal reflexes and absent extraocular movement, yet the pupils are reactive.

The eyes should be examined while at rest. The examiner should note the position of the eyelids and whether they are completely closed. The lids may be gently raised and allowed to close; slow and incomplete closure is associated with deep coma. The corneal reflexes should be tested. There should be a brisk direct and consensual response. If the patient's eyes are open it is possible to evaluate the visual fields by making a threatening gesture with the hands on one side and repeating the procedure on the other side and noting if the patient shows reflex blinking. The position of the eyes at rest should be noted. Complete paralysis of the third nerve produces abduction of the affected eye. Bilateral sixth nerve palsies may occur with increased intracranial pressure, and this sign is of no localizing value as an isolated phenomenon and does not necessarily indicate brain stem damage. Fixed conjugate deviation of the eyes indicates an ipsilateral destructive lesion, a contralateral irritative lesion of the frontal lobe, or a destructive lesion of the contralateral brain stem. Ocular bobbing is associated with an upper brain stem lesion, while skew deviation of the eyes indicates a severe pontine lesion.

The fundus should be examined in all comatose patients. The retina and optic nerves should be carefully evaluated for the presence of papilledema, hemorrhages, hypertensive or diabetic change, or spasm of the retinal arteries. Subarachnoid hemorrhage is often accompanied by a subhyaloid hemorrhage, which appears as a blotlike hemorrhage on the surface of the retina (see Figure 2–1).

Reflex eye movements should be tested in all comatose patients provided there is no evidence of a fracture of the cervical spine. Reflex eye movements are elicited by briskly turning the head to the right followed by turning it to the left and flexing and extending the head. If the patient's brain stem reflexes are intact, the eyes move in conjugate fashion in the opposite direction to the head movement and the "doll's eye" movements are said to be present. It is usually not possible to elicit this reflex in the conscious, alert patient as visual fixation overrides the reflex response. Reflex eye movements become increasingly difficult to elicit with progressive brain stem dysfunction. Paralysis of reflex eye movements will be total when the connections between the vestibular nuclei and the sixth nerve are disrupted at the level of the pontomedullary junction. In damage to the paramedian pontine reticular formation, the eyes move in conjugate fashion but fail to cross the midline when the examiner moves the head. In lesions of the medial longitudinal fasciculus (MLF) there is abduction of one eye but failure of adduction of the other eye on the side of the MLF lesion.

Caloric testing is used to augment the information obtained when testing reflex eye movements or when the possibility of a cervical spine fracture prohibits movement of the neck. The supine patient should be positioned with the head flexed forward 30 degrees, which places the horizontal semicircular canals in a horizontal position. The external canal should be free of cerumen, and the tympanic membrane should be intact. A slow injection of 20 ml of iced water should be made into the external canal. In the normal situation the eyes will slowly deviate to the ipsilateral side with a quick corrective return to the midline. Under these conditions, nystagmus is named by the fast component, injection of the left ear with iced water produces a right nystagmus. If warm water is injected, the slow phase will be toward the opposite side, and warm water injection into the left ear produces a left nystagmus. In patients with dysfunction of the cerebral hemispheres there is an ipsilateral tonic deviation of the eyes following injection of iced water, while injection of warm water produces a contralateral tonic deviation. Absence of response to caloric stimulation indicates total disruption

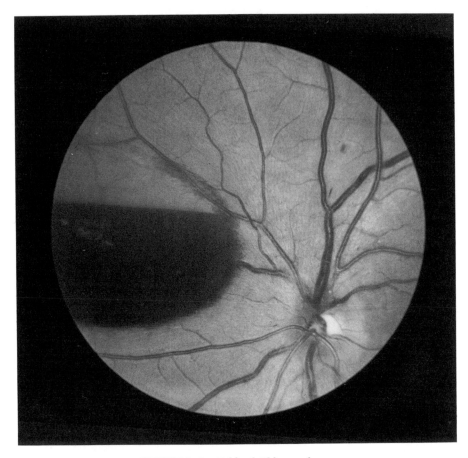

FIGURE 2–1.   Subhyaloid hemorrhage.

of the connections between the vestibular nuclei and sixth nerve nucleus.

Absence of reflex eye movements with preservation of caloric responses indicates the potential for a good outcome in the comatose patient. Absence of both reflex eye movements and caloric responses, however, indicates a poor prognosis (1). Absence of caloric responses and lack of pupillary light reflexes indicates a fatal outcome in all cases of coma (2).

In the absence of cervical fracture the head should be flexed forward onto the chest to detect the presence of nuchal rigidity. Tests for the presence of Kernig and Brudzinski signs should be performed. Nuchal rigidity suggests the possibility of encephalitis, meningitis, or subarachnoid hemorrhage. A lumbar puncture (LP) is indicated in patients who have nuchal rigidity. A magnetic resonance (MR) or computed tomography (CT) scan should be obtained before an LP is per-

formed if equipment is available to rule out the presence of a rapidly expanding supratentorial lesion.

The position of the limbs should be noted and the tone of each compared. In acute hemiplegia the upper limb is flaccid and the lower limb is flaccid and externally rotated. The stretch reflexes should be evaluated for the presence of any asymmetry. It is not unusual to find a bilateral extensor plantar response in a deeply comatose patient. A unilateral response suggests the presence of a contralateral, supratentorial mass lesion. The response of the patient to painful stimuli should be noted. The examiner may press upon the supraorbital notch, squeeze the trapezius or any muscle mass, or prick the skin. The patient may either wince in pain and attempt to withdraw from the stimulus, assume a decorticate or decerebrate posture (see Figure 2–2), or remain unresponsive, indicating deep coma.

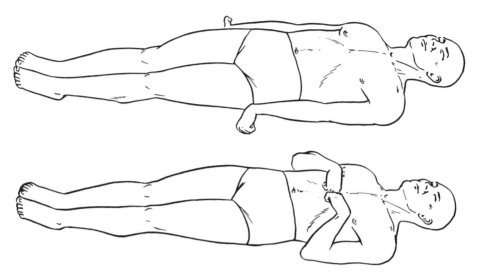

FIGURE 2–2.   Decerebrate versus decorticate posturing in the comatose patient.

The neurologic status of the patient should be repeatedly evaluated and the responses systematically recorded for later comparison.

Complications

Deterioration of the neurologic status may indicate incipient or ongoing herniation. Five types of herniation are of clinical importance.

1. Rostral-caudal deterioration when there is pressure on the brain stem from above by an expanding mass with progressive loss of brain stem function in a caudal direction (Table 2–2).

2. Uncal herniation with pressure on the brain stem caused by a herniation of the medial aspect of the temporal lobe over the free edge of the tentorium cerebelli.

Uncal herniation differs from rostral-caudal deterioration in that there is no diencephalic stage in uncal herniation. Coma develops rapidly and is preceded by unilateral dilatation of the pupil on the side of the uncal herniation that shows poor, then eventual absence of response to light due to pressure on the third nerve by the herniating mass. This is followed by lateral deviation of the eyes leading to external ophthalmoplegia on the affected side as the oculomotor fibers are paralyzed, then coma, bilateral decerebrate rigidity (Figure 2–2), and eventual total flaccidity. Hemiplegia associated with a fixed and dilated pupil is usually contralateral since uncal herniation usually occurs on the same side as an acute supratentorial mass lesion. However, if the mass shifts the brain stem so

that the contralateral cerebral peduncle is compressed against the tentorium (Kernohan-Woltman's notch), the hemiplegia will be ipsilateral to the mass lesion. In the more common central diencephalic syndrome of rostral-to-caudal deterioration with central pressure from above on the brain stem, there are no localizing pupillary signs.

Further deterioration in brain stem function is similar to the pontine and medullary stages in Table 2–2 except that the dilated fixed pupil remains larger on the side of the uncal herniation.

3. Cingulate herniation. In cingulate herniation the cingulate gyrus may herniate underneath the falx. This may be associated with compression of the anterior cerebral arteries followed by ischemia and infarction in the region of the paracentral lobules.

4. Upward cerebellar herniation. In posterior fossa lesions cerebellar hemorrhage or infarction may produce coma due to direct pressure on the brain stem or by upward herniation. There may be premonitory headache, vertigo, nausea, and vomiting followed by unreactive or poorly reactive pinpoint pupils, paralysis of upward or conjugate lateral gaze, and bilateral cerebral rigidity followed by flaccid quadriplegia.

5. Cerebellar tonsillar herniation. Posterior fossa lesions may also produce herniation of the cerebellar tonsils through the foramen magnum. This situation is associated with increasing occipital headache, nuchal rigidity, flexion of the head toward the side of the cer-

ebellar tonsillar herniation, and cardiac and respiratory arrest due to pressure on the medulla (see Figure 2–3).

Persistent Vegetative State

An occasional comatose patient stabilizes in a condition of incomplete recovery. A persistent vegetative state is said to be present when responsiveness is limited to postural and reflex movements of the extremities and eyes with absence of cortical function of more than two weeks duration. The electroencephalogram (EEG) shows several patterns and is of no value in predicting outcome. Brain stem auditory evoked potentials are normal. However, medial somatosensory evoked responses show prolonged central conduction time and an increasing delay may indicate further brain deterioration and approaching death (3).

Treatment

Increased intracranial pressure is defined as a mean cerebrospinal fluid pressure of more than 200 mm of water (15 mm of mercury). This in itself is not dangerous but when the increased pressure is associated with the presence of a mass lesion, distortion and pressure on other structures of the brain stem are always present and may decompensate with catastrophic results. Consequently, when a mass lesion is present the mass should be removed whenever possible. In those cases in which surgical decompression is not indicated or is going to be delayed, the treatment is aimed at reducing edema, thus decreasing the likelihood of shifts in pressure and herniation. Vasogenic edema is characterized by increased permeability of brain capillary endothelial cells and major involvement of white matter and is associated with mass lesions such as tumors and abscesses. Corticosteroids and osmotherapy have a beneficial effect in the treatment of this type of edema. Cytoxic edema, which is characterized by cellular swelling, involves both gray and white matter and is a complication of hypoxia following asphyxia or cardiac arrest, hypoosmolality, and severe hypoglycemia. Cytoxic edema responds only to osmotherapy.

Controlled Hyperventilation. Increase of the PCO_2 of the arterial system has a potent vasodilatory effect which in turn increases intracranial pressure. Controlled hyperventilation, which maintains the PCO_2 between 25 and 30, helps to decrease intracranial pressure.

Corticosteroid Therapy. Corticosteroid therapy can be administered using dexamethasone (Decadron) 12 mg initially, followed by 4 mg q6h. Response usually occurs within 12 to 24 hours. Dexamethasone stabilizes cellular membranes and also decreases CSF production. Beneficial effect of large dosages (16–32 mg q6h) remains to be established.

Osmotherapy. Osmotherapy has the advantage of acting very quickly. However, it decreases the amount of edema only in those

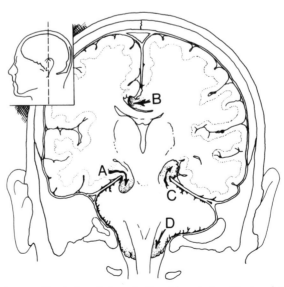

FIGURE 2–3. Types of brain herniation. A, Uncal herniation; B, cingulate herniation; C, upward cerebellar herniation; D, cerebellar tonsillar herniation.

areas with intact cellular membranes and vasculature. The effects are short-lived and can be associated with a rebound in intracranial pressure. In vasogenic edema, associated with trauma or mass lesions, mannitol is probably the best of the hyperosmolar agents available and should be administered in doses of 0.25 g/Kg q3h or 0.5 to 1.0 g/Kg q6h in a 20 percent solution over 20 minutes IV. In the absence of intracranial pressure monitoring a serum osmolality ranging from 305 to 315 mOsm/L is recommended. Constant elevation of the serum osmolality to levels greater than 320 mOsm can result in diffusion of osmotically active particles into the brain which can exacerbate edema. Excessive use of mannitol may also result in reduction of cardiac output and renal perfusion. This must be avoided. Glycerol, another osmotic agent, may be administered orally in a dosage of 1.5 g/Kg/day as a 50 or 75 percent solution in divided doses q6h.

Barbiturate Coma. When all attempts to control increased intracranial pressure are unsuccessful, barbiturate coma may be induced. Pentobarbital (Nembutal) and sodium thiopental (Pentothal) are the most frequently used barbiturates. If barbiturate coma therapy is to be used there must be a means of measuring intracranial pressure, arterial pressure, and pulmonary hemodynamics. A well-equipped, well-staffed intensive care unit is a necessity. Barbiturate coma has been shown to be most effective in reducing intracranial pressure due to head injury and encephalitis. The drugs are given in a loading dose of 5 to 30 mg/kg over one hour in 50 to 100 mg increments followed by a continuous maintenance infusion of 1 to 4 mg/kg/hr with the pentobarbital or thiopental dissolved in either 5 percent dextrose in water or 0.9 percent sodium chloride. The infusion is titrated to produce a burst suppression pattern in the electroencephalogram. (See treatment of status epilepticus, pages 79–80).

Intracranial Pressure Monitoring. It is now possible to monitor the intracranial pressure directly and continuously using an intraventricular catheter or a cranial bolt. This method has the advantage of detecting an early rise in intracranial pressure, thus avoiding the complications of herniation. As intracranial pressure rises there is a point of vascular decompensation with a loss of autoregulation and a sudden rise in pressure producing the plateau wave that may last for 5 to 20 minutes, accompanied by signs of neurologic deterioration such as pupillary dilatation or decerebrate posturing. This phenomenon indicates an urgent need for the use of measures to decrease intracranial pressure. A constant intraventricular pressure of 40 mm of mercury or more may indicate the need for urgent treatment to avoid impending herniation. Continuous intracranial pressure monitoring is also useful in assessing the effectiveness of osmotherapy and in predicting the need for an additional infusion of mannitol. It is often possible to "titrate" the dosage of mannitol to prevent the rebound of intracranial pressure that follows the single infusion of mannitol and to maintain intracranial pressure at a safe level.

REFERENCES

1. Ringel, R. A.; Riggs, J. E.; *et al.* Reversible coma with prolonged absence of pupillary and brainstem reflexes. Neurology 38:1275–1278; 1988.
2. Mueller-Jenson, A.; Neunzig, H-P.; *et al.* Outcome prediction in comatose patients: Significance of reflex eye movement analysis. J. Neurol. Neurosurg. Psychiatry. 50:389–392; 1987.
3. Hansotia, P. L. Persistent vegetative state. Review and report of electrodiagnostic studies in eight cases. Arch. Neurol. 42:1048–1052; 1985.

CHAPTER 3

CONGENITAL DISORDERS

DEVELOPMENTAL DEFECTS OF THE SPINAL CORD

Developmental defects of the spinal cord may be due to failure of closure of the neural tube, abnormalities in development of the spinal cord, or abnormalities in the development of the spinal ganglia and spinal nerves.

The developmental abnormalities occur within the first few weeks of life, and a number of etiologic factors have been identified, including genetic predisposition; viral infections, possibly rubella and other viruses; drugs; and irradiation during early pregnancy.

Neural Tube Defects

Definition. Neural tube defects are the most common birth defects in the United States and are due to failure of the neural tube to develop normally.

Etiology and Pathology. The etiology is uncertain at this time. Neural tube defects occur during early embryonic development at the time of closure of the neural tube. Failure of closure of the cephalic portion of the tube results in anencephaly. Failure of closure at other sites produces variable degrees of cranium bifidum or spina bifida.

Approximately 50 percent of neural tube defects result in anencephaly. Spina bifida occulta, which is the commonest defect involving the spinal canal, is characterized by failure of fusion of the vertebral laminae,

although the skin and superficial tissues are intact. A spinal meningocele consists of a cyst-like protrusion of meninges through the vertebral defect without involvement of the spinal cord. In myelomeningocele the cyst-like protrusion contains spinal cord and/or spinal nerves. Complete rachischisis consists of failure of fusion of the posterior spinal cord meninges and severe malformation of the spinal cord.

Dermal cysts are midline structures that develop when the dermis is included during closure of the midline structures. Dermoid cysts often occur in the lower lumbar area and are often connected to the spinal canal by a sinus tract. This is a potential channel for introduction of infection.

Clinical Features. Two out of every 1,000 babies born in the United States have a neural tube defect. Most anencephalic infants are either stillborn or die shortly after birth. In 80 percent of cases of spina bifida, there is an associated defect in the skin. Many of these infants are hydrocephalic and retarded and have no bladder or bowel control and a flaccid paralysis of all limbs. Twenty percent of children with spina bifida have a "closed" lesion in which the defect is covered by skin. These infants are usually of normal intelligence and have few or no physical handicaps.

Diagnostic Procedures. Neural tube defects are associated with an increased amount of alpha-fetoprotein (AFP) in the maternal circulation and in amniotic fluid. A series of screening tests should be performed to reduce the number of false-positive results. Defects such as anencephaly or hydrocephalus can be recognized by ultrasonography at a relatively early stage of fetal development.

Treatment. *Prevention.* The most effective means of decreasing the incidence of infants born with neural tube defects is by early detection and therapeutic abortion. A woman who has had one child with a neural tube defect has a 5 percent chance of having another.

Surgical Repair. Surgical treatment of a myelomeningocele should be carried out within 48 hours of birth to reduce the risk of infection. Many of these children will need subsequent treatment for hydrocephalus by ventriculoperitoneal shunting. All children should be followed closely with regular measurement of head circumference to detect the development of hydrocephalus, which can be confirmed by magnetic resonance (MR) or computed tomography (CT) scanning.

Children who survive but have paraparesis and/or impairment of bladder/rectal function may need additional surgical treatment later in life such as orthopedic correction of deformities of the lower limbs, the performance of an ileal loop procedure, or a colostomy. Children with severe cranial deficits are unlikely to survive, and surgery to repair the spinal developmental defect is not recommended.

Diastematomyelia

Definition. Complete duplication of the cord (dystomyelia) is extremely rare, while diastematomyelia, in which there is a cleft of the spinal cord, is occasionally encountered (1).

Etiology and Pathology. The etiology is unknown. The spinal cord is divided in the anteroposterior plane by a fibrous or cartilaginous band, which is attached to a bony septum on the wall of the spinal canal. The spinal cord may show various degrees of reduplication. Diastematomyelia is occasionally associated with a meningocele or congenital dermal cysts.

Clinical Features. The defect is usually associated with a heavily pigmented area of skin in the lumbar area and a growth of dark, coarse, or downy hair. The condition usually produces some degree of atrophy and weakness of the muscles in the lower limb and foot deformity. Sensory impairment may occur, and there may be joint deformities or ulceration of the feet. Sphincter control is impaired and occasionally lost. Examination of the spine reveals skin abnormality and kyphoscoliosis.

Diagnostic Procedures. X-rays of the spine reveal widening of the spinal canal and the presence of a bony septum. There may be associated abnormalities of the vertebra. The cleft of the spinal cord can be demonstrated by MR scan or CT metrizamide myelography.

Treatment. Removal of the midline septum is said to produce improvement in some cases. Other cases require orthopedic correction of deformities in the lower limbs and urologic treatment for sphincter problems.

Klippel-Fiel Syndrome

Definition. The Klippel-Fiel syndrome is a condition in which there is fusion of one or more vertebrae in the cervical area with shortening of the cervical spine.

Etiology and Pathology. The etiology is unknown. One or more of the cervical vertebrae are fused, and there may be absence of intervertebral disks at several levels. The condition is associated with incomplete closure of the dorsal arch in a number of cases.

Clinical Features. The patient has an abnormally short neck and low hair line, and there may be folds of skin that extend from the ears to the shoulders. Active and passive head movements are reduced. Associated abnormalities such as kyphoscoliosis and Sprengel's deformity occur. Patients may present with:

1. Synkinetic or mirror movements of the limbs, which are said to result from failure of adequate decussation of the corticospinal tracts in the medullary pyramids.
2. Progressive spastic quadriparesis, which should raise a suspicion of an associated Arnold-Chiari malformation.
3. Later development of syringomyelia.
4. Deafness in about 30 percent of cases due to malformation of the middle or inner ear.
5. Association with a number of systemic congenital abnormalities, including congenital heart disease and renal anomalies such as agenesis of the kidney, horseshoe kidneys, or hydronephrosis.

Treatment. Decompressive surgery is indicated when there is evidence of progressive neurologic deficit involving the cervical cord.

Sacrococcygeal Dystrophy

Definition. Sacrococcygeal dystrophy is a defect in the development of the sacrum and coccyx that is often associated with congenital abnormalities of the lumbosacral spinal cord.

Etiology and Pathology. The etiology is unknown. The absence of the sacrum and coccyx produces narrowing of the pelvis and congenital dislocation of the hips.

Clinical Features. There may be flaccid paralysis of the muscles of the pelvic girdle and lower limbs, sensory impairment in the lower limbs, and absence of sphincter control. There may be marked deformities of the joints of the lower limbs, including arthrogryposis multiplex congenita.

Treatment. Urologic treatment is necessary for sphincter problems.

DEVELOPMENTAL DEFECTS OF THE CRANIAL-CERVICAL JUNCTION

Arnold-Chiari Malformation

Definition. The Arnold-Chiari malformation is a condition in which there is abnormal development of the hindbrain, the base of the skull, and the upper cervical canal.

Etiology and Pathology. The etiology is unknown, but the Arnold-Chiari malformation probably represents a failure of harmonious development of the brain stem, cerebellum, and upper cervical region. The theory that the malformation is the result of "tethering" of the spinal cord to the sacrum by the filum terminale is unacceptable.

Two types of malformation are recognized: Chiari type I malformation and Arnold-Chiari malformations.

Chiari Type I Malformation. In the Chiari type I malformation there is herniation of the cerebellar tonsils below the foramen magnum. There are no other abnormalities, and the condition is not associated with a spinal myelomeningocele (see Figure 3–1).

Arnold-Chiari Malformation. In the Arnold-Chiari malformation the vermis of the cerebellum extends into the upper cervical canal along with the medulla and the fourth ventricle. The medulla is often folded upon itself in an S-shaped fashion. There is an associated meningocele or myelomeningocele in the lumbosacral area, and hydrocephalus is present with dilatation of the entire ventricular system of the brain. Hydrocephalus may be due to an associated aqueductal stenosis or an obstruction of the flow of the cerebrospinal fluid at the level of the base of the brain. Other congenital abnormalities of the central nervous system are not unusual and include microgyria, fusion of the corpora quadrigemina, cysts of the foramen of Magendie, upward herniation of the cerebellum through an abnormally large tentorial notch, enlargement of the massa intermedia, fusion of the thalami, hydromyelia, and syringomyelia.

Clinical Features. The Chiari type I malformation may be asymptomatic or may cause cerebellar signs and progressive spastic quadriplegia at any time during life. These symptoms may be delayed until adult life. Occasionally, syncope on exertion occurs due to a transient increase of intracranial pressure.

The Arnold-Chiari malformation usually presents in infancy with progressive enlargement of the head due to hydrocephalus. There is often an associated spinal meningomyelocele. When the diagnosis is delayed, compression of the spinal cord at the cervical medullary junction produces spasticity of the lower limbs with increased deep tendon reflexes and extensor plantar responses. Cerebellar involvement produces ataxia, which predominantly affects the lower limbs with later involvement of the upper limbs. Compression of the lower brain stem at the cervical medullary junction produces downbeat nystagmus (2), weakness and atrophy of the muscles of the tongue, the sternocleidomastoid, and the trapezius. There may be periodic venous congestion in the medulla with laryngeal stridor or respiration obstruction, which may be fatal.

Older children and adults may remain asymptomatic for many years and later present with pain in the suboccipital area, neck, and upper extremities, which is aggravated by head movement. There is an associated headache in the suboccipital area, which is increased on exertion. This is followed by weakness and spasticity involving all four limbs, ataxia of gait, and dysphagia. The association of the Arnold-Chiari malformation and syringomyelia in adult life is not unusual.

Diagnostic Procedures.

1. MR Imaging. The MR scan is the study of choice to demonstrate caudal displacement of cerebellar tissue including herniation of the vermis and cerebellar tonsils. Medullary herniation, inferior displacement of the aqueduct and fourth ventricle, and elongation and inferior displacement of the brain stem are usually present (3,4).
2. CT Scanning. CT scanning of the area following injection of contrast material into the subarachnoid space will also reveal the abnormality.

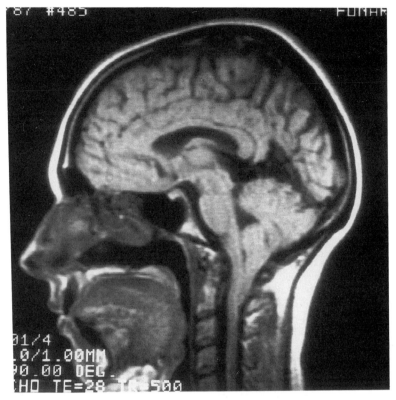

FIGURE 3–1.   Chiari Type 1 malformation. MR scan showing significant herniation of cerebellar tonsils down to the level of the second cervical vertebrae.

3. Myelography. If MR or CT scanning are not available, a myelogram may reveal herniation of the cerebellar tonsils below the foramen magnum.
4. Arteriography. A vertebral arteriogram shows abnormal displacement of the posterior inferior cerebellar artery below the foramen magnum. Films taken during the venous phase show the vermian veins, which lie on the surface of the cerebellum, below the foramen magnum.

Treatment. The myelomeningocele and hydrocephalus should be promptly treated in the affected infant. When signs of progressive neurologic deficit develop later in life, pressure may be reduced by suboccipital decompression and laminectomy.

Platybasia

Definition. Platybasia is an upward invagination of the foramen magnum which causes flattening of the base of the skull and distortion of the contents of the posterior fossa.

Etiology and Pathology. The condition occurs as a developmental abnormality but can be acquired later in life as a result of rickets, osteomalacia, or Paget's disease of the bone

Clinical Features. Pressure on the upper cervical spinal cord and medulla produces a progressive spastic quadriparesis occasionally accompanied by wasting of the tongue and dysphagia. Involvement of the cerebellum and cerebellar connections produces ataxia and nystagmus.

Diagnostic Procedures. A lateral x-ray of the skull or laminogram of the foramen magnum should be taken. The angle subtended by a line drawn from the glabella to the midpoint of the pituitary fossa and from this point to the anterior margin of the foramen magnum should be constructed. This angle is usually less than 140 degrees under normal circumstances but is increased in platybasia with invagination of the base of the skull.

Treatment. Laminectomy, removal of the posterior lip of the foramen magnum, and decompression of the cervical cord and the lower brain stem is advised.

Basilar Impression

Definition. Basilar impression or basilar invagination is an upward extension of the odontoid process through the foramen magnum producing compression of the lower brain stem and upper cervical cord.

Etiology and Pathology. The etiology is unknown in congenital cases. The condition may occur as an acquired disease in association with the acquired form of platybasia. The effects of compression of the brain stem in platybasia may well be due to impairment of blood supply rather than direct compression by the odontoid process.

Clinical Features. See platybasia, above.

Diagnostic Procedures. Lateral x-rays of the upper cervical region and the foramen magnum demonstrate projection of the odontoid process into the posterior fossa. This can be confirmed by constructing McGregor's line—a line drawn from the posterior aspect of the hard palate to the external surface of the most inferior portion of the occipital bone behind the foramen magnum. Under normal circumstances the odontoid process is usually below and not more than 3 mm above McGregor's line. The tip of the odontoid process lies more than 6 mm above McGregor's line in platybasia (5).

Treatment. The treatment is that of platybasia. In addition, some surgeons remove the odontoid process through an anterior approach with fusion of the upper two cervical vertebrae.

DEVELOPMENTAL DEFECTS OF THE BRAIN STEM

Mobius Syndrome

Mobius syndrome is a condition characterized by congenital weakness of the facial muscles associated with bilateral failure of abduction of the eyes. The condition is occasionally familial, but many cases are sporadic. The etiology is unknown. The condition may be due to a congenital abnormality of the neurons of the sixth and seventh cranial nerve nuclei in the brain stem or the result of a primary neuropathy involving the facial and extraocular muscles.

There are bilateral facial weakness and wasting with an inability to abduct the eyes on either side. Some cases show additional features of complete opthalmoplegia and/or wasting and paralysis of the pharynx and tongue. Occasionally, wasting of the pectoralis major, syndactyly, club feet, and mental retardation have been described in association with Mobius syndrome.

Cerebellar Dysgenesis

Many forms of congenital abnormality of the cerebellum have been described. These may occur as sole defects or in association with abnormalities involving brain stem and cerebral hemispheres (6). Children with cerebellar abnormalities may present with ataxia dating from birth. About 50 percent of these cases have a genetic disorder while others are examples of ataxic cerebral palsy. In some familial cases cerebellar ataxia is associated with mental retardation and additional findings of atrophy of the inferior olives, pons, restiform body, thalamus, and microcephaly (7). Many cases of congenital cerebellar dysgenesis remain undiagnosed and present as an incidental finding during life or at autopsy.

Dandy-Walker Syndrome

Definition. The Dandy-Walker syndrome is a condition in which there is maldevelopment of the roof of the fourth ventricle associated with failure of development of the cerebellar vermis.

Etiology and Pathology. The etiology is unknown. The posterior fossa is enlarged, and the internal occipital protuberance is elevated. The fourth ventricle is dilated and forms a cystlike protrusion between the cerebellar hemispheres. The brain shows signs of hydrocephalus.

Clinical Features. The condition may present with hydrocephalus in infancy or early childhood. Other cerebral brain stem or cerebellar anomalies are not unusual and visceral, particularly cardiac abnormalities, occur in a significant number of cases (8).

Diagnostic Procedures. Either MR or CT scanning will demonstrate the presence of a midline cystic mass in the posterior fossa, which extends between the cerebellar hemispheres, and diffuse dilation of the ventricular system due to hydrocephalus (9) (see Figure 3–2).

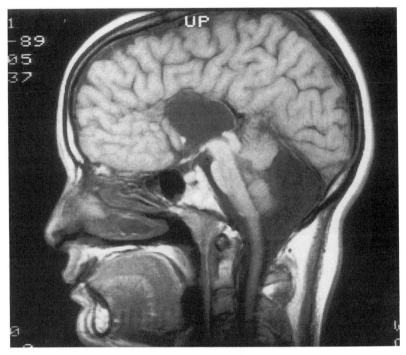

FIGURE 3-2. Dandy-Walker Syndrome. MR scan showing a large cyst replacing most of the cerebellum including the vermis and posterior portions of the hemispheres. The scan shows an additional abnormality—agenesis of the corpus callosum.

Treatment. The condition responds to a ventricular peritoneal shunting procedure.

Congenital Nystagmus

Definition. Congenital nystagmus is a familial condition, often inherited as a sex-linked recessive or an autosomal dominant trait in which nystagmus is present from birth.

Etiology and Pathology. It is postulated that the nystagmus is due to inequality in the activity of the vestibular reflex mechanisms responsible for saccadic eye movements.

Clinical Features. Nystagmus may be either pendular, in which the amplitude and rate of nystagmus is equal in the two directions, or it may be a jerk nystagmus, in which there is a slow and fast component to the nystagmus.

Nystagmus is usually present at rest and always increases in amplitude on lateral gaze. The condition is usually obvious at birth; when it is not, it typically appears in early infancy. In later life there may be associated rhythmic movements of the head. There is more than a chance association of other congenital abnormalities involving the central nervous system, particularly strabismus.

Diagnostic Procedures. The diagnosis is based on the history and physical examination.

Treatment. Treatment is usually not required.

Duane's Syndrome

Definition. Duane's syndrome is a congenital disorder of ocular movement inherited as an autosomal dominant trait in a minority of cases.

Etiology and Pathology. The etiology is unknown. A number of different pathologic changes have been described, including abnormalities in the neurons of the oculomotor nerves and myopathy affecting the lateral rectus nerves.

Clinical Features. The syndrome can be detected only on eye movement and is characterized by limitation of abduction, widening of the palpebral fissure and protrusion of the eye on attempted abduction, and narrowing of the palpebral fissure and retraction of the eye into the orbit on adduction. A downward and inward deviation of the eye may accompany adduction. Duane's syndrome has been described in association with many other congenital abnormalities.

Spasmus Nutans

Definition. Spasmus nutans is an uncommon congenital abnormality characterized by nystagmus and head tilting.

Etiology and Pathology. The etiology is unknown. The condition is said to occur in children who have been kept indoors for an undue period of time in dark or dimly illuminated surroundings. Pathologic changes are unknown.

Clinical Features. The condition usually begins between 16 and 18 months of age with the development of a horizontal, vertical, rotary, mixed, or monocular nystagmus. The development of nystagmus is accompanied by head nodding, which is usually intermittent and abolishes the nystagmus. Head tilting occurs in 50 percent of patients. There are no other abnormalities on neurologic examination.

Diagnostic Procedures. All children with monocular nystagmus should have a CT or MR scan to rule out a glioma of the optic nerve or optic chiasm (10).

Treatment. Treatment is not necessary since spasmus nutans shows spontaneous resolution six months or one year after onset.

DEVELOPMENTAL DEFECTS OF THE SKULL

There are several developmental defects of the skull, among them:

1. Cranium bifidum occultum is the mildest developmental defect of the skull. There is a deficiency in the midline fusion of bones of the skull, which usually occurs in the parietal occipital area. The condition is asymptomatic.
2. Meningoceles of the skull usually occur in the parietal occipital area. The bony defect is associated with protrusion of a sac consisting of dura and arachnoid and contains cerebrospinal fluid. This defect occasionally occurs in other sites, including the frontal area, nasal area, and nasopharynx. In a meningoencephalocele the sac also contains neural tissue.
3. Iniencephaly is a rare malformation of the posterior fossa involving the foramen magnum and upper cervical vertebrae. Deformities include retroflexion of the head, malformation of the brain, and malformation of many other organs of the body. Most patients die shortly after birth.
4. Complete rachischisis occurs when there is failure of fusion of the skull associated with failure of development of the rostral portion of the neural tube resulting in anencephaly. The brain may be represented by a mass of undifferentiated nervous tissue.
5. Dermal sinuses usually occur in the midline parietal occipital area. They may or may not be associated with a dermoid cyst that communicates with the subarachnoid space. This affords a tract between the surface and the subarachnoid space and may be the cause of recurrent meningitis. The dermoid cyst may occasionally discharge highly irritating sebaceous material into the subarachnoid space, which may cause a severe chemical meningitis.
6. Craniosynostosis is a condition characterized by premature fusion of one or more of the cranial sutures. The disorder appears to result from a failure of development of bones at the base of the skull with failure of transmission of forces through the dura to the calvarium. Two forms are recognized: primary craniosynostosis, in which there is failure of one or more of the cranial sutures to remain open, and secondary craniosynostosis, which occurs with diseases such as rickets, vitamin D-resistant rickets, and hypophosphatasia, and following excessive replacement of thyroid hormone in infantile cretinism.

Many syndromes have been associated with craniosynostosis. Some are inherited as autosomal dominant traits, while others occur as autosomal recessive traits. There is an association with mental retardation and increased intracranial pressure in some cases. The commonest condition is Crouzon syndrome. Other forms of craniosynostosis include scaphocephaly, brachycephaly, and trigonocephaly. These conditions are not usually associated with neurologic abnormalities.

Treatment is indicated only if the child develops increased intracranial pressure and for cosmetic restoration of normal cranial and facial appearance when the deformity is severe. Hydrocephalus should be treated with ventriculoperitoneal shunting.

Craniocleidodysostosis

This condition is due to failure of development of the membranous bones of the face, clavicles, and cranial vault. There is a typical facial appearance with a depressed nasal bridge and high arched palate. The clavicles are rudimentary or only partially developed, and the anterior and posterior fontanelles remain open. There is frequently some abnormality in the underlying brain, particularly involving the frontal lobes and the anterior portion of the corpus callosum. Mental retardation and seizures are common.

The x-ray of the skull is quite characteristic in this condition and shows partial ossification of the frontoparietal and occipital bones with persistence of the frontanelle. The appearance resembles a hot cross bun.

Achondroplasia

Definition. Achondroplasia is a condition in which there is abnormal development of cartilaginous bone.

Clinical Features. Patients have the typical appearance of an achondroplastic dwarf with a small face, depressed nasal bridge, and short extremities. There is marked lumbar lordosis and anterior flaring of the sacrum. Neurologic manifestations include a mild degree of mental retardation, hydrocephalus, and late development of progressive spastic paraparesis due to platybasia or spinal cord compression caused by herniation of one or more intervertebral disks or spondylosis. Sudden death can occur from brain stem compression (11).

Diagnostic Procedures.

1. Hydrocephalus can be diagnosed by radioactive cisternography.
2. The diagnosis of platybasia has already been discussed on page 59.

Treatment.

1. Hydrocephalus may be relieved by ventriculoperitoneal shunting.
2. Platybasia, spinal cord, or cauda equina compression from spinal stenosis with progressive neurologic deficit will require surgical intervention (12).

Microcephaly

A small skull is associated with a small brain, but this does not necessarily imply neurologic abnormality; approximately 2 percent of people with an unusually small brain or microcephaly have normal intelligence.

Microcephaly may be caused by the following:

1. A primary genetically determined condition that is inherited as an autosomal recessive trait accounts for 20 to 25 percent of cases of microcephaly.
2. A known chromosomal abnormality such as Down's syndrome.
3. Secondary microcephaly resulting from intrauterine infection by known viruses such as rubella or cytomegalovirus.
4. Asphyxia neonatorum.
5. Neonatal trauma.
6. Postpartum meningitis or encephalitis.

Intrauterine diagnosis of microcephaly by ultrasound may not be accurate since some microcephalics have normal head circumference at birth with slowing of head growth after birth (13).

Macrocrania

An enlarged skull is not necessarily associated with an enlarged brain. The commonest cause is hydrocephalus. The condition has also been described in benign intracranial hypertension and in bony abnormalities including osteogenesis imperfecta and craniocleidodysostosis. Asymmetrical enlargement of the skull may develop when subdural hematomas and hygromas occur in infants.

Megencephaly

Megencephaly, or enlargement of the brain, is occasionally seen in conditions affecting the parenchyma of the brain, such as the lipidoses and leukodystrophies.

Hypertelorism

Hypertelorism is a disproportionate enlargement of the lesser wings of the sphenoid bone associated with decrease in size of the greater wings of the sphenoid bone and an excessive distance between the orbits. The condition is seen in many mentally retarded individuals but may occur in perfectly normal individuals.

DEVELOPMENTAL DEFECTS OF THE FOREBRAIN

Anencephaly is a condition in which there is complete absence of development of the forebrain, which is usually represented by a mass of undifferentiated neural tissue. This condition may or may not be associated with failure of development of the skull. When the skull forms normally, the area normally occupied by the hemispheres contains cerebrospinal fluid. This is called hydranencephaly, which can be demonstrated by transillumination of the infant's head.

Severe deformities of the forebrain, or prosencephaly, are often associated with abnormalities involving the basal ganglia, thalamus, spinal cord, and marked deformities of the face, including cyclopia. Most of these conditions are incompatible with life.

Abnormalities of the gyri are usually associated with mental retardation and seizures. These abnormalities include absence of tyri (lissencephaly), numerous small gyri (microgyria), or wide irregular gyri (pachygyria).

A porencephalic cyst is a condition that occurs when there is failure of development of one hemisphere or part of one hemisphere and is often caused by a failure of development of a normal blood supply. This condition is often associated with contralateral hemiparesis and some degree of mental retardation. Seizures are not unusual. Less severe defects involving the hemispheres include schizencephaly in which there are clefts communicating with the ventricular system. Inclusions of gray matter in white matter are not uncommon and may give rise to seizures later in life, particularly when the inclusions occur in the temporal lobes. A number of developmental abnormalities are of no clinical significance, and these include the presence of a central cavity in the septum pellucidum, cavum septum pellucidi, or a more posterior cavity, cavum virgii.

One of the commonest malformations of the brain is partial failure of development of the corpus callosum. Agenesis of the corpus callosum is asymptomatic and does not lead to any problems later in life. However, the condition is often associated with other developmental defects, such as the G syndrome, that cause some degree of mental retardation and seizures (14).

The diagnosis of agenesis of the corpus callosum can be established by MR or CT scanning demonstrating wide separation of the lateral ventricles, dilatation of the occipital horns of the lateral ventricles, and a high position of the third ventricle.

DEVELOPMENTAL DEFECTS OF THE OPTIC NERVE AND RETINA

The most frequently encountered developmental defect of the optic nerve is of no clinical significance and consists of myelinated fibers which extend out from the edge of the optic nerve onto the retina. The optic nerve and retina have a normal appearance in patients with congenital absence of rods and cones. A midline coloboma or retinal defect occurs when there is failure of fusion of the optic vesicles. This midline cleft may involve the optic disk, as well as the retina, and may extend into the iris.

Pigmentary Degeneration of the Retina

In addition to retinitis pigmentosa a number of conditions are associated with pigmentary degeneration of the retina. The appearance of the retina is not always comparable to that of retinitis pigmentosa. Pigmentary degeneration of the retina may occur in association with spinocerebellar degeneration, hereditary spastic ataxia and spastic paraparesis, the Laurence-Moon-Biedl syndrome, heredopathia atactica polyneuritiformis (Refsum's disease), Kearn-Sayre syndrome, and a rare condition called homocarcinosis, in which there are spastic paraplegia, progressive mental retardation, and pigmentary degeneration of the retina.

CEREBRAL PALSY

Cerebral palsy is a nonprogressive disturbance of brain function due to prenatal factors in the majority of cases. The nature of the prenatal factors remains unknown. Perinatal factors such as asphyxia and birth trauma are responsible for less than 10 percent of cases (15, 16, 17) and these children all show the presence of abnormal neonatal neurologic findings such as decreased level of consciousness and disturbances of tone, sucking, swallowing, and respiration, with seizures and coma in the more severely affected (18). The risk of cerebral palsy is low in the asymptomatic newborn even after complicated delivery (19). Seven of every 10,000 children are born with cerebral palsy. Of these, one will die, three will always be dependent on others for their care, and three will be able to lead independent lives. Cerebral palsy is classified according to the clinical presentation. Five types are now recognized: spastic diplegia, hemiplegic cerebral palsy, athetotic cerebral palsy, ataxic cerebral palsy, and complex plegia.

Etiology and Pathology. The most common etiology factor is prematurity. One identifiable factor is bilateral symmetrical hemorrhage of the subependymal germinal matrix.

Spastic Diplegia

Definition. Spastic diplegia is one of the most common forms of cerebral palsy and is due to bilateral damage of the corticospinal tracts that control lower limb functions.

Etiology and Pathology. The most common etiology factor is low birth weight suggesting that some prenatal factor is responsible for spastic diplegia (18). The majority of these children are premature but some are born full term with normal birth weight. This latter group show a higher proportion of severely retarded infants. One identifiable factor is bilateral symmetrical hemorrhage of the subependymal germinal matrix. The hemorrhage dissects into the corticospinal tracts; hemorrhage into the ventricles is fatal. Pathologic examination is characterized by periventricular leukomalacia. Spastic diplegia also occurs in immature infants who suffer dehydration and thrombosis of the superior sagittal sinus with damage to the paracentral lobule of the brain bilaterally.

Clinical Features. There is usually a history of prematurity, birth weight less than 2,000 g, and a delay in reaching such motor milestones as sitting, standing, and walking. Signs of corticospinal tract damage develop and include hypertonia, adductor spasm, increased tendon reflexes, and bilateral extensor plantar responses. Patients have a typical "scissor" gait. There is a high incidence of associated strabismus or squint. Mental retardation, if present, is usually less severe in spastic diplegia than in other forms of cerebral palsy. Twenty-seven percent of patients develop a seizure disorder.

Hemiplegic Cerebral Palsy

Definition. Hemiplegic cerebral palsy is a common form of cerebral palsy and usually results from damage to the sensorimotor cortex that controls one side of the body.

Etiology and Pathology. The cause is multifactorial and head trauma at birth, anoxia, and embolism are now believed to be unlikely causes of hemiplegic cerebral palsy.

Clinical Features. The hemiparesis is usually not apparent at birth, and it may not be until much later that the child develops difficulty. Typically the hemiparesis involves the upper extremity more than the lower, and there is growth arrest of the affected limbs. This is usually most evident when comparing the size of the thumbnails on the two sides. Sensory deficits are of a cortical nature. This form of cerebral palsy is associated with the mildest mental retardation of all forms; however, 50 percent of these children develop a seizure disorder.

Athetotic Cerebral Palsy

Athetotic cerebral palsy is characterized by involuntary choreoathetoid movements due to damage to the extrapyramidal system. The factor or factors producing damage to the basal ganglia are unknown and asphyxia neonatorum with anoxia is no longer considered a factor. Similarly, kernicterus, damage to the basal ganglia due to deposition of bilirubin, was a leading cause of athetotic cerebral palsy in the past but is unusual now. These children are usually hypotonic at birth and develop generalized choreoathetoid movements after one year of age. The speech is severely dysarthric, but 45 percent of patients with athetotic cerebral palsy have an IQ greater than 90.

Ataxic Cerebral Palsy

Ataxic cerebral palsy is a rare form of cerebral palsy characterized by cerebellar ataxia. The condition most commonly occurs in children with cerebellar hemorrhage. Motor development and walking are delayed due to cerebellar ataxia. Speech is dysarthric. In most cases intelligence is normal.

Complex Plegia

Complex plegia is a form of cerebral palsy in which corticospinal, extrapyramidal, and/or cerebellar function are impaired. Children frequently have unilateral or bilateral motor involvement with spasticity and/or involuntary movements. Additional difficulties, including mental retardation, limb and truncal ataxia, and seizures, frequently occur.

Diagnostic Procedures.

1. Affected children should be screened for metabolic abnormalities such as hypoglycemia, hypothyroidism, and aminoacidurias.
2. CT or MR scanning will demonstrate developmental defects and areas of infarction, contusion, or hemorrhage. Three distinct types of CT scan are seen in hemiplegic cerebral palsy: a) cavity in the cerebral cortex and subcortical white matter suggesting an infarction in the distribution of the middle cerebral artery, b) ventricular enlargement and paraventricular cavity, and c) normal scan suggesting the possibility of brain stem involvement (20).

3. Psychological testing should be obtained as soon as possible to assess educational potential.
4. Urodynamic assessment to determine the cause of lower urinary tract dysfunction should lead to more rational treatment of the more than one-third of children with cerebral palsy who have voiding problems (21).
5. Ultrasonography through the anterior fontanelle is useful in demonstrating hemorrhage or paraventricular leukomalacia in newborn infants who fail to thrive (22).

Treatment of Cerebral Palsy. The key to success in treatment of cerebral palsy is teamwork with a planned approach to the individual child's problem. The child, parents, pediatrician, neurologist, psychologist, physical therapist, and school authorities should be involved. Educational programs must be tailored to the needs of the child. Many children with cerebral palsy have normal intelligence and should not be penalized because of dysarthria or involuntary movements. Conversely, many parents develop unrealistic expectations of children who have moderate to severe mental retardation. These cases require tactful handling, and realistic goals should be set.

REFERENCES

1. Simpson, K. R.; Rose, J. E. Cervical diastematomyelia: Report of a case and review of a rare congenital anomaly. Arch. Neurol. 1987, 44:331–335; 1987.
2. Bronstein, A. M.; Miller, D. H.; et al. Down beating nystagmus: Magnetic resonance imaging and neuro-otological findings. J. Neurol. Sci. 81:173–184; 1987.
3. El Gammal T.; Mark E. K.; et al. MR imaging of Chiari II malformation. A.J.R. 150:163–170; 1988.
4. Yuh, W. T. C.; Segall, H. D.; et al. MR imaging of Chiari II malformation associated with dysgenesis of cerebellum and brain stem. J. Comput. Tomogr. 11:188–191; 1987.
5. Adam, A. M. Skull radiograph measurements of normals and patients with basilar impression: Use of Landzert's angle. Surg. Radiol. Anat. 9:225–229; 1987.
6. Young, I. D.; Moore, J. R.; et al. Sex-linked recessive congenital ataxia. J. Neurol. Neurosurg. Psychiatry. 50:1230–1232; 1987.
7. Robain, D.; Dulas, O.; et al. Cerebellar hemispheric agenesis. Acta. Neuropathol. (Berl.) 74:202–206; 1987.
8. Golden, J. A.; Rorke, L. B.; et al. Dandy Walker syndrome and associated anomalies. Pediat. Neurosci. 13:38–44; 1987.
9. Narayaran, H. S.; Gandhi, D. H.; et al. Neurocutaneous melanosus associated with Dandy Walker syndrome. Clin. Neurol. Neurosurg. 89:197–200; 1987.
10. Hoyt, C. S. Nystagmus and other abnormal ocular movements in children. Pediatr. Clin. North. Am. 34:1415–1423; 1987.
11. Hecht, J. T.; Francomano, C. A.; et al. Mortality in achondroplasia. Am. J. Hum. Genet. 41:454–464; 1987.
12. Shikata, J.; Yamamuro, T.; et al. Surgical treatment of achondroplastic dwarfs with paraplegia. Surg. Neurol. 29:125–130; 1988.
13. Jaffe, M.; Terosh, E.; et al. The dilemma in prenatal diagnosis of idiopathic microcephaly. Dev. Med. Child. Neurol. 29:187–189; 1987.
14. Neri, G.; Genuardi, G.; et al. A girl with G syndrome and agenesis of the corpus callosum. Am. J. Med. Genet. 28:287–291; 1987.
15. Pharoah, P. O. D.; Cooke, T.; et al. Effects of birth weight, gestational age, and maternal obstetrical history of birth prevalence of cerebral palsy. Arch. Dis. Child. 62:1035–1040; 1987.
16. Stanley, F. J.; Watson, L. The cerebral palsies in Western Australia: Trends 1968 to 1981. Am. J. Obstet. Gynecol. 158:89–93; 1988.
17. Stanley, F. J. The changing face of cerebral palsy. Dev. Med. Child. Neurol. 29:263–265; 1987.
18. Nelson, K. B.; Ellenberg, J. H. Antecedents of cerebral palsy: Multivariant analysis of risk. N. Engl. J. Med. 315:81–86; 1986.
19. Nelson, K. B.; Ellenberg, J. H. The asymptomatic newborn and risk of cerebral palsy. Am. J. Dis. Child. 141:1333–1335; 1987.
20. Molteric, B.; Oleari, G.; et al. Relation between CT patterns, clinical findings and etiological factors in children born at term affected by congenital hemiparesis. Neuropediatrics. 18:75–80; 1987.
21. Decter, R. M.; Bauer, S. B.; et al. Urodynamic assessment of children with cerebral palsy. J. Urol. 138:1110–1112; 1987.
22. Graham, M.; Trounce, J. Q.; et al. Prediction of cerebral palsy in very low birth weight infants: Prospective ultrasound study. Lancet 2:593–596; 1987.

CHAPTER 4

EPILEPSY

Definition

Epilepsy is a condition characterized by abnormal, recurrent, and excessive discharges from neurons.

Under normal circumstances neuronal discharge is rhythmic and represents the interplay of excitatory and inhibitory influences. The summation of neuronal discharge is recorded in the electroencephalogram (EEG). In epilepsy a group of neurons generate a sudden uncontrolled high voltage discharge which may or may not spread depending upon the influence of excitatory or inhibitory mechanisms on other neuronal populations. Such mechanisms are probably mediated by neurotransmitters such as the inhibitory effect of gamma aminobutyric acid (GABA) or the excitatory effect of excess glutamate-aspartate. If the discharge spreads to involve all of the brain, a generalized seizure will be the result. When the discharge does not spread, the seizure will be focal or partial. In partial seizures the clinical manifestations are determined by the area of the brain involved. All areas of the brain are potentially epileptogenic; consequently, many different seizure patterns are possible. Epilepsy may be classified according to the clinical presentation of the seizure (see Table 4–1).

Etiology and Pathology

It is important to emphasize that seizures result only from the electrical discharge of living cells. Necrotic tissue and scar tissue, though not the origin of epileptic activity, frequently irritate adjacent neurons.

Hereditary Factors and Seizures. Fifty percent of patients with epilepsy have no demonstrable underlying neurologic disorder. These "idiopathic" cases have a strong genetic background and experience primary generalized seizures. Family studies have shown that the patient and approximately 30 percent of siblings and children of the patient have similar EEG abnormalities. The gene penetrance of this trait is about 14 percent in early childhood, rising to over 50 percent in middle childhood and then decreasing to low levels in adult life.

Seizures are not unusual concomitants of some of the rare hereditary diseases, including the leukodystrophies, lipidoses, and aminoacidurias. Tuberous sclerosis and Sturge-Weber disease are frequently accompanied by a seizure disorder. The hypoglycemia that results from several of the glycogen storage diseases and other hereditary hypoglycemias such as leucine-sensitive hypoglycemia frequently produce seizures in affected children. Some of the chromosomal abnormalities such as trisomy D are accompanied by intractable seizure activity.

Prenatal and Perinatal Factors and Seizures. A number of infections may be passed transplacentally from mother to fetus, often producing brain damage and seizure activity (see Table 4–2). These infections include syphilis, toxoplasmosis, rubella, cyto-

TABLE 4–1. Classification of Epilepsy

I. Focal (Partial Local) Seizures
   A. Simple focal seizures
      1. Motor—focal motor, focal motor with march (Jacksonian), versive, postural, phonatory
      2. Sensory—somatosensory, visual, auditory, olfactory, gustatory, vertiginous
      3. Autonomic—epigastric sensation, pallor, sweating, flushing, piloerection, pupillary dilatation
      4. Psychic—dysphasic, dysmnesic, cognitive, affective, illusions, hallucinations
   B. Complex focal seizures
      1. Simple focal seizures followed by impairment of consciousness
      2. With impaired consciousness at onset and in some cases automatisms
   C. Any focal seizures may evolve to a secondary generalized seizure

II. Generalized Seizures
   A. Absence seizures
      1. Absence seizures—usually impairment of consciousness only but may show mild clonic component, atonic component, tonic component, automatism, autonomic components
      2. Atypical absence
   B. Myoclonic seizures
   C. Tonic seizures
   D. Tonic-clonic seizures
   E. Atonia (astatic) seizures

III. Unclassified seizures which cannot be classified into one of the above categories

---

megalovirus, and *Herpes simplex*. The regular use of certain drugs including alcohol and trimethadione, in the prenatal period, has been implicated as the cause of brain damage in the fetus and subsequent seizure activity. Ir-

TABLE 4–2. Common Causes of Neonatal Seizures

1. Hypoglycemia
2. Hypocalcemia and/or hypomagnesemia
3. Hyponatremia, usually water intoxication
4. Hypoxic encephalopathy
5. Intracranial hemorrhage
6. Drug withdrawal
7. Infections, sepsis, meningitis
8. Inborn errors of metabolism
   a. Pyredoxine dependency
   b. Aminoacidurias
      1) Phenylketonuria
      2) Maple syrup urine disease

---

radiation in the early months of gestation can also produce brain damage, cerebral maldevelopment, and seizures.

Traumatic insults to the brain during parturition may have a number of effects. There may be direct damage to the brain. Excessive molding of the head as it passes through the birth canal may lead to herniation of the medial aspect of the temporal lobe over the free edge of the tentorium cerebelli. Although this condition resolves as soon as the head is born, the herniation is sufficient to produce ischemia of the medial aspect of the temporal lobe with subsequent gliosis. The area of incisural sclerosis may become epileptogenic later in life and is one of the causes of complex focal seizures (psychomotor or temporal lobe seizures). Perinatal trauma has a number of indirect effects, including cerebral anoxia and cerebral venous thrombosis. Both conditions may be associated with later seizure activity.

Perinatal anoxia has many causes. The basic problem lies in failure to establish spontaneous respirations at birth. This can occur in prematurity and in excess maternal sedation during labor. Anoxia is also a potent cause of liver cell damage and kernicterus, which leads to cerebral damage in about 25 percent of surviving infants, with subsequent development of microcephaly, mental retardation, choreoathetosis, and seizures.

Toxic, Metabolic, and Nutritional Causes of Seizures. Numerous toxins and drugs are epileptogenic. Commonly encountered toxic causes include alcohol withdrawal; sudden withdrawal of barbiturates or phenytoin in the epileptic; high doses of psychotropic drugs, particularly chlorpromazine (Thorazine) and butyrophenones; poisoning with carbon monoxide, lead, mercury, or antihistamines; and intravenous injection of heroin or cocaine (1).

Electrolyte disturbances, hyponatremia, hypernatremia, hypocalcemia, and hypomagnesemia produce neuronal irritability and seizures. Seizures frequently accompany uremic encephalopathy and other chronic metabolic encephalopathies.

Pyridoxine deficiency is a rare but potent cause of neonatal and infantile seizures and should always be considered in the investigation of seizures in this age group. Pyridoxine dependency occurs in infants who receive diets deficient in pyridoxine.

Infectious Causes of Seizures. Seizures are not unusual during the early stages of acute bacterial meningitis and acute encephalitis, particularly in children. More chronic infections such as neurosyphilis, tuberculosis, and fungal and parasitic infestation may also be accompanied by seizures.

Head Trauma, Cerebral Anoxia, and Seizures. Severe head trauma is often followed by seizures. The early onset of seizures within one to seven days post injury carries a better prognosis than a later onset. Posttraumatic seizures are discussed on page 336.

Anoxic encephalopathy can occur at any age and is frequently accompanied by seizures. An increasing number of patients suffer anoxia or hypoxia and are successfully resuscitated following cardiac or respiratory arrest.

Vascular and Neoplastic Causes of Seizures. Seizures occur in about 15 percent of patients with chronic cerebrovascular disease. Patients who suffer infarction or hemorrhage frequently develop a seizure disorder. The rarer arteritides, particularly polyarteritis nodosa, may be associated with the late onset of seizures.

All brain tumors are potentially epileptogenic, and the sudden onset of seizures in adult life should always raise the possibility of neoplasia; 40 to 60 percent of tumors produce seizures.

Degenerative and Demyelinating Causes of Seizures. All patients with degenerative diseases of the brain have an increased risk of seizure activity. Seizures are not uncommon during the course of Alzheimer's disease. Ten to 15 percent of patients with multiple sclerosis will have seizure activity some time during the course of their disease.

Clinical Features

Epidemiology. Epilepsy has a prevalence of 1 to 2 percent, which means there are from 2 million to 4 million people who suffer from epilepsy in the United States. The condition occurs in all races and has an equal distribution in males and females. Epilepsy occurs in all age groups, but there is a marked difference in incidence in relation to age. Two-thirds of all epileptic patients develop their seizure disorder in childhood or adolescence (see Table 4–3). Less than 2 percent of all epileptic patients have their first seizure after the age of 50.

Signs and Symptoms. The most frequently encountered seizure types, their clinical features, EEG characteristics, and the drugs of choice in treatment are as follows:

Tonic-Clonic Seizures (Grand Mal, Major Motor). Tonic-clonic seizures occur at any

TABLE 4–3. Common Causes of Seizures in Children

1. Febrile seizures
2. Hypertension—nearly all cases are uremic
3. Lead encephalopathy
4. Electrolyte disturbances—particularly hyponatremia
5. Meningitis
6. Encephalitis
7. Cerebral malformations, particularly tuberous sclerosis

age. The seizure is abrupt in onset with no prodromal symptoms. The total neuronal population is involved with simultaneous loss of consciousness and symmetric, tonic contractions of all voluntary muscles. If the vocal cords are closing as the diaphragm and intercostal muscles contract, the patient will make an audible sound, often a high-pitched cry. The patient drops to the ground in a decerebrate posture with all muscles in tonic contraction. During this state, which lasts from a few seconds to three minutes, there is absence of respiratory movement and cyanosis. The tonic phase is followed by a clonic phase, which is accompanied by violent expiratory contractions with expulsion of saliva. This stage may be accompanied by tongue biting, on the sides of the tongue, which results in blood-stained saliva. Urinary incontinence is not unusual if the bladder is full. The clonic movements gradually decline in frequency and cease. The patient remains in coma with no reaction to painful stimuli, fixed nonreactive pupils, flaccid limbs, and bilateral extensor plantar responses. Arousal is possible after several minutes, but the patient is typically combative, is extremely confused, and usually lapses into sleep. If awakened, the patient complains of severe headache, muscle aches, and extreme fatigue and appears irritable. Full recovery may occur in several hours, but many patients feel mentally dulled for several days after the seizure.

An accurate history is particularly important in these patients. One should always try to get a complete and accurate description of the seizures. It is imperative to distinguish those patients with focal seizures and secondary generalization of seizure activity from those with primary "idiopathic" seizures. In cases of a focal onset the patient may describe an aura or have evidence of a Todd's paralysis, both of which indicate a focal onset and the possibility of underlying brain damage. A Todd's paralysis is a hemiplegia or monoplegia which may persist from days to as long as a week after a seizure.

The interictal neurologic examination is usually normal. The interictal EEG is normal in 50 percent of patients. Other patients show short bursts of generalized spike and wave activity, often accentuated by hyperventilation. Isolated spikes or spike and wave activity occur in some cases.

The drugs of choice are carbamazepine, valproic acid, or phenytoin. Phenobarbital and primidone are also effective.

Absence (Petit-Mal). Absence occurs in children aged 2 to 10 years. The seizure is sudden in onset and brief; the attack lasts from a few seconds to less than 30 seconds. The child stares, and there may be a brief upward movement of the eyes. All activities, including speaking, eating, and gesturing, come to a sudden halt. The patient is nonresponsive if addressed. The attack terminates abruptly, there is no postictal confusion, and the patient continues previous activities. Most patients stop having seizures by the age of three; however, some go on to develop tonic-clonic seizures.

There are several variants of the "simple" absence described above, these include:

1. Absence with clonic components. The patient suffers myoclonic jerks involving the eyelids, face, or other muscles in addition to absence.
2. Absence with atonic components. The head may drop forward onto the chest and there is rarely more extensive involvement with a generalized loss of tone and falling.
3. Absence with tonic components. There may be tonic contraction or a tonic posture of the head or trunk or one or more limbs during the absence seizure.
4. Absence with automatisms. Some patients have automatisms such as lipsmacking, fumbling with clothing, or aimless wandering during a period of absence. It is important to distinguish absence with automatisms from complex focal seizures as the treatment is different.
5. Absence with autonomic components. It is unusual to see autonomic features such as changes in respiratory or heart rate, pallor, flushing, or enuresis.

The interictal neurologic examination is normal. The electroencephalogram recorded during a seizure is characterized by bilateral synchronous 3 hertz spike and wave activity.

There is a marked tendency to provocation or accentuation by hyperventilation.

Atypical Absence Seizures. This type of seizure presents with signs similar to absence seizures as outlined above but the EEG is more heterogeneous with irregular spike wave activity occurring bilaterally and symmetrically, and an abnormal background activity of paroxysmal spike or spike wave complexes (2).

The drug of choice in treatment is ethosuximide. Valproic acid, clonazepam, and trimethadione are also effective.

Atonic Seizures (Drop Attacks, Akinetic Seizures, Astatic Seizures). Atonic seizures occur only in children. There is usually a loss of tone, which may be generalized or confined to the neck. In a generalized atonic seizure the patient collapses to the ground. Other cases present with a sudden loss of tone in the neck, and the head falls forward onto the chest. The drop attack may be preceded by a myoclonic jerk in some cases.

The interictal neurologic examination is usually abnormal. The EEG during an attack is characterized by 1.5 to 2 hertz spike and wave activity.

The drug of choice is clonazepam. Valproic acid or clorazepate (Tranxene) is also effective. Patients frequently suffer other seizure types and are already receiving phenytoin or carbamazepine.

Tonic Seizures. Tonic seizures occur in children and are characterized by the sudden onset of sustained contraction of axial and limb musculature with loss of consciousness.

The interictal neurologic examination is abnormal in mentally retarded children. It is important to differentiate tonic seizures from the intermittent decerebrate rigidity due to severe and often acute disease of the cerebral hemispheres.

Focal (Partial Local) Seizures. Focal seizures may occur at any age and are characterized by focal epileptic activity without impairment of consciousness. The clinical features depend on the area of the brain involved. There are many variants and these include focal seizures with:

1. Motor seizures
   a. Focal motor seizures. There is clonic activity involving a strictly focal area of the body, usually the thumb, fingers, or face. The seizure may continue for hours or days (epilepsia partialis continua).

b. Focal motor with march (Jacksonian). There is clonic activity that begins focally and spreads in an orderly fashion to involve other structures on the same side of the body; spread corresponds to the relationship of representative neurons in the motor cortex, for example, thumb, fingers, wrist, forearm (see Figure 4-1).

c. Versive seizures. Involuntary movement of the head and trunk occurs in contraversive fashion (e.g., the head turns toward the involved arm), indicating the presence of an epileptic focus in the contralateral frontal or temporal lobe (3).

d. Postural seizures. There is a sudden tonic contraction of the muscles in a limb with the assumption of an abnormal posture in a hand or foot.

e. Phonatory seizures. These are characterized by brief involuntary vocalizations or, more commonly, brief speech arrest.

2. Autonomic Seizures. There is a sudden onset of anxiety, tachycardia, sweating, piloerection, borborygmi, and so forth—sometimes called autonomic diencephalic epilepsy.

3. Sensory Seizures
   a. Somatosensory seizures. There is a sudden onset of tingling affecting a strictly focal area of the body.
   b. Visual seizures. This usually consists of elementary visual phenomena such as flashes of light or colored balls of light in contrast to the more complex visual symptoms described in some cases of partial complex seizures.
   c. Auditory seizures. There may be a sudden onset of ringing, buzzing, or bell-like sounds.
   d. Olfactory seizures. A sudden intense hallucination of smell occurs that is usually unpleasant, often described vividly as "burnt blood" or "rotting material."
   e. Vertiginous seizures. There is a sudden onset of intense vertigo.

4. Psychic Seizures
   a. Aphasic seizures. A sudden failure of comprehension and inability to com-

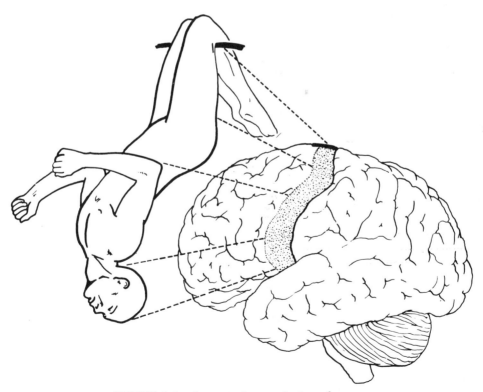

FIGURE 4-1. Somatotopic organization of cor-tex.

municate may occur with focal seizure activity confined to discrete areas of the dominant hemisphere.

b. Dysmnesic seizures. This typically consists of déjà vu, which is a sudden intense feeling of familiarity with a place, person, object, or situation. It is often described as having "lived it all before" or "been there before."

c. Cognitive seizures. There is an abrupt intrusion of a single thought or train of thoughts into consciousness with exclusion of other thought processes.

d. Affective seizures. The patient experiences fear or anger without an appropriate stimulus.

e. Seizures with illusions. In these cases there is distortion of an object's size or shape.

f. Seizures with structured hallucinations. The affected individual experiences the same hallucination with each seizure. The hallucination is complex (e.g., a rural scene or a human figure).

The interictal neurologic examination may be abnormal in cases with focal seizures of recent origin. There is increased tone and increased stretch reflexes on the affected side. The interictal EEG may reveal a focal spike discharge. It is important to rule out the existence of a treatable structural lesion. All focal seizures have the potential to develop into secondary generalized seizures.

The drug of choice is carbamazepine or valproic acid. Phenytoin and primidone are also effective.

Complex Focal Seizures (Partial Complex Seizures, Psychomotor Epilepsy, Temporal Lobe Epilepsy). Complex focal seizures may occur at any age. The important feature of complex focal seizures is the occurrence of some alteration of consciousness which may occur at the onset of the seizure or during the seizure. The alteration of consciousness may take the form of a "dreamy state" in which the patient recognizes that something unusual is happening but appreciates the phenomenon in a detached sense in much the same way as an individual "observes" a dream. However, in some cases the patient has no recollection of events that occurred during the seizure. The alteration of consciousness may be the onset manifestation of a complex focal seizure or there may be additional features which include:

1. Cognitive disturbances. An abrupt onset of a feeling of unreality, a sense of detachment, or depersonalization may occur. There may be distortion of time, impairment of memory, or forced thinking with the sudden intrusion of a single thought or a series of thoughts that dominate the thinking process. Déjà vu, a feeling of intense familiarity with a new situation, or jamais vu, a feeling of unfamiliarity with a known situation, are not uncommon.

2. Psychomotor activity. During the period of altered consciousness there may be automatic stereotyped behavior. This may take the form of lipsmacking, masticator movements, picking at clothing, or simple gestures such as scratching or stroking. Unilateral tonic posturing, dystonic posturing of a limb on the opposite side to the seizure discharge, or head and body turning may occur (4). Occasionally there is continuation of one action already in progress at the onset of the seizure. More complex acts such as walking, running, disrobing, or searching with the hands are less common. Some patients appear fearful and adopt defensive attitudes to escape or avoid danger. More complex acts such as driving a car or walking several blocks are occasionally reported. This may resemble transient global amnesia (see page 154).

3. Psychosensory phenomena. Two types of disturbances may occur: hallucinations or perceptual disorders. Visual hallucinations are usually elementary and consist of flashes or balls of light. Occasionally the patient experiences complex stereotyped visual phenomena such as a landscape or a human figure. Auditory hallucinations usually take the form of hissing or ringing, but the hallucinatory experience may present as the voice of persons known or unknown and the patient is often able to remember the details of the conversation after the attack. Hallucinations of smell are usually intense and often unpleasant. Hallucinations of movement, particularly vertigo, occur in some cases. Perceptual disorders usually take the form of distortion of body size and objects may appear to be larger or smaller during an attack.

4. Affective disturbances. An intense feeling of fear or dread is not unusual in complex partial seizures and may be associated with appropriate psychomotor activity. This is a stereotyped phenomenon and recurs during each attack experienced by the patient. Expressions of anger are rare. About 20 percent of children with autisms have epilepsy which is usually of the complex focal seizure type (5).

5. Autonomic activity. Many patients ex-

perience epigastric sensations such as borborygmi, a feeling of palpitation, or abdominal distress at the beginning of complex focal seizures. These symptoms are sometimes the only manifestation of a seizure. Other autonomic symptoms occasionally accompany a seizure, including pallor, flushing, sweating, piloerection, pupillary dilatation, or constriction and excessive salivation.

6. Speech disturbances. Vocalization of sound is not uncommon in complex focal seizures; normal speech may occur in some cases while speech arrest, dysphasia, dysarthria, and nonidentifiable speech can occur ictally or postictally (6).

7. Secondary generalized seizures may develop in patients with complex focal seizures at any time during an episode of seizure activity.

Patients may experience one or more of the major components of a complex focal seizure. Attacks may vary in one individual from a relatively brief episode with few symptoms to an extremely complex constellation of symptoms. Complex focal seizures are the main cause of accidents in epileptic drivers (7).

The interictal neurologic examination is often normal. Some patients show a slight increase in stretch reflexes on the side opposite to the epileptic focus. Patients with complex focal seizures are said to show a marked facial asymmetry which appears on involuntary facial movements such as smiling. The EEG may show focal spikes, polyspikes, and episodic high voltage slow waves occurring in one or both temporal regions. All cases of complex focal seizures of recent onset in adolescents and adults should be fully investigated. About 50 percent of children and adults experience school difficulties and behavior problems (8).

The drug of choice is carbamazepine (9) or valproic acid (10). Phenytoin, clonazepam, and primidone are also effective.

Myoclonic Seizures. Myoclonus consists of brief nonrepetitive shock-like contractions of muscles or muscle groups. Myoclonus can arise from electrical discharges at many levels in the central nervous system and occasionally occurs in normal individuals when falling asleep (nocturnal myoclonus) or on awakening in the morning. Myoclonus is also seen in metabolic encephalopathies, including hypoxia and hepatic and uremic encephalopathy, and in many infections and degenerative diseases of the brain, brain stem, and spinal cord.

Myoclonus occurring in epileptic patients and associated with paroxysmal discharges in the electroencephalogram is termed "myoclonic epilepsy." This condition is usually associated with other types of seizure, particularly the Lennox-Gastaut syndrome. Myoclonus can occur in children or adults with generalized tonic-clonic seizures who experience single or multiple myoclonic jerks within the first two hours of awakening in the morning. These myoclonic jerks may fling an object from the patient's hand or occasionally throw the patient to the ground.

The drug of choice is valproic acid. Clonazepam is also effective. Trimethadione is helpful in some cases.

The symptomatic myoclonus of metabolic infections or generative disorders of the nervous system is believed to result from depression of 5-hydroxytryptamine (serotonin) levels in the nervous system. Treatment is directed toward elevation of serotonin levels in the brain and spinal cord by administration of L-5-hydroxytryptamine, 500 to 2,500 mg/day, combined with carbidopa 100 to 300 mg/day. Fluoxetine has also been reported to be effective in controlling myoclonus.

Lennox-Gastaut Syndrome (Petit Mal Variant). The Lennox Gastaut syndrome is a recognized form of myoclonic seizure which begins in childhood before the age of six years.

This syndrome occurs in moderately or severely retarded children. The seizure patterns are variable and include episodic clouding of consciousness that is gradual in onset and termination. Some children experience lapses of posture with head flexion, others have akinetic drop attacks. Tonic seizures are not infrequent and tend to occur during sleep. Tonic-clonic, clonic, and myoclonic seizures are also seen in the syndrome. Most affected children have a mixed seizure pattern with frequent attacks. Tuberous sclerosis is the commonest recognizable cause. There are many other causes, but the common factor is severe brain damage.

The interictal neurologic examination is abnormal. The majority of affected children are moderately or severely retarded. The interictal EEG reveals a characteristic pattern of generalized slow spike waves 1 to 5 or 2 to 5 hertz occurring in runs, which is activated by sleep. A full evaluation should be undertaken to detect the underlying disease.

The patient often requires polydrug therapy. The drug of first choice is valproic acid. Clonazepam is also effective and trimethadione may be helpful in some cases.

Infantile Spasms (Hypsarrhythmia, Salaam Seizures). Infantile spasms occur in childhood during the first years of life, often as early as three months of age. A typical attack consists of sudden spasm of the flexor muscles of the neck, trunk, and limbs. This results in flexion of the head onto the chest accompanied by flexion of the trunk and limbs. Each episode is brief and is followed by relaxation to a normal posture. Hundreds of seizures may occur in one day. Extension rather than flexion may occur in some cases. Hemispasms or more complicated movements have been described.

Chronic encephalitis; cerebral malformations, particularly lissencephaly; and degenerative diseases of the brain such as tuberous sclerosis are frequently associated with infantile spasms. Rare conditions that may be remedied include pyridoxine dependency, hypoglycemia, and phenylketonuria. In some cases the patient's past history is entirely normal. Once the disorder appears, the patient shows rapid deterioration with loss of previously attained developmental levels.

The interictal neurologic examination is abnormal. The EEG associated with the spasms has a unique appearance of random high voltage and polyspike and wave activity on a background of mixed delta and theta activity.

It is important to delineate those cases which can be treated. An injection of 50 mg of pyridoxine (vitamin B_6) should be given intravenously during the EEG recording to detect pyridoxine dependency. In those cases there will be a dramatic improvement in the EEG. Hypoglycemia and phenylketonuria should be ruled out.

The drug of choice is adrenocorticotropic hormone (ACTH) or a corticosteroid. ACTH has been recommended in doses varying from 20 to 120 IU in 24 hours, and methylprednisolone from 0.3 to 1.0 g/Kg/day.

Valproic acid in doses of 15 to 60 mg/Kg/day is probably the most effective anticonvulsant medication. A ketogenic diet may be of benefit.

The prognosis is usually poor. Only 10 to 20 percent of children function at a normal or near normal intellectual level. Infantile spasms usually evolve to other seizure types, and the pattern may eventually resemble the Lennox-Gastaut syndrome.

Febrile Seizures. Febrile seizures occur in children between the ages of six months and three years. The seizure is generalized tonic-clonic in type and occurs during a fever associated with an acute, systemic infectious disease. The majority of children do not have a recurrence. Only 2 percent of patients develop a chronic seizure disorder. This small susceptible group consists of children who have abnormal neurologic findings or who have one or more predisposing factors. These include a history of nonfebrile seizures in parents or siblings, a first seizure with focal features or of prolonged duration, and multiple seizures during the first episode.

In most cases the interictal neurologic examination and EEG are normal. It is important to rule out an infection of the central nervous system.

The treatment of febrile seizures is controversial. In the majority of cases the seizure is self-limited. If the seizure is prolonged, greater than 5 to 10 minutes' duration, it should be terminated with intravenous phenobarbital or diazepam. Long-term prophylaxis with phenobarbital is recommended in those patients with abnormal neurologic findings and one or more of the predisposing factors mentioned above.

Neonatal Seizures. Neonatal seizures occur in the neonatal period. They are usually irregular, focal, clonic movements, sometimes associated with brief tonic components. There may be an associated alteration of posture, deviation of the eyes, and/or apnea. The common causes of neonatal seizures are given in Table 4–2.

The interictal neurologic examination is usually abnormal. Neonatal seizures indicate a severe disturbance of brain activity and are associated with a fatal outcome in about 15 percent of cases. The EEG reveals fragmentary spike wave activity with shifting foci. Treatment consists of immediate correction of cause. Immediate seizure control can be obtained with diazepam 1 mg/kg by slow intravenous injection. Repeated seizures require intravenous phenobarbital.

Seizures in Children. There are many types of seizures in children that are discussed under each category in this chapter. The commonest causes of seizures in children are listed in Table 4–3. The key to diagnosis is the history, which must be obtained from the parent and the older child in great detail. The commonest mistake is to misdiagnose complex focal seizures (psychomotor seizures), which are common in childhood, as absence (petit mal), a rare form of childhood seizure disorder. Incorrect diagnosis leads to inappropriate therapy and failure on seizure control.

Diagnostic Procedures and Differential Diagnosis

The history, with an accurate description of the seizure, and the neurologic examination are the most important factors in evaluation of the patient with epilepsy. The patient with a suspected seizure disorder should have:

1. Complete history, general physical examination, and neurologic examination. It is important to get an accurate description of the seizure from the patient and an observer and to inquire about the presence or absence of the factors discussed under "Etiology and Pathology."
2. EEG. In the majority of cases the interictal EEG is normal. Characteristic EEG findings are discussed under the particular seizure type. Hyperventilation, photic stimulation, and sleep deprivation are useful procedures to unmask a seizure disorder.
3. Blood should be drawn for electrolytes (Na+, K+, CA++, Mg++), blood urea nitrogen (BUN), creatinine, glucose, liver function, and thyroid function. Further studies—for example, toxicology screen, alcohol level—depend on clinical suspicion.
4. Further diagnostic procedures including skull x-rays, lumbar puncture, arteriography, and evaluation for cerebral metastases depend on clinical suspicion. Magnetic resonance (MR) scanning is particularly sensitive in detecting temporal lobe lesions including mesial temporal sclerosis and gliosis in patients with intractable seizures (11) (see Figure 4–2).
5. When a patient is already on medication but the diagnosis of a seizure disorder is doubtful, the following evaluation should be performed: If the initial EEG is normal, anticonvulsant medication should be withdrawn slowly and the EEG repeated. If the EEG remains normal and the patient has had no seizures, a sleep deprivation EEG should be obtained. If this is normal a 24-hour EEG recording is advised. If this remains normal and the patient has had no seizures, it is unlikely that the patient requires treatment.
6. It is important to recognize patients with hysterical seizures. This problem is frequently complicated by the occurrence of hysterical seizures in patients with a genuine seizure disorder. Patients who have hysterical generalized seizures are more likely to bite the tip of their tongue than

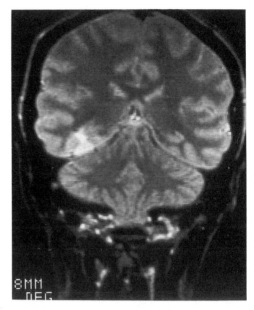

FIGURE 4–2. MR scan showing the presence of a glial scar inferomedial aspect right mid-temporal lobe in a patient with chronic complex focal seizures.

the side; there is no urinary incontinence, the patient responds to deep pain during the seizure, attempts to open the eyes are actively resisted, the pupils react to light, and there is a plantar flexor response. The patient is able to recall events that occurred during the seizure, the postictal EEG reveals no slowing, and a postictal creatine phosphokinase (CPK) level is normal in contrast to the elevated levels found following a tonic-clonic seizure.

Medical Treatment of Epilepsy

Every effort should be made to identify and treat the cause of epilepsy. All seizures of adult onset should be thoroughly investigated for the possible presence of a brain tumor (see page 224). Drug therapy for symptomatic treatment of seizures is determined by the identification of the type of seizure and EEG findings. Anticonvulsant therapy is the mainstay of treatment, and control of seizures is important since repetitive seizures may result in injury and deterioration of intellect. The following principles should be followed when attempting to obtain seizure control:

1. The appropriate drug for the seizure type should be selected.

2. The treatment should be initiated with one anticonvulsant and the dosage increased until the plasma levels are in the therapeutic range. The use of two drugs at the beginning of treatment does not convey any advantage in seizure control.

3. If the seizures are not controlled by one anticonvulsant when the plasma levels are in the therapeutic range, a second anticonvulsant should be added and increased until plasma levels are in the therapeutic range. A second anticonvulsant should not be added until the plasma level of the first anticonvulsant is in therapeutic range and appears to be in a "steady state."

4. There is no standard dose of any anticonvulsant. The patient requirement is the amount necessary to achieve a plasma level within the therapeutically effective range.

5. When a second drug is added, the plasma levels of both drugs should be monitored since the new drug may alter the plasma level of the first drug. When phenobarbital or primidone is added to phenytoin, the plasma level of phenytoin will drop. Similarly, phenytoin depresses carbamazepine levels.

6. The dosage in children is based on body weight. The treatment should be initiated at the lower limit of the calculated requirements and built up to the dose required to maintain a therapeutic plasma level.

7. Dosage schedules must take into account the half-life of the anticonvulsant so that plasma levels do not fluctuate and periodically fall below levels necessary for effective control (see Table 4–4).

8. When seizure control is inadequate using two anticonvulsants, the addition of a third anticonvulsant should precede the withdrawal of one of the two original drugs. Polydrug therapy should be avoided whenever possible.

9. Administration of two drugs of similar chemical composition—for example, primidone and phenobarbital—should be avoided.

10. Regular monitoring for blood dyscrasias or liver dysfunction is required when using some anticonvulsants. (See following discussion.)

11. If psychotropic drugs are required, the following choices of drugs are advised:
    a. Inappropriate behavior—thioridazine (Mellaril), up to 300 mg/day
    b. Psychosis—thioridazine (Mellaril); fluphenazine (Prolixin), 2.5 to 10 mg/day
    c. Depression—imipramine (Tofranil), 100 to 200 mg/day.

Drug Dosage

Since there is no standard dose of any anticonvulsant, the selected drug should be administered in sufficient amounts to achieve a therapeutic plasma concentration (see Table 4–4). In many cases it is prudent to begin

TABLE 4–4. **Pharmacologic Profile of Commonly Used Anticonvulsants**

Drug	Half-Life	Adult Dose (mg/day)	Child Dose (mg/Kg/day)	Therapeutic Levels (μg/ml)
Phenytoin (Dilantin)	24 hr ± 12 hr	300 to 700	3 to 10	10 to 20
Carbamazepine (Tegretol)	12 hr ± 6 hr	800 to 1,600	10 to 30	4.5 to 11
Phenobarbital	96 hr ± 12 hr	90 to 200	3 to 10	20 to 40
Primidone (Mysoline)	12 hr ± 6 hr	750 to 1,500	10 to 25	5 to 15 / 15 to 25 Phenobarbital
Clonazepam (Clonopin)	20 to 40 hr	1.5 to 2.0	0.01 to 0.1	5 to 70 ng/ml
Valproic acid (Depakene)	12 hr ± 6 hr	1,500 to 4,500	15 to 30	80 to 100
Ethosuximide (Zarontin)	30 hr ± 6 hr	750 to 2,000	20 to 40	60 to 120
Trimethadione	12 hr ± 4 hr	900 to 1,800	20 to 25	20 to 40

treatment with small doses of an anticonvulsant to avoid side effects, usually drowsiness. This is particularly important when using phenobarbital, primidone, and clonazepam. Plasma concentrations should be determined when the drug level has reached a steady state, which is generally four half-lives of the drug. Once a steady state has been achieved, a decision to maintain, increase, or decrease the dosage can be determined from the plasma concentration. If seizure control is achieved at levels below the therapeutic plasma level for the administered drug, it is not necessary to increase the dosage. Similarly, if seizure control is not achieved at the upper level of the therapeutic plasma range, the drug dosage may still be increased until control is achieved or until signs of toxicity occur. Failure of control due to systemic toxicity or neurotoxicity usually occurs early in the treatment period.

Determination of plasma levels of anticonvulsants should be made throughout the course of treatment as follows:

1. Seven days after beginning treatment
2. Seven days after each change in dosage
3. Seven days after the addition or withdrawal of a new anticonvulsant
4. If there is a recurrence of or increase in seizure activity
5. If signs of toxicity occur
6. At six-month intervals in controlled patients.

Carbamazepine (Tegretol) Action: resembles that of phenytoin but exact electrophysiologic and biochemical actions are unknown.

Drug Administration: q8h

Available In: tablets 200 mg

Side Effects: blurred vision, photophobia, anorexia, nausea, drowsiness, dizziness, depression with anxiety, allergic skin rashes, dry mouth, bone marrow suppression, kidney damage.

Valproic Acid (Depakene) Action: augments GABA-mediated postsynaptic inhibition; increases concentration of GABA in the brain by competitive inhibition of GABA transaminase, succinic semialdehyde dehydrogenase, and stimulation of enzymes that synthesize GABA, including glutamic acid dehydrogenase (12).

Drug Administration: q8h

Available In: capsules 250 mg; syrup 250 mg/5 ml

Side Effects: alopecia, nausea and vomiting, pancreatitis, bone marrow suppression, edema, elevated liver enzymes. Hepatic failure is rare, particularly in those receiving monotherapy (13).

Phenytoin (Dilantin) Action: controls spread of epileptic activity by preventing sodium influx into neurons and promoting sodium efflux, thus tending to stabilize the membrane threshold. The drug also increases the concentration of the inhibitory transmitters GABA and 5-HT.

Drug Administration: q12h

Available In: capsules 30 mg and 100 mg; tablets 50 mg; suspension 125 mg/5 ml, 30 mg/5 ml; injections 100 mg/2 ml, 250 mg/5 ml

Side Effects: ataxia, nystagmus, hirsutism, gingival hyperplasia, lethargy, dysarthria, blurred vision, diplopia, nausea and vomiting, bone marrow suppression, serum folate decrease (14), and megaloblastic anemia

Clonazepam (Clonopin) Action: limits spread of epileptic activity but does not suppress activity of epileptic focus; acts by augmenting inhibition in presynaptic and postsynaptic GABA-mediated systems

Drug Administration: q8h, q6h

Available In: tablets 0.5 mg, 1 mg, 2 mg

Side Effects: drowsiness, dizziness, dysarthria, ataxia, depression, rashes, irritability, personality changes, thrombocytopenia

Phenobarbital Action: limits spread of seizure activity possibly by augmenting postsynaptic inhibitory response to GABA

Drug Administration: q12h

Available In: tablets 15 mg, 30 mg, 60 mg, 100 mg; elixir 20 mg/5 ml; injection 130 mg/ml

Side Effects: drowsiness, nystagmus, paradoxic hyperactivity in children

Primidone (Mysoline) Action: as for phenobarbital. Drug rapidly metabolized into three active components

Drug Administration: q8h

Available In: tablets 50 mg, 250 mg; suspension 250 mg/5 ml

Side Effects: sedation, hyperactivity, vertigo, nausea and vomiting, anemia, personality changes

Ethosuximide (Zarontin) Action: unknown

Drug Administration: q12h

Available In: capsules 250 mg; syrup 250 mg/5 ml

Side Effects: lethargy, photophobia, headache, dizziness, skin rashes, nausea and vomiting, hiccups, bone marrow suppression

Surgical Treatment of Epilepsy

Surgical treatment of epilepsy is carried out at relatively few centers in the United States at this time because of the complexity of patient selection and operative procedures that are necessary to obtain optimum surgical results. Patients require assessment by a neurologist, an electroencephalographer, and a neuropsychologist during pre-operative evaluation. In many cases dural recording and depth recording are necessary in addition to the standard scalp EEG (15).

There are clear indications for surgical treatment of epilepsy:

1. The presence of a clearly identified surgical lesion, for example, tumor, arteriovenous malformation, cicatrix
2. Failure of medical treatment, which must include the use of adequate anticonvulsant medication
3. Cases in which seizure control can be obtained only with excessive toxicity from anticonvulsant medication.

Surgical treatment is not recommended in psychotic or severely mentally retarded patients. Current surgical treatment includes local excision of an epileptic focus, lobectomy, and partial hemispherectomy. Procedures such as stereotactic surgery and stimulation techniques are still largely experimental. Commissurotomy should be reserved for patients with severe epileptic disorders where there is clear evidence of propagation of epileptic activity from a severely damaged hemisphere to a relatively healthy hemisphere (16).

The Team Approach to the Treatment of Epilepsy

The chronic epileptic is a seriously disadvantaged individual who frequently fails to attain educational and employment levels comparable to those commonly achieved by individuals of equal intellectual development in the nonepileptic population. The epileptic patient suffers from the direct effects of the epileptic process and from the social and psychologic effects of a chronic disease that has traditionally received little sympathy from the public. It is not surprising, therefore, that the epileptic patient is frequently unable to cope with the pressures of the disease and the various problems that epilepsy poses in everyday life. In an effort to reduce the impact of the disease on the epileptic patient, many centers have developed a team approach to the treatment of chronic epilepsy. Members of the team should include a neurologist, neu-

rosurgeon, neuropsychologist, electroencephalographer, social worker, and psychiatrist. The contributions of individuals from several disciplines result in a better balance in the treatment program. Treatment is designed to control epileptic seizures, while dealing with the more chronic problems of the psychological concomitants and the social implications of the disease. Many patients who are thought to be unemployable can be restored to useful productive existence by this type of team treatment.

Pregnancy and Epilepsy

The pregnant epileptic patient presents several different considerations in treatment. The pregnant epileptic patient is twice as likely to have a multiple birth, more likely to require artificial rupture of membranes or cesarean section, and more likely to suffer pre-eclampsia. The neonatal mortality of the pregnant epileptic is three times that of the normal population.

Pregnancy decreases the brain's seizure threshold, possibly by causing electrolyte imbalance, hormonal alterations, or emotional stress. Pregnancy also results in decreased serum anticonvulsant levels due to decreased intestinal absorption and increased metabolism. Approximately 45 percent of pregnant epileptic patients will experience an increased seizure frequency. This is particularly true in patients who had greater than one seizure per month prior to conception.

Certain anticonvulsants have been shown to be teratogenic. Phenytoin administration was linked to the "fetal hydantoin syndrome" but it is now believed that the syndrome is not specific for any anticonvulsant or combination of anticonvulsants. The syndrome consists of craniofacial abnormalities (low, flat nasal bridge; hypertelorism; short, upturned nose; ptosis and/or strabismus; and a wide mouth with prominent puckered lips), limb defects (hypoplasia of distal phalanges, fingerlike thumb), deficiency in growth (small stature, low birth weight), and mild to moderate mental retardation. Trimethadione may produce the following defects: developmental delay, speech disturbances, V-shaped eyebrows, low-set ears, palatal abnormalities, and irregular teeth. Diazepam administered early in pregnancy may result in cleft palate. Phenobarbital usage results in withdrawal signs in the infant. The child may later become hyperactive or show evidence of minimal brain dysfunction. Valproic acid has been associated with a neural tube defect with an incidence of about 1 percent. The condition can be detected by ultrasonography and confirmed by the presence of alpha fetoprotein in the amniotic fluid. Fetuses who are exposed to phenytoin, phenobarbital, or trimethadione may develop drug-induced vitamin K deficiency.

The treatment of the pregnant epileptic is as follows:

1. Optimum seizure control should be established in an epileptic woman who is contemplating pregnancy. As few anticonvulsants as possible should be used. Trimethadione should be avoided.
2. The patient should be followed monthly, and anticonvulsant dosage should be adjusted appropriately according to plasma levels.
3. The newborn infant should be carefully examined for the congenital malformations associated with the anticonvulsant to which it was exposed. Phytonadione (vitamin K) 1 mg should be administered and clotting factors carefully monitored.
4. The anticonvulsant dosage of the postpartum patients may not drop to preconception levels for several months. The patient should be monitored monthly until a stable plasma level is attained.

Status Epilepticus

Definition. A condition in which a patient has a series of seizures without total recovery of consciousness between seizures.

An alternative definition would include the following:

1. Epileptic seizures that are so frequently repeated or so prolonged so as to create a fixed and lasting epileptic condition or
2. A seizure that is repeated frequently enough to produce a fixed and enduring epileptic condition lasting at least 30 minutes.

The combination of these definitions covers both generalized status epilepticus and focal status epilepticus.

Etiology and Pathology. Fifty percent of patients are chronic epileptics in whom the commonest cause is noncompliance in the use of anticonvulsant medication. The other 50 percent are patients with severe central nervous system disease as outlined in Table 4–5.

Treatment

1. The airway should be maintained by insertion of an endotracheal tube. All pharyngeal and bronchial secretions should be cleared by frequent suctioning.

TABLE 4–5. **Some Causes of Status Epilepticus**

Symptomatic 70 to 80 percent, Idiopathic 20 to 30 percent

Congenital abnormalities of the brain
Perinatal anoxia
Acute head trauma
Posttraumatic encephalopathy
Postcraniotomy
Viral encephalitis
Acute purulent meningitis
Tubercular meningitis
Alcohol withdrawal
Toxic bronchodilator drugs
Brain tumor

Cerebrovascular disease

Multiinfarct state
Arteriovenous malformation
Acute infarction
Intracerebral hemorrhage
Subarachnoid hemorrhage

Degenerative conditions

Multiple sclerosis
Alzheimer's disease
Unverricht-Lafora

2. Blood should be drawn and sent for electrolytes (Na+, K+, Ca++, Mg++), BUN, creatinine, glucose, and anticonvulsant levels if there is a history of previous seizures.
3. An intravenous infusion should be established.
4. Diazepam 2 to 10 mg may be administered intravenously. In the majority of cases the seizures will cease. The effect of diazepam lasts 15 to 20 minutes and the injection can be repeated if seizures should recur. The use of diazepam is occasionally complicated by hypotension and/or respiratory arrest. If respiratory arrest should occur the patient should be intubated immediately and given mechanical respiration.
5. Since the effect of diazepam is brief, phenytoin (Dilantin) should be administered to prevent a recurrence of seizure activity. A loading dose of 18 mg/kg may be administered by intravenous injection at the rate of 50 mg/min. The phenytoin may be complicated by hypotension, cardiac dysrhythmias, and cardiac or respiratory arrest. The blood pressure, pulse, and respiratory rate should be evaluated every minute during the first five minutes of injection. It is recommended that intravenous (IV) infusion of phenytoin always be

carried out with electrocardiographic monitoring whenever it is possible.

6. For patients who fail to respond to the use of benzodiazepines and phenytoin, and in whom status epilepticus continues, the induction of general anesthesia should be considered. It is critical that this decision to use general anesthesia be made within 60 minutes of status epilepticus if permanent neurologic sequelae or death is to be avoided. There is evidence indicating that permanent cell damage to the hippocampus, amygdala, cerebellum, thalamus, and middle cerebral cortical layers occurs after 60 minutes of status epilepticus. In addition, secondary metabolic complications including lactic acidosis, an increase in cerebrospinal fluid pressure, hypoglycemia, hypothermia, excessive diaphoresis with dehydration, and eventually shock may develop after 60 minutes of status epilepticus. The most appropriate pharmacologic agent for induction of general anesthesia is an intravenous barbiturate. The pharmacologic rationale for the use of a barbiturate anesthesia rests on the ability of barbiturates to depress neuronal excitation by enhancing the effects of GABA, to lower the metabolic rate of oxygen utilization, and to blunt the increase in intracranial pressure accompanying status epilepticus.

Prior to the initiation of barbiturate therapy the patient should be transferred to an intensive care unit, intubated, and given assisted ventilation. Continuous monitoring of the electrocardiogram is mandatory and frequent monitoring of the EEG is necessary during induction of barbiturate anesthesia and during barbiturate coma. An arterial line for measurement of blood gases and arterial pressure is required. Patients should be catheterized to permit accurate assessment of urinary output.

The primary goal of barbiturate anesthesia is the control of clinical seizure activity and the appearance of a burst suppression pattern in the EEG (17). A loading dose of 10 mg/Kg of pentobarbital is recommended given at a rate of 25 mg/minute until the seizures stop (18). This should be followed by a continuous maintenance infusion of pentobarbital 2.5 mg/Kg/hr (19). The maintenance infusion should, however, be titrated to achieve the electroencephalographic response of a burst suppression pattern (20). Intravenous solution should be prepared with 5 percent dextrose in water or 0.9 percent sodium chloride.

If breakthrough seizures occur a bolus of 50 mg pentobarbital (25 mg/minute) should be given and the maintenance infusion increased to 3.0 mg/Kg/hr.

The optimum duration of barbiturate anesthesia remains to be determined. Continuous therapy for as long as 13 days has been reported. One approach is to allow 24 hours of seizure control following which the infusion can be reduced every four to six hours by 1 mg/Kg/hr if the pentobarbital level is above 50 μg/ml or reduced by 0.5 mg/Kg/hr if the level is below 50 μg/ml. If seizures recur during tapering a bolus of 50 mg pentobarbital (25 mg/minute) should be given and the maintenance infusion increased to the closest preseizure dose.

Adverse effects of barbiturate anesthesia include hypotension, decreased myocardial contractility, hypothermia, and hypersensitivity reactions. Patients should be repositioned frequently to avoid decubitus ulcers.

7. In cases of prolonged status epilepticus, cerebral anoxia may result in cerebral edema and increased intracranial pressure. Dexamethasone (Decadron) 12 mg IV followed by 4 mg q6h may be useful in reducing cerebral edema.

Focal status should be treated in a similar fashion since prolonged focal seizure activity can lead to permanent neurologic deficits.

REFERENCES

1. Choy-Kwang, M.; Lipton, R. B. Seizures in hospitalized cocaine users. Neurology 39:425–427; 1989.
2. Holmes, G. L.; McKeever, M.; et al. Absence seizures in children: clinical and electroencephalographic features. Ann. Neurol. 21:268–273; 1987.
3. McLacklau, R. S. The significance of head and eye turning in seizures. Neurology 37:1617–1619; 1987.
4. Kotagal, P.; Luders, H.; et al. Dystonic posturing in complex partial seizures of temporal lobe onset: a new lateralizing sign. Neurology 39:196–201; 1989.
5. Olsson, I.; Steffenberg, S.; et al. Epilepsy in autism and autistic-like conditions. A population-based study. Arch. Neurol. 45:666–668; 1988.

6. Gabr, M.; Luders, H.; *et al.* Speech manifestations in lateralization of temporal lobe seizures. Ann. Neurol. 25:82–87; 1989.

7. Gastaut, H.; Zifkin, B. G. The risk of automobile accidents with seizures occurring while driving: relation to seizure type. Neurology 37:1613–1616; 1987.

8. Kotogel, P.; Rothrer, A. D.; *et al.* Complex partial seizures of childhood onset. Arch. Neurol. 44:1177–1180; 1987.

9. Carbamazepine's place in antiepileptic drug therapy. Epilepsia (Suppl) 3:S1–S87; 1987.

10. Bourgeois, B.; Beaumanoir, A.; *et al.* Monotherapy with Valproate in primary generalized epilepsies. Epilepsia (Suppl 2) 28:S8–S11; 1987.

11. Kuznecky, R.; De La Sayette, V.; *et al.* Magnetic resonance imaging in temporal lobe epilepsy: pathological considerations. Ann. Neurol. 22:341–347; 1987.

12. Marks, W. A.; Morris, M. P.; *et al.* Gastritis with valproate therapy. Arch. Neurol. 45:903–905; 1988.

13. Dreifuss, F. E.; Langer, D. H.; *et al.* Valproic acid hepatic fatalities. U.S. experience since 1984. Neurology 39:201–207; 1989.

14. Berg, M. J.; Finchan, R. W.; *et al.* Decrease of serum folates in healthy male volunteers taking phenytoin. Epilepsia 29:67–73; 1988.

15. So, N.; Olivier, A.; *et al.* Results of surgical treatment in patients with bitemporal epileptiform abnormalities. Ann. Neurol. 25:432–439; 1989.

16. Spencer, S. S.; Spencer, D. D.; *et al.* Corpus callosotomy for epilepsy—I. seizure affect. Neurology 38:19–24; 1988.

17. Rashkin, M. C.; Youngs, C.; *et al.* Pentobarbital in refractory status epilepticus. Neurology 37:500–503; 1987.

18. Shaner, D. M.; McCurdy, S. A.; *et al.* Treatment of status epilepticus: a prospective comparison of diazepam and phenytoin versus phenobarbital and optional phenytoin. Neurology 38:202–207; 1988.

19. Osorio, I.; Reed, R. C. Treatment of refractory generalized tonic-clonic status epilepticus with pentobarbital anesthesia after high-dose phenytoin. Epilepsia 30:464–471; 1989.

20. Lowenstein, D. H.; Aminoff, M. J.; *et al.* Barbiturate anesthesia in the treatment of status epilepticus. Clinical experience with 14 patients. Neurology 38:395–400; 1988.

CHAPTER 5

HEADACHE

A headache is a pain or discomfort that occurs over the superior portion of the head and occasionally spreads into the face, teeth, jaws, and neck. Pain-sensitive structures in the cranial cavity include the venous sinuses and their cortical tributaries; the large arteries at the base of the brain; the dura lining the floor of the anterior and posterior fossa; the fifth, ninth, and tenth cranial nerves, and the first three cervical nerves. These structures contain pain-sensitive nerve endings, which may be stimulated by traction, inflammation, pressure, neoplastic infiltration, and as yet unidentified biochemical substances that are liberated in certain types of headaches. Stimulation of pain-sensitive structures above the tentorium cerebelli tends to produce headaches in the frontotemporoparietal area. Stimulation of pain-sensitive structures in the posterior fossa produces pain in the occipital and suboccipital areas. Although intracranial pain-sensitive structures are limited in number, all of the tissues of the scalp, face, and neck appear to be sensitive to painful stimulation. Headaches can also occur in diseases of the eye and orbital contents, the nasal cavity and paranasal sinuses, the teeth, and the external and middle ears.

In summary, headaches may be caused by:

1. Traction on or displacement of the venous sinuses and their cortical tributaries
2. Traction, dilatation, or inflammation involving intracranial or extracranial arteries
3. Traction, displacement, or diseases of the fifth, ninth, and tenth cranial nerves and the first three cervical nerves
4. Changes in intracranial pressure
5. Disease of the tissues of the scalp, face, eye, nose, ear, and neck.

Migraine

Definition. Migraine is a condition characterized by recurrent headache which may be unilateral or bilateral and associated with personality change, prostration, and nausea and vomiting. The headache may be preceded by or associated with neurologic disturbances.

Etiology. The vascular hypothesis that migraine is the result of an initial vasospasm followed by vasodilatation is under critical review (1), and while there is no doubt that vascular changes occur there is a growing consensus that such changes may be a secondary phenomenon or epiphenomenon in migraine.

The possibility that a migraine attack may be initiated by spreading depression is an attractive alternative (2). This condition is a transient disruption of neuronal activity in the brain accompanied by a flux of sodium, calcium, and chloride ions into the cells. This results in a brief burst of electrical activity followed by electrical silence which progresses as an expanding concentric wave through the brain at the same rate as a developing migraine aura. The pain of migraine could result from the release of substance P in sensory ganglia with stimulation of pain fibers in the trigeminal and facial nerves (3); the vascular changes of constriction and dilatation could result from stimulation and inhibition of noradrenergic nerves supplying intracranial and extracranial arteries. Such a complex situation would depend upon the periodic activity of some central source in the brain that has the necessary anatomical connections to the cerebral cortex and the brain stem to orchestrate the several changes which constitute the migraine attack (4).

There is a positive family history in migraine in about 60 percent of cases, which suggests the presence of a hereditary factor; some studies indicate that it is inherited as an autosomal dominant or an autosomal recessive trait. Alternatively, migraine is a common complaint, and its presence in several family members may be no more than a chance occurrence. There is an impression that migraine affects people of superior intelligence in the higher socioeconomic groups and in professional occupations. This erroneous concept can probably be explained by the tendency for patients in this category to seek medical help. There is ample evidence that migraine is not related to intelligence and that this type of headache occurs with equal frequency in all socioeconomic groups. Psychological studies show that people with migraine are more likely to be psychoneurotic, to be more introverted, and to have higher levels of hostility with inadequate emotional expression.

There appears to be a relationship between attacks of migraine and the menstrual cycle; many women experience migraine at the onset of each menstrual period. Oral contraceptive use and estrogen therapy exacerbate migraine symptoms in some cases, and there may be an exacerbation during the menopause. Some women experience freedom from attacks during pregnancy, while others experience exacerbation of headaches during the early months of pregnancy. The relationship between migraine, the menstrual cycle, and pregnancy suggests that some cases of migraine may be triggered by endocrine or electrolyte changes that occur during the menstrual cycle and pregnancy.

Migraine can also occur in response to stress, particularly those situations which result in frustration and tension. In addition, a number of other stress factors appear to be related to the onset of migraine, including fatigue, exposure to bright lights, meteorologic change, exposure to high altitudes, use of various drugs such as vasodilators and reserpine, and repeated mild head trauma. Many patients report the development of migraine during a period of hunger. Investigation shows that this is not related to hypoglycemia, suggesting that more complex metabolic factors are involved and that there may be a so-called hunger factor in some cases of migraine.

Migraine has also been associated with ingestion of certain foods, including chocolate, cheese, citrus fruits, smoked fish, and alcohol (5). Some of these foods have a high tyramine content, and it is possible that dietary migraine occurs in patients who have a deficiency of tyramine-*o*-sulfatase. The excess tyramine could be responsible for the release of catecholamines and could initiate the vasoconstrictive stage of migraine.

Many patients with migraine show hyperaggregability of platelets when free from headache. This platelet aggregation is increased during the prodromal stage of migraine. The reason for this is not clear, but it could be related to an increase in epinephrine, thrombin, or arachidonic acid in the circulation in response to anxiety, stress, hunger, smoking, ingestion of tyramine-containing foods, or ingestion of alcohol. The platelet hyperaggregability is unlikely to be a primary or triggering effect in migraine and is generally regarded as an epiphenomenon.

Clinical Features. The following are the more common types of migraine headaches.

Classic Migraine. A classic migraine headache is preceded by visual symptoms known as an aura. The attack of classic migraine begins with an aura in which the patient may experience scintillating scotomata, streaks of light, or scotomata with regular projecting and reverse angles resembling the bastions and walls of a fortified city sometimes termed fortification spectra (6). Occasionally large central or paracentral field defects or homonymous hemianopia may occur. Olfactory hallucinations are a less frequent aura preceding the headache in some cases (7).

Approximately 20 minutes after the aura begins the patient develops a headache. The headache is usually bifrontal, but it may be unilateral and can occur in any part of the cranial cavity. In about 50 percent of cases it is bilateral. The pain is pulsatile initially but increases in severity and becomes a continuous, intense ache. The patient may feel that the entire head is involved and the pain may spread down into the neck and face. There is marked systemic upset, nausea is common, and vomiting is not infrequent. The patient is photophobic and prefers to lie quietly in a darkened room. The condition gradually subsides over a period of hours in the majority of cases but occasionally lasts all day and is terminated only after sleep. In a few cases the headache may be present for two or three days. Prolonged headache produces considerable prostration, and vomiting may contribute to dehydration. When the headache resolves, the patient is left with a feeling of heaviness and aching in the head, the scalp may be tender, and there may be considerable fatigue and listlessness for several days. The termination of the attack is often accompanied by a marked diuresis.

Common Migraine. A common migraine headache is a migrainous headache without a preceding aura. The attack of common migraine begins with the headache. This is usually a dull ache. It may be bifrontal or confined to one side and, as with classic migraine, it can occur in other parts of the head. It is usually accompanied by nausea and occasionally by vomiting. An attack often lasts longer than classical migraine and may last for several days in some cases.

Hemiplegic Migraine. This is a rather unusual form of headache in which the patient experiences symptoms of numbness and/or weakness preceding the onset of the headache. The weakness and numbness involve a hand or upper limb, which spreads in some cases to the whole of one side of the body. The symptoms may be accompanied by dysphasia or aphasia if the dominant hemisphere is involved. The headache usually begins within 60 minutes after the onset of the prodromal symptoms. The headache is typically migrainous and similar to that described in classic migraine. The weakness and numbness may last for several days but usually resolve. Permanent deficits have been recorded, however, presumably due to infarction during the height of vasoconstriction (8,9). This complication is fortunately rare.

Two types of hemiplegic migraine have been recognized.

1. Familial hemiplegic migraine. The symptoms are similar in all affected members of the family and they rarely have migraine of any other types.

2. Nonfamilial hemiplegic migraine. In this condition the affected members have occasional attacks of classic migraine or common migraine without hemiplegic symptoms.

Basilar Migraine. In this type of migraine the headache may be preceded or accompanied by symptoms of vertigo, ataxia, dysarthria, bilateral visual field defects, or motor weakness of the hemiparetic type. There may be some impairment of consciousness. The patient appears to be confused, restless, and sometimes incoherent and dysphasic. This stage is occasionally followed by a period of stupor. The migraine headache is usually bilateral and occipital. Symptoms and neurologic deficit may persist for several hours following the onset of headache. The electroencephalogram (EEG) may be normal or show paroxysmal activity including spike wave complexes. In the absence of clinical seizure activity these cases may respond to antimigraine therapy (10).

Basilar migraine has also been described following hyperextension-flexion (whiplash) injury to the neck. The condition will respond to antimigraine medication and physical therapy (11).

Ophthalmoplegic Migraine. Ophthalmoplegic migraine is a form of migraine in which the patient develops ipsilateral ophthalmoplegia at the height of the migraine headache. Ophthalmoplegia is believed to be due to compression of the third nerve and occasionally compression of the fourth and sixth nerves and the ophthalmic division of the fifth nerve in the lateral wall of the cavernous sinus by a dilated internal carotid artery. Patients with ophthalmoplegic migraine typically give a history of common or classic migraine without oculomotor involvement of many years' duration before the development of ophthalmoplegia. The ophthalmoplegia and headache are always unilateral and occur on the same side. It is rare for patients to experience attacks that move from one side to the other. One of the features of ophthalmoplegic migraine is that the headache always precedes the oculomotor deficit by several hours or even days in some cases. Paresis always outlasts the pain, and rare cases have been reported in which there is a partial permanent oculomotor deficit.

Migrainous Psychosis. Migrainous psychosis is migraine associated with emotional, intellectual, or personality change. The patient may appear to be confused; may exhibit abnormal behavior, anxiety, fear, or hallucinations; may express a total loss of contact with surroundings; and occasionally may lapse into stupor. A number of cases occur in families where other family members suffer from similar migrainous attacks. When these symptoms occur without headache (see "Migraine Equivalents"), or when the patient is dysphasic and unable to complain of headache, migrainous psychosis may mimic an acute encephalopathy.

Complicated Migraine. Migraine is usually regarded as a benign condition associated with vasoconstriction and profound reduction of cerebral blood flow. Occasionally, this reduction of blood flow is sufficient to produce infarction, and the patient can develop permanent neurologic deficits. These deficits usually take the form of hemiparesis or hemisensory loss, but cardiac arrhythmias and respiratory arrest are possible complications of basilar migraine.

Migraine Equivalents. Prodromal symptoms of migraine may occur without subsequent development of headache. The commonest migraine equivalent is the scintillating scotoma of classic migraine, and it is not unusual for these visual symptoms to occur as an isolated symptom in a migraine sufferer. Other neurologic deficits, including transient hemiparesis or hemisensory symptoms, cause concern or alarm to patients and physicians when the expected headache fails to develop. However, the patient will usually admit to a slight headache or dull ache at the time of the expected migraine headache.

Abdominal Migraine. This condition occurs in children who have episodes of midline abdominal pain occuring on awakening in the morning, lasting all day, and relieved by sleep. The pain is accompanied by pallor, headache, anorexia, and nausea and vomiting. Some affected children have migraine headaches and there is usually a strong family history of migraine. Prophylactic treatment with small doses of propranolol is effective in most cases (12).

Migraine in Children. Migraine is not unusual in children. It has been estimated that about 5 percent of children aged 11 years have migraine. Many of these children have an antecedent history of periodic cyclic vomiting and episodic vertigo or transient neurologic deficits such as hemiparesis, ptosis, diplopia, or ataxia without headache. Migraine is often precipitated by fatigue, anxiety, exercise, menses, and illness. Minor head trauma is a potent cause of migraine in children. Attacks occur once or twice per month and last two to six hours. Complex migraine with transient neurologic deficits is not uncommon (13).

Migraine often presents as a bilateral headache in children. It is only later in life that the child develops a unilateral headache. Some children develop migrainous headaches in the later afternoon after school hours. These attacks are probably precipitated by fatigue. Prostration is very prominent in childhood migraine, with rapid recovery after the attack. Ergotamines are often successful in aborting an attack. Propranolol is most effective in prophylaxis. Calcium channel blockers or cyproheptadine can be used in propranolol resistant cases.

Differential Diagnosis. In addition to the conditions listed in Table 5–1 the differential diagnosis of migraine headaches includes:

1. Seizures. Migraine attacks can usually be differentiated from seizures without difficulty.
   a. The prodromal stages are quite different, the prodromal stage in migraine being much longer than that of partial seizures.
   b. The EEG is totally different in the two conditions.
   c. Migraine does not respond to anticonvulsants.
   d. Epilepsy does not respond to vasoconstrictor drugs.
2. Transient Ischemic Attacks. Patients who have migraine and who occasionally have prominent auras without the development of headache may be misdiagnosed as having transient ischemic attacks. A careful history that includes a detailed description of the attack and an account of previous attacks of migraine should alert the examiner to the correct diagnosis of a migraine equivalent.

Diagnostic Procedures. In most cases the diagnosis of migraine can be established by history alone. The neurologic examination is normal and further diagnostic procedures are unnecessary and may occasionally lead to confusion. For example, the EEG is usually normal between attacks of migraine but may show focal slowing if taken during an attack of migraine or shortly after an attack. This EEG abnormality may create the impression of a possible space-occupying lesion or infarction and lead to a series of further procedures unless the EEG changes in migraine are appreciated.

Treatment. The treatment of migraine headaches includes:

1. Analgesics. Although most patients use simple analgesics such as aspirin, aspirin with

TABLE 5–1. Differential Diagnosis of Headache

Headache Type	Epidemiology	Location	Signs and Symptoms	Treatment
Migraine	Family history Children, young adults, F > M	Bifrontal, may be unilateral	Nausea, vomiting, may be neurologic deficits	Ergots Propranolol Amitriptyline Verapamil
Tension	F > M	Bilateral, generalized, or occipital	Long duration Anxiety Depression	Anxiolytics Antidepressants
Cluster	Adolescent and adult, M > F	Unilateral, orbitofrontal	Lacrimation Unilateral nasal congestion	Ergots Propranolol Amitriptyline Lithium
Hypertensive	Family history	Bilateral, occipital, or frontal	Hypertensive retinopathy, may be papilledema	Treatment of hypertension
Increased intracranial pressure		Varies	Nausea, vomiting, papilledema	Treatment of elevated intracranial pressure, steroids, mannitol, surgery
Temporal arteritis	Adults	Unilateral, temporal	Tender temporal artery Impairment of vision Elevated sedimentation rate	Corticosteroids
Subarachnoid hemorrhage, meningitis		Bilateral, occipital	Sudden onset with subarachnoid hemorrhage Nuchal rigidity Fever	Treatment of meningitis or subarachnoid hemorrhage

codeine, propoxyphene hydrochloride (Darvon), or acetaminophen to alleviate headache, there is delayed absorption of oral medications from the stomach in a migraine attack and simple analgesics are usually ineffective.

2. Many patients prefer to retire to a quiet, darkened room and lie with a cold compress applied to the head. The attack will usually terminate if the patient manages to sleep for several hours. Sleep may be induced by the use of amobarbital sodium (Amytal sodium), 65 to 200 mg, and the patient awakens free from headache in most cases.

3. Ergotamine preparations are still widely used for the treatment of migraine. Since ergotamine is a vasoconstrictor, the drug should be given during the prodromal stages of the attack in an effort to prevent subsequent vasodilatation and headache. Ergotamine tartrate 1 mg is conveniently combined with caffeine, 100 mg, in tablet form (Cafergot). Two of these tablets are taken orally and may be repeated in 30 minutes should the patient develop headache. An-

other two tablets may be taken 30 minutes later if necessary. Sublingual tablets of ergotamine tartrate 2 mg are also available and because of rapid absorption into the bloodstream are probably more effective than the oral preparations. Sublingual tablets should be placed beneath the tongue at the onset of the warning symptoms. The dose may be repeated in 30 minutes if the headache develops. Patients suffering from severe nausea and vomiting may use ergotamine suppositories at the time of the aura or at the very beginning of the headache.

4. Migraine Status: Patients experiencing migraine of several days duration frequently become dehydrated and may develop electrolyte imbalance from repeated vomiting. Treatment consists of intravenous fluids and the injection of 0.5 to 1.0 mg dihydroergotamine intravenously every six hours. Metoclopramide 10 mg can be given IV slowly before the dihydroergotamine to minimize vomiting.

5. Prevention of Migraine (see Table 5–2)

TABLE 5–2.   Treatment of Migraine and Cluster Headaches

Headache Type	Drug Class	Drug
Migraine	Vasoconstrictors	ergotamine, dihydroergotamine
	Beta Blockers	propranolol, nadalol, atenolol, timolol, metoprolol
	Tricyclics	amitriptyline, nortriptyline, doxepin
	Antiinflammatory Agents	naproxen
	Antiserotoninergics	cyproheptadine, methysergide
	Autonomic Inhibitors	Bellergal
	MAO Inhibitors	phenelzine
	Calcium Channel Blockers	verapamil, nifedipine
	Vasodilators	papaverine
Cluster Headache	Vasoconstrictors	ergotamine
	Antiserotoninergics	methysergide, cyproheptadine
	Steroids	prednisone
	Lithium	lithium carbonate
	Antiinflammatory Agents	indomethacin

a. Beta-adrenergic blocking agents are effective in the prevention of migraine. Propranolol (Inderal) is effective in some patients beginning with 20 mg t.i.d. and increasing by 20 mg increments to as high as 240 mg if necessary. Convergence to long-acting preparations of Inderal can be made at the appropriate time during the build-up of the dosage (14). The drug should not be used in patients who are suffering from chronic bronchitis, chronic obstructive pulmonary disease, or asthma. There are few side effects, but patients should be monitored for bradycardia and hypotension.

b. Tricyclic antidepressants are also effective to treat migraine. Amitryptyline 25 mg h.s. is slowly increased until effective or to a maximum of 150 mg in divided doses in 24 hours. The side effects of drowsiness, dryness of the mouth, and excessive perspiration are troublesome in some cases.

c. Calcium channel blockers such as verapamil beginning at 80 mg q8h and increasing to as high as 480 mg per day are also effective in the prevention of migraine.

d. Cyproheptadine (Periactin), a histamine and serotonin antagonist, is occasionally effective if given in doses of 4 mg q.i.d. Again, the most prominent side effect is drowsiness.

e. Methysergide (Sansert), another serotonin antagonist, is given in a dose of 2 mg q.d., increasing slowly to a total of 3 or 4 tablets q.d. (maximum 8 mg). The dosage should be increased only when the patient is free from side effects including drowsiness,

ataxia, and nausea. Methysergide should not be used for more than six months because of the risk of retroperitoneal fibrosis. Pleuropulmonary and cardiac fibrosis following long-term use of methysergide have also been occasionally reported.

f. Naproxen, an antiinflammatory drug, may be an effective preventive in doses of 375 to 500 mg b.i.d (15).

Cluster Headaches

Definition. Cluster headaches are severe unilateral headaches of relatively short duration which occur daily or several times a day for a period of several weeks. The condition then resolves for a period of several months and is followed by recurrence of another cluster of headaches.

Etiology and Pathology. The etiology is unknown. Cluster headaches are associated with vasodilatation that occurs in the distribution of one external carotid artery. There is marked intraocular vasodilatation and increased intraocular pressure on the same side. Platelet levels of histamine and serotonin parallel the course of cluster headaches. They increase during occurrence and drop during improvement. The increased association between peptic ulcer and cluster headaches suggests that there is a hypersensitivity to histamine in those who suffer cluster headaches.

Clinical Features. Cluster headaches occur predominantly in males between the ages of 20 and 50 years. Headaches are often precipitated by ingestion of alcohol but, once established, occur spontaneously. Attacks occur once or several times a day, often awakening the patient at night and lasting from 30 to 120 minutes. An episode of cluster headaches lasts from 4 to 12 weeks, followed by remission which may last for months or years.

Cluster headaches occur without any preceding symptoms. The onset is sudden with an excruciating pain, which is strictly localized to one orbit and frontotemporal region. An attack is associated with extreme distress, photophobia, lacrimation, unilateral nasal congestion, and occasionally Horner's syndrome.

A rare, chronic form of cluster headaches has been described where attacks occur almost daily without any remission. Another variant known as "lower half headache" consists of pain in the cheek and lower jaw, often accompanied by Horner's syndrome and frequently associated with peptic ulceration.

Differential Diagnosis. The differential diagnosis of cluster headache should also include:

1. Acute glaucoma. This condition can be differentiated by the presence of visual loss, the "steamy" appearance of the cornea, and the presence of raised intraocular pressure in glaucoma.

2. Temporal arteritis. Temporal arteritis tends to occur in older patients, but the headache can be paroxysmal and mimic cluster headaches. The sedimentation rate is elevated in temporal arteritis, and a temporal artery biopsy establishes the diagnosis.

3. Ophthalmoplegic Migraine. See page 84.

4. Tolosa Hunt Syndrome. See below.

Treatment

1. The patient should avoid any known precipitating factor such as alcohol.
2. Suppositories containing 1 or 2 mg of ergotamine can be taken every 8 to 12 hours and are often effective in preventing cluster headaches. Treatment should be continued for 10 days and then stopped. If the cluster headaches return, another 10-day course of treatment is indicated.
3. Methysergide (Sansert) beginning 2 mg q.h.s. and increasing by one tablet every three days to a total of two tablets q.i.d. is often an effective prophylactic.
4. Corticosteroids such as methylprednisolone (Medrol) 80 mg q.d. in a single dose may produce dramatic relief from cluster headaches in some cases.
5. Cyproheptadine (Periactin) 4 mg q.i.d. has been effective in some cases.
6. Propranolol (Inderal) beginning 20 mg t.i.d. and increasing to as high as 240 mg is also reported to be effective.
7. Chronic cluster headaches may respond to lithium carbonate beginning with 300 mg q.h.s. and gradually increasing the dose to produce a serum level of 1 to 2 mEq/L.
8. Indomethacin, 25 mg b.i.d., increasing by 25 mg increments to 150 mg per day, if necessary, is also effective in cluster headaches.

Tolosa-Hunt Syndrome

Definition. The Tolosa-Hunt syndrome is a unilateral headache involving one orbit associated with ophthalmoplegia, which develops several days later.

Etiology and Pathology. There is some evidence that the Tolosa-Hunt syndrome results from an acute arteritis involving the temporal portion of the carotid artery and the walls of the cavernous sinus.

Clinical Features. There is severe headache involving the orbit on the affected side associated with ophthalmoplegia, which develops several days after the onset of the headache. The ophthalmoplegia usually presents with a third nerve paralysis followed by involvement of the fourth, sixth, and ophthalmic division of the fifth cranial nerve. Horner's syndrome due to involvement of the carotid sympathetic plexus is not unusual. Optic neuritis has been described in some cases. The condition typically persists for several days but eventually remits spontaneously in most cases.

Treatment. The Tolosa-Hunt syndrome shows a good response to corticosteroids with rapid resolution of symptoms. Methylprednisolone (Medrol), 80 mg q.d. with progressive reduction of the dosage as response occurs, is effective.

Tension Headache

Definition. Tension headaches are a very common type of headache that occur in patients subject to stress, anxiety, and/or depression.

Etiology. The headache is probably a direct result of sustained contraction of the skeletal muscles of the scalp, face, neck, and shoulders.

Clinical Features. The headaches are usually generalized and of long duration. The patient experiences constant pain with temporary relief after analgesics and sleep. The condition is often described in dramatic terms, using such adjectives as "viselike," "constant pressure," "bursting," or "crushing." There is frequent radiation of the pain into the neck and shoulders. The headaches often last for several days, and many patients state that they rarely experience freedom from headaches. Nevertheless, the appearance of the patient is usually normal with no outward signs of suffering, even though the patient indicates that the headache is present at the time of examination.

Diagnostic Procedures. The patient should be subjected to a minimum of diagnostic procedures since the diagnosis can be established by a good history. Nevertheless, it is important to conduct a general physical and neurologic examination in all cases.

Treatment. The physician should attempt to identify the stress or emotional problem underlying the headache. The cause should be explained to the patient. The patient should then be reassured that the condition does not indicate an underlying disease based on the adequate general physical and neurologic examination that has already been performed. Anxiety may be controlled by the regular use of a mild tranquilizer. Depressed patients may benefit from a tricyclic antidepressant such as imipramine (Tofranil) or amitriptyline (Elavil). When sleep is disturbed, it is important to establish a normal sleep pattern using short-acting hypnotic agents.

When tension headaches are symptomatic of a severe emotional problem, the patient should be referred for psychiatric evaluation and treatment.

Headache in Cerebrovascular Diseases

Hypertensive Encephalopathy. Generalized headache is a prominent feature of hypertensive encephalopathy and usually precedes the onset of seizures. Patients have a sustained high blood pressure and hypertensive retinopathy. Papilledema, which indicates the presence of cerebral edema, is present in most cases (16). Hypertensive encephalopathy is a medical emergency and should be treated with intravenous antihypertensive agents to lower the blood pressure to acceptable levels as quickly and safely as possible (see p. 147).

Subarachnoid Hemorrhage. The headache in subarachnoid hemorrhage is one of the most severe pains experienced by man (17). Conscious patients complain of the sudden onset of generalized headache which is often maximal in the occipital area and radiates into the neck. There is marked nuchal rigidity. The headache of subarachnoid hemorrhage requires regular doses of narcotics such as meperidine hydrochloride (Demerol) 100 mg q4h or morphine sulfate 15 mg q4h.

Unruptured Cerebral Aneurysms. Large aneurysms of the terminal internal carotid artery or of the circle of Willis may produce a chronic, dull unilateral headache when there is pressure on the parasellar structures. A sentinel headache is a frequent antecedent of a subarachnoid hemorrhage. In about 50 percent of cases the headache (thunderclap headache) is sudden in onset, severe, and unlike any headache experienced previously (18). It is usually focal in the frontal, occipital, or retroorbital areas and may be accompanied by vomiting, neck pain, syncope, visual symptoms, or focal, motor, or sensory symptoms. The headache subsides after several hours to days (19).

The chronic, dull unilateral headache is usually a retrospective complaint following subarachnoid hemorrhage, and it is possible that the "sentinel headache" is the result of leakage of a minute amount of blood through a small tear in the wall of the aneurysm (20).

Arteriovenous Malformation. Unilateral headaches resembling common migraine have been reported in a number of cases of arteriovenous malformation. These headaches occur over the site of the malformation and probably result from dilatation of the extracranial and intracranial arteries that supply the malformation.

Cerebrovascular Insufficiency. Patients with cerebrovascular insufficiency often complain of chronic headache. This occurs in the frontotemporal area in cases of internal carotid artery insufficiency and is probably due to the development of collateral circulation through the external carotid system. Dull occipital headache is not unusual in vertebral basilar insufficiency and is often exacerbated following a transient ischemic episode. This suggests that the headache is caused by vasodilatation and is possibly related to the development of collateral circulation. However, a number of cases of vertebral basilar insufficiency and occipital headache are probably experiencing discomfort from an associated cervical spondylosis.

Cerebral Arteritis. Inflammation of the branches of the superior temporal artery, temporal arteritis (giant cell arteritis), produces severe unilateral headache. The inflamed vessels are usually, but not always, tender on palpation. Temporal arteritis should be considered in every elderly individual who has recent onset of headaches. Pain may occur in the temple or in the frontal vertex or occipital areas and may be unilateral, bilateral, or generalized (21). The sedimentation rate is elevated. The condition shows a dramatic response to cortiocosteroid therapy (see p. 152).

Headache in Anemia

The occurrence of headache in anemia may be related to increased cerebral blood flow and decreased cerebrovascular resistance.

Headache in Polycythemia

There is marked reduction of cerebral blood flow in polycythemia. The headache that occurs in this condition may be the result of chronic cerebral ischemia.

Headache Due to Meningeal Inflammation

The headache of bacterial meningitis or viral encephalitis is the result of inflammation of the meninges at the base of the brain and in the posterior fossa. The inflammatory process also involves nerve roots in the cervical area, producing reflex contraction of the neck muscles. The headache often begins in the occipital area but becomes generalized in most cases of meningitis and encephalitis and is accompanied by pain and stiffness in the neck, which is increased when the head is flexed. All patients with recent onset of headache should be tested for the presence of nuchal rigidity.

Headache Due to Decreased Intracranial Pressure

A postlumbar puncture headache should be an unusual experience and most cases can be avoided by reassuring the patient before the examination is performed. A few patients will experience headache several hours after a lumbar puncture, which is presumed to be due to a leakage of cerebrospinal fluid at the site of the needle puncture. Most cases will resolve if the patient is placed in a prone position in bed and given extra oral fluids and adequate analgesics. When headache persists, resolution may occur after a short course of fludrocortisone acetate (Florinef) 0.1 mg q12h.

Headache Due to Increased Intracranial Pressure

Increased intracranial pressure from any cause will produce stretching of the nerve endings in the meninges and pressure on the blood vessels at the base of the brain. This often results in a generalized headache, which increases in severity with increasing intracranial pressure. Reduction of increased intracranial pressure to normal levels produces prompt resolution of headache.

Headache in Brain Tumor

The headache in brain tumor is often focal prior to the development of increased intracranial pressure. Therefore, in a case of suspected brain tumor without papilledema:

1. The headache is likely to be unilateral and on the same side as the tumor.
2. The headache tends to be occipital in subtentorial tumors.
3. The headache is located in the frontal or temporal regions in supratentorial tumors.

Posttraumatic Headaches

There are at least three types of headache occurring in the posttraumatic period.

1. Constant, dull headaches of generalized distribution due to contraction of the skeletal muscles in the scalp and cervical area. These headaches are similar to tension headaches.
2. Unilateral, throbbing headaches similar to common migraine or classic migraine. These headaches may be provoked by trivial head injury in susceptible individuals (22).
3. Dysautonomic headaches due to injury to the neck and damage to sympathetic nerves. This condition is characterized by unilateral frontotemporal headache, ipsilateral mydriasis, facial hypohidrosis, ptosis, and miosis. There is a good response to propranolol (Inderal), 20 mg t.i.d., with increase in dosage to as high as 240 mg q.d. in divided dosages.

Headache in Systemic Disease

Headaches frequently accompany an infectious process. In many cases this is probably due to an increase in cerebral blood flow associated with an elevated temperature. However, certain infectious diseases such as influenza, malaria, typhus, and typhoid are associated with severe headache, probably caused by a circulating toxin, which produces further dilatation of the intracerebral vessels. It is not unusual to find some degree of neck stiffness in children with fever and headache. This condition of meningismus is often mistaken for early meningitis, and the diagnosis must be clarified by lumbar puncture. This procedure should also be performed in any patient with a febrile illness who has severe headache and who develops abnormal neurologic signs suggesting an early encephalitis or meningitis.

Episodic headaches of rapid onset with severe bilateral throbbing are a feature of phaeochromocytoma due to release of adrenalin or noradrenalin into the circulation. The blood pressure is very high at the onset of the headache and the urine contains excessive catecholamines.

Headache in Obstructive Pulmonary Disease

Impaired respiratory exchange with retention of carbon dioxide causes cerebral vasodilatation and chronic headache. Headache is a feature of chronic emphysema and may also occur in patients who suffer from hypoventilation due to extreme obesity (pickwickian syndrome). Headaches due to carbon dioxide retention can be relieved by improving pulmonary function.

Headache in Hypoglycemia

Although headaches are a feature of hypoglycemia, this condition is all too frequently and erroneously cited as a cause of headache in patients with tension headaches or headaches due to psychological stress. The demonstration of hypoglycemia should not depend upon a single casual blood glucose determination but rather on adequate study of the problem. Patients with headache due to hypoglycemia respond to appropriate treatment (see page 313).

Headache in Heat Exhaustion

Headache is a feature of heat stroke and heat exhaustion and probably results from increased cerebral blood flow secondary to temperature elevation. Additional factors may be dehydration and lowered cerebrospinal fluid pressure, which produces increased traction on pain-sensitive structures within the cranial cavity. The complications and the headache respond to appropriate correction of fluid and electrolyte imbalance.

Toxic Causes of Headache

Hangover Headache. The "hangover" headache, which is a throbbing generalized headache, resembles common migraine and is also the result of vasodilatation. Ingestion of alcohol may precipitate migraine in certain individuals. In most cases hangover headache is the result of ingestion of small quantities of aromatic substances which are contained in alcoholic beverages rather than the alcohol itself. Treatment consists of rest, fluid replacement, and the use of simple analgesics, but in many cases relief is obtained only after a period of sleep.

Carbon Monoxide Poisoning. Carbon monoxide poisoning results in a reduction of arterial oxygen saturation, which produces vasodilatation. While acute carbon monoxide poisoning causes loss of consciousness, chronic poisoning produces severe paroxysmal headaches, which resolve when the source of carbon monoxide is removed.

Headaches Following Ingestion of Medication. A number of medications produce vasodilatation and headache. Thus, headache is often common after ingestion of amylnitrate, amonitrate, or nitroglycerin. Sudden headache may occur in patients receiving monoamine oxidase inhibitors who eat cheese or drink red wine, both of which have a high tyramine content.

Chinese Restaurant and Hot Dog Headaches. Ingestion of foods containing monosodium glutamate, which is used abundantly in Chinese food or foods containing nitrites such as cured meats and hot dogs, may cause throbbing headache in susceptible individuals.

Headache in Diseases of the Eye. It is a common assumption that headaches are caused by refractory errors, but this is a rather uncommon event. Occasionally hypermetropic children complain of headache toward the end of the school day. This can be corrected by prescription of suitable glasses.

Infections involving the superficial structures of the eye or the tissues surrounding the eye frequently produce periorbital headache. This includes conjunctivitis, dacryocystitis, and keratitis. Pain is particularly severe in *Herpes zoster* ophthalmicus. Orbital cellulitis will also produce pain and discomfort in the orbit and frontotemporal area. Headache also accompanies inflammation within the eye, for example, uveitis, iritis, and endo- or panophthalmitis. Acute optic neuritis often presents with acute onset of pain in and around the eye and frontal headache. The pain is exacerbated by eye movement and is associated with sudden dimness or loss of vision.

Acute glaucoma produces severe unilateral headache, vomiting, and prostration, and the condition resembles an acute and severe attack of migraine. However, the cornea is steamy, the pupil is dilated, and the diagnosis can be quickly established by ophthalmologic examination. Chronic glaucoma is a cause of intermittent frontal headache. Visual symptoms are often minimal, but the diagnosis can be established by determination of intraocular pressure.

Headaches in Diseases of the Nose and Paranasal Sinuses

Acute sinusitis may produce frontal headache, particularly if the ethmoidal or sphenoidal sinuses are involved. Patients are febrile and toxic and have an elevated white count. The condition responds to antibiotics and analgesics.

Chronic sinusitis is a rare cause of headache (23). Patients with chronic sinus infection may experience problems with changes in atmospheric pressure as occur during flying. There may be a failure to equalize pressure in a congested sinus during the descent of an aircraft, with the sudden occurrence of severe pain over the affected sinus. The condition is relieved by nasal decongestants.

Tumors of the paranasal sinuses produce chronic headache or facial pain, which tends to be referred to the site of the involved sinus. Tumors of the maxillary sinus produce pain over the cheek and upper teeth, often associated with epistaxis, and followed by the later development of headache on the same side. Ethmoidal sinus tumors cause pain over the bridge of the nose. Frontal sinus tumors produce unilateral frontal headache. Nasopharyngeal tumors can cause unilateral nasal obstruction with headache; epistaxis; pain in the throat on the affected side, which is often referred to the ipsilateral ear; and some decrease in hearing on that side. Tumors in the nasopharyngeal area can also involve the maxillary and mandibular divisions of the fifth cranial nerve, producing constant pain in the maxillary and mandibular areas of the face. Early nasopharyngeal tumors can be difficult to diagnose, and the nasopharynx should always be examined when patients complain of unilateral facial pain, pharyngeal pain, or pain in the ear.

Miscellaneous Causes of Headache

Cervical Spondylosis and Cervical Osteoarthritis. Patients with degenerative disease of the cervical spine often complain of headache in the occipital region. This may be caused by:

1. Compression of cervical nerve roots and involvement of the greater occipital nerves

2. Prolonged contraction of skeletal muscle in the neck and posterior scalp
3. Referred pain from diseased joints in the cervical spine in cervical disk disease or spondylosis (24).
4. Compression of the vertebral arteries by osteophytes in the neck producing vertebrobasilar insufficiency and occipital headache.

Headache During the Menopause. The menopause is not a cause of headache. Although it is possible that headache could develop because of hormonal changes, this cause is unlikely and most cases can be related to tension and depression.

Headache Following Sexual Activity. The occurrence of headache during or immediately following sexual activity is probably due to contraction of muscles in the neck, jaw, and scalp during sexual intercourse. Patients may be reassured that this is a benign condition.

Cough Headache. The occurrence of severe generalized headache following a bout of coughing is probably due to a sudden rise in intracranial pressure. Some of these patients have herniation of the cerebellar tonsils into the spinal canal (Chiari type I malformation) and may require surgical decompression to relieve this symptom.

Lancinating Ocular Headache. Patients occasionally complain of a sudden intense pain passing through the eyeball, which is often described dramatically as the passage of a needle through the eye. The condition is benign, and the cause is unknown. There is no effective treatment.

Ice Pick Headaches. Sudden intensely painful stabbing pains in the scalp are sometimes experienced by patients who are known to suffer from migraine. Symptoms last only for several seconds and occur without warning between migraine attacks. Ice pick headaches occasionally occur without a preceding history of migraine. The condition is benign, the cause unknown, and there is no effective treatment.

Ice Cream Headaches. This condition is also benign and consists of the sudden development of intense unilateral headache affecting the orbit and frontal areas following the ingestion of substances at low temperature. The condition resolves very rapidly as soon as the patient ceases to swallow the frozen substance. Ice cream headache tends to recur under similar conditions, and afflicted individuals should learn to avoid rapid ingestion of extremely cold substances.

REFERENCES

1. Olsen, T. S.; Friberg, L.; *et al.* Ischemia may be the primary cause of neurologic deficits in classical migraine. Arch. Neurol. 44:156–161; 1987.
2. Pearce, J. M. S. Is migraine explained by Leao's spreading depression? Lancet 2:763–766; 1985.
3. Secuteri, F.; Renzi, D.; *et al.* Substance P and enkephalins: a creditable tandem in the pathophysiology of cluster headache and migraine. Adv. Exp. Med. Biol. 198B:145–152; 1986.
4. Welch, K. M. A. Migraine. A biobehavioral disorder. Arch. Neurol. 44:323–327; 1987.
5. Littlewood, J. T.; Gibb, C.; *et al* Red wine as a cause of migraine. Lancet 1:558–559; 1988.
6. Plant, G. T. The fortifications spectra of migraine. Br. Med. J. (Clin. Res.) 293:1613–1617; 1986.
7. Schreiber, A. O.; Calvert, P. C. Migrainous olfactory hallucinations. Headache 26:513–514; 1986.
8. Lane, P. L.; Ross, R.; Rothrock, J. F.; Walicke, P.; *et al.* Migranous stroke. Arch. Neurol. 45:63–67; 1988.
9. Anderson, A. B.; Freberg, L.; *et al.* Delayed hyperemia following hypoperfusion in classical migraine. Arch. Neurol. 45:154–159; 1988.
10. Jacome, D. E.; Risko, M. The non-epileptiform basilar artery migraine. Headache 26:447–450; 1986.
11. Jacome, D. E. Basilar artery migraine after uncomplicated whiplash injuries. Headache 26:515–516; 1986.
12. Symon, D. N. K.; Russell, G. Abdominal migraine: a childhood syndrome defined. Cephalalgia 6:223–228; 1986.
13. Rothner, A. D. The migraine syndrome in children and adolescents. Pediatr. Neurol. 2:121–126; 1986.
14. Olerud, B.; Gustausson, C. L.; *et al.* Nadolol and Propranolol in migraine management. Headache 26:490–493; 1986.
15. Welch, K. M. A.; Ellis, D. J.; *et al.* Successful migraine prophylaxis with Naproxen Sodium. Neurology 35:1304–1310; 1985.
16. Hauser, R. A.; Lacey, M.; *et al.* Hypertensive encephalopathy: magnetic resonance imaging demonstration of reversible cortical and white matter lesions. Arch. Neurol. 45:1078–1083; 1988.
17. Linnik, M. D.; Sakas, D. E.; *et al.* Subarachnoid blood and headache: Altered trigeminal tachykinin gene expression. Ann. Neurol. 25:179–184; 1989.
18. Day, J. W.; Rashin, N. H. Thunderclap headaches: symptoms of unruptured cerebral aneurysm. Lancet 2:1247–1248; 1986.
19. Gorelick, P. B.; Hier, D. B.; *et al.* Headache in acute cerebrovascular disease. Neurology 36:1445–1450; 1986.
20. Verwey, R. D.; Wijdicks, E. F. M. Warning headaches in aneurysmal subarachnoid hemorrhage. Arch. Neurol. 45:1019–1020; 1988.
21. Solomon, S.; Cappa, K. G. The headache of temporal arteritis. Geriatr. Soc. 35:163–165; 1987.
22. Haas, D. C.; Lourie, H. Trauma induced migraine: an explanation for common neurological attacks after minor head injury. J. Neurosurg. 68:181–188; 1988.
23. Faleck, H., Rothner, A. D.; *et al.* Headache and subacute sinusitis in children and adolescents. Headache 28:96–98; 1988.
24. Edmeads, J. The cervical spine and headache. Neurology 38:1874–1878; 1988.

CHAPTER 6

MOVEMENT DISORDERS

A number of neurologic disorders are characterized by the presence of conspicuous involuntary movements. Although these movements occur in many different unrelated pathologic conditions, their appearance permits convenient clinical classification. Involuntary movements have certain common properties.

1. In most cases the type of movement is recognized by observation.
2. Involuntary movements are often accentuated by stress.
3. Involuntary movements disappear during sleep.

The following terms are used in describing involuntary movements:

Chorea: Abrupt, spasmodic, irregular movements of short duration involving the fingers, hands, arms, face, tongue, or head.

Athetosis: Irregular, slow, sinuous movements usually involving the hands and fingers.

Choreoathetosis: A combination of choreiform and athetoid movements.

Dystonia: An abnormal sustained movement or posture due to a disturbance of muscle tone in agonists and antagonists.

Myoclonus: Sudden shocklike contractions of a muscle or a group of muscles.

Palatal myoclonus (syn palatal nystagmus): Rapid, rhythmic contractions of one side of the palate producing a rhythmic movement of

the uvula, which is usually accompanied by synchronous movements of the pharynx. (The condition occasionally spreads to involve the face, tongue, platysma, shoulders, and diaphragm).

Myokymia: Persistent irregular twitching of muscle producing a quivering "bag of worms" appearance, often seen in the periorbital region (facial myokymia).

Fasciculations: Irregular contractions and relaxations of muscle fascicles, innervated by the same motor unit, which are visible through the skin.

Tic: Repetitive spasmodic movements that occur in an irregular fashion and resemble volitional movements.

Habit spasm: A tic of long duration

Clonus: A rhythmic movement produced by rapid contraction and relaxation of muscle, usually seen with increased muscle tone.

Tremor: A rhythmic movement of short amplitude.

CHOREA

Rheumatic (Sydenham's) Chorea

Definition. Rheumatic chorea is believed to be a delayed manifestation of infection with group A beta-hemolytic streptococci. It occurs most commonly in the 5- to 15-year-old age group.

Etiology and Pathology. Rheumatic chorea probably represents the cerebral form of rheumatic fever. Rheumatic fever is a systemic disease characterized by inflammation, degeneration, and fibrosis of collagen. The heart and arterial system are particularly susceptible to rheumatic involvement. The exact etiology of rheumatic fever is still unclear, but the condition is believed to be an abnormal immune response involving group A streptococci.

Rheumatic chorea is associated with a vasculitis and occasionally an exudative necrosis of the smaller cerebral arteries. There is a perivascular cellular infiltration around the affected arteries and neurons in the cerebral cortex, basal ganglia, and cerebellum.

Clinical Features. The duration between the attack of rheumatic fever and the detection of chorea varies from two to nine months. The onset is insidious and the affected child often appears to be clumsy before involuntary movements develop. Choreic movements involve the fingers and hands initially, followed by gradual involvement of the upper limbs and spread to the face and tongue. Examination may reveal a mild fever and tachycardia, and the patient presents with choreiform movements that are increased by excitement or stress. When the tongue is protruded it suddenly jerks back into the mouth. The hands show a typical posture when the arms are outstretched with flexion of the wrist, extension of the metacarpophalangeal and interphalangeal joints, and extension and abduction of the thumb. The wrist is pronated when the arms are held above the head. In severe cases there may be continuous movements with flinging of the limbs. The speech is dysarthric with an irregular, explosive quality due to sudden contractions of the respiratory muscles. Constant movements of the head may lead to loss of hair over the occipital area. Involvement of the pharyngeal muscles produces dysphagia and increases the risk of aspiration pneumonia.

There is generalized hypotonia and muscle weakness, and coordination is slowed and impaired with irregular overflinging during rapid alternating movements. The stretch reflexes are normal, but the knee jerks are pendular. There is a bilateral plantar flexor response. Sensation is normal. Evidence of systemic rheumatic involvement (e.g., fever, carditis, polyarthritis, erythema marginatum) may be present. Chorea usually lasts for about four to six weeks, but prolonged episodes up to 12 months have been observed. Persistence is rare.

Diagnostic Procedures.

1. The sedimentation rate is usually elevated.
2. The antistreptolysin O (ASO) test is the best available serologic test; however, by the time chorea appears, the antibody titers may have declined.
3. The antistreptozyme test, a hemagglutination reaction to streptococcus Ag, is very sensitive but not widely available.
4. Other serologic tests which may be helpful in documenting the infection include antistreptokinase (ASK), antideoxyribonuclease B (anti-DNaseB), anti-NAD-ase, and antihyaluronidase.
5. Lumbar puncture. The cerebrospinal fluid (CSF) is normal.

Differential Diagnosis.

1. Viral encephalitis. The patient typically presents with headache followed by alteration in level of consciousness. Corticospinal tract involvement and extensor plantar responses are usually present. The CSF is abnormal.
2. Postinfectious encephalomyelitis. Brain, spinal cord, and corticospinal tract are involved, with extensor plantar responses and sensory deficits.
3. Lupus erythematosus LE. The LE preparation, antinuclear antibodies (ANA), and rheumatoid factor are usually positive.
4. Anoxic encephalopathy. There is typically a history of an anoxic episode and evidence of diffuse damage to the central nervous system (CNS).
5. Drug-induced chorea. Chorea may occur as a side effect of certain drugs such as phenothiazines and carbamazepine (Tegretol).

Treatment. The treatment consists of:

1. Bed rest.
2. The head and limbs should be protected from trauma when there are severe involuntary movements.
3. Chlorpromazine, beginning 10 mg t.i.d., gradually increasing until the choreiform are controlled, is very effective in most cases.
4. A short course of corticosteroids produces dramatic improvement in many cases. Prednisone 60 mg q.d. for 7 to 14 days is usually effective.
5. Severe cases will respond to haloperidol (Haldol) beginning 1 mg q12h and in-

creasing slowly until adequate response occurs.

6. Carbamazepine can be used as an alternative in difficult cases (1).
7. Pimozide may be effective in refractory cases (2).
8. Prophylaxis. About 50 percent of patients with rheumatic chorea develop overt signs of rheumatic carditis. This may be prevented with prophylactic penicillin given as benzathine penicillin G 1.2 million units intramuscularly (IM) every month or oral penicillin G 250,000 units q12h until age 21 years.

Prognosis. Good. Neurologic complications of rheumatic chorea are very rare. A few children show minor intellectual impairment or emotional lability which requires special attention on returning to school. Recurrence is rare.

Chorea Gravidarum

Chorea gravidarum is a rare condition related to rheumatic fever since many patients report attacks of chorea when not pregnant, one-third give a history of rheumatic heart disease, and one-third show clinical evidence of heart disease. However, with the decline of rheumatic fever, most cases seen today are secondary to systemic lupus erythematosus or possibly Huntington's disease.

Acute psychosis with anxiety, delirium, or mania is the most important complication of chorea gravidarum. This may become permanent in some cases. Speech disturbances which may be dysphasic or dysarthric have been reported. Chorea gravidarum may recur during subsequent pregnancies (3).

Senile Chorea

Chorea is occasionally seen in elderly patients and occurs with or without dementia. Senile chorea with dementia is probably due to neuronal degeneration of the basal ganglia in patients with Alzheimer's disease. A few cases may be due to late onset of Huntington's disease. Cases without dementia are rare and are probably due to degenerative changes or multiple lacunar infarcts confined to the basal ganglia.

Hemichorea

Choreiform movements involving one limb are occasionally seen following a mild stroke. These patients usually exhibit pronounced sensory changes in the affected limb, suggesting the presence of a lesion in the posterior ventrolateral nucleus of the thalamus.

Symptomatic Chorea

Chorea is occasionally seen during acute encephalitis and is a rare finding in more chronic diseases including systemic lupus erythematosus, multiple sclerosis, and the leukodystrophies. Chorea has been observed in a number of metabolic conditions including hyperthyroidism, hypocalcemia, and hypernatremia. Choreiform movements have been described during treatment with phenothiazines, phenytoin (Dilantin), carbamazepine (Tegretol), anticholinergic drugs, amphetamine-like drugs, digoxin, cimetidine, methylphenidate, cyclizine, and oral contraceptives. The presence of chorea has also been recorded in blood dyscrasias, including polycythemia vera and sickle cell disease. Chorea and dystonia can occur as a remote effect of carcinoma. Pimozide or tetrabenazine may be effective in senile chorea, hemichorea or symptomatic chorea.

Benign Hereditary Chorea

This is a rare condition in which the symptoms of chorea appear in late infancy or early childhood. The chorea affects the upper limbs more than the lower limbs. There is associated generalized hypotonia and the condition remains unchanged without significant progression into adult life. There is no mental deterioration. Improvement has been reported with corticosteroids but the relatively benign nature of the chorea hardly warrants long-term steroid therapy (4).

Familial Amyotrophic Chorea with Acanthocytosis

This rare condition is characterized by the onset in adult life of a progressive neurologic deficit consisting of choreiform movements, seizures, buccolingual dyskinesia, orofacial tics, neurogenic muscular atrophy with areflexia, and acanthocytosis. The serum creatine kinase level is elevated but betalipoprotein levels are normal (5). Haloperidol will decrease the involuntary facial movements.

Familial Calcification of the Basal Ganglia

This condition is occasionally associated with the presence of chorea which is nonprogressive. Diagnosis is established by the demonstration of calcification of the basal ganglia.

ATHETOSIS

The common athetotic syndromes are discussed under "Cerebral Palsy" (see page 65).

Athetosis is occasionally encountered in a number of genetically determined conditions with metabolic defects including the aminoacidurias, in particular phenylketonuria; disorders of lipid metabolism including the lipidoses and leukodystrophies; the Lesch-Nyhan syndrome, a genetically determined disorder of purine metabolism; and a genetically determined disorder of copper metabolism, hepatolenticular degeneration. Athetosis is not unusual in degenerative diseases of the brain, including tuberous sclerosis, Hallervorden-Spatz disease, ataxia telangiectasia, and the dementias, in particular Alzheimer's disease.

Paroxysmal Choreoathetosis

Definition. Paroxysmal choreoathetosis is a condition characterized by sudden paroxysms of choreoathetosis. Two distinct types have been recognized. In paroxysmal kinesiogenic choreoathetosis the choreoathetosis is precipitated by sudden movement, whereas in paroxysmal dystonic choreoathetosis the choreoathetosis occurs spontaneously.

Etiology and Pathology. Paroxysmal choreoathetosis is related to the epilepsies, and some cases are inherited as an autosomal dominant or recessive trait. The cause is usually unknown but it has been described in progressive supranuclear palsy after a head injury (6) and following thalamic infarction (7).

Clinical Features. The clinical features are as follows:

Paroxysmal Kinesiogenic Choreoathetosis. The condition begins in childhood with the development of sudden paroxysms of choreoathetoid movements which may occur several times a day. The attacks are precipitated by sudden voluntary movement or by movement after a prolonged period of immobility. The paroxysm begins in the distal limbs and spreads rapidly to involve the proximal muscles, the trunk, and the neck. This produces a bizarre contortion, coupled with writhing movements, and the patient may collapse to the floor. There is no loss of consciousness. Paroxysms may be confined to one side of the body in some cases. There may be brief choreiform movements of the fingers and feet between attacks. Some patients can abort attacks by a voluntary act such as clenching the fist or flexing the toes and arching the feet. The relationship to epilepsy is established by the precipitation of attacks by hyperventilation and the beneficial effect of anticonvulsant medication. The neurologic examination,

including mentation, is normal between attacks, and there is no effect on intellect.

Paroxysmal Dystonic (Nonkinesiogenic) Choreoathetosis. This condition is rare. The symptoms are similar to the kinesiogenic form of the disease, but the movements occur spontaneously without warning and are not precipitated by sudden movement.

Diagnostic Procedures. Magnetic resonance (MR) and computed tomography (CT) scanning are usually normal (8). High voltage paroxysmal discharges have been reported in the electroencephalogram during hyperventilation.

Differential Diagnosis. Characterized by choreoathetosis, listed in Table 6–1.

Treatment. Phenytoin (Dilantin) in therapeutic doses will usually control these attacks. Other drugs such as haloperidol (Haldol), carbamazepine (Tegretol), levodopa (L-dopa), phenobarbital, primidone (Mysoline), and valproic acid (Depakene) have been reported to give relief in phenytoin-refractory cases.

Hallervorden-Spatz Disease

Definition. Hallervorden-Spatz disease is a rare familial condition that begins in infancy or childhood and is associated with progressive neurologic deficits. It is inherited as an autosomal recessive trait.

Etiology and Pathology. The condition is the result of cysteine accumulation locally in the globus pallidus due to an enzymatic block in the metabolic pathway from cysteine to taurine (9). Microscopic examination shows neuronal loss, axonal swelling, iron deposits, and gliosis.

Clinical Features. The condition begins in infancy or childhood usually between the ages of 7 and 12. Progressive mental deteri-

TABLE 6–1. Choreoathetosis

Hereditary

1. Huntington's disease
2. Familial paroxysmal choreoathetosis
3. Wilson's disease (hepatolenticular degeneration)
4. Lesch-Nyhan syndrome
5. Hallervorden-Spatz disease
6. Familial calcification of the basal ganglia

Acquired

1. Infarction of caudate nucleus of putamen
2. Drug induced—lithium, phenytoin, carbamazepine, amphetamines (62)

oration associated with emotional disorders of the pseudobulbar types, spasticity, dysarthria, dystonia, and choreoathetotic movements of the limbs are typically present. About 50 percent of cases show pigmentary degeneration of the retina and optic atrophy.

Diagnostic Procedures. MR and CT scanning reveal anterior enlargement of the lateral ventricles and flattening of the caudate nuclei. There is prominent atrophy of the cortex and brain stem.

Treatment. There is no treatment at this time. The condition is progressive with death usually occurring from intercurrent infection 10 to 20 years after onset.

Huntington's Disease (Huntington's Chorea)

Definition. Huntington's disease is a hereditary degenerative disease characterized by involuntary choreoathetotic movements and chronic dementia. The genetic abnormality has been localized to chromosome 4.

Etiology and Pathology. The brain shows cortical atrophy, most prominent in the frontal lobes, and ventricular dilatation, which is more marked in the frontal horns of the lateral ventricles, resulting from atrophy of the caudate nucleus. Microscopic examination shows a profound loss of medium sized spiney neurons which make up 80 percent of the neurons in the caudate nucleus and putamen with sparing of the larger neurons. There is a reactive gliosis in the basal ganglia with the presence of prominent, characteristic astrocytes. It should be realized, however, that Huntington's disease is a generalized neuronal atrophy, and there is neuronal loss of lesser extent in most of the gray matter of the cerebral hemispheres and cerebellum. There are a number of biochemical deficiencies in Huntington's disease. Gamma aminobutyric acid (GABA), acetylcholine, substance P, and dynophin are all decreased in the caudate nucleus and putamen. The dopaminergic nigrostriatal pathway and dopamine concentrations are preserved and an imbalance between dopamine, GABA, and acetylcholine may account for the involuntary movements of Huntington's disease. The cause of the dementia, however, remains unexplained (10,11).

Clinical Features. *Epidemiology.* Huntington's disease is seen in all races and has a prevalence of approximately 6.5 cases per 100,000 population. It is inherited as an autosomal dominant trait.

Signs and Symptoms. The mean age of onset ranges from 35 to 42 years, but 6 percent develop symptoms before 21 years and 3 percent before 15 years of age. In some cases choreiform movements begin as late as the sixth to eighth decade. The progression of the disease is slow in such cases (12). Initially, the patient appears restless; this eventually progresses to irregular choreoathetoid movements affecting the fingers and wrists, with later involvement of the more proximal muscle groups of the upper limbs. The gait is ataxic in the fully developed state and has a bouncing quality due to irregular choreoathetoid movements. Choreoathetoid movements of the face and tongue result in nonrepetitive facial and mouth movements, and the patient is dysarthric. There is a slowly progressive dementia, which presents as a loss of memory coupled with impairment of judgment and insight. Many patients develop depression and suicidal thoughts. The disease progresses relentlessly and the patient eventually becomes bedridden.

There are two notable variants of Huntington's disease. There are:

1. Variant I (Westphal). This more rapid form of Huntington's disease consists of the development of rigidity beginning with the trunk and proximal limb musculature and gradually involving all muscle groups. There is rapid dementia, and death occurs within a few years of the onset of the disease. Examination shows masklike facies, generalized rigidity, and evidence of corticospinal trace involvement with increased reflexes and bilateral extensor plantar responses.
2. Variant II (Juvenile). This variant occurs in children and adolescents. Progressive rigidity, ataxia, and dementia with seizures are followed by death within a few years of onset.

Diagnostic Procedures.

1. MR or CT scan shows ventricular dilatation with flattening of the caudate nuclei in established cases (see Figure 6–1). It should be realized that ventricular dilatation may not be present in early cases of Huntington's disease. Late cases show the presence of cortical atrophy.
2. Electroencephalography shows progressive loss of background alpha activity and the appearance of slower frequencies in all leads.
3. CSF GABA is said to be reduced.
4. Serial neuropsychologic testing shows progressive deterioration of intellectual

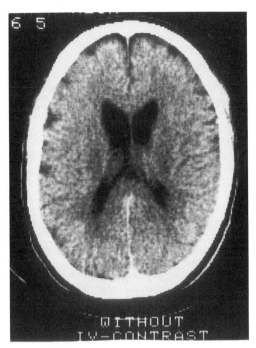

FIGURE 6-1. Huntington's Disease. CT scan showing loss of normal concavity, a lateral wall, lateral ventricle in presence of atrophy of the caudate nucleus.

functioning. Testing of siblings may reveal cases of Huntington's disease since serial testing will show a progressive deterioration of performance IQ (13).

5. Predictive testing for Huntington's disease is now feasible with the discovery of a DNA marker linked to Huntington's disease gene. Such testing raises many ethical questions which should be discussed with a genetic counselor before testing is requested (14).

Treatment. The treatment of Huntington's disease is as follows:

1. In the early stages of the disease choreoathetoid movements may be controlled with a phenothiazine. This may require up to 150 mg q.d. of chlorpromazine (Thorazine) in divided dosages.
2. Reserpine beginning 1 mg per day, and increasing slowly to as high as 15 mg per day if necessary, is very effective in controlling choreiform movements.
3. Haloperidol (Haldol) 3 to 6 mg q.d. is probably the most effective drug in established cases of Huntington's disease and will control choreoathetoid movements in most patients.

4. Tetrabenazine 50 mg t.i.d. has been reported to be effective in some cases (15).
5. Other drugs which have been used include amantadine, bromocriptine, thiopropazate, and lithium.
6. There is a high risk of depression with suicidal tendencies in patients with Huntington's disease, and the physician and the patient's family should be aware of this. Depressed patients may benefit from a tricyclic antidepressant such as amitriptyline (Elavil) or imipramine (Tofranil), beginning with 50 mg of either drug at night and increasing until effective.

Prognosis. The disease is fatal and in most cases death occurs between 10 to 15 years after onset. A few patients have a more chronic course and will survive beyond 20 years.

Hepatolenticular Degeneration (Wilson's Disease)

Definition. Hepatolenticular degeneration is a disorder of copper metabolism which is inherited as an autosomal recessive trait and results from genetic expression of a locus on chromosome 13 (16).

Etiology and Pathology. There is increased absorption of copper from the intestinal tract, failure of copper to bind with apoceruloplasmin, and decreased formation of the bound product ceruloplasmin. This results in elevated free serum copper levels, deposition of copper in the tissues, and increased excretion of copper in the urine.

Pathologic changes consist of deposition of copper in liver cells which eventually produces cirrhosis of the liver. Deposition of copper in kidney cells produces damage to renal tubules and consequent aminoaciduria, alkaline urine, low serum uric acid, and low serum phosphate levels in chronic cases. Copper is deposited in Descemet's membrane of the cornea which produces the characteristic Kayser-Fleischer ring. Deposition of copper in the brain produces damage in the caudate nucleus and putamen which may show cavitation. The globus pallidus is shrunken but rarely cavitated. Lesions are also seen in the subthalamic nucleus, thalamus, red nucleus, claustrum, blood vessels, myelinated fiber bundles, and there are minor cortical changes. Microscopic examination reveals neuronal loss; surviving neurons are pyknotic. Vascular changes consisting of capillary swelling and proliferation, swelling of arterial endothelium, and perivascular thickening occurring in the basal ganglia.

Clinical Features. Hepatolenticular degeneration occurs in childhood, adolescence, and adult life up to the age of 40. The condition affects both sexes, and there is often a marked similarity in the presentation of the illness in members of affected families. First symptoms may be psychiatric, neurologic, or hepatic (17). Psychiatric symptoms consisting of depression, emotional lability, and personality changes are the initial presentation in about 30 percent of patients who may receive psychiatric treatment before the diagnosis of hepatolenticular degeneration is established.

There are two types of neurologic presentation:

1. The choreoathetotic form, probably the commonest form of Wilson's disease, is characterized by the appearance of choreoathetotic movements of the fingers and hands which spread to involve the more proximal muscles of the upper limbs, followed by involvement of the lower limbs, trunk, and head. There is a mild progressive dementia, and the patient has a typical facial appearance with a fixed, vacant smile. The speech is dysarthric but later becomes aphonic. Dysphagia and drooling occur. Constant choreoathetotic movements give the gait a peculiar dancing quality. The disease progresses and the victim becomes bedridden and the limbs become fixed with contractures. Death occurs from intercurrent infection.

2. The dystonic form is rare and is characterized by generalized muscle rigidity and bradykinesis. The gait has a festinant quality resembling that seen in parkinsonism. The patient is severely dysarthric and may have some absence of facial expression. Liver disease consisting of cirrhosis, liver failure, or hepatitis is the first manifestation of hepatolenticular degeneration in about 15 percent of cases. All patients eventually develop Kayser-Fleischer rings. Initially, crescents appear in the superior and inferior aspects of the cornea at the corneoscleral junction. Crescents gradually extend and eventually join to form a complete ring. The color is usually brownish-red or brownish-green and should not be confused with arcus senilis, a much commoner condition. A definitive diagnosis can be made by slit lamp examination.

Diagnostic Procedures.

1. Ceruloplasmin levels are reduced below 20 mg percent.
2. Serum copper levels are usually elevated in Wilson's disease about 80 to 150 mg/dl.
3. Urinary copper excretion is increased to more than 100 mg/24 hr.
4. The presence of Kayser-Fleischer rings can be confirmed by slit lamp examination in early cases. Alternatively, the copper content of the cornea can be measured by x-ray excitation spectometry.
5. Chronic cases of Wilson's disease show the presence of aminoaciduria, glycosuria, and alkaline urine.
6. Cirrhosis of the liver is usually mild in Wilson's disease. Excess copper concentrations can be demonstrated on liver biopsy.
7. In very early cases the diagnosis of Wilson's disease can be established with a radioactive copper kinetic study using Cu^{64} or Cu^{67}.
8. MR scans are usually abnormal with lesions in T2 weighted scans presenting as an increased signal or atrophy. Sites of involvement include the basal ganglia; white matter of the frontal, temporal, and occipital lobes; the centrum semiovale, midbrain, and pons; and the deep cerebellar nuclei. There may be generalized atrophy and ventricular dilation. Basal ganglia lesions are usually symmetric; white matter lesions, multiple and asymmetric. Dystonia correlates with lesions of the putamen, dysarthria with lesions of the putamen and caudate nucleus (18). Computed tomography scanning may reveal degenerative changes in the lentiform nuclei.

Treatment. The object of treatment is to decrease the absorption of copper from the intestinal tract and promote excretion of copper from the tissues into the urine. This can be accomplished by:

1. Reduction of dietary copper to below 1 mg/day.
2. Binding of dietary copper by potassium sulfide given in 40 mg doses with each meal.
3. Use of chelating agents to remove copper from the tissues. The most effective chelating agent is D-penicillamine, which is given in doses of 1 to 4 g/day in divided doses on an empty stomach. Supplementary vitamin B_6 should be given during the

administration of D-penicillamine to minimize the risk of optic neuritis. Side effects include fever, morbilliform rashes, bone marrow suppression, and systemic lupus erythematosus. When necessary, these reactions can be minimized by concomitant administration of oral corticosteroids, and penicillamine therapy can be continued. All members of a family at risk should be investigated for low ceruloplasmin levels and/or elevated hepatic copper content. Those found to have metabolic abnormalities suggesting Wilson's disease, although asymptomatic, should be treated with D-penicillamine.

Prognosis. Untreated cases usually die within four years of the appearance of symptoms. However, survival for 10 years or more has been described in some cases. The prognosis has been improved significantly with D-penicillamine therapy.

Spasmodic Torticollis

Definition. Spasmodic torticollis is a form of dystonia characterized by intermittent and recurrent involuntary movements of the head due to contraction of the neck muscles.

Etiology and Pathology. The condition may be inherited as an autosomal dominant or autosomal recessive trait. Other causes include congenital abnormalities in one sternocleidomastoid muscle, congenital anomalies of the cervical spine, hemiatlas or hypoplasia of the atlas, neurovascular compression of the 11th cranial nerve by the vertebral artery or posterior inferior cerebellar artery; unilateral lesions of the mesencephalon or diencephalon following viral encephalitis, and a bilateral breakdown of the normal metabolic relationships between the thalamus and basal ganglia.

Clinical Features. Spasmodic torticollis may begin in adolescence or adult life. There is often a history of preceding trauma to the neck. The onset is usually gradual with intermittent rotation and flexion of the head to one side. This gradually increases in severity, and in severe cases there may be prolonged periods of dystonic deviation of the head. In most cases the head movement is intermittent and is associated with periodic irregular contractions of the neck musculature. Bilateral involvement is rare but has been described with extension of the head (retrocollis). The movement can often be decreased by counterpressure on the side of the head using the hand or resting the head against a wall. Some patients experience increasing cervical pain due to progressive cervical arthritic changes with nerve root compression secondary to the involuntary head movement. Spasmodic torticollis is occasionally complicated by blepharospasm, oromandibular dystonia, and writer's cramp (19).

Diagnostic Procedures.

1. Electromyography shows persistent muscle contraction in the affected neck muscles including the sternocleidomastoid, spleneus capitus, and trapezius muscles.
2. Thyroid function tests should be obtained since there may be more than a chance association between hyperthyroidism and spasmodic torticollis. Some improvement may occur if the patient is restored to the euthyroid state.
3. X-rays of the cervical spine should be obtained when there is severe neck pain.

Treatment. There is no one drug that is effective in the treatment of spasmodic torticollis.

1. Mild cases may respond to benzodiazepines such as diazepam (Valium) 10 to 40 mg q.d. or lorazepam (Ativan) 3 to 6 mg q.d. in b.i.d. or t.i.d. dosage.
2. High doses of trihexyphenidyl (Artane) 24 to 40 mg per day are usually effective in patients with tonic rather than phasic head turning (20).
3. Haloperidol (Haldol) 0.5 mg b.i.d., increasing to as high as 5 mg q.d. may be effective.
4. Baclofen (Lioresal) up to 100 mg per day has produced improvement in some cases.
5. Sensory feedback methods have produced some benefit in a few cases.
6. Implanted spinal cord stimulators have been used with some successful results.
7. Section of the 11th cranial nerve with or without anterior rhizotomy of the upper cervical nerves is still used occasionally (21).
8. Neurovascular decompression of the spinal accessory (11th cranial) nerve is indicated in selected cases (22).
9. Thalamotomy is reported to be of benefit in severe cases but should be reserved for those who do not respond to drug therapy since bilateral thalamic lesions may be necessary to produce improvement.
10. Injection of botulinum toxin into af-

fected neck muscles produces temporary relief (23).

Prognosis. The condition is not life threatening, and many patients can now be controlled adequately with one or a combination of the drugs listed above.

Dystonia Musculorum Deformans (Torsion Spasm)

Definition. Dystonia musculorum deformans is a condition characterized by progressive dystonic involvement of the axial and limb musculature which may be inherited as an autosomal dominant or recessive trait.

Etiology and Pathology. There is no known biochemical abnormality. Autopsy reveals atrophy of the caudate nucleus, putamen, and globus pallidus with microscopic loss of neurons and a reactive gliosis.

Clinical Features. The condition usually begins with difficulty in gait due to intermittent dystonic posturing of the feet. If the patient is carefully observed there will also be intermittent dystonic posturing of the hand at the wrist at this stage. The dystonic movements gradually become more frequent and involve the whole of the lower limb. The patient tends to present with a moment-to-moment variation in the position of the limbs and trunk due to the unpredictable occurrence of dystonia.

In the fully developed case, limb and axial muscles on both sides are involved and the patient is no longer able to walk. The body is in constant dystonic motion producing unpredictable contortions of the trunk, limbs, and head, with involvement of the neck muscles. The head may be moved in any direction and the speech becomes dysarthric.

Examination of the patient reveals normal mentation and dystonic involvement of muscle groups with absence of other neurologic abnormality.

Diagnostic Procedures. The diagnosis presents no difficulty in advanced cases. Early cases are missed unless the patient is observed carefully, particularly during walking.

The electroencephalogram (EEG) is said to show diffuse slowing in advanced cases. There are no focal features.

Treatment. Trihexyphenidyl (Artane) is often effective but requires high dosage. Treatment should commence with 2 mg daily gradually increasing by 2 mg increments until the dystonia is controlled or side effects prevent further increase in dosage (24).

Prognosis. Spontaneous remissions often occur. If patients do not respond to therapy they may be permanently disabled by this condition and either confined to a wheelchair or bedridden. In partial cases the condition does not affect the life span. Patients with a complete dystonia musculorum deformans often die from intercurrent infection. Neurosurgical treatment including thalamotomy should be considered in severe cases that fail to respond to medical measures.

Ballism

Definition. Ballism is an unusual condition characterized by the abrupt onset of violent flinging movements affecting the limbs, neck, and trunk, often on one side of the body (hemiballism) or involving a single limb (monoballism).

Etiology and Pathology. The majority of cases are due to a lesion involving the contralateral subthalamic nucleus or affecting the efferent or afferent connections of the subthalamic nucleus. There have been rare examples of ballism in which lesions were confined to the contralateral globus pallidus, putamen, caudate nucleus, or thalamus. Most cases are associated with occlusion of a small artery producing a well-circumscribed infarct. Other rare causes include focal hemorrhage from an arteriovenous malformation, embolism, metastatic tumor, abscess tuberculoma, encephalitis, multiple sclerosis, phenytoin intoxication, stereotactic thalamotomy, and hypoglycemia (25).

Clinical Features. The onset is usually abrupt, and the patient presents with almost continuous violent, flinging movements affecting the proximal muscles of the shoulders, arms, pelvis, and thighs. There may be contraction of the neck muscles producing violent movements of the head and an associated facial grimacing. The movements of the limbs are essentially nonrepetitive and represent completely uncoordinated contractions of agonist and antagonist muscles.

The movements cease during sleep but are extremely exhausting and many elderly patients succumb from progressive exhaustion and intercurrent infection, particularly pneumonia. In some cases spontaneous remission occurs approximately six weeks following onset of the movements.

Diagnostic Procedures. Once ballistic movements are controlled, every effort should be made to determine and treat the etiology of the lesion.

Treatment.

1. Protective measures should be taken to prevent damage to the limbs by placing the patient in a bed with a heavily padded headboard, footboard, and siderails. The affected limbs can be restrained until there is a response to treatment.
2. Most cases will respond to a slow intravenous infusion of diazepam (Valium) given at the rate of 1 mg every 10 seconds. The patient should be watched carefully during infusion of diazepam to avoid respiratory arrest. In the majority of cases once the movements are controlled by intravenous diazepam, good control can be maintained with oral diazepam.

Prognosis. Since most cases of ballism can now be controlled, the prognosis becomes that of the underlying disease.

Myoclonus

Myoclonus has been associated with a large number of neurologic conditions and may, for example, be seen in:

1. Infections of the nervous system including acute encephalitis, acute purulent meningitis, chronic encephalitis, subacute sclerosing panencephalitis, and Jakob-Creutzfeldt disease.
2. Metabolic abnormalities such as the lipidoses or leukodystrophies.
3. Degenerative conditions, dyssynergia cerebellaris myoclonica, myoclonic epilepsy of Unverricht-Lafora.
4. Anoxic encephalopathy.
5. Lesions of the brain stem (palatal myoclonus).
6. Lesions of the spinal cord.

A number of these conditions have been discussed elsewhere.

Progressive Familial Myoclonic Epilepsy (Unverricht-Lafora)

Definition. Progressive familial myoclonic epilepsy is a progressive degenerative condition beginning with generalized seizures in childhood and progressing to generalized myoclonus and dementia. It is inherited as an autosomal recessive trait.

Etiology and Pathology. The characteristic pathologic change consists of the presence of intracellular and extracellular Lafora bodies in the central nervous system. These bodies consist of a complex of protein surrounded by polyglucosan and probably de-velop within neurons and to a lesser extent in astrocytes and other glial cells. They stain with hematoxylin and are probably the result of an as yet unidentified metabolic abnormality. Lafora bodies have also been described in the retina, heart, liver, peripheral nerves, and striated muscle.

Clinical Features. The symptoms begin with the development of generalized seizures in childhood or adolescence followed by the appearance of myoclonus. There is progressive dementia, and the course is one of steady deterioration over a 10-year period.

Examination reveals dementia, dysarthria, and myoclonus; some cases show rigidity or choreoathetosis. In others there are signs of cerebellar involvement including hypotonia, intention tremor, and truncal ataxia. Some cases show evidence of corticospinal tract involvement with increased stretch reflexes. There is progressive visual loss and the terminal stage consists of severe dementia and blindness with continuous epileptic activity.

Diagnostic Procedures.

1. The electroencephalogram shows progressive deterioration with loss of alpha background activity and replacement by slower rhythms. Periodic bursts of spike and wave activity may occur and this epileptic activity may be activated by light, sound, or tactile stimulation.
2. The diagnosis is established by liver biopsy or brain biopsy with demonstration of typical Lafora bodies.

Treatment. Seizure activity should be controlled with adequate anticonvulsant medication. Anticonvulsant treatment does not affect the course of the disease.

Prognosis. Death occurs within 10 years of onset.

Dyssynergia Cerebellaris Myoclonica

This rare hereditary degenerative disorder appears to be a variant of Friedreich's ataxia with late development of myoclonus. These myoclonic movements may be very violent; and the patient may be flung to the ground or fall from a chair or bed. The myoclonus may be precipitated by movement.

Myoclonus Following Anoxic Encephalopathy

Generalized myoclonus may be associated with anoxic encephalopathy. The condition may be transient or permanent when it is associated with severe brain damage (26). Myoclonus and/or seizures can be expected to occur in approximately 50 percent of adult survivors of cardiopulmonary resuscitation. Myoclonic jerks are frequently induced by voluntary motor activities (action myoclonus) following recovery of consciousness (27).

Treatment.

1. L-5 hydroxytryptophan. This drug is the precursor of 5-hydroxytryptamine (serotonin), which is depleted in some conditions associated with myoclonus. Patients should be treated with 100 to 300 mg q.d. of alpha-methyldopa hydrazine (Carbidopa) beginning two days before the administration of L-5-hydroxytryptophan and continuing during the treatment with this drug. This will reduce the peripheral effects of 5-hydroxytryptamine. L-5-hydroxytryptophan is administered in capsules with meals beginning with 10 mg/kg of body weight q.d. and increasing slowly until the myoclonus is controlled or until side effects make further administration unacceptable. These side effects include nausea, vomiting, anorexia, and toxic psychosis.
2. Clonazepam and valproic acid are also effective in the treatment of myoclonus.

Hereditary Essential Myoclonus (Paramyoclonus Multiplex)

This rare condition consists of the appearance of myoclonus during childhood or adolescence which persists throughout life. The condition is benign. It does not affect the life span and it is not associated with any other neurologic abnormality.

TICS—TIC DISEASES

Tics may occur under two conditions:

1. When there is no evidence of organic disease, nonorganic tics
2. When there is evidence of organic disease, organic tics, for example:
   a. Tick convulsif (Gilles de la Tourette syndrome)
   b. Hemifacial spasm

Nonorganic tics are extremely common and often begin in childhood. It is often assumed that tics are a response to an emotionally stressful situation. It is not uncommon, however, to find other members of the family with tics, and it is possible that some hereditary trait predisposes the patient to develop these conditions. Most tics occur in the region of the head and neck and involve the eyes, face, nose, lips, tongue, pharynx, and muscles of the neck and shoulders. A variety of treatments including psychotherapy and hypnosis have been employed in the past with only limited success.

Tic Convulsif (Gilles de la Tourette Syndrome)

Definition. Tic convulsif is a genetically determined metabolic disorder associated with generalized tics.

Etiology and Pathology. Tic convulsif is thought to be a disorder of purine metabolism or caused by an imbalance between the centrally located neurotransmitters, dopamine, and 5-hydroxytryptamine. The pathologic changes are unknown.

Clinical Features. The first manifestation of the disease consists of the development of tics involving the face or neck. The movements increase, with involvement of the shoulders and upper limbs, followed by involvement of the lower limbs. Respiration and phonation become involved, and the patient develops a vocal component consistent of grunting or barking. The expulsion of air imparts an explosive quality to the speech with occasional associated hissing sounds. Some patients develop repetitive verbal expressions, often of obscene sexual character (coprolalia). The patient is unable to control this unfortunate symptom, which may be uttered in a loud voice, causing considerable embarrassment. In addition to coprolalia, patients may show echolalia, in which there is repetition of words, and echopraxia, in which there is repetition of acts.

Examination of patients with tic convulsif often reveals only minor neurologic abnormalities. Many patients are left-handed or ambidextrous.

Diagnostic Procedures. The electroencephalogram is abnormal in many cases, although there is no definite pattern to the abnormality.

Treatment.

1. Pimozide, beginning with 0.5 mg daily and increasing by 0.5 mg increments to as high as 9 mg daily if necessary, is effective in 80 percent of cases. Side effects include sedation, weight gain, depression, and restless legs (28).
2. Haloperidol should be used in those patients who fail to respond to pimozide. The risk of long-term side effects such as tardive dyskinesia is less with pimozide than haloperidol.
3. Trifluoperazine or thiothixene are effective in refractory cases (29).

4. A combination of neuroleptics may be needed.

Prognosis. Treatment with pimozide or haloperidol has made a great deal of difference to patients with tic convulsif, many of whom are now restored to full activity in the community. The disease does not in any way affect the life span of the patient.

Hemifacial Spasm
See page 357.

Exaggerated Startle Reaction
An exaggerated startle reaction is not unusual in conditions where there is increased excitability of the brain stem reticular formation. This may be seen in toxic, metabolic, and degenerative conditions, including delirium tremens; withdrawal from long-term drug therapy including barbiturates, diazepam, and analeptic drugs; high-dosage steroid therapy; and in the lipidoses and leukodystrophies. Exaggerated startle reactions have also been described as familial conditions.

Jumping Frenchmen of Maine
This condition was first recognized in French Canadians and may be inherited as an autosomal recessive trait. An exaggerated startle reaction appears in childhood and persists throughout life. The reaction occurs in response to an unexpected sound or visual stimulus which is followed by a single, violent startle reaction so that the patient appears to jump from the ground. The jump may be accompanied by an involuntary exclamation or reiteration of a verbal command. The neurologic examination is normal. This condition, or a variant, has been described in a number of countries and is known as Myriachin in Siberia and Latah in Malaya.

Restless Legs Syndrome
This disturbing syndrome usually occurs in middle age but has been described in adolescence. It may be associated with diabetic or uremic neuropathies, but the cause cannot be determined in most cases. Symptoms consist of a sensation of creeping, crawling, prickling, or burning dysesthesias in the lower extremities, worse in the evening, and relieved by movement. There is a good response to carbidopa/Levodopa (Sinemet) 10/100 (30) or Bromocriptine (31) taken at bedtime. An opioid such as codeine 30 mg is also effective.

TREMOR

Parkinson's Disease
Parkinson's disease is a syndrome characterized by rigidity, tremor, and bradykinesis. The triad of symptoms composing the parkinsonian syndrome is seen in a variety of disorders:

1. Paralysis agitans or idiopathic parkinsonism
2. Postencephalitic parkinsonism
3. Arteriosclerotic parkinsonism
4. Drug-induced parkinsonism
5. Parkinsonism secondary to infectious diseases
6. Toxic parkinsonism, following exposure to manganese, carbon monoxide, or carbon disulfide
7. Parkinsonism following anoxic encephalopathy
8. Parkinsonian features in Alzheimer's disease and other chronic neurologic conditions

The signs and symptoms of parkinsonism are related to a reduction in the activity of the neurotransmitter dopamine in the basal ganglia. There may be a failure of release of dopamine from the nigrostriatal axons, a reduced output by these axons, or a failure of binding of dopamine by dopaminergic receptors in the basal ganglia. The failure of the dopaminergic nigrostriatal system results in a relative overactivity of other receptor dependent systems in the basal ganglia. This imbalance influences other portions of the brain via the thalamus and thalamic connections. The ultimate effect is felt at the level of the final common pathway of the motor system, the anterior horn cell, where there are two basic defects:

1. Increased inhibition of the gamma motor neuron
2. Increased alpha motor neuron activity.

The cardinal symptoms of parkinsonism (i.e., tremor, rigidity, and bradykinesis) may be explained as follows:

1. Tremor is due to inhibition of gamma motor neuron activity. This inhibition leads to loss of gamma circuit sensitivity resulting in a decrease in the fine control of motor movement. This lack of control permits the appearance of involuntary movements generated at other levels in the CNS. The tremor of parkinsonism is probably initiated by rhythmic discharges of the alpha motor neuron under the influ-

ence of impulses generated in the ventral lateral nucleus of the thalamus. This activity is normally suppressed by action of the gamma motor neuron circuit but can appear as tremor when this circuit is inhibited.

2. Rigidity is due to increased tone in both antagonists and protagonists, and there appears to be a failure of inhibition of motor neuron activity in both protagonists and antagonists during movement. The increased alpha motor neuron activity in both protagonists and antagonists results in rigidity which is present throughout the full range of movement in the affected limb.

3. Bradykinesis is the end result of a disorder of integration of optic, labyrinthine, proprioceptive, and other sensory impulses in the basal ganglia. This results in an alteration in reflex activity influencing the gamma and alpha motor neurons.

Idiopathic Parkinsonism (Paralysis Agitans)

Definition. Idiopathic parkinsonism is the most common form of Parkinson's disease and occurs in middle-aged or elderly individuals. The prevalence varies between 60 and 120 per 100,000.

Etiology and Pathology. The etiology is unknown. Evidence for a viral etiology is unsubstantiated at this time. Sections of the midbrain show marked diminution or absence of melanin in the area of the substantia nigra. Microscopic examination reveals a loss of neurons in the zona compacta; the surviving neurons are abnormal and contain intracytoplasmic hyaline inclusion (Lewy bodies). Pathologic changes are not confined to the substantia nigra. There is a diffuse neuronal loss involving the whole of the brain and brain stem with particular involvement of the cerebral cortex, basal ganglia, thalamus, oculomotor nuclei, locus caeruleus, and dorsal motor nucleus of the vagus.

Clinical Features. The following are the clinical characteristics of idiopathic parkinsonism:

1. Tremor. The tremor of Parkinson's disease often appears unilaterally and may be confined to one upper limb for months or even years. The tremor is first seen in the fingers and thumb, and there may be a characteristic apposition of forefinger and thumb of 6 hz, producing the so-called pill-rolling tremor. The tremor eventually spreads to involve the entire affected limb and appears in the opposite limb. In severe cases the tremor involves all four limbs; the head and neck, producing titubation; and the facial musculature, tongue, and jaw. The tremor is markedly increased by tension or exertion and disappears during sleep.

2. Rigidity. Rigidity is an increased response to muscle stretch that appears in both antagonists and agonists. Both muscle groups contract and their tendons may be visible during movement. The muscles contract without recruitment during passive movements so that the activation of one motor unit is associated with the deactivation of another, maintaining uniform tension in the muscle. Rigidity usually appears unilaterally and proximally in an upper limb, spreading later to involve all of the muscles of that limb and eventually involving the opposite side and muscles of the neck and trunk. One of the earliest signs of rigidity is loss of associated movements of the arms when walking. More advanced cases show extension of the wrist, flexion of the metacarpophalangeal joints, and hyperextension of the interphalangeal joints.

3. Bradykinesia. The bradykinesia of Parkinson's disease is not related to rigidity and is probably the result of biochemical dysfunction in the basal ganglia, which produces an alteration in the inhibitory reflexes impinging on the motor neurons of the cranial nuclei and spinal cord. The patient shows loss of facial expression, slowing of lip and tongue movements during talking, loss of fine movements in writing and in handling small objects, and difficulty in rising from a chair and initiating gait.

4. Weakness and fatigue. Most patients with idiopathic parkinsonism experience weakness and easy fatigue once the disease becomes generalized. This compounds bradykinesia and increases immobility.

5. Dystonia. Although dystonia is frequently encountered as a complication of therapy, dystonic postures may be seen in hands and feet in early cases of Parkinson's disease before the diagnosis is established (32). Dystonia does not negate the diagnosis of Parkinson's disease (33).

6. Parkinsonian facies. The typical facial

appearance of patients with idiopathic parkinsonism is caused by bradykinesia. The face is "masklike" with infrequent blinking and lack of expression. In addition, there is a somewhat "greasy" appearance to the skin of the face and occasional drooling due to loss of the swallowing movements that normally dispose of saliva.

7. Micrographia. The gradual development of small cramped writing is characteristic of idiopathic parkinsonism when the dominant hand is involved. This is the first symptom in some cases.

8. Festinant gait. Bradykinesia results in the typical small steps seen in Parkinson's disease. In the fully developed state the patient has a flexed posture with the head flexed on the chest, the shoulders bent forward, the back arched forward, and the arms held immobile at the sides when walking. Muscle rigidity prevents rapid compensation for loss of balance, and many patients show propulsion, an "inability to catch up with their center of gravity," and quicken their pace if propelled forward. This may result in a fall. Similarly, if suddenly unbalanced, the patient may display lateropulsion or retropulsion and eventually fall. Serious injury can occur in these falls.

9. Freezing. This phenomenon is seen in more advanced cases of Parkinson's disease when the patient will suddenly stop and have trouble resuming walking. This is particularly troublesome when walking through a confined space such as a doorway or in turning.

10. Speech. Rigidity and bradykinesia of the respiratory muscles, vocal cords, pharyngeal muscles, tongue, and lips result in the slow monotonous speech of poor volume so characteristic of Parkinson's disease. In some cases the voice is reduced to a slowed whisper.

11. Ocular movements. The established Parkinsonian shows infrequent blinking, impaired upward gaze, poor convergence, and defective voluntary and following eye movements which are saccadic in quality. An exaggerated blink reflex (glabellar reflex) can be obtained by rhythmical percussion of the forehead just above the root of the nose.

12. Pain. Many patients with idiopathic parkinsonism experience discomfort or actual pain which is usually poorly local-

ized but may be cramplike and situated in either the axial muscles or the limbs. Some patients experience paresthesias in the extremities.

13. Autonomic dysfunction. There may be signs of autonomic dysfunction due to a progressive loss of neurons in the sympathetic ganglia. This results in excessive sweating; excessive salivation; sphincter problems, particularly incontinence; and disabling orthostatic hypotension.

14. Sialorrhea. Many patients have excessive salivary secretions which may produce a troublesome drooling in some cases.

15. Hypotension. Orthostatic hypotension is often a feature of advanced parkinsonism and may be enhanced by drug therapy.

16. Depression. Depression may further impede the restricted activities of the parkinsonian. Significant depression occurs in at least 50 percent of cases and should be recognized and treated. Referral to a psychiatrist or psychologist is appropriate in cases of severe depression. Tricyclic antidepressants may enhance the effect of levodopa (see page 109).

17. Dementia. There is a generalized neuronal loss in Parkinson's disease, and 50 percent of patients show a progressive dementia. This may be associated with delusions and visual or auditory hallucinations. Dementia may antedate parkinsonism by months or years in some cases (34).

Diagnostic Procedures. The history and physical examination are diagnostic and few tests are needed after the full initial clinical evaluation. At each office visit the patient should have:

1. The blood pressure recorded lying and standing in order to detect orthostatic hypotension which may be aggravated by medication.

2. An assessment of response to stress. Patients may appear to respond well to treatment until they are subject to mild stress. The patient should be given a simple task such as standing with the arms extended, asked rapidly to open and close the fingers on one side and at the same time count back from 100. This stress is usually sufficient to produce increased tremor and/or rigidity in the other limb when the patient is not fully responding to medication.

3. Measurement of functional activity. The patient should be asked to write his or her name and the date on the top of a large

sheet of paper. This should be followed by writing a simple sentence and drawing concentric circles with both the right and left hands. This should be attached to the patient's clinical notes and is a graphic measurement of functional activity which can be compared at each visit.

4. Optional studies. Electroencephalography may show progressive generalized slowing as the disease progresses. MR or CT scanning will show diffuse cortical atrophy with widening of the sulci and hydrocephalus ex vacuo in advanced cases.

Treatment. See page 109.

Prognosis. Although there has been considerable improvement in the survival of patients with Parkinson's disease following the introduction of levodopa, Parkinson's disease does significantly reduce life span in most patients who have developed the generalized form of the disease in their fifties or sixties. Since there is a progressive neuronal loss, the condition continues to progress despite response to medication. Ultimately, the effect of medication decreases and the patient deteriorates, becomes bedridden, and dies from intercurrent infection.

Postencephalitic Parkinsonism

Definition. Postencephalitic parkinsonism was first described during the epidemic of encephalitis lethargica from 1917 to 1928. Encephalitis lethargica (Von Economo) was a putative viral encephalitis of worldwide distribution. Some cases of parkinsonism were parainfectious. The majority were postinfectious with an interval of many years or decades between infection and overt symptoms. Consequently, postencephalitic parkinsonism may be regarded as a "slow virus" disease. The population with postencephalitic parkinsonism related to encephalitis lethargica has largely disappeared because of the passage of time. However, sporadic cases of postencephalitic parkinsonism still occur due mainly to the effects of viral encephalitis such as Eastern Equine or Japanese B virus infections.

Etiology and Pathology. There is marked pallor of the substantia nigra and locus caeruleus corresponding to a severe loss of neurons in these structures. Surviving neurons show Alzheimer's neurofibrillary tangles. Neuronal loss and fibrillary changes are also seen in the basal ganglia and hypothalamus.

Clinical Features. Patients show the tremor, rigidity, and bradykinesis of parkinsonism with additional features which include:

1. Changes in mentation including hallucinations, psychoses, and dementia
2. Oculogyric crises; tonic deviation of the eyes usually in a vertical plane, lasting from several minutes to an hour or more
3. Smooth conjugate eye movements replaced by coarse saccadic movements
4. Blepharospasm or lid retraction
5. Nystagmus
6. Cranial nerve palsies
7. Irregular respiratory movements
8. Autonomic disturbances including excessive perspiration, excessive salivation with drooling, disturbance of bladder function, postural hypotension.

Diagnostic Procedures

1. On EEG there is a reduction of background alpha activity and gradual replacement with slower frequencies recorded symmetrically from both hemispheres.
2. MR or CT scans show ventricular dilation and diffuse brain atrophy in advanced cases.
3. Serial neuropsychological testing indicates a progressive loss of intellectual functioning over a period of several years.

Treatment. See page 109.

Prognosis. Postencephalitic parkinsonism is a slowly progressive condition which results in total disability and considerable reduction in life span in many cases. Death usually occurs from intercurrent infection.

Arteriosclerotic Parkinsonism

Etiology and Pathology. Arteriosclerotic parkinsonism is due to infarction of the brain which damages the substantia nigra, the nigrostriatal pathways, or the basal ganglia, producing disruption of dopaminergic systems in the brain.

The brain shows gross evidence of atrophy and numerous lacunar infarcts in the brain stem and basal ganglia. Larger areas of infarction may be present in one or both hemispheres.

Clinical Features. Patients show the tremor, rigidity, and bradykinesis of parkinsonism with additional features, including:

1. History of repeated transient ischemic attacks
2. History and physical findings compatible with one or more episodes of infarction
3. Dementia

4. Pseudobulbar emotional responses, usually pseudobulbar crying.

Diagnostic Procedures. The metabolic, cardiac, and cerebral abnormalities of ischemic cerebrovascular disease can be demonstrated (see pages 137–138).

Treatment. The treatment is as follows:

1. For parkinsonism, see below.
2. For ischemic cerebrovascular disease, see page 139.

Prognosis. Poor. There is a high risk of further episodes of cerebral infarction and a high risk of myocardial infarction.

Drug-Induced Parkinsonism

The blocking of dopamine receptors by drugs of the phenothiazine or butyrophenone group results in rigidity, masklike facies, bradykinesis, and less frequently parkinsonian tremor. Dopaminergic drugs and dopamine agonists are not effective treatment since receptor sites are blocked. Anticholinergic drugs alleviate some symptoms by suppression of the uninhibited central cholinergic systems. Symptoms of parkinsonism may completely diappear when the causative drug is withdrawn.

Parkinsonism Secondary to Infectious Diseases

Parkinsonian symptoms occasionally occur in patients recovering from viral encephalitis. Parkinsonian features have also been described in treated neurosyphilis, arrested tuberculosis, meningitis, sarcoidosis, and chronic meningoencephalitis due to fungi and yeast.

Toxic Parkinsonism

Signs of parkinsonism with rigidity and bradykinesia rather than tremor can occur in susceptible individuals engaged in the mining, crushing, and smelting of manganese ores or exposure to manganese containing fungisides (35). Parkinsonian symptoms have occurred following recovery from carbon monoxide poisoning, hypoxia, exposure to toxic solvents such as carbon disulfide, and use of MPTP, a toxic byproduct of the illicit synthesis of meperidine (36).

Parkinsonian Features in Chronic Neurologic Conditions

Parkinsonism can occur in any degenerative condition that is associated with neuronal loss in the substantia nigra and impairment of nigrostriatal function. Parkinsonian features are not unusual in Alzheimer's disease which is often misdiagnosed as Parkinson's disease. The other conditions that often show rigidity and bradykinesia of parkinsonism during the course of the disease include Huntington's disease, Wilson's disease, oliopontocerebellar degeneration, Shy-Drager syndrome, progressive supranuclear palsy, Jakob-Creutzfeldt disease, and the parkinsonian-dementia complex.

Treatment

Parkinsonism may be regarded as a condition in which there is a relative insufficiency of dopamine in the CNS. Cerebral dopaminergic systems are depressed and there is an imbalance of activity and interaction between dopaminergic systems and other biochemically dependent systems in the brain. At this time therapy is directed toward the restoration of dopaminergic systems in the brain in the following manner:

1. Levodopa (L-Dopa). Levodopa crosses the blood-brain barrier and enters the CNS where it undergoes enzymatic conversion to dopamine. Dopamine inhibits the activity of neurons in the basal ganglia which are also influenced by the activity of an excitatory cholinergic system. The failure of the inhibitory dopaminergic nigrostriatal system is reduced by the increased amounts of dopamine and the balance between inhibitory dopaminergic and excitatory cholinergic systems is restored.

   Levodopa is indicated in the treatment of idiopathic Parkinson's disease, postencephalitic parkinsonism, arteriosclerotic parkinsonism, and toxic parkinsonism. Levodopa is less effective in other chronic neurologic disorders with parkinsonian features (37).

   Levodopa is contraindicated in narrow-angle glaucoma, when the patient has been using monoamine oxidase inhibitors in the last two weeks, and when the patient has a melanoma (levodopa may induce malignancy).

   Levodopa should be used with caution when the patient has severe heart disease, obstructive pulmonary disease, renal or hepatic disease, an active peptic ulcer, a history of psychosis or suicidal tendencies, or if there is suspicion of a pituitary tumor (levodopa increases production of growth hormone).

   Vitamin preparations containing pyridoxine hydrochloride (B₆) should not be given since B₆ reverses the therapeutic action of levodopa. Phenothiazines, reserpine, and butyrophenones act by blocking dopamine receptors and antagonize the effects of levodopa.

Levodopa is available in tablets or capsules of 0.25 g, 0.5 g, and 1.0 g. The initial dosage is 0.25 to 0.5 g b.i.d. with food and should be increased slowly by increments of not more than 0.75 g every three to seven days. The dosage is often limited by development of side effects; it should not exceed 8 g q.d. Levodopa therapy has been superseded by the use of carbidopa/levodopa in most cases.

2. Carbidopa/levodopa (Sinemet). The actions are the same as levodopa. Carbidopa inhibits peripheral decarboxylation of levodopa to dopamine. Dopamine and carbidopa do not cross the blood-brain-barrier. Therefore, more levodopa is available to cross the blood-brain barrier for conversion to dopamine in the brain.

Sinemet is available in three strengths, 10/100, 25/100, and 25/250. The initial dosage is 10/100 t.i.d. slowly increased to effect. Most patients require medication every three to four hours during the day. A dose increase should be begun with the first dose of the day with the addition of increments progressively through the day at three-to five-day intervals. This method allows earlier saturation of the peripheral dopa decarboxylase and increases the effect of smaller doses of Sinemet later in the day. The effect of Sinemet can be prolonged by the use of a low protein diet at breakfast and lunch (38). Most patients will experience side effects during levodopa or Sinemet therapy (39).

a. Nausea, vomiting, and abdominal distress are very common with levodopa therapy, less so with Sinemet.
b. Postural hypotension is common. The blood pressure should be recorded supine and standing at each office visit.
c. Cardiac arrhythmias may occur. This side effect is due to the beta adrenergic effect of dopamine on the conducting system of the heart and can be treated with beta adrenergic blocking agents such as propranolol (Inderal).
d. Involuntary movements. About 80 percent of patients develop choreoathetosis after months, or in some cases, years of treatment. The patient may not notice mild movements which are usually tolerated by the family. Severe movements can be reduced only by lowering the dose of Sinemet and accepting some return of Parkinsonian symptoms.
e. On-off phenomenon. Some patients experience sudden change from immobility to normal function or severe dyskinetic movements. This "on-off" phenomenon is often disabling and can be controlled by a low protein diet at breakfast and lunch, and a change to smaller frequent doses of Sinemet (40).
f. Psychosis and abnormal behavior. Mild symptoms of anxiety and agitation can occur during the induction period. The dose of Sinemet should be reduced to the minimum and increased slowly, that is, once a week with small increments. At the same time the physician should encourage the patient to persist with medication since rejection is rarely followed by acceptance in the future.

Hallucinations are quite common and are often more acceptable to the patient, who often finds them pleasant, than they are to the family. Consequently, mild benign hallucinations should be accepted rather than lowering the dose of Sinemet, producing an increase in Parkinsonian symptoms.

More serious symptoms of confusion, paranoid delusions, and dementia are more likely to occur in patients who show obvious dementia before starting treatment.
g. Sleep disturbance. Sinemet may induce drowsiness or insomnia. A reversal of the sleep cycle can occur with excessive sleeping during the day and insomnia at night.
h. Depression. The tendency to depression may be enhanced by Sinemet. The condition can be treated with small doses of amitriptyline beginning with 10 to 25 mg a day and increasing by 10 mg increments every two weeks until the symptoms are relieved or side effects are unacceptable.
i. Disturbances in walking. Hesitancy in initiation of walking or sudden im-

mobility in a confined space such as a doorway (freezing) usually develop after prolonged Sinemet therapy. There is no response to changes in medication and the patient must be taught to initiate a step by counting when walking, marching (left-right-left-right), or stepping over an object or an imaginary object.

The introduction of a controlled release Carbidopa/levodopa preparation will both delay the onset and reduce the severity of side effects encountered during Sinemet therapy (41,42).

3. Anticholinergic drugs. The anticholinergic drugs act by inhibiting the cholinergic system in the basal ganglia. The cholinergic system is normally inhibited by the nigrostriatal dopaminergic system, but the lack of inhibitory input results in overactivity of the excitatory cholinergic system. Anticholinergic drugs are more effective in the treatment of Parkinsonian tremor than rigidity or bradykinesis, and may have an additive effect when taken concurrently with Sinemet. Ethopropazine (Parsidol) is probably the most effective anticholinergic for control of tremor (10 mg daily with increments of 10 mg every three days). Trihexyphenidyl HCl (Artane), benztropine (Cogentin), and biperiden (Akineton) are also useful for control of tremor and are the only drugs that are effective in drug-induced parkinsonism due to the use of phenothiazines or butyrophenones. The anticholinergic drugs do not usually show additional benefit when given more than three times a day.

Dry mouth, constipation, and urinary retention are the commonest complications of the anticholinergic drugs. Impairment of memory, judgment, and insight can occur. Hallucinations may be troublesome, particularly in demented patients (43).

4. Antihistamines. The action of the antihistamines in the treatment of Parkinson's disease is not fully understood. Most antihistamines have mild anticholinergic properties which may account for some of the benefits of these drugs. Antihistamines are used in the control of tremor. They may be used alone in the early stages of the disease or as adjuvant therapy in more advanced cases that show only partial response to levodopa and/or bromocriptine.

Orphenedrine (Disipal), diphenhydramine (Benadryl), and chlorphenoxamine (Phenoxene) are useful preparations. The initial dosage of any of the antihistamine drugs is 50 mg q.h.s. with a gradual increase to 50 mg t.i.d. in order to reduce unpleasant drowsiness. Tolerance develops quickly.

5. Bromocriptine. Bromocriptine is a dopamine receptor agonist. It is indicated when there is poor or incomplete response to Sinemet therapy, severe dyskinesia on Sinemet therapy, or when the "on-off" phenomenon persists on Sinemet therapy (44). It is also preferred by some physicians to initiate therapy in early cases of mild Parkinson's disease (45). The initial dose is 1.25 mg daily increasing by 1.25 mg every week until the patient experiences maximum benefit or unacceptable side effects. A low dose initially followed by low dose increments every week reduces the risk of side effects and increases patient acceptance (46). There is usually a good response when the dosage exceeds 25 mg daily but may not be achieved until doses of 45 to 50 mg daily are administered. The side effects are the same as those for levodopa. When bromocriptine is added with the intention of replacing Sinemet, the Sinemet should be reduced as the bromocriptine is increased. It can be used with other antiparkinsonian drugs including anticholinergics, antihistamines, and amantadine. Bromocriptine should not be given to patients with severe dementia because of the risk of increasing confusion and agitation. Bromocriptine will increase postural hypotension and may cause peripheral edema.

6. Pergolide mesylate is a potent dopamine receptor agonist acting at both D_1 and D_2 receptor sites. Therapy should begin with a daily dose of 0.05 mg for two days. The dose is then increased by 0.1 mg daily in divided doses three times a day for the next 12 days. This can be followed by an increase of 0.25 mg daily every three days until optimum therapeutic results are obtained. Concurrent carbidopa/levodopa therapy should be reduced slowly. The usual dose of pergolide is 3.0 mg per day.

Side effects associated with the use of pergolide are not uncommon and include dyskinesia, dizziness, hallucinations, confusion, somnolence, insomnia, nausea, constipation, diarrhea, dyspepsia and rhinitis (47).

7. Amantadine (Symmetrel). Amantadine probably releases residual dopamine from presynaptic storage sites of the nigrostriatal pathway in the basal ganglia. It is a useful adjuvant and may produce further improvement in patients who cannot tolerate higher dosages of levodopa or bromocriptine. It is available in capsules of 100 mg and the initial dosage is one capsule b.i.d. Higher doses do not produce additional benefit. The side effects include livido reticularis and edema involving the lower extremities. Insomnia and vivid dreams or nightmares are occasionally troublesome. Severe psychiatric symptoms are unusual. Postural hypotension, heart failure, and urinary retention are rare.

8. Extra decarboxylase inhibitors. Patients with marked fluctuation in response from Sinemet may benefit from extra carbidopa or the addition of a second decarboxylase inhibitor benserazide.

9. Blocking dopamine re-uptake. An enhanced effect of dopamine can be obtained by using pemoline in some cases.

10. Enhanced release of dopamine. Tricyclic antidepressants may have a modest effect with improvement of rigidity in some cases.

11. Inhibition of dopamine metabolism. The monoamine oxidase-B (MAO-B) inhibitor deprenyl 5 mg b.i.d. has some beneficial effect by inhibition of dopamine metabolism and may delay the progression of the disease (48,49).

12. Neuroleptic drugs such as thioridazine, chlorpromazine, or haloperidol may help in some cases with severe dyskinesia or hallucinations, but carry the risk of increasing Parkinsonian symptoms (50).

13. Lithium is reported to reduce receptor supersensitivity with reduction of the severity of "on-off" periods.

14. Clonazepam 0.25 to 0.5 mg per day is effective in improving hypokinetic dysarthria in some cases and may also reduce tremor (51). Higher doses are less effective.

15. Primidone is occasionally effective in reducing parkinsonian tremor.

16. Beta blockers such as propranolol will reduce the drenching sweats that occur in some cases of chronic parkinsonism.

17. Fludrohydrocortisone 0.1 mg q am will reduce postural hypotension. The dosage can be increased by 0.1 mg increments to as high as 0.2 mg b.i.d. if necessary.

18. Adrenal cell implants. This method of placing cells obtained from the patient's own adrenal medulla into the basal ganglia has shown equivocal results but may be a possible re-introduction of surgery for Parkinson's disease (52).

Benign Familial (Essential) Tremor

Definition. Benign familial tremor is characterized by a bilateral symmetric tremor which begins in the fingers and hands. It is inherited as an autosomal dominant trait.

Etiology and Pathology. The disorder is believed to result from an imbalance of neurotransmitter substances in the basal ganglia; the noradrenergic system, particularly β-1 receptors, are believed to be hyperactive. There are no characteristic pathologic changes.

Clinical Features. The tremor typically appears in the young adult or in aged individuals. It characteristically involves the fingers, hands, and head, and the lower extremities are not usually involved. The tremor is exacerbated by emotional upset such as anger or excitement. Mild cerebellar signs may be present.

Differential Diagnosis (see Table 6-2).

Treatment.

1. Propranolol (Inderal). Propranolol 10 to 40 mg t.i.d. is recommended. In those patients who cannot tolerate propranolol, for example, those with asthma, metoprolol (Lopressor) is advised. The initial dose is 25 mg b.i.d. with 25 mg increments q.d. to effect or until a maximum of 50 mg t.i.d. is reached.

2. Primidone (Mysoline). Primidone, 125 mg daily increasing to 250 mg t.i.d. if necessary, is almost as effective as propranolol and should be used in patients who cannot take beta blockers.

3. Clonidine. This alpha adrenergic agent is also effective in essential tremor in doses of 0.1 mg to 0.9 mg daily.

Involuntary Movements Complicating Phenothiazine Therapy

The phenothiazines are major tranquilizers which decrease muscle tone and diminish motor activity. Drugs of the phenothiazine group have antipsychotic properties, probably due to blocking of dopamine receptors in the CNS. There are several involuntary

TABLE 6–2. Differential Diagnosis of Tremor

Tremor	Symptoms	Signs	Treatment
Benign (essential) also physiologic	Occurs at rest or with movement Exacerbated by emotion	6 to 12 cps°—involves UE† and head	Propranolol (Inderal) or metoprolol (Lopressor) Diazepam (Valium)
Intention (action)	Increases with movement	3 to 5 cps—involves UE	Propranolol (Inderal) Diazepam (Valium)
Resting (Parkinson's)	Present at rest Exacerbated by emotion	3 to 7 cps (typically 6)—involves extremities and head in characteristic "pill-rolling"	Dopamine agonist (e.g., L-dopa, bromocriptine) Anticholinergics
Metabolic	Symptoms of basic disorder	10 to 20 cps—involves UE† and head, signs of metabolic disorder (hyperthyroidism, liver disease, etc.)	Correct disturbed metabolic state
Alcohol withdrawal	Appears 8 to 12 hr after last ingestion of alcohol	6 to 10 cps—involves extremities and head	Chlordiazepoxide (Librium) Diazepam (Valium)

° cps = cycles per second
† UE = upper extremities

movements that complicate the use of phenothiazines (53):

1. Acute dystonic reaction. This is characterized by sudden onset of dystonic movements of the face, torticollis, and tonic deviation of the eyes and/or opisthotonus after ingestion or injection of a phenothiazine. The condition is frequently misdiagnosed as a conversion (hysterical) reaction. Parenteral injection of benztropine (Cogentin) 2 mg or diphenhydramine (Benadryl) 25 mg produces a dramatic response. A seven-day course of benztropine given at the onset of high potency neuroleptic therapy significantly reduces the risk of an acute dystonic reaction (54).
2. Parkinsonism. A gradual development of rigidity, tremor, and akinesia may occur during administration of a phenothiazine. The dosage should be lowered if possible and an anticholinergic agent such as benztropine used daily.
3. Akathisia. The patient experiences increasing restlessness with a feeling that he cannot sit still for more than a short period of time and must continuously stand or walk. The dosage should be lowered if possible. If symptoms persist, propranolol 40 to 120 mg per day is most likely to be effective. Anticholinergic drugs and benzodiazapines singly or in combination are a second choice.
4. Tardive dyskinesia.
5. Tardive dystonia.
6. Malignant neuroleptic syndrome.
7. Rabbit syndrome.

Tardive Dyskinesia

Definition. Tardive dyskinesia is repetitive involuntary movements of the mouth, lips, and tongue, occasionally accompanied by dystonic posturing or choreoathetotic movements of the trunk and limbs.

Etiology. The etiology is not clear. The favored hypothesis is denervation supersensitivity. In this theory, chronic dopamine receptor blockade results in a rebound receptor supersensitivity.

Tardive dyskinesia is a syndrome. Most cases begin during the administration of phenothiazines and may become more evident when the medication is stopped. The syndrome is also seen following administration of other antipsychotic drugs and antihistamines. It may be a feature of chronic alcohol abuse or degenerative brain disease, including Alzheimer's disease and cerebrovascular disease.

Clinical Features. Tardive dyskinesia is a late complication of neuroleptic therapy occurring in 10 to 20 percent of patients treated for more than one year with antipsychotic medications. It is not dose related and occurs in older patients, particularly women.

The first indication is the appearance of brief repetitive movements of the lips and eyes. The fully developed syndrome consists of sucking movements, lip-smacking, or sudden withdrawal of the lips exposing the teeth. The jaw may be retracted or moved laterally. The tongue is often thrust forward or rolled in the mouth. Each patient develops a stereotyped pattern sometimes accompanied by a grunting expiratory sound. The extremities and trunk are held in a dystonic posture or exhibit choreoathetoid movements. About one-third of the patients have features of parkinsonism. The onset may be accompanied by a depressive episode, and some patients have a pseudodementia which resolves on withdrawal of phenothiazines. Complications of tardive dyskinesia include:

1. Some patients lose weight and become dehydrated because of inability to sustain nutrition.
2. Parkinsonism may restrict movement and the patient may become bedridden with increased susceptibility to infection.
3. Jaw movements may become extremely painful. Dislocation has been reported.
4. Anticholinergic agents, alcohol, oxazepam, diazepam, and levodopa increase the movements of tardive dyskinesia.
5. A Tourette-like syndrome has been reported to occur concurrently with tardive dyskinesia and the term tardive-tourette-like syndrome has been used to describe this condition. The syndrome is treated as tardive dyskinesia (55).

Differential Diagnosis.

1. Parkinson's disease. Patients with Parkinson's disease may have a head and neck tremor, but other parkinsonian signs are present and the dyskinesias respond to dopaminergic agents.
2. Essential tremor. A positive family history and improvement of the movements with alcohol or propranolol are typical.
3. Orofacial dyskinesia (Meige's disease) is characterized by blepharospasm, photophobia, oromandibular dystonia, and exacerbation with physostigmine.
4. Palatal myoclonus. In palatal myoclonus there are rhythmic movements of the palate and occasionally of the eyes and head which respond to serotonergic agents and clonazepam (clonopin).
5. Choreiform movements of the face can occur in Huntington's disease, Sydenham's chorea, Wilson's disease, and with the use of carbamazepine (Tegretol), phenytoin (Dilantin), ethosuximide (Zarontin), dopaminergic drugs, oral contraceptives, and imipramine (Tofranil).
6. Cerebellar or labyrinthine disease. Dyskinesias of the head may occur with cerebellar or labyrinthine disease.
7. Hemifacial spasm. In this condition only one-half of the face is involved.
8. Facial tics. Facial tics are essentially repetitive, stereotyped movements.

Diagnostic Procedures. Elevated 24-hour urinary-free cortisol levels and low thyroid-stimulating hormone levels may occur.

Treatment.

1. Agents that block dopamine receptors (dopamine antagonists) are effective in some cases. Haloperidol (Haldol) 1 mg daily increasing to 2 mg q8h may be effective, although the effect is often temporary.
2. Catecholamine-depleting agents (reserpine, tetrabenazine) are also temporarily effective. Reserpine may cause severe depression.
3. Baclofen 20 to 80 mg per day, a GABA mimetic, has been used with success in the treatment of tardive dyskinesia.
4. Verapamil, a calcium channel blocker, 80 mg q.i.d., which is known to influence release of dopamine in the basal ganglia, is effective in some cases of tardive dyskinesia (56).
5. Antiserotonin agents such as cyproheptadine and some of the tricyclics have been reported to be effective.
6. Other drugs including alphamethyldopa (Aldomet), alphamethylparatyrosine, oxiperomide, sulpiride, valproic acid (Depakene), and apomorphine may produce some improvement in particularly difficult cases.

Prognosis. Many drugs are temporarily effective in tardive dyskinesia. Improved control may be obtained by regularly changing medications known to produce temporary benefit in a particular patient. Some cases show resolution after withdrawal of neuroleptic drugs. In others, symptoms increase or remain unchanged for many months, then subside. A few continue indefinitely.

Tardive Dystonia

This late onset complication involves sustained, often painful, involuntary contractions of muscles which may be focal, segmental, and rarely generalized. It is probably related to tardive dyskinesia. Baclofen, up to 60 mg per day, is the treatment of choice in tardive dystonia (57). If Baclofen is not effective, treat as for tardive dyskinesia (58).

Malignant Neuroleptic Syndrome (Neuroleptic Induced Extrapyramidal Symptoms with Fever)

This rare but potentially fatal condition is characterized by severe rigidity and fever with autonomic dysfunction during the course of neuroleptic therapy. The presence of hypertension, dehydration, agitation, and confusion has been recorded in many cases. Creatine phosphokinase (CPK) levels are often elevated (59).

Most patients respond to a reduction in neuroleptic dose and to the use of anticholinergics or dopaminergic drugs (bromocriptine up to 60 mg p.o. per day; carbidopa/levodopa, 25/100 mg t.i.d. to 50/200 mg q.i.d.). There must be concurrent correction of dehydration and electrolyte imbalance and prompt treatment of infection.

Dantrolene, amantadine, and lorazepam are also effective in the treatment of this condition.

The Rabbit Syndrome

This late complication of neuroleptic therapy consists of a fine rhythmical pouting of the lips accentuated by finger tapping just above the upper lip. The condition is often associated with drug-induced Parkinsonism. The symptoms improve with anticholinergic medication (60).

Orofacial Dyskinesia (Meige's or Breugel's Disease)

A condition resembling tardive dyskinesia but without a history of exposure to neuroleptic drugs can occur in middle aged and elderly individuals. The dyskinesia consists of blepharospasm and dystonic movements involving the facial muscles and tongue. While many cases are idiopathic, some patients ultimately develop signs of Alzheimer's disease (61). Physostigmine exacerbates the condition, while haloperidol (Haldol) and the dopamine-depleting agents tetrabenazine or reserpine result in improvement.

Blepharospasm

Involuntary closure of the eyelids may occur as an isolated phenomenon in middle aged or elderly individuals, but many patients ultimately develop additional signs of orofacial dyskinesia.

Periodic injection of botulinum toxin into the muscles of the eyelids has been of value in some cases (38).

REFERENCES

1. Roig, M.; Monserrat, L.; et al. Carbamazepine: an alternative drug for the treatment of non-hereditary chorea. Pediatrics 82(3 pt 2):492–495; 1988.
2. Harris-Jones, R.; Gibson, J. G. Successful treatment of refractory Sydenham's chorea with Pimozide. J. Neurol. Neursurg. Psychiatry 48:390–391; 1985.
3. Ghanem, Q. Recurrent chorea gravidarum in four pregnancies. Can. J. Neurol. Sci. 12:136–138; 1985.
4. Robinson, R. O.; Thornett, C.E.E. Benign hereditary chorea—Response to steroids. Dev. Med. Child. Neurol. 27:814–816; 1985.
5. Goss, K. B.; Sterwanek, J. A. Familial amyotrophic chorea with acanthocytosis. New clinical and laboratory investigations. Arch. Neurol. 42:753–756; 1985.
6. Richardson, J. L. Kinesiogenic choreoathetosis due to brain injury. Canad. J. Neurol. Sci. 14:626–628; 1987.
7. Drake, M. E. Paroxysmal kinesiogenic choreoathetosis in hyperthyroidism. Postgrad. Med. J. 63:1089–1090; 1987.
8. Gilroy, J. Abnormal computed tomograms in paroxysmal kinesiogenic choreoathetosis. Arch. Neurol. 39:779–781; 1982.
9. Perry, T. L.; Norman, M. C. Cysteine accumulation and cysteine dioxygenase deficiency in the globus pallidus. Ann. Neurol. 18:482–489; 1985.
10. Martin, J. B.; Gusella, J. F. Huntington's disease. Pathogenesis and management. New. Engl. J. Med. 315:1267–1276; 1986.
11. Young, A. B.; Penney, J. B.; et al. PET scan investigation of Huntington's disease: cerebral metabolic correlations of neurological features and functional decline. Ann. Neurol. 20:296–303; 1986.
12. Folstein, S. E.; Leigh, R. J., et al. The diagnosis of Huntington's disease. Neurology 36:1279–1283; 1986.
13. Jason, G. W. Presymptomatic neuropsychological impairment in Huntington's disease. Arch. Neurol. 45:769–773; 1988.
14. Farrer, L. A.; Connolly, P. M. Predictability of phenotype in Huntington's disease. Arch. Neurol. 44:109–113; 1987.
15. Jankovic, J.; Orman, J. Tetrabenazine therapy of dystonia, chorea, tics and other dyskinesias. Neurology 38:391–394; 1988.

16. Frydman, M.; Bonne-Tamer, B.; *et al.* Assignment of the gene for Wilson's disease to chromosome 13: linkage to the Esterase D locus. Proc. Natl. Acad. Sci. USA 82:1819–1821; 1984.

17. Dobyns, W. B.; Goldstein, N. P.; *et al.* Clinical spectrum of Wilson's disease (hepatolenticular degeneration). Mayo. Clinic Proc. 54:35–42; 1979.

18. Starosta-Rubinstein, S.; Young, A. B.; *et al.* Clinical assessment of 31 patients with Wilson's disease. Correlations with structural changes on magnetic resonance imaging. Arch. Neurol. 44:365–370; 1987.

19. Lowenstein, D. H.; Aminoff, M. J. The clinical course of spasmodic torticollis. Neurology 38:530–532; 1988.

20. Gaulhier, S. Idiopathic spasmodic torticollis: pathophysiology and treatment. Can. J. Neurol. Sci. 13:88–90; 1986.

21. Lee, E. H.; Kang, Y. K.; *et al.* Surgical correction of muscular torticollis in older children. J. Pediatrics Orthop. 6:585–589; 1986.

22. Colbassani, H. J., Jr.; Wood, J. H. Management of spasmodic torticollis. Surg. Neurol. 25:153–158; 1986.

23. Tsui, J. K. C.; Eisen, A.; *et al.* Double blind study of botulinum toxin in spasmodic torticollis. Lancet 2:245–247; 1986.

24. Long, A. E. High dose anticholinergic therapy in adult dystonia. Canad. J. Neurol. Sci. 13:42–46; 1986.

25. Manorama, T. K.; Kumar, D.; *et al.* Hemiballismus and intracranial metastases. Acta. Neurol. (Napoli) 8:491–494; 1986.

26. Krumholz, A.; Stern, B. J.; *et al.* Outcome from coma after cardiopulmonary resuscitation: relation to seizures and myoclonus. Neurology 38:401–405; 1988.

27. Fahn, S. Posthypoxic action myoclonus. Adv. Neurol. 43:157–169; 1986.

28. Regeur, L.; Pakkenberg, B.; *et al.* Clinical features and long-term treatment with Pimozide in 65 patients with Gille de la Tourette syndrome. J. Neurol. Neurosurg. Psychiatry 49:791–795; 1986.

29. Mesulam, M. M.; Peterson, R. C. Treatment of Gille de la Tourette syndrome: Eight-year practice-based experience in a predominantly adult population. Neurology 37:1828–1833; 1987.

30. Brodeur, C.; Montplaisir, J.; *et al.* Treatment of restless leg syndrome and periodic movements during sleep with L-Dopa: a double blind controlled study. Neurology 38:1845–1848; 1988.

31. Walters, A. S.; Hening, W. A.; *et al.* A double blind crossover test of bromocriptine and placebo in restless leg syndrome. Ann. Neurol. 24:455–458; 1988.

32. LeWitt, P. A.; Buons, R. S.; *et al.* Dystonia in untreated parkinsonism. Clin. Neuropharmacol. 9:293–297; 1986.

33. Poewe, W. H.; Lees, A. J.; *et al.* Dystonia in Parkinson's disease: clinical and pharmacological features. Ann. Neurol. 23:73–78; 1988.

34. Gilbert, J. J.; Kish, S. J.; *et al.* Dementia, parkinsonism and motor neuron disease: Neuroanatomical and neuropathological correlates. Ann. Neurol. 24:688–691; 1988.

35. Ferraz, H. B.; Bertolucci, P. H. F.; *et al.* Chronic exposure to the fungiside monab may produce symptoms and signs of CNS manganese intoxication. Neurology 38:550–553; 1988.

36. Snyder, S. H.; D'Amato, R. J. MPTP: a neurotoxin relevant to the pathophysiology of Parkinson's disease. The 1985 George C. Cotzios lecture. Neurology 36:250–258; 1986.

37. Lees, A. J. L-dopa treatment and Parkinson's disease. Quart. J. Med. 59:535–547; 1986.

38. Tsui, J. K.; Ross, S.; *et al.* The effect of dietary protein on the efficacy of L-dopa: a double blind study. Neurology 39:549–552; 1988.

39. Wooten, G. F. Progress in understanding the pathophysiology of treatment-related fluctuations in Parkinson's disease (Editorial). Ann. Neurol. 24:363–365; 1988.

40. Riley, D.; Long, A. E. Practical application of a low protein diet for Parkinson's disease. Neurology 38:1026–1031; 1988.

41. Hutton, J. T.; Morris, J. L.; *et al.* Treatment of chronic Parkinson's disease with controlled-release carbidopa/levodopa. Arch. Neurol. 45:861–864; 1988.

42. Goetz, C. G.; Tanner, C. M.; *et al.* Controlled-release carbidopa/levodopa (CR4-Sinemet) in Parkinson's disease patients with and without motor fluctuations. Neurology 38:1143–1146; 1988.

43. Kurlan, R. Drug induced parkinsonism. Arch. Neurol. 45:356–357; 1988.

44. Schlechte, J. A. Bromocriptine—An update. Iowa Med. 76:133–135; 1986.

45. Kurlan, R. International symposium on early dopamine agonist therapy of Parkinson's disease. Arch. Neurol. 45:204–208; 1988.

46. Staal-Schreinemachers, A. L.; Wesseling, H.; *et al.* Low-dose bromocriptine therapy in Parkinson's disease: Double-blind placebo controlled study. Neurology 36:291–293; 1986.

47. Walters, E. C.; Calne, D. B. Recent advances in pharmacotherapy: Parkinson's disease. Canad. Med. Ass. J. 140:507–514; 1989.

48. Golbe, L. L.; Lieberman, A. N.; *et al.* Deprenyl in the treatment of symptom fluctuations in advanced Parkinson's disease. Clin. Neuropharmacol. 11:45–55; 1988.

49. Sonsalla P. K.; Golbe, L. I. Deprenyl as prophylaxis against Parkinson's disease? Clin. Neuropharmacol. 11:500–511; 1988.

50. LeWitt, P. A. New perspectives in the treatment of Parkinson's disease. Clin. Neuropharmacol. 9:537–546; 1986.

51. Biary, N.; Pimental, P. A.; *et al.* A double-blind trial of clonazepam in the treatment of parkin-

sonian dysarthria. Neurology 38:255–258; 1988.

52. Lindvall, O.; Backlund, E. O.; *et al.* Transplantation in Parkinson's disease: Two cases of adrenal medullary grafts to the putamen. Ann. Neurol. 22:457–468; 1987.

53. Ruben, E. H.; Zodemski, C. F. Clinical and neurological implications of antipsychotic-induced movement disorders. Compr. Therapy 12:61–67; 1986.

54. Winslow, R. S.; Stillner, V.; *et al.* Prevention of acute dystonia reaction in patients beginning high potency neuroleptics. Am. J. Psychiatry 143:706–710; 1986.

55. Jeste, D. V.; Wisniewski, A. A.; *et al.* Neuroleptic-associated tardive syndromes. Psychiatr. Clin. North Am. 9:183–192; 1986.

56. Barrow, N.; Childs, A. An anti-tardive dyskinesia effect of Verapamil. Am. J. Psychiatry 143:11; 1986.

57. Rosse, R. B.; Allen, A.; *et al.* Baclofen treatment in a patient with tardive dystonia. J. Clin. Psychiatry 47:474–475; 1986.

58. Keepers, G. A.; Casey, D. E. Clinical management of acute neuroleptic-induced extrapyramidal syndromes. Cur. Psychiatr. Ther. 23:139–157; 1986.

59. Levinson, D. F.; Simpson, G. M. Neuroleptic-induced extrapyramidal symptoms with fever. Arch. Gen. Psychiatry 43:839–848; 1986.

60. Yassor, R.; Lal, S. Prevalence of the rabbit syndrome. Am. J. Psychiatry 143:656–657; 1986.

61. D'Alessandro, R. The prevalence of lingual-facial-buccal dyskinesia in the elderly. Neurology 36:1350–1351; 1986.

62. Rhee, K. J. Choreoathetoid disorders associated with amphetamine-like drugs. Am. J. Emerg. Med. 6:131–133; 1988.

CHAPTER 7

MULTIPLE SCLEROSIS

Definition

Multiple sclerosis is a disease produced by an environmental agent, almost certainly a virus, in a genetically susceptible individual, resulting in an alteration in immune mechanisms within the central nervous system (CNS) (1).

Etiology and Pathology

While the cause of multiple sclerosis remains elusive, there is increasing evidence from epidemiologic and immunologic studies that the disease is a slow virus infection. The effect of the infection is an alteration of immunity within the CNS producing a periodic autoimmune response directed against the oligodendrocyte resulting in irregular areas of demyelination (2–4).

Antibodies against many viruses have been found in the serum and cerebrospinal fluid of patients suffering from multiple sclerosis, but results are inconsistent. The most likely and logical candidate in the list of viral agents which might cause multiple sclerosis is a retrovirus of the human T-cell lymphotropic virus (HTLV) group, but the presence of such a virus has yet to be confirmed.

The pathologic changes in multiple sclerosis vary with the age of the demyelination plaque. In the acute stage, there is active demyelination and the area shows the presence of sudanophilic myelin breakdown products. There is surrounding edema, and the blood vessels show perivascular lymphocytic cuffing. The condition then proceeds to either restoration of myelin or gliosis. If there is restoration of the myelin, the plaque will eventually have a normal appearance. In the alternative situation, gliosis, the end result is a glial scar or plaque and destruction of the axons.

Epidemiology

The natural history of multiple sclerosis has been studied extensively, and there are now more than 200 reports on this subject. Multiple sclerosis is distributed throughout the world within three zones with high, medium, and low prevalence rates. High frequency prevalence rates, more than 30 per 100,000 population, occur in areas lying between latitudes 45 and 65 degrees north or south. This includes northern Europe, southern Canada, northern United States, New Zealand, and southern Australia. These areas of high frequency are bounded by areas of medium frequency with prevalence rates of 5 to 25 per 100,000 and include southern Europe, southern United States, and most of Australia. Tropical areas of Asia, Africa, and South America have low prevalence rates of less than 5 per 100,000 population.

Multiple sclerosis predominantly affects white populations. In the United States, American black males are far less likely to develop multiple sclerosis when compared to

118

white males in the same geographic area. Studies in Japan and Korea indicate a very low prevalence rate for populations in these countries. Similarly, oriental populations in the United States also show a low prevalence rate. An individual who migrates from one area to another before the age of 15 tends to assume the risk of the indigent population in the new area of residence.

Although further studies on the epidemiology of multiple sclerosis are indicated, current information tends to indicate that multiple sclerosis is an acquired and probably transmittable disease. In addition, there is evidence for a relationship between the human leukocyte antigen (HLA) system and multiple sclerosis indicating a genetic susceptibility to the disease. In Northern Europeans the main association is with HLA-DR2, but this genetic pattern is not as clear in other parts of the world (5).

Clinical Features

The diagnosis of multiple sclerosis is based on the clinical demonstration of patchy involvement of the CNS. Symptoms may be grouped under several headings (6).

Sensory Symptoms. Sensory symptoms are the commonest symptoms experienced by patients with multiple sclerosis. These symptoms are often forgotten or ignored by both patient and physician. Even prolonged sensory symptoms fail to evoke concern, in contrast to the almost immediate response that occurs with weakness or paralysis. Consequently, many patients date the onset of multiple sclerosis from the first appearance of a weakness, visual loss, or other symptoms of dramatic onset rather than forgotten or poorly recorded sensory symptoms.

Sensory symptoms include impairment of sensation (anesthesia), tingling (paresthesias), and uncomfortable sensations (dysesthesias) often referred to as "burning." All patients with suspected multiple sclerosis should be carefully questioned about the occurrence of previous sensory symptoms.

Motor Symptoms. Paralysis or paresis of the upper or lower limbs is the most common presenting symptom in patients with multiple sclerosis.

Visual Symptoms. Optic neuritis presents with sudden visual loss and pain on eye movement, which may be followed by a rapid progression to total loss of vision in the affected eye (see Figure 7–1).

Recovery is variable. Many patients experience no further problems for several years and then develop symptoms of brain and/or spinal cord involvement indicating multiple sclerosis. About 50 percent of adolescents and young adults who present with sudden onset of optic neuritis subsequently develop multiple sclerosis. Those with a large time interval between the optic neuritis and the development of additional symptoms have a better prognosis than patients with more florid forms of multiple sclerosis. The clinician should always inquire about the possibility of preceding symptoms in any patient who presents with optic neuritis, since the presence of symptoms some years prior to the more dramatic motor or visual problems might indicate a more benign course.

Bladder Symptoms. A number of patients with multiple sclerosis give a history of repeated urgency of micturition prior to the diagnosis of multiple sclerosis. Most of these patients have been diagnosed and treated for "bladder infection," and the improvement following the use of antibiotics seems to confirm the diagnosis. However, the improvement is due to the natural remitting picture of multiple sclerosis rather than cure of any infection. Many patients have urgency of micturition early in multiple sclerosis. Progressive involvement of bladder function in multiple sclerosis leads to extreme urgency with occasional incontinence and finally to total incontinence. Urinary retention is unusual but can occur.

Spinal Cord Symptoms. Most established cases of multiple sclerosis have signs of spinal cord involvement. These signs include some degree of spastic paraparesis with increased tone in both lower limbs, bilateral ankle clonus, increased stretch reflexes, and bilateral extensor plantar responses. It is not unusual to see progression of paraparesis with increasing disability. This does not necessarily indicate progression of the disease but is due to progressive gliosis of plaques in the spinal cord. This scarring produces increasing traction on and destruction of axons descending from higher centers in the nervous system and results in increasing spasticity and paraparesis.

Brain stem Symptoms. Many patients with multiple sclerosis develop signs of brain stem involvement. These include diplopia and internuclear ophthalmoplegia due to involvement of interaxial fibers connnecting the oculomotor nuclei; sensory loss over the face due to involvement of the afferent fibers entering the pons from the trigeminal nucleus; facial weakness due to involvement of

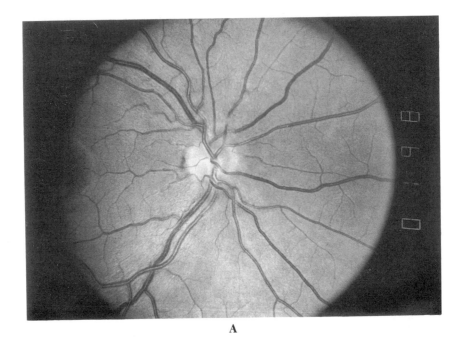

A

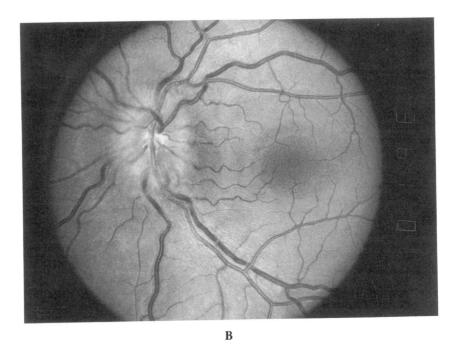

B

FIGURE 7–1.   Acute optic neuritis in a patient with multiple sclerosis.
A. Unaffected right eye showing a distinct disc margin.
B. Swollen left optic head of acute optic neuritis.

the seventh nerve in the pons; episodic dysarthria and dysphagia due to involvement of the vagal nerve in the medulla; and dysarthria due to involvement of the hypoglossal nerve in its course through the medulla. Involvement of the corticospinal tracts in the brain stem can produce a progressive spastic quadriparesis, while involvement of the cerebellar connections results in progressive limb and truncal ataxia.

Cerebellar Symptoms. The majority of cerebellar symptoms, which include dysarthria, ataxia, dysmetria, and dysdiadochokinesis, are due to involvement of the cerebellar connections in the brain stem and spinal cord.

Dementia. Fifty percent of patients with multiple sclerosis show some deterioration in intellectual functioning as the disease progresses over a period of many years. The disease can, however, remain predominantly spinal or bulbar in form with little involvement of the white matter in the cerebral hemispheres and preservation of intellect. Patients with demyelination in the periventricular white matter of the brain often show an explosive emotional response with inappropriate laughter or occasional crying during conversation. This condition results from interruption of an inhibitory dopaminergic pathway connecting the thalamus and the frontal lobe. Despite the laughter which has been incorrectly termed euphoria, many patients are depressed and are often embarrassed by the inability to control this often incongruous response.

Miscellaneous Symptoms. Patients with chronic multiple sclerosis may develop almost any abnormal neurologic sign. The interruption of the connections to and from the basal ganglia may produce involuntary movements including chorea, athetosis, or even ballistic-type movements. Pupillary abnormalities, including hippus, are not uncommon. Optic neuritis and optic atrophy are associated with the Marcus-Gunn phenomenon (see page 21), while involvement of the tectum of the midbrain may produce a classic Argyll-Robertson pupil. Severe involvement of the spinal cord results in the clinical picture of transverse myelitis with severe spastic paraplegia and total bladder incontinence. This condition combined with acute, bilateral optic neuritis has been termed Devic's disease.

Flexion of the head may result in an electric-like shock passing down the spine and out of the limbs (L'hermitte sign). This phenomenon, while not pathognomonic, is highly suggestive of multiple sclerosis and may also preceed the development of other symptoms by months or years in some cases.

Classification of Multiple Sclerosis

Although multiple sclerosis can affect white matter anywhere in the CNS, it is possible to recognize four types of disease:

1. Chronic relapsing remitting multiple sclerosis. This is the classical form of multiple sclerosis that often begins in the late teens or 20s, with a severe attack followed by incomplete recovery. Further attacks occur at unpredictable intervals each followed by increasing disability. The relapsing remitting pattern tends to change into the chronic progressive form of the disease in the late 30s.

2. Chronic progressive multiple sclerosis. The disease runs a steady deteriorating course which may be interrupted by periods of quiescence without improvement. The rate of progression is variable; at its most severe, this form of multiple sclerosis can terminate in death within a few years. In contrast, the more chronic form of progressive multiple sclerosis is similar to the benign form of the disease. Multiple sclerosis may present in the chronic progressive form of the disease, or the pattern may develop in the late stages of the chronic relapsing remitting form or spinal form of the disease.

3. Spinal form of multiple sclerosis. This form of multiple sclerosis presents with symptoms and signs of predominantly spinal cord involvement from the beginning and maintains this pattern. There may be a clear cut pattern of relapse and remission initially followed by chronic progressive form of the disease after several years, or the presentation may be one of steady deterioration from the onset.

4. Benign form of multiple sclerosis. About 15 percent of cases have the benign form of multiple sclerosis. This may be defined as multiple sclerosis in which the patient is able to function at the level of full employment or provide care of home and family independently 10 years after the appearance of the first symptoms. It is extremely unlikely that these patients will ever be incapacitated by the disease and they should continue to live a full life span

with only occasional minor symptoms (7, 8).

The existence of a benign form of multiple sclerosis increases the importance of recording the date of the first symptom in patients who appear to have few residual abnormal signs several years after the onset of the disease. These patients may be informed that they have a benign form of multiple sclerosis and may be told the implication of this diagnosis in the years ahead.

Diagnostic Procedures.

1. The diagnosis of multiple sclerosis is established by careful interpretation of clinical signs and symptoms. These indicate a patchy involvement of the CNS. The diagnosis may be strengthened by interpretation of other findings discussed below but remains a matter of clinical judgment (9).

2. Magnetic resonance imaging (MRI) or computed tomography (CT) scanning. Magnetic resonance imaging can be expected to show multiple areas of increased T2 signal density in the periventricular white matter of the brain in approximately 80 percent of cases (Figure 7–2). These areas may be dis-

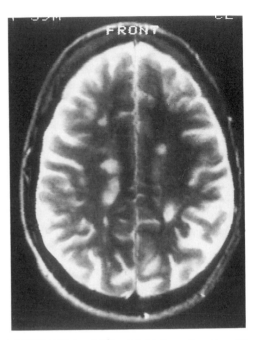

FIGURE 7–3. MRI. Multiple sclerosis. T2 weighted image showing multiple discrete areas of increased signal in the centrum semiovale. This patient had severe disabling disease. MR scans with equivalent signal changes may be seen in patients with minimal clinical signs.

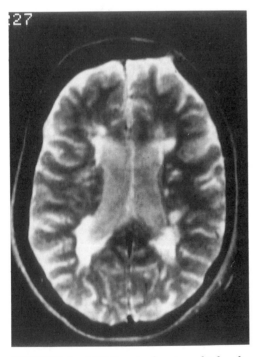

FIGURE 7–2. MRI Scan in chronic multiple sclerosis. Note the confluent periventricular plaques and the moderate ventricular dilatation.

crete or confluent and are frequently accompanied by similar abnormalities which appear to cover the horns of the ventricles. The abnormalities may show rapid change, and serial MR scans may be helpful in assessing the course of the disease (Figure 7–3). Computed tomography scanning does not possess the sensitivity of MRI, which is the primary mode of scanning of multiple sclerosis if available. Furthermore, it has been postulated that the total lesion area of cerebral lesions defined by MRI may be an indication of the degree of cognitive dysfunction in multiple sclerosis (10–16).

3. Visual evoked potentials are positive in about 80 percent of patients with multiple sclerosis. Many of these cases have not had any visual symptoms. Similarly, auditory evoked potentials are positive in about 70 percent of cases with multiple sclerosis, and a number of these cases do not show clinical signs of brain stem involvement. Somatosensory evoked potentials are positive in about 60 percent of cases of multiple sclerosis. The

presence of abnormal evoked potentials provides additional objective evidence of patchy involvement of the CNS.

4. Examination of the cerebrospinal fluid (CSF). Acute exacerbations of multiple sclerosis may be accompanied by a lymphocytic or polymorphonuclear pleocytosis in the CSF. This is short-lived and does not usually exceed a hundred cells/cubic millimeter. The CSF protein is elevated, particularly in early cases and during acute exacerbations. This rarely exceeds 100 mg/dl. Gamma globulin elevation is seen in many cases and exceeds 15 percent of the total protein content. Elevation of IgG and IgM and oligoclonal bands are seen with electrophoresis. Elevation of myelin basic protein is present in approximately 80 percent of cases of acute multiple sclerosis or multiple sclerosis in exacerbation (17).

5. Neuropsychological testing. Neuropsychological testing is useful and may reveal unexpected involvement of the cerebral hemispheres. Serial psychological testing is valuable.

Differential Diagnosis. Multiple sclerosis can mimic almost any chronic disease affecting the CNS. The diagnosis is usually not difficult in well-established cases with evidence of multiple areas of involvement in the nervous system, but early cases are often a problem in diagnosis (18). The following conditions can be confused with multiple sclerosis:

1. The leukodystrophies. The adult form of metachromatic leukodystrophy and leukodystrophy with diffuse rosenthal fiber formation can present with progressive deterioration and evidence of multiple areas of involvement of the nervous system. There is a peripheral neuropathy with slowing of nerve conduction velocities in metachromatic leukodystrophy which is not present in multiple sclerosis. The demonstration of metachromatic material and low levels of aryl sulphatase A will establish the diagnosis. The diagnosis of leukodystrophy with diffuse rosenthal fiber formation can be made only by brain biopsy.

2. The spinocerebellar degenerations. Sporadic cases of olivopontocerebellar degeneration and Friedreich's ataxia may resemble multiple sclerosis. The diagnosis is usually established by continued observation of the patient. Although the spinocerebellar degenerations are progressive, additional neurologic deficits do not appear.

3. Syphilis. Both meningeal and vascular syphilis may mimic multiple sclerosis. The diagnosis is established by abnormalites in the CSF and a positive serologic test for syphilis.

4. Subacute combined degeneration of the spinal cord may resemble multiple sclerosis, particularly if there is an associated dementia and optic atrophy. Serum B_{12} levels are low in this condition.

5. Brain tumor. The persistence of a fixed single neurologic deficit in a young adult should always suggest the possibility of a brain tumor rather than multiple sclerosis. The diagnosis is established by MR or CT scanning.

6. The arteritides. Both polyarteritis nodosa and systemic lupus erythematosus can produce multiple lesions of the CNS. However, they often involve the organs and cause peripheral neuropathy within an elevated sedimentation rate, abnormal nerve conduction velocities, and a positive nerve biopsy. The presence of an abnormal lupus erythematosus (LE) preparation, antinuclear antibodies (ANA), anti-DNA antibodies, and reduced complement levels is characteristic of lupus erythematosus.

7. Transverse myelitis. Multiple sclerosis is a relatively rare cause of transverse myelitis (see Table 12-2, page 185). Unless there is definitive evidence of multiple areas of involvement of the CNS, other conditions of transverse myelitis should be considered.

8. Leber's optic atrophy. The delayed development of cerebellar ataxia in a case of optic atrophy suggests multiple sclerosis. The differentiation from Leber's optic atrophy may not be possible until the development of additional signs of involvement of the CNS.

9. Sjögren's syndrome. There is a marked similarity in the clinical presentation of multiple sclerosis and Sjögren's syndrome with CNS involvement (19). Both conditions may have optic neuritis, spinal cord involvement, psychiatric manifestations, abnormal evoked potentials, similar CSF profiles, and indistinguishable abnormalities in CT or MRI. Features which may distinguish Sjögren's syndrome include the sicca complex of xerophthalmia, xerostomia, or recurrent salivary gland enlargement, peripheral neuropathy, vasculitis in skin or muscle, elevated sedimentation rate, abnormal antinuclear antibody, positive rheumatoid factor, anti-RO(SS-A), or LA(SS-B) antibodies, and decreased complement.

Treatment.

1. Bed rest. Patients with acute multiple sclerosis or an acute exacerbation of multiple sclerosis benefit from complete bed rest. Patients who are removed from the necessity of self-care and the added worries of the home environment improve with rest. The period of rest need not be protracted in the majority of cases. Once the patient shows improvement, the institution of a graded program in physical therapy becomes paramount.

2. Corticosteroids. There is evidence that high doses of intravenous corticosteroids may arrest the progress of multiple sclerosis (20). The medication can be given as methyl prednisolone succinate 1 g IV piggyback over three hours each day for five days followed by oral methyl prednisolone on alternate days beginning with 80 mg and reducing by 8 mg q.o.d. In the majority this regimen will result in at least six months' remission and several months or even years more in many cases. The treatment can be repeated if relapse occurs. Side effects are infrequent but insomnia or hypomanic behavior may occur. Both symptoms will resolve immediately once treatment is stopped.

3. Immunosuppressive drugs. The results of long-term treatment with immunosuppressive drugs such as azathioprine, cyclophosphamide, or cyclosporin have been equivocal. Patients receiving immunosuppressant drugs of this type must be monitored carefully with a complete blood count and platelet count weekly (21).

4. Other forms of therapy include plasmaphoresis, interferon, and poly(I,C)-LC. All are currently under investigation.

5. Physical therapy. All patients with multiple sclerosis should be evaluated by a physiatrist and should be placed in a graded program of physical therapy. This program should be under constant review so that it can be modified as the results of corticosteroid treatment and physical therapy are appreciated.

6. Treatment of spasticity. Increased muscle tone, exaggerated tendon reflexes, clonus, and spontaneous muscle spasms are often present in patients with advanced multiple sclerosis. Spasticity may be treated with the following:

a. Baclofen (Lioresal) is the most effective drug for the treatment of spasticity resulting from lesions of the spinal cord, where it acts as a gamma aminobutyric acid (GABA) agonist at the presynaptic level. Baclofen is especially effective in decreasing the frequency and severity of painful flexor or extensor spasms and in decreasing protracted, tonic flexor states of the lower extremities in patients with spinal spasticity. It has little effect on spasticity in patients with cerebral lesions but is not as likely as diazepam or dantrolene to produce sedation or generalized weakness. The initial dosage of 5 mg b.i.d. may be increased by 5 mg every three days to effect or to a maximum dosage of 100 mg per day. Severe spastic paraparesis or paraplegia can be treated by continuous infusion of baclofen into the spinal subarachnoid space. This method requires the use of a subcutaneous pump device with catheter placement into the subarachnoid space. Small doses of baclofen are effective when given by this method.

b. Diazepam (Valium). Benzodiazepines enhance GABA action probably by potentiating its postsynaptic effects and by enhancing its endogenous release. Diazepam is useful alone or as adjunct therapy for spasticity in patients with spinal cord lesions. Side effects include somnolence, lightheadedness, and increased muscle weakness. Long-term therapy may be associated with insomnia, anxiety, hallucinations, hostility, increased spasticity, and addiction. The initial dosage of 2 mg b.i.d. can be increased slowly until side effects become unacceptable or to a maximum dosage of 20 mg t.i.d.

c. Dantrolene (Dantrium) acts directly on the contractile mechanisms within muscle. It is particularly useful for treatment of spasticity in nonambulatory patients with severe prolonged muscle contraction who will not be adversely affected by the decrease in voluntary muscle power associated with the use of this drug. Side effects include damage to the liver, drowsiness, and lightheadedness. The initial dosage of 25 mg per day may be increased by 25 mg twice per week to a maximum dosage of 100 mg per day.

Other patients fail to respond to drug treatment of spasticity. Under these circumstances a full evaluation using multiple channel electromyography may be helpful. In ambulatory patients the study of the electromyographic responses may indicate possible benefit from other forms of treatment. Methods available include peroneal electrical stimulation to reduce ankle clonus and spinal cord stimulation to produce improvement in motor control of both lower limbs. In non-ambulatory patients with severe paraparesis, the problems of spontaneous flexor-extensor spasm often interfere with nursing care, transfer to a wheelchair, and the maintenance of posture in a wheelchair. Multiple channel electromyographic studies may indicate that relief may be obtained by the injection of selected muscles at the motor point with a 40 percent alcohol in water solution. When muscle hypertonia is confined to the muscles supplied by one nerve, a nerve block may be performed using a 6 percent solution of phenol in water. When muscle spasms are more generalized in the lower limbs, reduction of spasm can be achieved by chemical rhizotomy using a phenol solution injected in the subarachnoid space via a lumbar puncture. This latter procedure requires considerable skill to produce the desired effect without damage to other nerves in the lumbosacral area.

7. Management of bladder problems. Urinary bladder symptoms of urgency and frequency of micturition are very common in patients with multiple sclerosis and probably affect as many as 70 percent of established cases. Symptomatic treatment of these symptoms is often unsuccessful, and it is recommended that all patients with urinary bladder symptoms should receive full evaluation by a urologist. The diagnosis of bladder dysfunction in patients with multiple sclerosis is classified as follows:

Failure to store
a. Uninhibited detrusor contractions
b. Small capacity bladder
c. Sphincter dysfunction
Failure to empty
a. Detrusor dysfunction
b. Outlet obstruction
A combination of the above

It should be noted that the combined failure to store and failure to empty, which is usually a bladder-external sphincter dyssynergia, is a very common condition in patients with severe signs of spinal cord involvement. Patients who have simple failure to store can be treated with anticholinergic drugs such as propantheline 50 mg orally four times a day, oxybutynin chloride 5 mg t.i.d., or imipramine 100 mg q.h.s. When this is unsuccessful, the male may use an indwelling catheter. Failure to empty can be treated with bethanechol chloride 25 mg q.i.d. or by intermit-

tent self-catheterization. Patients with bladder-external sphincter dyssynergia can be treated with a combination of propantheline plus intermittent self-catheterization. When any of these programs fails, the choice of an indwelling catheter or urinary diversion should be made. In general, urinary diversion should be reserved for cases with repeated urinary tract infection, formation of calculi, or inability to retain an indwelling catheter.

8. Community services. Patients with severe multiple sclerosis who are unable to continue their employment or who become increasingly dependent upon others face the prospect of increasing pressures in their home and in the community. However, most patients are ill-equipped to cope with the stresses of chronic illness and should be given the benefit of social service consultation and advice whenever possible. This results in a smoother transition from hospital to home, better development of home conditions to suit the patient, and improved support for family members in identification of community resources available to the multiple sclerosis patient. There is an increased incidence of bipolar or unipolar affective disorders in multiple sclerosis, and many patients have an unsuspected depression or marital problems, which are often unexpressed by the patient and recognized only by the experienced social worker (22). This type of problem can be dealt with appropriately by referral to a marriage counselor, psychologist, or psychiatrist.

9. Simple prophylactic measures. All patients with multiple sclerosis should be advised to:

a. Avoid excessive prolonged contact with direct sunlight. Patients with multiple sclerosis experience considerable weakness and appearance of previous symptoms if exposed to a hot environment, in particular after prolonged exposure to sunlight. The patient should be reassured that the symptoms will disappear when the ambient temperature decreases.

b. Combat infections. Many patients recognize that relapse occurs after an infection. It is prudent, therefore, to treat all infections in multiple sclerosis patients seriously and to resort to the early use of antibiotics.

c. Avoid fatigue. Some patients note relapse following periods of unexpected fatigue. Ambulatory patients with multiple sclerosis should be told to avoid sudden unexpected athletic activities or prolonged exertion. Multiple sclerosis patients should gradually develop any program involving this type of activity.

Prognosis. The prognosis in multiple sclerosis has improved in the last decade. The mean survival is now 22 to 25 years. This can be attributed to better treatment and control of infections in debilitated patients. The physician should be frank with the patient and relatives in discussing prognosis. Multiple sclerosis resembles a chronic infectious disease in presentation and prognosis. Consequently, multiple sclerosis may be mild, chronically relapsing and remitting, chronically progressive, severely disabling, or fatal. In general, patients who present with mild symptoms and who have several mild relapses tend to remain in a mild category and do not become severely disabled. Patients who remain fully active and fully employed 10 years after the diagnosis of multiple sclerosis are considered to have a benign form of the disease and can be informed that they will not be disabled by multiple sclerosis. However, these patients must also be informed that mild exacerbation of multiple sclerosis will continue at unpredictable times well past the fiftieth birthday.

The prognosis of multiple sclerosis can be improved by avoiding known precipitating factors. Patients should be advised to avoid unusual physical or emotional stress, infection, and prolonged exposure to sunlight. All infections should be treated promptly with early use of antibiotics. Patients with chronic multiple sclerosis who are bedridden or confined to a wheelchair often experience slow deterioration that is not appreciated by the patient or relatives. The prognosis can be improved in these cases by regular reevaluation at six-month intervals followed by prompt attention to obvious areas of deterioration. Patients with urinary tract problems should have frequent reevaluation. Loss of function in a limb calls for prompt reinstitution of physical therapy, and paraparesis should not render a patient bedridden. Prescription of the correct type of wheelchair and instruction in the proper transfer from bed to chair permit broader contacts with friends and relatives, improve morale, and improve the long-term outlook for the patient.

Pregnancy is associated with clinical stability in most cases, but the postpartum period carries a risk for exacerbation of multiple sclerosis at about two or three times the expected relapse rate. Patients should be told that there is some increased risk of multiple sclerosis in offspring if one parent has the disease, but the actual risk is small (23).

REFERENCES

1. Koprawski, H.; DeFreitas, E. C.; Harper, M. E.; *et al.* Multiple sclerosis and human T-cell lymphotrophic retroviruses. Nature 318:154–160; 1985.
2. Rivera, V. M. Multiple sclerosis. Is the mystery beginning to unfold? Postgrad. Med. 79:217–232; 1986.
3. McDonald, W. I. The mystery of the origin of multiple sclerosis. J. Neurol. Neurosurg. Psychiatry 49:113–123; 1986.
4. Marx, J. L. Indications of a new virus in M.S. patients. Science 230:1028; 1985.
5. Kinnunen, E.; Juntunen, J.; *et al.* Genetic susceptibility to multiple sclerosis. A co-twin study of a nationwide series. Arch. Neurol. 45:1108–1111; 1988.
6. Sanders, E. A. C. M.; Bollen, E. L. E. M.; Vander Velde, E. A. Presenting signs and symptoms in multiple sclerosis. Acta. Neurol. Scand. 73:269–272; 1986.
7. Engell, T. Neurological disease activity in multiple sclerosis patients with periphlebitis retinae. Acta. Neurol. Scand. 73:168–172; 1986.
8. Thompson, A. J.; Hutchinson, M.; Brazil, J.; *et al.* A clinical and laboratory study of benign multiple sclerosis. Quart. J. Med. 58:69–80; 1986.
9. Sanders, E. A. C. M.; Ruelen, J. P. H.; *et al.* The diagnosis of multiple sclerosis. Contribution of non-clinical tests. J. Neurol. Sci. 72:273–285; 1986.
10. Honig, L. S.; Siddharthan, R.; *et al.* Multiple sclerosis: correlation of magnetic resonance imaging with cerebrospinal fluid findings. J. Neurol. Neurosurg. Psychiatry 51:277–280; 1988.
11. Farlow, M. R.; Markand, O. N.; Edwards, M. K.; *et al.* multiple sclerosis: Magnetic resonance imaging, evoked responses, and spinal fluid electrophoresis. Neurology, 36:828–831; 1986.
12. Jacobs, L.; Kinhal, W. R.; Palachini, I.; *et al.* Correlations of nuclear magnetic resonance imaging, computerized tomography, and clinical profile in multiple sclerosis. Neurology 36:27–34; 1986.
13. Sheldon, J. J.; Siddharthan, R.; Tobias, J.; *et al.* MR imaging of multiple sclerosis: comparison with clinical and CT examination in 74 patients. Amer. J. Radiol. 145:957–964; 1985.
14. Smith, A. S.; Weinstein, M. A.; Modic, M. T.; *et al.* Magnetic resonance with marked T2-weighted images. Improved demonstration of brain lesions, tumor, and edema. Amer. J. Radiol. 145:949–955; 1985.
15. Willoughby, E. C. V.; Grochowski, E.; *et al.* Se-

rial magnetic resonance scanning in multiple sclerosis: a second prospective study in relapsing patients. Ann. Neurol. 25:43–49; 1989.

16. Rao, S. M.; Leo, G. J.; *et al.* Correlation of magnetic resonance imaging with neuropsychological testing in multiple sclerosis. Neurology 39:161–166; 1989.

17. Thompson, A. J.; Hutchinson, M.; Martin, E. A.; *et al.* Suspected and clinically defined multiple sclerosis: the relationship between CSF immunoglobulins and clinical course. J. Neurol. Neurosurg. Psychiatry 48:989–994; 1985.

18. Rudick, R. A.; Schiffer, R. B.; Schwetz, K. M.; *et al.* Multiple sclerosis. The problem of incorrect diagnosis. Arch. Neurol. 43:578–583; 1986.

19. Alexander, E. L.; Malinov, K.; *et al.* Primary Sjögren's syndrome with central nervous system disease mimicking multiple sclerosis. Ann. Int. Med. 104:323–330; 1986.

20. Durelli, L.; Cocito, A.; *et al.* High dose intravenous methylprednisolone in the treatment of multiple sclerosis. Neurology 36:238–243; 1986.

21. Hughes, R. A. C. Immunological treatment of multiple sclerosis. J. Neurol 233:66–68; 1986.

22. Schiffer, R. B.; Weitkamp, L. R.; *et al.* Multiple sclerosis and affective disorder. Family history, sex and HLA-DR antigens. Arch. Neurol. 45:1345–1348; 1988.

23. Birk, K.; Rudick, R. Pregnancy and multiple sclerosis. Arch. Neurology 43:719–726; 1986.

CHAPTER 8

CEREBROVASCULAR DISEASE

Cerebrovascular disease is one of the major causes of morbidity and death in the United States. The condition has an increased incidence and prevalence with increasing age but is not, as usually thought, a disease confined to the elderly. The incidence appears to be 0.5 per thousand at age 40, rising to more than 10 per thousand at age 40, and to approximately 70 per thousand at age 70. At present there are about 12,500 cases of cerebrovascular disease in a community of one million.

In the same community of one million persons, there will be approximately 2,500 new cases each year, including:

1. 250 cases of subarachnoid hemorrhage with 50 percent mortality within 30 days
2. 375 cases of intracerebral hemorrhage with 80 percent mortality within 30 days
3. 1,875 cases of cerebral infarction with 40 percent mortality within 30 days.

For each 100 survivors, 10 are able to return to work without impairment, 40 have mild residual disability, 50 have more severe disability requiring special services in a home case situation, and 10 need permanent institutional care. Of the 12,500 persons with cerebrovascular disease, community resources will be expected to provide special care services for 6,250 cases at home and institutional care for 1,250 cases.

Anatomy of the Blood Supply to the Brain

The brain is supplied by two paired arteries, the internal carotid arteries anteriorly and the vertebral arteries posteriorly. The vertebral arteries unite to form the basilar artery. These two arterial systems form the circle of Willis at the base of the brain, a unique anastomotic system, which gives rise to all of the vessels supplying the cerebral hemispheres (see Figure 8–1).

Internal Carotid Artery. The internal carotid artery arises in the neck as one of the two branches of the common carotid artery. It ascends in the neck and enters the carotid canal in the petrous temporal bone, where it ascends, loops forward and medially, then ascends again to enter the cranial cavity. The artery enters the cavernous sinus and passes forward, closely related to the sella and hypophysis medially and to the third, fourth, sixth, and ophthalmic and maxillary division of the fifth cranial nerve laterally. The terminal portion of the internal carotid ascends and pierces the dura medial to the anterior clinoid process, where the artery is closely related to the optic nerve. The cavernous and terminal portions of the internal carotid artery are frequently referred to as the carotid siphon.

The branches of the internal carotid include:

1. Petrous portion
   a. Caroticotympanic   artery—supplies

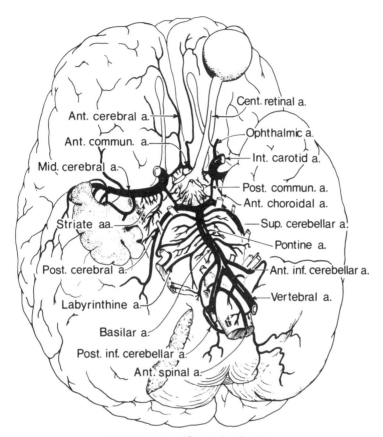

FIGURE 8–1.   The circle of Willis.

the anterior and part of the medial wall of the middle ear.

2. Cavernous portion
   a. Cavernous arteries—small vessels supplying the hypophysis and walls of the cavernous sinus
   b. Hypophyseal arteries—supply the hypophysis
   c. Semilunar artery—supplies the trigeminal (semilunar) ganglion.
   d. Anterior meningeal artery—supplies the dura of the anterior cranial fossa.
3. Supraclinoid portion
   a. Ophthalmic artery
   b. Anterior choroidal artery
   c. Posterior communicating artery
4. Terminal portion
   a. Anterior cerebral artery
   b. Middle cerebral artery

Ophthalmic Artery. The ophthalmic artery arises from the supraclinoid portion of the internal carotid artery, pierces the dura, and accompanies the optic nerve through the optic foramen into the orbit. The artery passes medially, superior to the optic nerve, to the roof of the orbit, where it divides into the supratrochlear and dorsal nasal arteries. Branches of the ophthalmic artery anastomose with branches of the external cartoid system. This anastomosis may supply blood to intracranial structures following insufficiency or occlusion of the internal carotid artery.

The branches of the ophthalmic artery include:

1. Central retinal artery—arises from the ophthalmic artery and enters the optic nerve close to the eye. The artery emerges from the center of the optic disk in the optic cup and divides into several branches supplying the optic disk and retina.
2. Ciliary arteries—several in number, which supply the sclera, choroid, lens, and conjunctiva of the eye.
3. Lacrimal artery—arises from the ophthalmic artery near the optic foramen and

runs laterally along the upper border of the lateral rectus muscle to supply the lacrimal gland.

4. Supraorbital artery—arises from the ophthalmic artery and passes above the eye to join the supraorbital nerve. The artery supplies the skin, muscle, and other structures over the forehead and anastomoses with branches of the superficial temporal artery.
5. Ethmoidal arteries—supply the ethmoidal sinuses, the nasal cavity, and the dura of the anterior fossa.
6. Dorsal nasal artery—distributed to the outer surface of the nose and anastomoses with the angular artery.
7. Frontal artery—supplies the medial aspect of the forehead.
8. Superior–inferior palpebral arteries—encircle the eylids near the face margins.
9. Muscular branches—supply the extraocular muscles.

Anterior Choroidal Artery. The anterior choroidal artery arises from the terminal portion of the internal carotid artery and passes posteriorly along the optic tract to reach the lateral geniculate body. The artery then enters the choroidal fissure and supplies the choroid plexus in the inferior horn of the lateral ventricle. In its course, the artery supplies the optic tract, the cerebral peduncle, the lateral portion of the lateral geniculate body, the posterior two-thirds of the posterior limb of the internal capsule, the retrolenticular and infralenticular portions of the internal capsule, the optic radiation, the hippocampus, the choroid plexus, the tail of the caudate nucleus, and the amygdala.

Posterior Communicating Artery. The posterior communicating artery arises from the terminal portion of the internal carotid artery and passes posteriorly, immediately above the oculomotor nerve, to anastomose with the posterior cerebral artery. Branches of the posterior communicating artery supply the thalamus, subthalamus, internal capsule, mammillary bodies, optic chiasm, and optic tract.

Anterior Cerebral Artery. The anterior cerebral artery arises from the terminal portion of the internal carotid artery and passes anteromedially above the optic nerve to come into contact with the opposite anterior cerebral artery. The two arteries are connected by a short anterior communicating artery, then pass around the genu and body of the corpus callosum to anastomose with

branches of the posterior cerebral artery at the level of the parietooccipital fissure.

The branches of the anterior cerebral artery include:

1. Anterior communicating artery—supplies the optic chiasm and hypothalamus
2. Perforating branches—penetrate the anterior perforating substance and lamina terminalis to supply the rostrum of the corpus callosum and the septum pellucidum
3. Recurrent branch (medial striate artery, recurrent artery of Heubner)—is distributed to the head of the caudate nucleus and the anterior limb of the internal capsule.
4. Cortical branches
   a. Orbital branches—supply the orbital and medial surfaces of the frontal lobe
   b. Frontopolar branch—supplies the anterior portion of the medial aspect of the superior frontal gyrus and extends about one inch onto the superior lateral surface
   c. Pericallosal branch—supplies the cingulate gyrus and corpus callosum
   d. Callosomarginal branch—supplies the cingulate gyrus, the medial aspect of the superior frontal gyrus, and the paracentral lobule.

Middle Cerebral Artery. The middle cerebral artery should be regarded as the intracranial extension of the internal carotid artery.* Emboli entering the internal carotid artery inevitably enter the middle cerebral artery. The middle cerebral artery runs laterally in the lateral fissure between the frontal and temporal lobes (see Figure 8–2) to reach the surface of the insula, where it divides into several branches.

The branches of the middle cerebral artery include:

1. Lenticulostriate   arteries—perforating branches that arise close to the origin of the middle cerebral artery and penetrate the substance of the brain to supply the head of the caudate nucleus, putamen, globus pallidus, and internal capsule.
2. Cortical branches—radiate outward from the middle cerebral artery as it lies on the insula. Cortical branches that can be recognized by arteriography are the orbitofrontal, frontal, preRolandic, postRolandic, anterior parietal, and posterior parietal arteries. The angular branch follows the line of the lateral fissure and the

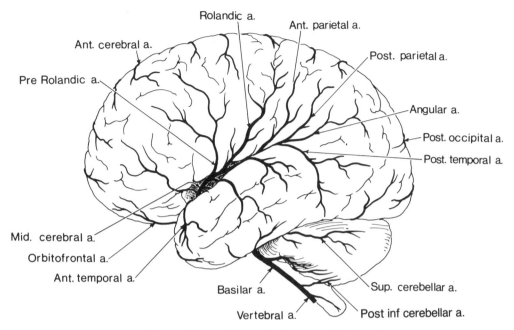

FIGURE 8-2. The middle cerebral artery and its branches.

anterior, middle, and posterior temporal branches extend over the surface of the temporal lobe.

Vertebral Artery. The vertebral artery arises from the first portion of the subclavian artery in the neck. The anatomic course can be considered in four parts:

First part—ascends posteromedially and enters the foramen of the transverse process of the sixth cervical vertebra

Second part—ascends through the foramina of the transverse processes of the upper six cervical vertebrae

Third part—curves backward in a groove behind the superior articular process of the atlas and passes through the foramen magnum

Fourth part—pierces the dura to lie on the ventral surface of the medulla, where it ascends to the lower border of the pons to unite with the vertebral artery from the opposite side forming the basilar artery.

The branches of the vertebral artery include:

1. Spinal branches—accompany the nerve roots into the spinal canal. Only one or two of these branches anastomose with the anterior spinal artery.

2. Muscular branches—supply the deep muscles of the neck.

3. Meningeal branches—arise from the vertebral arteries at the level of the foramen magnum and supply the dura of the posterior fossa and the falx cerebelli.

4. Anterior spinal artery—arises from the vertebral artery near its termination and descends over the ventral surface of the medulla to unite with the artery from the opposite side and form one anterior spinal artery. This artery lies in the ventral sulcus of the spinal cord and terminates as a fine vessel in the cauda equina. The anterior spinal artery supplies the medial and inferior portion of the medulla, including the medullar pyramids and all of the spinal cord except the posterior columns and posterior horns of the gray matter.

5. Posterior inferior cerebellar artery—arises from the fourth part of the vertebral artery and passes around the medulla onto the inferior surface of the cerebellum, where it divides into two branches. The posterior inferior cerebellar artery supplies the lateral portion of the medulla and the inferior cerebellar peduncle. The median branch supplies the inferior ver-

mis, the medial aspect of the cerebellar hemisphere, and the choroid plexus of the fourth ventricle. The lateral branch supplies the inferior surface of the cerebellar hemisphere. There is a well-developed anastomosis with the anterior inferior cerebellar and superior cerebellar arteries.

Basilar Artery. The basilar artery (see Figure 8–3) takes origin at the inferior border of the pons from the junction of the two vertebral arteries and ascends in the median groove to terminate at the upper border of the pons by dividing into the two posterior cerebral arteries.

The branches of the basilar artery include:

1. Pontine branches—supply the pons.
2. Internal auditory artery—accompanies the seventh and eighth cranial nerves into the internal auditory meatus and supplies the inner ear.
3. Anterior inferior cerebellar artery—arises just above the lower border of the pons and passes around the pons onto the inferior surface of the cerebellar hemisphere and anastomoses with the posterior inferior cerebellar artery.
4. Superior cerebellar artery—arises just below the terminating of the basilar artery and passes around the pons separated

from the posterior cerebral artery by the oculomotor nerve. The superior cerebellar artery supplies the superior and middle cerebellar peduncles, the pineal gland, the choroid plexus of the third ventricle, and the superior surface of the cerebellum.

Posterior Cerebral Artery. The posterior cerebral artery arises at the termination of the basilar artery, where it is separated from the superior cerebellar artery by the oculomotor nerve. The posterior communicating artery joins the posterior cerebral artery, which winds around the cerebral peduncle onto the tentorial surface of the occipital lobe.

The branches of the posterior cerebral artery include:

1. Posteromedial arteries—enter the posterior perforated substance to supply the medial surface of the thalamus and the wall of the third ventricle.
2. Posterior choroidal artery—runs beneath the splenium of the corpus callosum to supply the choroid plexus of the third ventricle.
3. Posterolateral arteries—supply the lateral thalamus and the midbrain.
4. Anterior temporal branches—supply the

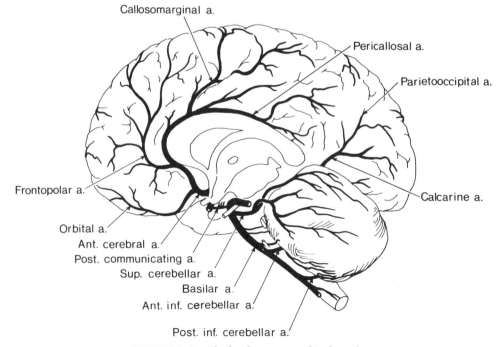

FIGURE 8–3. The basilar artery and its branches.

uncus and the fusiform gyrus of the temporal lobe.

5. Posterior temporal branches—supply the inferior temporal gyrus.
6. Calcarine branches—supply the medial surface of the occipital lobe with a short extension onto the superior lateral surface of the hemisphere and the occipital pole. The posterior cerebral artery anastomoses with the anterior cerebral artery at the level of the parietooccipital fissure on the medial surface of the hemisphere.

Arterial Circle of Willis. This unique anastomosis, which lies at the base of the brain, is derived from the internal carotid and vertebral arterial systems (see Figure 8–1). The anterior portion of the circle is formed by the two anterior cerebral arteries, derived from the internal carotid arteries, and connected by the anterior communicating artery. The posterior portion of the circle consists of the two posterior cerebral arteries, which are the terminal branches of the basilar artery. The posterior cerebral arteries are connected to the internal carotid arteries on each side by the posterior communicating arteries. The circle of Willis encloses the anterior perforating substance, the optic chiasm, the infundibulum, the tuber cinereum, the mammillary bodies, and the posterior perforating substance.

Anatomy of the Venous Drainage of the Brain

The cerebral venous system can be divided into two subdivisions, the superficial external venous drainage and the deep internal venous drainage. Both systems eventually drain into the venous sinuses.

The upper lateral surface of the cerebral hemisphere is drained by the superficial cerebral veins, which enter the superior longitudinal sinus. The superficial middle cerebral vein also drains the lateral surface of the cerebral hemisphere and passes forward in the lateral fissure to enter the cavernous sinus. The superficial middle cerebral vein communicates with the superior longitudinal sinus through the superior anastomatic vein of Trolard and with the transverse sinus through the inferior anastomotic vein of Labbé. The inferior cerebral veins drain the orbital surface of the frontal lobe, the lateral aspect of the temporal lobe, and the lateral aspect of the occipital lobe to empty into the cavernous and transverse sinuses. The veins over the insula unite to form the deep middle cerebral vein, which passes anteriorly deep in the lateral fissure to join the basal vein of Rosenthal. This latter structure arises in the anterior perforating substance by the union of the anterior cerebral vein and the veins of the corpus callosum. The basal vein is joined by the deep middle cerebral vein as it passes posteriorly in close relationship to the uncus and hippocampus. The basal vein then winds around the midbrain to unite with the basal vein from the opposite side at the origin of the great cerebral vein.

The deep internal group of cerebral veins drain the central structures of the cerebral hemispheres and are closely related to the ventricular system.

The terminal (thalamostriate) vein arises in the inferior horn of the lateral ventricle and follows the tail of the caudate nucleus into the body of the lateral ventricle lying between the caudate nucleus and the thalamus. The terminal vein runs forward to the interventricular foramen and is joined by the anterior caudate vein; the septal vein, which drains the septum pellucidum; and the choroidal vein, which drains the choroid plexus of the lateral ventricle to form the internal cerebral vein. This structure turns at its origin, forming the venous angle, and then passes along the roof of the third ventricle and through the velum interpositum to join with the opposite internal cerebral vein. The great cerebral vein of Galen is formed by the union of the internal cerebral veins and the junction of the basal veins of Rosenthal. After a short course, the great cerebral vein is joined by the inferior sagittal sinus to form the straight sinus.

The intracranial venous sinuses are thin-walled, endothelial-lined structures lying within the dura. The superior longitudinal sinus takes origin at the foramen cecum anteriorly and passes in the superior surface of the falx cerebri to the internal occipital protuberance, then turns to the right to form the right transverse sinus. The superior longitudinal sinus receives the superior cerebral veins. The walls of the sinus contain granulations, which are responsible for the absorption of cerebrospinal fluid into the venous system. The inferior longitudinal sinus arises in the free margin of the falx cerebri by the union of a number of small veins and runs posteriorly to terminate in the straight sinus at the junction of the falx cerebri and the tentorium cerebelli. The straight sinus is formed by the union of the great vein of Galen and the inferior longitudinal sinus and passes posteriorly in the junction of the falx cerebri and tentorium cerebelli. The straight sinus terminates at the internal occipital protuberance by becoming the left transverse sinus. The transverse sinuses arise at the internal occipital protuberance and run along the edge of the tentorium cerebelli to end at the base of the petrous temporal bone, where they become the sigmoid sinuses. The transverse sinuses receive most of the venous drainage from the cerebellum. The sigmoid sinuses are a direct continuation of the transverse sinuses, beginning at the base of the petrous temporal bone and terminating at the jugular foramen as the internal jugular vein.

The cavernous sinus arises anteriorly from the superior ophthalmic vein at the superior orbital fissure and passes posteriorly, close to the sella turcica, and terminates by dividing into the superior and inferior petrosal sinuses. The cavernous sinuses communicate with each other through the intercavernous sinuses and lie anteriorly and posteriorly to the sella turcica. The lateral walls of the cavernous sinus contain the third, fourth, and sixth nerves and the ophthalmic and maxillary divisions of the trigeminal nerve. The intracavernous portion of the internal carotid artery is contained within the cavernous sinus. The superior petrosal sinus arises from the cavernous sinus at the apex of the petrous temporal bone and passes along the edge of the tentorium cerebelli to terminate in the transverse sinus. The inferior petrosal sinus also arises at the apex of the petrous temporal bone and enters a groove lying in the junction of the petrous, temporal, and occipital bones to terminate in the jugular bulb of the internal jugular vein.

Transient Ischemic Attacks

Definition. Transient ischemic attacks (TIAs) are episodes of temporary focal ischemia involving the brain or brain stem. They are commonly 2 to 30 minutes' duration and by definition last less than 24 hours. The onset is sudden, and symptoms usually reach maximum intensity within two minutes. The episodes usually rapidly resolve with a 50 percent recovery in one hour and a 90 percent recovery in four hours (1). The frequency varies; some patients experience a single attack, while others experience multiple attacks at different intervals.

Etiology and Pathology. The causes of transient ischemic attacks can be considered under three major categories:

1. Diseases of the blood vessels
2. Abnormalities of the blood constituents

3. Reduced cerebral perfusion.

These three factors may act individually or in combination, but the end result is the same: a focal reduction in cerebral blood flow, which is of sufficient magnitude to cause a temporary interference with cerebral activity.

Diseases of the Blood Vessels. Diseases of the blood vessels include:

1. Artherosclerotic plaques. Most transient ischemic attacks occur in patients who have cerebral atherosclerosis. The process begins with endothelial injury of unknown cause and proliferation of collagen to produce fibrointimal thickening. This is followed by proliferation of muscle cells giving rise to the fibrous plaque. There is progressive encroachment on the lumen with the development of intraplaque hemorrhages. The breakdown of blood within the plaque leads to the presence of cholesterol which may form a cholesterol abscess. At this stage a further hemorrhage may rupture into the lumen of the artery or an abscess may discharge with embolization. In many cases this is asymptomatic but embolization can cause TIAs or more serious neurologic deficits and emboli may make a transient appearance in the retinal circulation (see Figure 8–4). The atheromatous ulcer formed by the discharge of cholesterol in blood presents an ideal surface for platelet adherence which is a further source of embolization. In some cases the ulcer will heal or rarely calcify. However, the material released from an atheromatous plaque is a powerful procoagulant and can lead to local thrombosis with partial or complete obstruction of the lumen.

Common sites of plaque formation are the origin of the internal carotid arteries, origin of the vertebral arteries, and origin of the middle cerebral arteries.

Factors that contribute to accelerated development of atherosclerosis include:

a. Hypertension. Chronic hypertension is a primary risk factor for stroke and appears to acccelerate the atherosclerotic process. There is a steady increase of the risk of stroke with increased levels of systolic blood pressure, and there is no dividing line between normotensive and hypertensive individuals. Many patients with chronic cerebrovascular disease have labile hypertension, and casual measurements of blood pressure may give an erroneous impression of normotensive levels. Such patients are nearly all susceptible to a

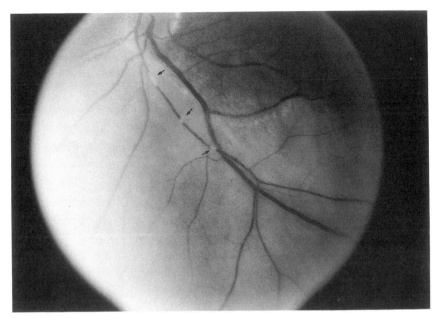

FIGURE 8–4. Carotid atherosclerotic embolism. Box car appearance of interrupted blood flow from presumed cholesterol emboli.

considerable rise in systolic blood pressure in response to stress and may have sustained periods of hypertension during the day, leading to accelerated atherosclerosis. Therefore, intermittent hypertension should be treated whenever identified.

b. Diabetes mellitus. Approximately 30 percent of patients with cerebral atherosclerosis have evidence of diabetes mellitus and the incidence of stroke is twice as high in diabetics as in nondiabetics with equivalent atherosclerotic vascular disease. The prevalence of high-grade carotid artery stenosis is also significantly higher in diabetics. The risk of stroke is increased when diabetes mellitus is associated with hypertension, hypercholesterolemia, and smoking. This combination appears to greatly accelerate atherosclerosis although there is no evidence to show that accelerated atherosclerosis is more common in the severe than in the mild diabetic or that strict control of diabetes mellitus reduces the risk of developing stroke. Nevertheless the coexistence of hypertension and poorly controlled diabetes is significant in the early recurrence of stroke (2).

c. Obesity. Both hypertension and overt diabetes mellitus are commoner in obese patients. In addition obesity has been shown to be one of the factors contributing to accelerated atherosclerosis, and obese patients should have a strict program of weight reduction.

d. Hyperuricemia. Several studies have shown a relationship between hyperuricemia and chronic cerebrovascular disease. Hyperuricemia is usually asymptomatic, and patients rarely have symptoms of gout. There is some evidence of increased predisposition to stenosis of extracranial vessels in the necks of patients with cerebrovascular disease and hyperuricemia. Consequently, hyperuricemia, whether symptomatic or asymptomatic, should be treated if detected.

e. Hypothyroidism. Some of the stoke population has shown a significant prevalence of hypothyroidism. Since this condition can contribute to atherosclerosis, all patients with cerebrovascular disease should be investigated for hypothyroidism.

f. Abnormal serum lipid levels. Patients in their late 30s, 40s, and early 50s who have transient ischemic attack or acute stroke often show evidence of hyperlipidemia. This condition is considered an important cause of generalized atherosclerosis and when detected should be treated appropriately. Lowering of serum triglycerides in elderly patients with symptoms of cerebrovascular disease and hypertriglyceridemia is effective in improving cerebral perfusion and cognition (3).

g. Smoking. The relationship between smoking and increased risk of cerebrovascular disease is well established. The combination of smoking, hypertension, diabetes mellitus, and hyperlipidemia is particularly hazardous (4).

2. Arteriosclerosis. Hypertrophic arteriosclerosis in chronic hypertension is not uncommon in the cerebral vessels. The reduplication of the elastic lamina and hyalinization of the vessel wall produce narrowing of the lumen, which may reduce cerebral blood flow.

3. Arteritis. Inflammation of the vessel wall from any cause (e.g., syphilis, sarcoidosis, polyarteritis nodosa) leads to a narrowing of the lumen with reduction of cerebral blood flow. About 5 percent of patients with TIA or infarction have syphilitic arteritis, which can cause a severe stroke in younger patients.

4. Fibromuscular dysplasia. This rare condition may produce significant stenosis of the carotid arteries.

5. Organ transplant recipients. The cerebral infarction and TIAs are the commonest neurologic complications of organ transplantation. Recipients older than 40 years, and those with diabetes mellitus, are at a greater risk.

Abnormalities of the Blood Constituents. Abnormalities of the blood constituents include:

1. Hypercoagulability. Abnormal platelet activation with a tendency to aggregation has been demonstrated in a number of young persons with TIAs and stroke (sticky platelets). In addition, polycythemia or activation of thrombin precursors predisposes to thrombosis.

2. Embolism.

a. Platelet emboli may originate on atherosclerotic plaques in the carotid or vertebral circulation and enter the small vessels of the brain, producing local transient ischemia.

b. Cholesterol discharged from cholesterol abscesses in atherosclerotic plaques can also occlude small vessels in the brain.

c. Thromboemboli may arise from thrombi which form over atherosclerotic plaques in any artery supplying blood to the brain. Thromboemboli may also arise as a complication of heart conditions including atrial arrhythmias, atrial myxoma, mitral valve prolapse, calcific aortic stenosis, myocardial infarction with mural thrombosis, hypertensive cardiomyopathy, infective endocarditis, and nonbacterial thrombotic endocarditis.

Reduced Cerebral Perfusion. Causes of reduced cerebral perfusion include:

1. Diminished effective cardiac output. Diminished cardiac output may be a significant factor in the production of focal ischemia in the brain when cerebral vessels are diseased and narrowed. Diminished cardiac output occurs in orthostatic hypotension, aortic valvular stenosis or insufficiency, subaortic stenosis, cardiac dysrhythmias, arteriosclerotic heart disease, and certain primary cardiomyopathies.

2. Steal syndromes. Steal syndromes may be extracranial or intracranial. The best known extracranial steal syndrome is the subclavian steal syndrome, in which blood flows normally up the vertebral artery toward the basilar artery, then flows down the opposite vertebral artery into the subclavian artery. The subclavian steal is caused by diminished pressure in the subclavian artery due to severe proximal stenosis of the vessel. Intracranial steal syndromes are not uncommon and depend upon the development of collateral circulation from one area of the brain to another area of diminished perfusion pressure. This may lead to diversion of blood from part of the brain sufficient to produce symptoms of transient ischemia.

3. Kinking and compression of extracranial vessels. The internal carotid and vertebral arteries occasionally undergo kinking or compression in the neck with head turning. This results in reduction or cessation of flow through the affected vessel. Arteriosclerotic vessels frequently lose elasticity and lengthen, resulting in the formation of redundant coils or kinks even with the head in normal position. The internal carotid can be narrowed or occluded by the lateral mass of the atlas when the head is turned to the opposite side. This may result in the production of carotid insufficiency. The vertebral arteries are sometimes compressed on head turning by osteophytes arising along the margins of the cervical vertebrae and interpeduncular joints. This osteophytic compression of the vertebral arteries, as they pass through the intervertebral foramina, produces vertebrobasilar insufficiency. These abnormalities can be detected by arteriography and many cases

can be corrected by appropriate surgical treatment.

Clinical Features. The symptoms of a transient ischemic attack depend upon the site of the focal ischemia in the brain. There are two categories of TIA: those that occur in response to ischemia in the carotid arterial system and those resulting from disturbed blood flow in the vertebral-basilar system.

Carotid Arterial Insufficiency. Carotid arterial insufficiency may produce:

1. Visual symptoms. Dimness of vision or loss of vision affecting the eye on the side of the carotid insufficiency (amaurosis fugax) may occur due to involvement of the ophthalmic arterial system. Homonymous hemianopia may result when there is cerebral hemisphere ischemia.

2. Language dysfunction. Dysphasia or aphasia may occur when there is ischemia of the dominant hemisphere.

3. Motor symptoms. Contralateral hemiparesis or hemiplegia occurs with hemispheric ischemia.

4. Sensory symptoms. Contralateral numbness, coldness, or paresthesias involving the hand, upper limb, lower limb, or both limbs may result from ischemia of the parietal lobe.

Vertebral Basilar Insufficiency. Vertebral basilar insufficiency may produce:

1. Visual symptoms. Dimness of vision, hemianopia, alexia without agraphia, color anomia, simple or complex visual hallucinations, visual perseveration, prosopagnosia are all due to occipital lobe ischemia.

2. Eye movement disorders. These include Parinaud's syndrome, vertical gaze paresis, paralysis of downward gaze, bilateral ptosis, blepharospasm, pupillary abnormalities, nystagmus, decreased blinking, internuclear ophthalmoplegia.

3. Cranial nerve deficits. Diplopia, facial numbness, facial weakness, tinnitus, vertigo, dysarthria, or dysphagia may result from brain stem ischemia. Isolated vertigo occurring in episodic fashion in an elderly patient is often the result of a TIA (5).

4. Motor symptoms. Paresis or paralysis of one or more limbs, Horner's syndrome, or decerebrate posturing may occur.

5. Coordination deficits. Ataxia or clumsiness of upper or lower limbs on one side or both sides, rubral tremor, hemiballismus, or choreoathetosis may result from cerebellar ischemia or ischemic involvement of cerebellar connections in the brain stem.

6. Sensory symptoms. Paresthesias of one or both sides of the face and upper or lower limbs, or thalamic pain can occur with ischemia in the territory supplied by the posterior cerebral arteries.

7. Drop attacks. Sudden loss of tone in the lower limbs may result from ischemia of the medullary pyramids.

8. Altered consciousness. This includes brief episodes of impaired or loss of consciousness, abulia, drowsiness, confusion, agitation, and altered sleep wake cycle.

9. A combination of any or all of the above. Numbers six and seven are unlikely to be caused by vertebral basilar insufficiency unless they are accompanied by one or more of the other manifestations of transient ischemia.

Diagnostic Procedures.

1. Complete blood count and sedimentation rate. These may reveal anemia, which contributes to ischemia by reducing oxygen transport to the brain; polycythemia, which reduces blood flow and oxygen availability; and elevated white count, which may indicate an unsuspected infection; or an elevated sedimentation rate, which suggests a vasculitis (arteritis).

2. Urinalysis. Urinalysis may show evidence of renal damage, which is not unusual in the chronic atherosclerotic patient, or the presence of glycosuria, which suggests diabetes mellitus.

3. Blood urea nitrogen (BUN) and serum creatinine. The BUN and creatinine are elevated in prerenal problems such as dehydration and in renal disease.

4. Fasting blood glucose. Two-hour postprandial blood glucose elevation suggests diabetes mellitus. This should be confirmed with a glucose tolerance test.

5. Cardiac evaluation. The relationship between cerebral vascular disease and cardiac disease is twofold:

a. Atherosclerosis of the cervicointracranial vessels is usually associated with coronary artery disease.

b. The heart is a frequent and often unsuspected source of emboli in patients with TIAs or stroke. Consequently, all patients with a TIA or stroke should receive a full cardiac evaluation. Although atrial myxoma is rare, cerebral embolism is a common complication of this tumor (6).

6. Serologic test for syphilis. Syphilitic arteritis is still an occasional cause of TIA and stroke.

7. Chest x-ray. Chest x-ray may reveal an unexpected tumor as the source of cerebral

metastases, which may mimic TIA. The heart is enlarged in chronic hypertension and heart disease.

8. Serum lipids, fasting cholesterol, triglycerides. A significant number of patients with TIA have hyperlipidemia, hypercholesterolemia, or hypertriglyceridemia.

9. Serum uric acid. Hyperuricemia occurs in about 30 percent of patients with cerebrovascular disease.

10. Thyroid function tests. Hypothyroidism is associated with accelerated atherosclerosis.

11. Antinuclear factor, LE preparation, LE anticoagulant, rheumatoid factor. These tests should be performed if the patient has symptoms suggesting a "collagen disease" or has an elevated sedimentation rate.

12. Platelet count and coagulation profile. A coagulation disorder may predispose to the development of a hemorrhagic infarction in the area of the ischemic infarction.

13. Electroencephalography. Focal slowing suggesting a focal structural lesion may be present in patients with an acute onset of hemiparesis when a computed tomography (CT) scan fails to demonstrate hemorrhage or infarction (7).

14. Magnetic resonance imaging (MRI) and CT scans may reveal the presence of an unexpected cerebral infarct or an unexpected subdural hematoma or tumor. The MRI is superior to CT scanning, which may not be abnormal for 7 to 10 days after an ischemic cerebral infarction. The superiority of MRI is most striking in brain stem infarction (8, 9).

15. Lumbar puncture. The need for lumbar puncture has decreased following the introduction of MRI and CT but there are indications for a lumbar puncture when the MRI or CT scan is negative but the patient has a focal neurologic deficit and nuchal rigidity (subarachnoid hemorrhage, encephalitis, meningitis).

16. Ophthalmic consultation. Patients with neovascular glaucoma without a precipitating fundus condition may have severe carotid artery stenosis leading to retinal ischemia and glaucoma. Ischemic optic neuropathy is generally associated with stenosis and occlusion of the ophthalmic artery rather than carotid stenosis.

17. Doppler ultrasound imaging. The Doppler method provides the opportunity to detect abnormalities in the carotid artery with a high degree of positivity but does not substitute for arteriography. Three-dimen-sional transcranial Doppler blood flow mapping can identify the circle of Willis and all major branches and demonstrate intracranial arterial stenosis with a high degree of reliability (10).

18. Real time B mode ultrasonography. This method is useful in imaging nonobstructive atheromatous plaques in the carotid bifurcation and can detect hemorrhage into or ulceration of plaque in symptomatic patients.

19. Ophthalmodynamometry. Ophthalmodynamometry will detect approximately 70 percent of cases with a significant unilateral carotid stenosis.

20. Arteriography. Intravenous digital subtraction angiography is useful and accurate in the detection of atherosclerotic plaques in the cervical carotid arteries but fails to detect intracranial vascular disease. Four-vessel conventional arteriography remains the standard procedure for the evaluation of cervical and intracranial vessels prior to a decision to recommend carotid endarterectomy.

21. LE anticoagulant. This acquired serum gamma globulin is associated with TIAs cerebral and ocular ischemia and infarction. Associated conductions include systemic lupus erythematosus in about one-third of the cases, noncerebral venous thrombosis, and hypertension. The partial thromboplastin time is prolonged and there may be a false positive venereal disease research laboratory (VDRL) test result (11).

Differential Diagnosis. The differential diagnosis of TIA includes:

1. Epilepsy. The recent onset of partial seizures in a middle-aged or elderly person may suggest transient ischemic attacks. This is particularly common in psychomotor seizures when the patient complains of transient loss of consciousness. A tonic-clonic seizure is unlikely to be mistaken for a transient ischemic attack, but the subsequent hemiparesis (Todd's paralysis) that occurs in some patients may be misdiagnosed if the history is not obtained.

2. Cardiac disorders. The majority of patients with cerebrovascular disease have some degree of cardiovascular disease and are therefore subject to sudden changes in cardiac rhythm such as paroxysmal fibrillation, paroxysmal tachycardia, and heart block. These disorders may be associated with temporary neurologic deficits. Myocardial infarction may produce a precipitous reduction in cardiac output with impairment of

cerebral circulation and transient neurologic deficits due to reversible anoxia.

3. Postural hypotension. The role of postural hypotension in the production of transient ischemic attacks has been overemphasized in the past. Nevertheless, the postural hypotension of Parkinson's disease, other degenerative diseases, syringomyelia, peripheral neuropathy, and idiopathic orthostatic hypotension may produce syncope resembling transient ischemic attacks.

4. Hypoglycemia. Hypoglycemia may be associated with transient neurologic deficits. The condition is not usually difficult to diagnose when the onset is sudden because of the prominence of autonomic symptoms. However, gradual development of hypoglycemia following an overdose of slow-release insulin preparations may produce clouding of consciousness and focal neurologic signs causing considerable difficulty in diagnosis.

5. Syncope. Fainting spells are not usually difficult to diagnose since they are frequently precipitated by a sudden stress. They may, however, occur with or without obvious precipitating factors in the presence of anemia or in debilitated persons and mimic a TIA.

6. Renal and hepatic failure. Transient clouding of consciousness is not unusual in established uremia and hepatic encephalopathy. The diagnosis is established by appropriate tests.

7. Electrolyte imbalance. Hyponatremia and hypokalemia may produce sudden neurologic deficits with clouding of consciousness and focal neurologic signs. There is considerable electrolyte imbalance in such cases.

8. Drugs. Alcohol, barbiturates, nonbarbiturate sleeping preparations, and tranquilizers may all produce nystagmus, slurring of speech, and clouding of consciousness of a temporary nature.

9. Migraine. The neurologic deficits accompanying certain migraine attacks (i.e., ophthalmoplegia, hemiplegia, aphasia, unilateral sensory loss, hemianopia, vertigo, dysarthria, and clouding of consciousness) may closely mimic transient ischemic attacks. The history of migraine and the accompanying headache usually clarifies the diagnosis. Migraine attacks occasionally occur with neurologic deficits and without subsequent headache. This situation may produce considerable difficulty in diagnosis.

10. Labyrinthian disorders. Middle-aged and elderly patients with acute onset of vertigo should receive a careful neurologic examination since many of them show additional signs of brain stem involvement indicating a transient ischemic attack and are erroneously diagnosed as labyrinthitis.

11. Ocular disturbances. Glaucoma, retinal vascular disease, and sudden changes in refraction in diabetic patients receiving insulin therapy may produce symptoms of transient blurring or dimness of vision and suggest cerebrovascular insufficiency.

12. Intracranial mass lesion. It is not unusual for intracranial mass lesions such as tumors, subdural hematomas, and cerebral abscesses to cause transient neurologic deficits suggesting transient ischemic attacks. The situation will be clarified as the patient is fully evaluated for either cerebrovascular disease or as a tumor suspect.

13. Psychiatric disorders. Transient impairment or loss of consciousness occurring in an emotionally disturbed individual with a conversion reaction may be mistaken for a transient ischemic attack. The lightheadedness and occasional syncope associated with hyperventilation in anxiety neurosis may also suggest transient impairment of cerebral circulation. In both cases a careful history will usually clarify the situation.

Treatment. Patients with TIAs are high-risk candidates for both cerebral infarction and myocardial infarction. Consequently, the treatment should include the following:

1. Any blood or metabolic abnormality identified in the evaluation process should be adequately treated.
2. Any cardiac abnormality identified in the evaluation process should be remedied.
3. Hypertension should be appropriately managed, but hypotensive episodes should be avoided. See page 147 for the management of hypertension.
4. Anticoagulants. There is no conclusive evidence that anticoagulants prevent the development of stroke in patients with TIA. Nevertheless, some physicians advise anticoagulants, particularly when patients are suffering repeated episodes of transient ischemia in a period of 24 to 48 hours. An MR or CT scan should be obtained to rule out intracranial bleeding followed by a partial thromboplastin time (PTT) and platelet count. If the results of PTT and platelet count are within normal limits, 5,000 units heparin intravenous (IV) bolus should be given followed by a slow mechanical infusion of 1,000 units

heparin each hour. The PTT should be repeated after four hours and the IV heparin dose adjusted according to results. If the patient shows signs of deterioration, intracranial bleeding should be considered. If bleeding occurs at any site, the infusion should be terminated. Effects of heparin can be reversed with protamine sulfate if necessary. In all cases the hemoglobin and hematocrit should be checked every 48 hours to detect occult bleeding. Once the patient stabilizes he or she should be converted to warfarin sodium (Coumadin). An initial dose of 40 mg q.d. should be given orally and the dose regulated according to daily prothrombin time (PT). When the PT is one and one-half times normal, the heparin should be discontinued and the Coumadin continued. Bleeding during Coumadin therapy can be controlled with vitamin K (phytonadione). The use of aspirin, phenylbutazone, and chloramphenicol should be avoided. Cholesterol embolization is occasionally enhanced by anticoagulation with warfarin when the drug interferes with plaque healing and showers of cholesteral emboli enter the circulation. Patients present with evidence of involvement of multiple cerebral arteries and there is a purple color on the palmar surfaces of the feet several weeks after the beginning of treatment. Other features include lividoreticularis, cyanosis, infarction of digits, fever, elevated sedimentation rate, evidence of visceral ischemia, and a rising creatinine. Diagnosis can be confirmed by the presence of retinal emboli or by skin biopsy. The syndrome has been seen in carotid and aortic surgery and cardiopulmonary bypass as well as anticoagulation.

5. Antiplatelet agents. Chronic use of acetylsalicylic acid (aspirin 325 mg) has been shown to reduce the incidence of stroke. Dipyridamole (Persantine) 50 mg t.i.d. has a significant antiaggregant effect on platelets. Ticlopidine 250 mg b.i.d. is an effective alternative and may be more effective in stroke prevention than aspirin (12).

6. Surgical treatment consisting of surgical excision of a cartoid plaque is controversial and studies have proved inconclusive or failed to prove effectiveness. If surgical complications of stroke and death can be kept below 3 percent it is possible that carotid endarterectomy is effective in symptomatic patients with severe ulceration of carotid plaques or high-grade stenosis (13, 14).

Prognosis. Many patients have had single or multiple episodes of transient ischemia before a stroke but fail to seek medical advice. Prospective studies of the natural history of TIA show differing figures for subsequent cerebral thrombosis depending on the age group, location, and race of the population studied.

The risk of stroke appears to be greatest in the first year following a TIA, and stroke tends to occur after a small number of TIAs with decreasing risk as the attacks continue. Between 10 and 25 percent of patients with TIA develop cerebral infarction within a year following the first TIA, and about 5 percent of patients per year each subsequent year. A TIA is a sign indicating a major risk of cerebral or brain stem infarction. Since vascular disease is not confined to one system, a TIA is a sign indicating a major risk of myocardial infarction.

Cerebral Infarction

Definition. Cerebral infarction occurs when there are ischemia and necrosis of an area of the brain following reduction of blood supply below the critical level necessary for cell survival.

Etiology. There are two major causes of cerebral infarction: thrombosis and embolism.

Thrombosis. The term "cerebral thrombosis" is only partially correct since infarction may result from thrombosis of the internal carotid or vertebral arteries as well as the cerebral arteries and their branches.

The majority of cases of cerebral infarction follow thrombosis of an atherosclerotic vessel. Consequently, cerebral thrombosis occurs in individuals who have one or more risk factors producing accelerated atherosclerosis (see page 134). Cerebral thrombosis also occurs as a complication of another disease, for example, arteritis affecting the cerebral (or cervical) arteries, or abnormalities of the blood and possibly following a critical fall in perfusion of the brain.

Cerebral Embolism. The commonest cause of cerebral embolism is a thrombotic embolus of the middle cerebral artery. Emboli originating in or passing through the heart have a much greater chance of entering the common carotid arteries than the vertebral arteries. An embolus in a common carotid artery tends to enter the internal carotid artery and pass into the middle cerebral artery, which is the largest branch and the anatomic continuation of the internal carotid artery. About 15 percent of all ischemic strokes and 30 percent of strokes in the elderly are associated with atrial fibrillation (15). In patients with atrial fibrillation embolism is more likely to occur at the onset of paroxysmal atrial fibrillation and within a year of the transition to chronic atrial fibrillation (16). The several causes of cerebral embolism are listed in Table 8–1.

Cerebral infarction will occur only when there is a critical reduction of blood flow to an area of the brain. The brain has a well-developed anastomotic system which affords considerable protection against reduction in blood flow, and there are no end arterial systems in the brain. The anastomotic potential begins with the arterial circle of Willis; in addition, the anterior, middle, and posterior cerebral arteries communicate with each other through numerous anastomotic connections. Infarction will occur only (a) when there is a failure of blood flow through a major vessel and (b) when there is a failure of flow through the anastomotic vessels supplying the ischemic area of the brain.

The site of infarction depends upon the effectiveness of anastomotic connections. For example, if there is gradual stenosis at the origin or an atherosclerotic middle cerebral artery with the development of adequate blood flow through anastomotic channels from the posterior or anterior cerebral circulations at the time of thrombosis of the middle cerebral artery, (a) infarction may not occur at all or (b) if infarction occurs, the infarct will be located close to the origin of the middle cerebral artery, which is at the edge of the area supplied by the anastomotic vessels. On the other hand, a sudden occlusion of a healthy middle cerebral artery might be followed by a large infarction in the middle cerebral artery territory because there has been no previous stimulation for the development of effective collateral circulation. Similarly, thrombosis of an atherosclerotic middle cerebral artery will be followed by major infarction if the anterior and posterior cerebral arteries are also atherosclerotic and incapable of supporting an adequate collateral circulation (see Figure 8–5).

Pathology. The earliest changes occur in neurons, which are more sensitive to hypoxia than glial cells. Neurons show Nissl degeneration and pyknosis which precede neuronal disintegration. This is followed by necrotic changes in astrocytic and white matter. The

TABLE 8–1. **Causes of Cerebral Embolism**

1. Cardiovascular sources of emboli
   a. Atherosclerotic plaques in major vessels supplying the brain
   b. Stumps of previously occluded vessels
   c. Trauma of neck vessels
   d. Aneurysm of ascending aorta
   e. Mural thrombus due to myocardial infarction, cardiac arrhythmias, postoperative heart surgery
   f. Valvular disease (i.e., rheumatic heart disease, prolapsed mitral valve, endocarditis)
   g. Congenital heart disease with right-to-left shunt
   h. Rarely, atrial myxoma, collagen disease, cardiomyopathies, endocardial fibrosis

2. Systemic sources of emboli
   a. Septic emboli from lung, abdomen, pelvis
   b. Fat emboli
   c. Air emboli
   d. Metastatic cells
   e. Foreign bodies

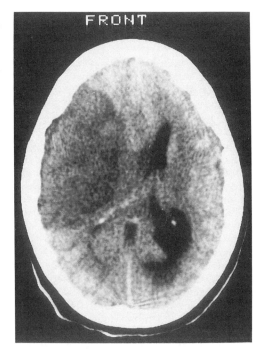

FIGURE 8–5. Acute cerebral infarction due to occlusion right middle cerebral artery. CT scan showing typical "trangular" appearance. There is marked right hemisphere edema and a right to left shift of the midline structures.

blood vessels penetrating the infarct are widely dilated, and the necrotic walls allow the passage of red cells into the infarcted area. This change is present to some extent in all cerebral infarcts but may be quite marked in some cases where there has been restoration of flow into damaged vessels, giving rise to a hemorrhagic infarction. The area surrounding the necrotic center of an infarct contains damaged but potentially viable neurons and glial cells. In the first 24 hours after infarction the blood vessels in this area contain polymorphonuclear cells, which migrate into the perivascular spaces and occasionally reach the subarachnoid space, producing a transient polymorphonuclear pleocytosis in the cerebrospinal fluid (CSF). The polymorphonuclears in the blood vessels are replaced by mononuclear cells, which migrate into the necrotic area of the infarct. Active phagocytosis of dead material proceeds over a period of several months. There are proliferation of astrocytes in the surrounding area and partial replacement of dead tissue by glia, but the center of an infarct often remains as a glial-lined cyst.

Clinical Features. Infarction of the brain in an area supplied by a cerebral artery tends to produce a clearly recognizable clinical syndrome. Each syndrome will be discussed separately.

Occlusion of the Internal Carotid Artery. The following features are characteristic of occlusion of the internal carotid artery:

1. Occlusion is preceded by transient ischemic attacks in about 50 percent of cases (see page 134).

2. Infarction usually occurs in the region of the brain supplied by the middle cerebral artery, producing contralateral signs including homonymous hemianopia, central type of facial paralysis, hemiparesis or hemiplegia, and hemisensory loss. Involvement of the dominant hemisphere produces dysphasia or aphasia, while involvement of frontal lobe produces deviation of the head and eyes toward the side of the infarction. Onset is usually followed by some impairment of the level of consciousness, which varies from drowsiness to coma, depending upon the degree of cerebral edema.

3. Occlusion of an internal carotid artery can be asymptomatic when the collateral circulation in the middle cerebral territory is adequate.

4. When the involved internal carotid artery supplies both anterior cerebral arteries,

the ipsilateral middle cerebral artery, and the posterior cerebral artery through the posterior communicating artery, an occlusion of the internal carotid artery may produce ischemia and infarction involving both frontal lobes and all of the hemisphere on the affected side. This usually results in severe cerebral edema, uncal herniation, brain stem compression, and death within a few days.

Occlusion of the Middle Cerebral Artery. Occlusion of the middle cerebral artery is characterized by the following:

1. Symptoms of occlusion of the middle cerebral artery are often indistinguishable from those of occlusion of the internal carotid artery. See above.

2. The commonest syndrome consists of the sudden onset of contralateral signs including homonymous hemianopia, central type of facial weakness, flaccid hemiparesis or hemiplegia, and hemisensory loss. The patient is dysphasic or aphasic if the dominant hemisphere is involved, and the head and eyes are often deviated toward the side of infarction and away from the side of weakness. The head and eye deviation usually resolves within a few days, and there is gradual improvement in the degree of weakness, which is much more apparent in the lower limb than in the upper limb. This improvement is associated with progressive spasticity, increased stretch reflexes, and an extensor plantar response on the affected side. The persistence of a homonymous hemianopia indicates a poor prognosis for recovery.

Occlusion of the Anterior Cerebral Artery. Involvement of the anterior cerebral artery may produce the following:

1. Occlusion of the recurrent branch (Heubner's artery) produces ischemia and infarction involving the anterior limb of the internal capsule and the anterior portion of the caudate nucleus and putamen. Involvement of these structures results in contralateral paralysis or paresis of the face and upper limb. There may be some rigidity or dystonia due to basal ganglia involvement.

2. Occlusion of distal cortical branches causes infarction of the paracentral lobule producing paralysis and sensory loss in the contralateral lower limb.

3. Complete occlusion of one anterior cerebral artery results in a combination of numbers 1 and 2 (i.e., contralateral hemiparesis and hemisensory loss). In addition, right-handed persons show dyspraxia of the left hand because of ischemia or infarction involving the corpus callosum.

4. Bilateral occlusion of the anterior cerebral arteries produces bilateral frontal lobe ischemia. There may be minimal limb weakness in survivors, but patients who are fully conscious show a remarkable apathy. There is an apparent indifference to surrounding activity and no interest in food, but the affected individual will chew and swallow if fed. This state is associated with lack of discrimination and acceptance of any material as food if it is fed to the patient. Language is intact, but it is extremely difficult to hold a conversation because of lack of motivation. The speech is monotonous and slowed. Patients with this condition are incontinent of bowel and bladder due to bilateral involvement of sphincter control centers lying on the medial aspect of the frontal lobes. This incontinence is a "neglect" situation, and the patient shows complete indifference to bladder emptying or bowel movement.

Occlusion of the Anterior Choroidal Artery. Occlusion of the anterior choroidal artery can cause infarction of the posterior limb of the internal capsule, thalamus, midbrain, temporal lobe, or lateral geniculate body depending upon the territory supplied by the vessel (17). The features follow:

1. The commonest sign is hemiplegia.
2. Hemisensory loss is usually transient.
3. Field defects including a homonymous upper quadrantinopia, hemianopia, or upper and lower quadrantinopia sparing a horizontal meridian. The latter indicates involvement of the lateral geniculate body.

Occlusion of the Posterior Cerebral Artery. Posterior cerebral artery occlusion may produce the following:

1. Occlusion of penetrating branches to the midbrain results in ischemia or infarction involving the cerebral peduncle, the third nerve, and the red nucleus. This produces contralateral hemiparesis; ipsilateral or contralateral cerebellar ataxia and tremor due to ischemia of the red nucleus, or involvement of fibers passing from the cerebellum to the ipsilateral or contralateral red nucleus; and ipsilateral third nerve paralysis.

2. Occlusion of penetrating branches to the subthalamic nucleus results in a contralateral ballism (hemiballismus) with involuntary flinging movements of the affected limb and severe hemiataxia.

3. Occlusion of the thalamostriate branches produces infarction of the posteriolateral ventral nucleus of the thalamus (see Figure 8–6). This results in severe contralateral sensory loss. The symptoms vary from

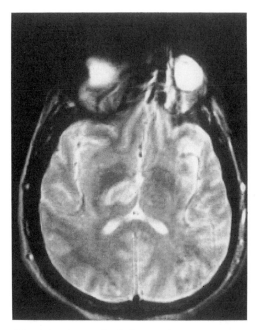

FIGURE 8–6.   Right thalamic infarct. MR scan T2 weighted image with a well circumscribed area of increased signal density in the region of the right thalamus.

sensory loss affecting the hand (useless hand syndrome) to complete hemisensory involvement (sensory stroke). The hemisensory loss is sometimes accompanied by a mild hemiparesis due to involvement of the internal capsule. This usually resolves with some residual spasticity and increased reflexes. After several months the affected limbs and trunk show some return of sensory function, sometimes accompanied by a severe burning pain, which is accentuated by mildly painful stimuli or even contact with clothing in extreme cases. This condition, the thalamic syndrome, is extremely distressing and debilitating.

4. Bilateral occlusion of the thalamostriate arteries can occasionally arise from occlusion of a single trunk of one posterior cerebral artery or from a basilar artery, which supplies all of the thalamus striate arteries, resulting in bilateral paramedian thalami infarction. The onset is sudden with somnolence or loss of consciousness followed by apathy, persistent amnesia resembling Korsakoff's syndrome, dementia, lack of spontaneity, slowness of thought, poor insight, confabulation, perseveration, dysgraphia, and impairment of downward gaze (18).

5. Occlusion of the distal branches that supply the occipital lobe results in a contralateral homonymous hemianopia (see Figure 8–7). Cortical blindness results if both posterior cerebral arteries are involved (19). Right-handed individuals with left occipital lobe infarction may show alexia without agraphia (inability to read with preservation of writing). This syndrome is the result of ischemia to the posterior portion of the corpus callosum, preventing the transfer of information from the surviving right occipital lobe for interpretation in the left hemisphere. Depression and obsessive thinking, anomia, and color anomia are features of dominant hemisphere infarction, and visual perseverating and metamorphosis may occur (20). Headache is not uncommon in posterior cerebral artery occlusion. Visual hallucinations including complex hallucinations are well recognized in posterior cerebral infarction (21,22).

6. Occlusion of the main trunk of the posterior cerebral artery is often sudden, suggesting an embolic cause. Signs consist of a homonymous hemianopia associated with one or more of the following: hemisensory loss, hemiparesis, dyslexia, unsteady gait, poor hand coordination, confusion, and poor memory when the hypocampal area of the dominant hemisphere is involved. It is not unusual to find a contralateral homonymous hemianopia without any other signs of neurologic deficit in complete occlusion of the posterior cerebral artery.

Occlusion of the Vertebral Artery. The following are characteristic of occlusion of the vertebral artery:

1. Occlusion of one vertebral artery may be asymptomatic because of adequate collateral circulation unless the opposite vertebral artery is small or severely atherosclerotic.

2. Vertebral artery occlusion may result in a small infarction in the medulla or pons when the collateral circulation is poor or when there is marked atherosclerosis of the basilar artery or its penetrating branches. This type of stroke is sudden in onset with the development of a number of possible symptoms including ataxia, diplopia, facial weakness, vertigo, dysarthria, dysphonia, and dysphagia. Many patients make a good recovery over a period of weeks or months.

3. Thrombosis of the fourth portion of the vertebral artery may present with symptoms of posterior inferior cerebellar artery thrombosis (see below).

4. Occlusion of a vertebral artery is occasionally followed by symptoms suggesting basilar artery thrombosis (see below).

Occlusion of the Posterior Inferior Cerebellar Artery (Lateral Medullary Infarction). This artery supplies the lateral portion of the medulla, the inferior surface of the cerebellum, and arterial occlusion may be followed by infarction in any portion or all of this region.

The onset is acute with intense vertigo due to involvement of the inferior vestibular nucleus and vomiting because of vestigulovagal and vestibulosympathetic stimulation. At the same time there may be complaints of unilateral facial pain or paresthesias due to irritation of the spinal tract of the fifth cranial nerve. These early symptoms tend to subside, but the patient is left with several deficits including:

a. Involvement of the nucleus ambiguous or the tenth nerve transversing the medulla results in an ipsilateral paralysis of the palate, larynx, and pharynx producing dysarthria, dysphonia, and dysphagia.

b. Infarction of the inferior cerebellar peduncle and/or cerebellum results in nys-

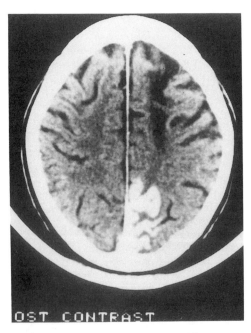

FIGURE 8–7. CT scan post-contrast showing enhancement of the gyri (gray matter enhancement) in the left occipital area compatible with recent infarction. There is an old infarct in the left frontal lobe.

tagmus, which is maximal on looking toward the side of the lesion, and an ipsilateral cerebellar ataxia.

c. Involvement of the descending sympathetic fibers in the medullary reticular formation usually causes a partial rather than a complete Horner syndrome with miosis and ptosis on the side of the lesion.

d. Infarction of the lateral spinothalamic tract produces a contralateral loss of pain and temperature sensation involving the limbs and trunk.

e. Involvement of the spinal tract of the fifth nerve results in an ipsilateral loss of pain and temperature sensation involving the face.

f. Inconsistent signs including mild ipsilateral facial weakness and mild contralateral hemiparesis are occasionally seen when the ischemia spreads beyond the usual boundaries of the lateral medullary infarct.

Occlusion of the Basilar Artery and Its Branches. This may produce the following:

1. Emboli arising from atheromatous plaques in the basilar artery (or vertebral artery) enter distal branches of the basilar artery and may give rise to single or multiple small strokes in the midbrain thalamus or occipital lobes. See "Occlusion of the Posterior Cerebral Artery" (p. 143).

2. Thrombosis of a small penetrating artery entering the pons produces a paramedian infarction in the brachium pontis with involvement of the corticobulbar and corticospinal trans, pontine nuclei, descending sympathetic fibers, and the fibers passing to the middle cerebellar peduncle. This results in contralateral hemiparesis, ipsilateral cerebellar signs, and a partial Horner's syndrome. Repeated thrombosis involving penetrating arteries on both sides of the midline results in accumulating neurologic deficits and eventually severe dysarthria, dysphagia, and quadriparesis.

3. Thrombosis of the short circumferential arches arising from the basilar artery results in infarction of the lateral or tegmental area of the pons.

a. Infarction in the lateral portion of the pons involves the root of the fifth cranial nerve, the medial lemniscus, and the middle cerebellar peduncle with involvement of the fibers in the corticospinal tract subserving the lower extremity. This results in an ipsilateral sensory loss over the face, cerebellar signs, and Horner's syndrome with contralateral hemiparesis with greater weakness and loss of vibration and position sense in the lower extremity.

b. An infarct in the tegmental area of the pons and the fifth, sixth, and seventh cranial nerves may produce ipsilateral loss of sensation over the face, facial weakness, and diplopia. There may also be some involvement of the medial longitudinal fasciculus and superior cerebellar peduncle. This will result in an internuclear ophthalmoplegia and ipsilateral cerebellar signs.

4. Complete thrombosis of the basilar artery is usually a catastrophic affair with rapid onset of coma and a high mortality. Survivors show signs of bilateral brain stem involvement including quadriparesis which may persist with return of consciousness, a condition aptly termed the locked-in syndrome (see page 155). This may be coupled with signs of occipital lobe infarction producing severe impairment of vision or permanent cortical blindness. Recovery may occur over a period of several months and is quite good in some survivors, while others show severe neurologic deficits including multiple bilateral cranial nerve involvement, impairment of ocular movements, nystagmus, loss of sensation over the face, facial paralysis, dysarthria, and dysphagia. Bilateral corticospinal tract involvement results in spastic quadriparesis. Involvement of the lateral spinothalamic tracts and medial lemnisci results in severe bilateral sensory loss. Pulmonary complications are the leading cause of death (23).

Occlusion of the Superior Cerebellar Artery. This artery supplies the midbrain, the superior cerebellar peduncle, and the superior surface of the cerebellum (see Figure 8–8). Infarction produces signs of ipsilateral or contralateral rubral tremor or myoclonus. This is a Horner's syndrome on the side of the lesion, and involvement of the spinothalamic tracts results in contralateral loss of pain and temperature sensation.

Occlusion of the Terminal Portion of the Basilar Artery. This condition usually results from embolism and has been termed "saddle embolism." This can occur by embolism arising from a mural thrombus following a myocardial infarction. Saddle embolism can occur in any cardiac condition associated with thrombosis including rheumatic heart disease, subacute bacterial endocarditis, and prolapsed mitral valve. Emboli occasionally arise more distally at the origin of the vertebral arteries in atherosclerotic individuals.

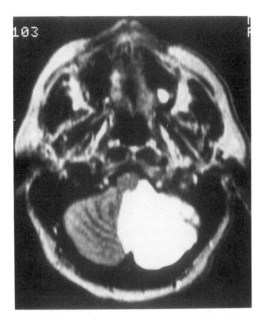

FIGURE 8–8. Cerebellar infarction. MR scan T2 weighted image showing increased signal in the left cerebellar hemisphere which is swollen and exerting pressure on the opposite hemisphere and brain stem.

Saddle embolus produces occlusion of both posterior cerebral arteries and, if extensive, will also produce occlusion of both superior cerebellar arteries.

Symptoms include cortical blindness due to involvement and infarction of both occipital lobes. It is not infrequent to find some sparing of small areas in the occipital lobes with visual field constriction and unusual visual field patterns such as altitudinal hemianopia. Occasionally there is extensive damage to the visual association areas in which patients develop anosognosia or denial of blindness (Anton's syndrome). These patients, although totally blind, will describe situations visually and supply answers to questions that require vision.

The Lacunar Syndrome. This condition is associated with small areas of infarction deep in the cerebral tissues or pons resulting from occlusion of a single perforating artery. Such cases occur in a 55 years old and older population and constitute 13 to 23 percent of all cerebral infarcts (24).

Four clinical syndromes can be recognized.

1. Pure motor stroke. A unilateral pure motor deficit affecting the face, or upper and lower limbs, or at least two of these areas

without any other demonstrable deficit. This is the most common presenting complaint in the Lacunar syndrome (25).

2. Pure sensory stroke. As above, with sensory rather than motor symptoms.

3. Sensory-motor stroke. A combination of numbers 1 and 2 above.

4. Ataxic hemiparesis. A combination of ipsilateral corticospinal and cerebellar dysfunction without other features localized to the posterior circulation. This includes the dysarthria/clumsy hand syndrome. Mortality is low, but recurrence of 12 percent in one year can be expected. Death occurs from complications of immobility such as pneumonia and pulmonary embolism or from heart disease.

Diagnostic Procedures. All patients should receive full evaluation for diseases of the blood vessels, abnormalities of the blood constituents, and reduced cerebral perfusion. These investigations have been outlined in the diagnostic procedures for transient ischemic attacks (see page 134). Future development of MRI, positron emission tomography (PET), and single photon emission computerized tomography (SPECT) will refine the location and extent of damaged cerebral tissue and may permit early identification of narrowed or occluded arteries.

Treatment of the Comatose Patient

1. Respiratory care. The airway should be established and maintained. Comatose patients require insertion of a short airway. There should be no hesitation in passing a low-pressure cuffed endotracheal tube if pharyngeal secretions are excessive and impede respiratory exchange.

All patients should be suctioned freuqently to clear the airway. This may be aided by turning the patient every two hours from right lateral to supine to left lateral positions. The drainage of pulmonary secretions into the pahrynx for suctioning is facilitated by elevating the foot of the bed. The chest should be examined frequently by auscultation, and suspected atelectasis or pneumonia confirmed by x-ray. Any infection should be treated promptly with antibiotics, and culture of secretions should be obtained for identification of organisms and sensitivity to antibiotics. The importance of respiratory care cannot be overemphasized particularly in those who are immobilized for long periods of time such as patients with "the locked in" syndrome (23).

2. Management of hypertension. Many patients are hypertensive on admission to the

hospital, but the hypertension resolves rapidly with rest, catheterization of a distended bladder, and removal of any impediment to respiratory exchange.

Those patients who show sustained severe hypertension, diastolic pressure above 140 mmHg, require urgent treatment using nitroprusside (Nipride) 10 μg/kg per minute IV. Nitroprusside should be given with the patient lying flat in bed, and any hypotension can be immediately controlled by elevating the foot of the bed. When the control of the hypertension is a less urgent requirement, that is, systolic pressure above 230 mmHg, diastolic pressure below 140 mmHg, an intravenous injection of labetalol 20 mg over two minutes should be given. This may be repeated every 20 minutes until a satisfactory reduction of blood pressure occurs.

Hypertension less than 200 mmHg systolic may be controlled by the use of diuretic agents such as furosemide (Lasix) 40 to 80 mg IV or IM or by oral labetalol beginning with 100 mg b.i.d. and increasing to 400 mg b.i.d. if necessary, or nifedipine 10 mg q6h. In a comatose patient, normotensive readings may be maintained by IV labetalol.

Comatose patients occasionally become hypotensive because of excessive use of antihypertensive agents or other drugs. There is usually a prompt response to a fluid challenge. Vasoactive agents such as dopamine (Isotropin) or isoproterenol may be required. When the response is poor, the failure to respond may be due to adrenal insufficiency. Therefore, all patients who fail to respond to pressor agents should receive intravenous corticosteroids such as hydrocortisone 100 mg q8h.

3. Care of the heart. An electrocardiogram should be obtained on admission and consultation requested for a cardiologist or internist if there is any electrocardiographic abnormality, congestive failure, or persistent arrhythmia. Acute myocardial infarction is not unusual in patients with acute cerebral infarction and many others suffer from arteriosclerotic heart disease.

4. Care of the bladder. The comatose patient frequently fails to empty the bladder, which becomes distended, and this situation may contribute to excessive rise in blood pressure. All comatose patients should be catheterized, and an indwelling catheter should be inserted. The risk of infection is high, and the bladder should be irrigated with an antiseptic solution or an antibiotic solution such as a polymyxin-neomycin mix-

ture, consisting of neomycin 100 mg, polymyxin 25 mg, and 1,000 ml of normal saline. Irrigation should be carried out with 250 ml every six hours.

Some comatose patients require prolonged catheterization. The catheter should be clamped and drained every two hours to prevent bladder contraction. As soon as the patient is conscious, an effort should be made to remove the bladder catheter, because the unnecessary use of bladder catheters leads to increased infections of the bladder, ureter, and kidneys, and also increases difficulty in regaining sphincter control.

5. Care of skin and joints. The comatose patient has a tendency to develop decubiti over the pressure points. This can be minimized by turning the patient every two hours as indicated above under number 1, "Respiratory Care." Pressure areas should be protected with suitable lambskin or soft plastic appliances. This applies particularly to the heels and the sacral areas. Any reddening of the skin should be treated promptly with removal of all pressure and application of tincture of benzoin. Patients with hemiparesis or quadriparesis develop ankylosis of joints in a few days unless these joints are moved through a full range of motion passively several times a day. The tendency to ankylosis is most apparent in the shoulder joints but can involve other joints, particularly when the limb is totally paralyzed. Thus, paralyzed or severely paretic limbs should be supported in the position of function. In the lower limb this entails maintaining the limb in a neutral position and the prevention of external rotation by the use of sandbags against the thigh. The foot should be placed in a functional position at the right angle to the ankle and maintained in that position with a suitable splint. This splint should be padded to protect the heels from pressure. As spasticity develops, the knee should be slightly flexed over a pillow and the knees should be separated by another pillow to prevent contact due to adductor spasticity. The upper limbs should be placed in a position of function with the arm slightly abducted and a pillow placed in the axilla to prevent adduction. The forearm and elbow should be placed on a pillow with the hand elevated above the elbow and the elbow elevated higher than the shoulder. This prevents the development of edema. The hand should be slightly extended at the wrist and the fingers should be placed around a handroll in a position of function. These positions should be maintained until the patient re-

gains consciousness and begins to move the affected limbs, at which time a graded program of physical therapy should be instituted.

6. Deep vein thrombosis and the accompanying risk of pulmonary thromboembolism warrant the use of subcutaneous heparin 5,000 units q8h.

7. Water and electrolyte balance. Comatose patients require intravenous fluids for at least 24 hours. Every effort should be made to make up water deficits, and if intravenous fluids are continued the average adult usually requires 3,000 ml per day. If electrolytes are normal, this should be given in a 5 percent solution of glucose with 0.3 N saline. Twenty mEq of potassium should be added to each 1,000 ml of fluid once satisfactory urinary output is established. Adequate intake and output records must be kept, and electrolytes should be measured every 24 hours. A nasogastric tube should be passed during the first two or three days, and the fluids should be given through the tube for a 24-hour period. This minimizes the risk of aspiration. After 24 hours a liquid diet can be given through the nasogastric tube. This is usually given in divided amounts to a total of 2,000 ml over 24 hours with an additional 1,000 ml of water again in divided amounts every two hours. Nasogastric feedings can be slowly discontinued as the patient recovers consciousness and begins to swallow. Finally, the tube should be removed when the patient can take sufficient nourishment and fluid by mouth. At that time attention should be given to supplementing the bulk of the diet to prevent the development of fecal impaction.

8. Acute infarction in conscious patients. During the first few days following a stroke conscious patients are often seriously ill and require care similar to that for comatose patients. Equal stress should be placed on the prevention of pulmonary or bladder infections and adequate attention to water and electrolyte balance. Conscious patients should be ambulated as soon as possible and placed in a program of physical therapy.

9. Treatment of cerebral edema in acute cerebral infarction. Patients with acute infarction develop cerebral edema. If the infarction is large, the addition of edema may lead to an increase in intracranial pressure. This will result in a decrease in the level of consciousness in the conscious patient and an increase in the level of stupor or coma in the unconscious patient with the development of signs of brain stem compression (see page 50). Every effort should be made to reduce cerebral edema in this situation, and the pa-

tient can be treated intravenously with hyperosmolar solutions such as mannitol, or glycerol orally (see page 55).

10. Cerebral embolism with infarction should be treated with anticoagulation beginning with IV heparin. This may be followed by long-term anticoagulation if indicated using warfarin sodium and maintaining the prothrombin time one and a half times normal control. Chronic anticoagulation is particularly important in rheumatic or nonrheumatic atrial fibrillation (26). The risk of converting an ischemic infarction into a hemorrhagic infarction is small (27) and is outweighed by the reduction in risk of further cerebral embolism obtained through anticoagulation.

11. Anticoagulants do not appear to be of benefit in the treatment of cerebral infarction of nonembolic origin (28).

12. Poststroke depression of a significant degree occurs in about 50 percent of patients. This debilitating problem may hinder physical therapy and rehabilitation (29). Appropriate antidepressant therapy and referral for psychotherapy should be obtained at an early stage.

13. Local intraarterial fibrinolytic therapy using an intraarterial infusion of urokinase or streptokinase delivered through an intraarterial catheter may lead to recanalization of an occluded artery and have some benefit if the technique is employed at an early stage following occlusion and infarction (30, 31).

14. Nimodipine 30 to 60 mg q6h may be effective in reducing mortality and morbidity in acute ischemic cerebral infarction if begun within 24 hours of onset of symptoms (32).

Prognosis. Survivors of cerebral infarction run a high risk of a second stroke or myocardial infarction, and approximately 50 percent of patients who have had cerebral infarction die from a subsequent myocardial infarction. In addition to age, the major risk factors, including hypertension, diabetes mellitus, and preexisting cardiovascular disease, are related to increased mortality in a patient who has had a stroke.

CEREBROVASCULAR CAUSES OF DEMENTIA

Multiinfarct Dementia

Definition. Multiinfarct dementia is an irregularly progressive dementia caused by repeated infarction.

Etiology and Pathology. Multiinfarct dementia, also called atherosclerotic or arteriosclerotic dementia, occurs in hypertensive and diabetic individuals who develop repeated infarcts in the cerebral hemispheres and brain stem. The basic pathology involves occlusion of multiple vessels in the brain resulting in the development of multiple infarctions (see Figure 8–9).

Clinical Features. There is a widespread misconception that all dementia in the elderly is the result of atherosclerosis. The most common causes of dementia in middle-aged and elderly people are Alzheimer's disease and multiinfarct dementia. Since the development of infarction is irregular, the symptoms show an irregular progression. Patients with multiinfarct dementia develop a stepwise intellectual deterioration, including impairment of judgment and lack of insight; impairment of memory; changes in personality, including irritability and apathy; and depression, the latter being more prevalent in multiinfarct dementia than Alzheimer's disease (33). Hemiparesis, ataxia of gait, pseudobulbar crying, dysarthria, dysphagia, increased deep tendon reflexes, extensor plantar responses, blepharospasm, impersistence of gaze, sucking and rooting reflexes, and grasp reflexes also develop in a progressive stepwise fashion.

Diagnostic Procedures. Diagnostic procedures should be performed to identify those factors which contribute to accelerated atherosclerosis. Patients should be fully investigated as outlined under "Transient Ischemic Attacks" (see page 134).

Treatment. Hypertension and smoking should be rigidly controlled, and any metabolic and cardiac abnormalities should be corrected. Improvement in cerebral blood flow may be associated with improvement in cognition in multiinfarct dementia (34).

Prognosis. Many patients die from myocardial infarction, while others die from a massive cerebral or brain stem infarction. The survivors show progression of the dementia and neurologic deficits and die from intercurrent infection once they are reduced to a bedridden state.

Binswanger's Disease (Subcortical Arteriosclerotic Encephalopathy)

Binswanger's disease is a form of dementia of presumed vascular etiology characterized by arteriosclerotic changes in the long penetrating vessels supplying the central white matter of the cerebral hemispheres. There is diffuse white matter loss with relative preservation of the cortex. The diagnosis is usually established by autopsy. Binswanger's disease occurs in both sexes with onset between 50 and 65 years of age. The clinical picture is characterized by a history of hypertension, systemic vascular disease, and the irregular occurrence of focal neurologic signs and symptoms over weeks or months. The disease may be quiescent for long periods of time. The gradual accumulation of neurologic deficits leads to prominent motor signs with spasticity and quadriparesis and the development of pseudobulbar palsy. MRI and CT scans show the presence of a characteristic leukoencephalopathy and hydrocephalus (35). Treatment should be directed to the control of hypertension.

Hypertensive Encephalopathy

Definition. Hypertensive encephalopathy is a syndrome characterized by marked elevation of blood pressure and evidence of increased intracranial pressure.

Etiology and Pathology. Most patients with hypertensive encephalopathy have a long history of essential hypertension. In other cases the elevation of blood pressure is

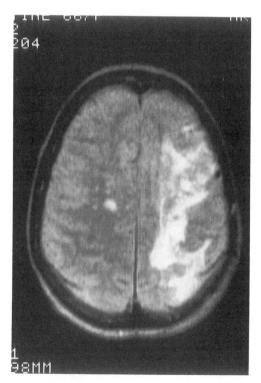

FIGURE 8–9.   MR scan showing increased signal within the left hemisphere compatible with gliosis secondary to a previous infarction. There is a white matter infarct present in the right hemisphere.

secondary to another disease process, such as acute glomerulonephritis, chronic nephritis, pheochromocytoma, Cushing's disease, or acute toxemia of pregnancy.

There is diffuse cerebral edema, and cerebral vasospasm may be present. Microscopic examination reveals petechial hemorrhages and fibrinoid necrosis of the arteries.

Clinical Features. The patient complains of severe headache with nausea and vomiting. Visual disturbances including blurring of vision and scotomata frequently occur. Confusion with progression to stupor, convulsions, and coma is seen in untreated cases. Examination of the fundi reveals papilledema and hypertensive retinal changes. Focal neurologic signs are not characteristic but may be seen as a postictal phenomenon or when intracranial hemorrhage occurs.

Diagnostic Procedures. Computed tomography reveals diffuse cerebral edema.

Treatment. Hypertensive encephalopathy is a medical emergency, and the blood pressure should be reduced as rapidly and safely as possible (page 147).

Prognosis. Untreated hypertensive encephalopathy is fatal. Follow-up care and appropriate long-term medication allow many patients to survive many years.

CEREBRAL ARTERITIS

A number of rare conditions produce inflammation of the cerebral arteries and may lead to thrombosis and infarction. The arteritides include syphilitic arteritis (see page 267); polyarteritis nodosa; systemic lupus erythematosus; giant cell arteritis; and thrombotic thrombocytopenic purpura. Both heparin and cocaine abuse may result in cerebral infarction caused by vasculitis in some cases (36).

Polyarteritis Nodosa

Definition. Polyarteritis nodosa is an inflammatory arteritis of unknown etiology affecting small- and medium-size arteries.

Etiology and Pathology. The etiology is unknown. Pathologic changes consist of inflammation involving all layers of the arterial wall with areas of necrosis and occasional aneurysm formation. Developing and healing lesions may coexist in affected vessels, and thrombosis is not unusual.

Clinical Features. Polyarteritis nodosa is commoner in males, with a male-to-female ratio of 3:1. The condition can present in many ways. Systemic signs and symptoms include fever, weakness, weight loss, arthral-gia, myalgia, and muscle cramps. Abdominal pain is not unusual and may indicate mesenteric thrombosis or pancreatic involvement. Peptic ulceration with hematemesis or melena may occur. Testicular pain is a common complaint in the male. Liver involvement is indicated by hepatic enlargement and jaundice. Skin lesions include erythema, purpura, and ulcers; livedo reticularis is quite common. Coronary artery involvement may lead to myocardial infarction. Pleuritic pain and pneumonia may be recurrent complaints.

Neurologic complications include a symmetric peripheral neuropathy in about 25 percent of cases due to involvement of the vasa nervorum. Mononeuropathies and mononeuritis multiplex may occur. Cerebral symptoms are rare and include cerebral infarction with hemiparesis and aphasia; intracerebral hemorrhage; seizures; cranial nerve palsies, particularly involving the eighth nerve with hearing loss; and subarachnoid hemorrhage. Spinal cord involvement may produce a transverse myelitis or an anterior spinal artery occlusion (see page 183).

Diagnostic Procedures. Diagnostic procedures include:

1. Complete blood count. The white blood count is usually elevated between 10 and 25,000/cu mm and there may be an eosinophilia.
2. The sedimentation rate is elevated.
3. A high proportion of cases show the presence of aneurysms on the renal arteries, which can be demonstrated by arteriography.
4. The diagnosis can be established my muscle biopsy and/or sural nerve biopsy.

Treatment. The disorder can be suppressed by corticosteroids beginning with prednisone 80 mg q.d. and converting to alternate day therapy when symptoms subside. The treatment may have to be continued for many months or years on an alternate day basis on the minimal amount of steroids to keep the patient symptom-free and the sedimentation rate normal.

Prognosis. Approximately 50 percent of cases are alive after five years of steroid therapy.

Systemic Lupus Erythematosus

Definition. Systemic lupus erythematosus (SLE) is a multisystem autoimmune disease in which antibodies against many cellular constituents including DNA nuclear protein and mitochrondria are formed.

Etiology and Pathology. The cause is unknown. There appears to be hereditary susceptibility to SLE; there is more than a chance association between SLE and specific human leukocyte antigens (HLA). There has been recent interest in a viral etiology following the isolation of certain viruses in patients with SLE. The development of numerous autoimmune antibodies in this disease suggests that there is a basic defect in the autoimmune system, probably in the T-lymphocyte population. The disease has been related to the use of certain drugs, including hydralazine, procainamide, phenytoin, reserpine, and isoniazid. It is probable that these drugs produce some change in the immune system.

The essential pathologic change consists of a vasculitis with necrosis and a deposition of fibrinoid material within vessel walls. The fibrinoid deposits contain immunoglobulins, DNA, fibrinogen, and the third component of complement (C_3). The deposition of this material in the subendothelial tissues produces narrowing of the vessel lumen and thrombosis in some cases. Affected vessels show perivascular lymphocytic infiltration.

Clinical Features. SLE is commoner in women than men, with a ratio of 9:1, and occurs predominantly in the 20- to 40-year-old age group. Patients with SLE usually have a number of the following signs: facial erythema, discoid lupus rash, Raynaud's phenomenon, alopecia, photosensitivity, oral or nasopharyngeal ulceration, recurrent arthritis without deformity, the presence of LE cells in the peripheral blood, a chronic false-positive serologic test for syphilis, proteinuria of more than 3.5 g/day, cellular casts in the urine, recurrent pleuritis or pericarditis, recurrent psychosis and convulsions, and the presence of leukopenia, hemolytic anemia, or thrombocytopenia.

Neurologic manifestations of SLE include seizures, progressive dementia, and intermittent psychosis including delusions, hallucinations, and paranoia. Episodic clouding of consciousness may occur, and the patient may develop focal neurologic signs including hemiparesis and aphasia secondary to cerebral infarction. Intracranial hemorrhage and subarachnoid hemorrhage have been reported. Brain stem involvement produces nystagmus, vertigo, and cerebellar ataxia. Chorea is not unusual in younger patients. Visual loss can occur from involvement of the optic nerve producing central scotoma or homonymous hemianopia when there is involvement of the optic pathways. Some patients show cortical blindness. Spinal cord involvement produces transverse myelitis (37). Peripheral neuropathy is a feature of SLE, and myopathy has been described. The multisystem involvement of the central nervous system (CNS) and the relapsing, remitting course frequently leads to consideration of multiple sclerosis (38).

Diagnostic Procedures.

1. Lumbar puncture. There is a pleocytosis with elevated protein content in patients with aseptic meningitis secondary to SLE. Red blood cells are present in subarachnoid hemorrhage and intracranial hemorrhage.

2. The complete blood count may show the presence of anemia, leukopenia, and thrombocytopenia.

3. The peripheral blood smear may show the presence of LE cells.

4. The diagnosis can be established by the demonstration of antinuclear antibodies in titers greater than 1:64 and there may be a false positive VDRL test result. Anticardiolipin antibodies are present in more than 50 percent of cases.

5. There may be evidence of a hypercoagulable state with decreased fibrinolysis, decreased plasminogen activation, and decreased tissue plasminogen activation.

6. Lupus anticoagulant may be present particularly in cases with systemic thrombosis.

7. Electroencephalography. The electroencephalogram (EEG) will be abnormal in patients with cerebral involvement including seizure discharges or focal slowing in the presence of infarction.

8. MRI and CT scan. The CT scan reveals cerebral infarction, intracerebral hemorrhage, or the gradual development of cerebral atrophy on serial studies. The MRI may also show white matter lesions which resemble findings in multiple sclerosis.

9. The complement level is often reduced in SLE.

Treatment. The use of high doses of corticosteroids has been equivocal in treatment of SLE. The occurrence of psychosis and myopathy has been attributed to the use of steroids rather than the disease in some cases. Purine antagonists, for example, azathioprine (Imuran); or alkylating agents, for example, cyclophosphamide (Cytoxan), chlorambucil (Leukeran), or cyclosporine, may be effective in refractory cases with life-threatening disease. Anticoagulants have been advised on cases with cerebral infarction and a hypercoagulable state (39).

Prognosis. Approximately 70 percent of patients with SLE are alive at five years and 60 percent at 10 years after the onset of the disease. Death is usually due to renal failure.

Giant Cell Arteritis

Definition. Giant cell arteritis is an inflammatory disease of blood vessels characterized by the presence of an inflammatory exudate including giant cells involving all layers of the vessel wall.

Etiology and Pathology. The etiology is unknown. Pathologic changes consist of internal proliferation with obliteration of the vascular lumen, an inflammation of all layers of the vessel wall, and the presence of typical giant cells. The inflammatory exudate contains lymphocytes, eosinophils, and polymorphonuclear cells. In chronic cases the larger vessels may show the presence of concentric fibrosis.

Clinical Features. Three distinct entities constitute the syndrome of giant cell arteritis: polymyalgia rheumatica, temporal arteritis, and aortic arch syndrome (Takayasu's disease, pulseless disease).

Polymyalgia rheumatica may precede the development of other forms of giant cell arteritis by many years. The condition consists of fluctuating episodes of muscle and joint pains associated with proximal muscle weakness, malaise, nausea, low-grade fever, and weight loss of many years' duration. The condition often disappears four to eight years after onset even if untreated.

Temporal arteritis occurs in elderly patients who usually develop unilateral headache in the supraorbital region associated with tenderness in the distribution of the superficial temporal artery. However, the headache of temporal arteritis may be generalized or occur in any part of the head (40). Intermittent claudication of the jaw muscles when chewing is virtually pathognomonic. Temporal arteritis should be considered in every elderly individual who begins to complain of headache. Sudden visual loss proceeding to blindness may occur in 50 percent of cases (see Figure 8–10). Alopecia and blanching of the tongue are frequent concomitants. Patients show signs of systemic disease with fever, arthralgias, and weight loss.

The aortic arch syndrome is a chronic form of giant cell arteritis in which there is progressive narrowing and occlusion of the major branches of the aorta. This may present with transient ischemic attacks, subclavian steal syndrome, angina, or aortic insufficiency. Hypertension may be secondary to stenosis of the renal arteries.

Diagnostic Procedures.

1. The complete blood count shows elevation of the white blood cell count.
2. The sedimentation rate is usually elevated but may be normal in about 5 percent of cases (41).
3. The diagnosis can be established by biopsy of the superficial temporal artery in the case of temporal arteritis.

Treatment. The condition responds well to corticosteroids. The patient should be started on 80 mg of prednisone q.d. and converted to alternate day therapy as symptoms subside. The dosage can then be reduced to the dosage that keeps the patient symptom-free with a normal sedimentation rate. This dosage may have to be continued for many years.

Prognosis. Polymyalgia rheumatica responds rapidly to prednisone 10 to 20 mg per day but frequently disappears even without treatment. Temporal arteritis can be adequately controlled with corticosteroid therapy; 50 percent of patients lose their sight in one or both eyes if untreated. The aortic arch syndrome may require reconstructive surgery but often continues to progress, with death from myocardial infarction or cerebral infarction.

Thrombotic Thrombocytopenic Purpura

Definition. Thrombotic thrombocytopenic purpura is a rare condition with the formation of multiple platelet thrombi in the brain and other organs.

Etiology and Pathology. The etiology is unknown. The condition may be a variant of SLE.

Pathologic changes consist of fibrinoid degeneration of subintimal collagen in the smaller blood vessels of the brain and other organs. The brain shows the presence of numerous small infarcts. The blood vessels are occluded by platelet thrombi.

Clinical Features. The disease occurs primarily in younger adults. Systemic symptoms consist of fever and weight loss associated with purpura, hemolytic anemia, thrombocytopenia, and jaundice.

Diffuse involvement of the brain produces progressive dementia, seizures, hemiparesis, dysphasia, visual deterioration, cranial nerve

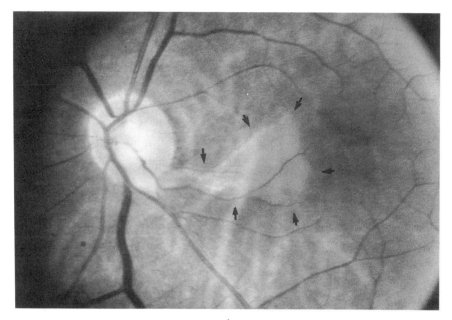

A

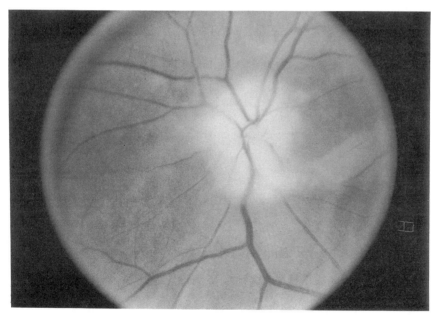

B

FIGURE 8–10. Temporal (giant cell) arteritis.
A. Retinal vessel occlusion showing infarcted area of the retina (arrows).
B. Complete infarction of the optic nerve three days later. This 66-year-old patient had experienced amourosis fugax in the opposite eye then visual loss in the ipsilateral eye followed by complete blindness three days later. The classical pale swollen appearance of the optic nerve head is the signal for temporal artery biopsy.

palsies, and dysarthria. Symptoms wax and wane as the disease takes a downhill course and is ultimately fatal. Intracerebral hemorrhage and subarachnoid hemorrhage have been reported.

Diagnostic Procedures.

1. The complete blood count shows the presence of microangiopathic hemolytic anemia and thrombocytopenia.
2. There is microscopic hematuria indicating renal involvement.

Treatment. There is no effective treatment for this disorder. Massive doses of corticosteroids, the use of heparin, and the use of platelet inhibitors (sulfinpyrazone) have been suggested. Exchange transfusion may provide temporary improvement.

Isolated Angiitis of the Nervous System

Definition. Isolated angiitis or granulomatous angiitis is a rare condition characterized by a vasculitis restricted to the nervous system.

Etiology and Pathology. The etiology is unknown. There is a vasculitis with a mononuclear cell infiltration and occasional granuloma formation involving the arteries and occasionally the veins in the CNS.

Clinical Features. The presenting symptom is usually severe headache resembling migraine followed by changes in mental status including memory failure and intellectual deterioration, and focal deficits such as hemiparesis, dysphasia, alexia, and partial seizures.

Isolated angiitis of the spinal cord has been described with progressive paraparesis, radicular pain, and bladder dysfunctions.

Diagnostic Procedures.

1. The routine laboratory studies such as CBC, sedimentation rate, LE cell preparation, antinuclear antibodies (ANA), rheumatoid factor, cryoglobulins, and circulating immune complex determinations are usually normal.
2. Cerebral angiography shows narrowing or beading of large intermediate or small arteries at multiple sites. Other causes of cerebral arteritis including herpes zoster, bacterial meningitis, syphilis tuberculosis, fungal infections, Hodgkin's disease, SLE, rheumatoid arthritis, scleroderma, systemic necrotizing vasculitis, Wegener's granulomatosis, lymphomatoid granulomatosis, vasculitis due to heroin, meth-

amphetamine, or allopurinal, and radiation vasculitis must be excluded.
3. The arteriogram may be normal in some cases.
4. Lumbar puncture. The cerebrospinal fluid may show a slight to moderate elevation in protein content.
6. Tissue biopsy is needed to establish the diagnosis in cases with spinal cord involvement and in those with normal arteriography where leptomeningeal biopsy is recommended.

Treatment. The response to corticosteroids is unpredictable but the method should be tried initially (42). If relapse occurs, a combination of daily cyclophosphamide and alternate day prednisone may induce a sustained clinical remission. Treatment may be necessary intermittently or continuously for many years.

Prognosis. The prognosis has been poor and was invariably fatal until the introduction of combined prednisone and cyclophosphamide therapy.

Neurologic Complications of Other Arteritides

Neurologic complications have, rarely, been described in other forms of arteritis, including Wegener's granulomatosis—diffuse symmetric peripheral neuropathy; Schölein-Henoch purpura—hemiplegia, seizures, chorea, subarachnoid hemorrhage, particularly in children; and the arteritis associated with rheumatoid arthritis—peripheral neuropathy and focal neurologic signs including hemiparesis. Scleroderma has not been reported to involve the central nervous system, but it may produce secondary neurologic symptoms due to hypertension or uremia following sclerodermic involvement of the heart, lungs, or kidneys. Involvement of the small intestine may produce malabsorption, vitamin B_{12} deficiency, and subacute combined degeneration of the spinal cord.

Transient Global Amnesia

Definition. Transient global amnesia is a syndrome characterized by sudden total amnesia lasting several hours, without other signs of neurologic involvement, followed by complete recovery.

Etiology and Pathology. The etiology is unknown. While it is not unusual to obtain a history of migraine or cerebrovascular disease the relationship is not established.

The onset is sudden and follows exertion

such as manual labor, athletic activity, sexual intercourse, or an intense emotional experience in many cases (43).

Clinical Features. Transient global amnesia occurs in middle-aged or elderly individuals who are apparently healthy. The onset is sudden, and there is a period of total amnesia lasting several hours. During that time the individual behaves in a normal or near-normal fashion. However, individuals who are acquainted with the patient can detect subtle changes in behavior. The attack usually terminates slowly, with the patient showing gradual improvement and identification of those around him. The rates of recurrence, subsequent stroke, and development of dementia are low (44).

Diagnostic Procedures. When signs of cerebral atherosclerosis are present the attack should be investigated as a transient ischemic attack (see pages 137–138).

Treatment. Any underlying disease (e.g., hypertension) should receive treatment.

Locked-In Syndrome

Definition. The locked-in syndrome is characterized by quadriparesis and lower bulbar palsy due to bilateral infarction of the ventral pons.

Etiology and Pathology. Most cases of this syndrome are due to basilar artery thrombosis with bilateral infarction of the ventral pons. The condition can occur following head and neck trauma with vertebral artery damage and occlusion (45). The syndrome occasionally occurs in multiple sclerosis and pontine gliomas that involve the ventral pons bilaterally (23).

Clinical Features. In the majority of cases with thrombosis of the basilar artery the onset is sudden with the development of acute hemiparesis, which rapidly progresses to quadriparesis. Initially, there may be severe dysarthria and dysphonia, which rapidly progress to a state of mutism. The patients are unable to handle oral-pharyngeal secretions, and aspiration pneumonia occurs at an early stage.

Examination shows complete quadriplegia with mutism and paralysis of all functions supplied by the cranial nerves bilaterally from the fifth to the 12th cranial nerves. There is impairment of horizontal eye movement, but vertical eye movements and blinking are preserved.

These patients give the superficial impression of coma because of quadriplegia and mutism. However, they are fully conscious and alert and can communicate via vertical eye movements and/or blinking.

Diagnostic Procedures. Arteriography is the definitive procedure in identifying basilar artery thrombosis.

Treatment. Patients with the locked-in syndrome should receive full supportive treatment as many have recovered from this seemingly hopeless condition. See treatment of cerebral infarction (page 146).

Prognosis. Approximately 20 percent of patients will survive if given adequate care. Improvement occurs beginning anywhere from a week to three months after the onset of the illness. Many patients have been able to return home when control of bowel and bladder and recovery of swallowing mechanisms occur. There is usually residual dysarthria. Some patients eventually are able to walk without assistance.

Cerebral Infarction Due to Cerebral Venous or Dural Sinus Thrombosis

Definitions. This is a thrombosis in the cerebral venous system followed by cerebral infarction.

Etiology and Pathology. Cerebral venous thrombosis and dural sinus thrombosis may be caused by infection following otitis media, mastoiditis, acute sinusitis, or furunculosis of the face. Noninfectious thrombosis may be associated with head trauma, sickle cell disease, neoplasia, the immediate postpartum period, and the presence of lupus anticoagulant (46).

Clinical Features. The clinical features depend on the location of the venous thrombosis.

1. Superior saggital sinus thrombosis. The condition usually presents with generalized headache followed by seizures and progressive weakness of one or both lower extremities. The patient becomes obtunded or stuporous, and there are signs of increased intracranial pressure with papilledema and distention of scalp veins. Young children show bulging of the anterior fontanelle. Thrombosis of the posterior half of the superior sagittal sinus may result in benign intracranial hypertension.

2. Cerebral venous thrombosis. The condition is usually seen in the immediate postpartum period. The patient experiences increasing headache and seizures, followed by the development of hemiparesis.

3. Transverse sinus thrombosis and cav-

ernous sinus thrombosis. These are usually caused by infection. Transverse sinus thrombosis may be asymptomatic or associated with papilledema, headache, neck pain, nausea, vomiting, and ataxia (47). Cavernous sinus thrombosis is usually characterized by edema of the orbit and eyelids with ptosis, chemosis, and orbital edema. The third and fourth and the ophthalmic division of the fifth and sixth cranial nerves may be involved.

Diagnostic Procedures.

1. Electroencephalogram (EEG). The EEG shows focal slowing often associated with intermittent spike wave activity on the side of the infarction.
2. MR or CT scanning may show an area or areas of increased density in the cerebral hemispheres in patients with hemorrhagic infarction.
3. Arteriography. The venous stage of an angiogram demonstrates lack of filling of the affected vessel.
4. Lupus anticoagulant can be demonstrated in some cases.

Treatment.

1. Seizures should be controlled with adequate dosage of anticonvulsants.
2. Patients with increased intracranial pressure of sufficient magnitude to produce papilledema should receive intracranial monitoring and appropriate treatment with dexamethasone (Decadron) and hyperosmolar agents.
3. Patients with lupus anticoagulant respond to anticoagulants and prednisone.

Prognosis. In most cases residual neurologic deficits cannot be predicted. Seizure disorder may require long-term anticonvulsant therapy.

Sickle Cell Disease

Definition. Sickle cell disease is a genetically determined hemoglobinopathy in which abnormal "sickling" of red cells occurs.

Etiology and Pathology. Three abnormal states have been recognized:

1. Sickle cell disease, a homozygous condition in which red cells contain hemoglobin S.
2. Sickle cell trait, a heterozygous condition in which the red cells contain hemoglobin S and normal hemoglobin.
3. Sickle cell hemoglobin C disease in which red cells contain hemoglobin S and hemoglobin C.

Hemoglobin S reduces the life span of the red cell and produces hemolytic anemia. In addition, hemoglobin S forms a gel under low oxygen tension. This alters the shape of the red cell, which assumes a sickle shape and blocks the microcirculation.

Occlusion of blood vessels by sickle cells may be followed by distal embolization resulting in cerebral infarction or cerebral hemorrhage. The most extensive areas of infarction involve the border zone between the anterior cerebral and middle cerebral arteries (48).

Clinical Features. Sickle cell disease is a systemic disease, and affected individuals are usually of short stature with a dorsal kyphosis and lumbar lordosis. There is chronic ulceration of the legs.

Examination shows a moderate to severe anemia, cardiomegaly, hepatomegaly, and splenomegaly. During sickle cell crisis, in which there is obstruction of blood vessels in many organs, patients develop acute abdominal pain, arthritic pain, severe bone pain, and hematuria. Neurologic complications occur in about 25 percent of patients and include hemiparesis, subarachnoid hemorrhage, seizures, and meningeal irritation. Optic neuritis may occur followed by optic atrophy. Sudden deafness may also occur due to bilateral involvement of the cochlear nucleus and/or auditory nerve. Other cranial nerve and spinal nerve palsies have been described. Infarction of the spinal cord may produce sudden paraplegia.

Many patients with neurologic symptoms show repeated episodes of cerebral infarction, which ultimately result in dementia. Sickle cell disease in children may present with occlusion of the main branches of the circle of Willis and increasingly severe neurologic deficits.

Diagnostic Procedures.

1. Sickling of red cells can be demonstrated by the in vitro slide test under reduced oxygen tension.
2. X-rays of the skull show thickening of the diploë and fine radial striations. X-ray of the long bones may show irregular areas of infarction and sclerosis.
3. Hemoglobin electrophoresis will demonstrate the presence of hemoglobin S.
4. MRI or CT scans will reveal multiple infarcts in the border zones between ante-

rior and middle cerebral arteries and between middle and posterior cerebral arteries.

Treatment. There is no specific treatment for sickle cell disease. Patients often experience severe pain during crisis and require adequate doses of narcotics. Exchange transfusion is often beneficial. It is possible that hyperbaric oxygenation will reduce the tendency to sickle cell formation and improve microcirculation in affected organs.

Sickle Cell Trait and Sickle Cell Hemoglobin C Disease

These conditions are usually benign but carry an increased risk of cerebral infarction, central retinal artery occlusion, retinal detachment, and chorioretinal infarction. Patients are said to have an increased incidence of complicated migraine.

Neurologic Complications of Drug Abuse

The repeated intravenous injection of illicit drugs may produce a number of cerebrovascular complications.

1. Chronic heroin and cocaine users may develop a cerebral arteritis with cerebral infarction or subarachnoid hemorrhage.
2. Repeated intravenous injections without sterile precautions may lead to subacute bacterial endocarditis and the subsequent development of embolism and mycotic aneurysms. The presence of mycotic aneurysms may be complicated by subarachnoid hemorrhage or cerebral infarction.

Cerebrovascular Complications of Migraine

This is a benign condition in a great majority of cases, but occasionally patients with more complex forms of migraine will develop cerebral infarction. The infarctions and angiographic abnormalities are usually in the distribution of the posterior cerebral artery (49).

REFERENCES

1. Wernelin, L.; Juhler, M. The course of transient ischemic attacks. Neurology 38:677–680; 1988.
2. Sacco, R. L.; Foulkes, M. A.; *et al.* Determinants of early recurrence of cerebral infarction the stroke data bank. Stroke 20:983–989; 1989.
3. Rogers, R. L.; Meyer, J. S.; *et al.* Reducing hypertriglyceridemia in elderly patients with cerebrovascular disease stabilizes or improves cognition and cerebral perfusion. Angiology 40:260–264; 1989.
4. Rogers, R. L.; Meyer, J. S.; *et al.* Additional predisposing risk factors for atherothrombotic cerebrovascular disease among treated hypertensive volunteers. Stroke 18:335–341; 1987.
5. Grad, A.; Balok, R. W. Vertigo of vascular origin. Clinical and electronystagmographic features in 84 cases. Arch. Neurol. 46:281–284; 1989.
6. Knepper, L. E.; Biller, J.; *et al.* Neurologic manifestations of atrial myxoma: a 12-year experience and review. Stroke 19:1435–1440; 1988.
7. Macdonell, R. A. L.; Donnan, G. A.; *et al.* The electroencephalogram and acute ischemic stroke. Arch. Neurol. 45:520–524; 1988.
8. Ross, M. A.; Beller, J.; *et al.* Magnetic resonance imaging in Wallenburg's lateral medullar syndrome. Stroke 17:542–545; 1986.
9. Beller, J.; Williams, T. C.; *et al.* Early diagnosis of basilar artery occlusion using magnetic resonance imaging. Stroke 19:297–306; 1988.
10. Niedenkom, K.; Myers, L. G.; *et al.* Three-dimensional transcranial Doppler blood flow mapping in patients with cerebrovascular disorders. Stroke 19:1335–1344; 1988.
11. Levine, S. R.; Welch, K. M. A. Cerebrovascular ischemia associated with lupus anticoagulant. Stroke 18:257–263; 1987.
12. Merz, B. Large trial finds trilopedine superior to aspirin in preventing stroke. JAMA 161:1541; 1989.
13. Patterson, R. H. Can carotid endarterectomy be justified? Yes. Arch. Neurol. 44:641–652; 1987.
14. Jonas, S. Can carotid endarterectomy be justified? Yes. Arch. Neurol. 44:652–654; 1987.
15. Halperin, J. L.; Hart, R. G. Atrial fibrillation and stroke: new ideas, persisting dilemmas. Stroke 19:937–941; 1988.
16. Peterson, P.; Godtfredsen, J. Embolic complications in paroxysmal atrial fibrillation. Stroke 17:622–626; 1986.
17. Helgason, C.; Caplan, L. R.; *et al.* Anterior choroidal artery territory infarction. Arch. Neurol. 43:681–686; 1986.
18. Meissner, I.; Sapir, S.; *et al.* The paramedian diencephalic syndrome—A dynamic phenomenon. Stroke 18:380–385; 1987.
19. Aldrich, M. S.; Allessi, A. G.; *et al.* Cortical blindness: etiology, diagnosis, and prognosis. Arch. Neurol. 21:149–158; 1987.
20. Fisher, C. M. The posterior cerebral artery syndrome. Can. J. Neurol. Sci. 13:232–239; 1986.
21. Pessin, M. S.; Lathi, E. S.; *et al.* Clinical features and mechanism of occipital infarction. Ann. Neurol. 21:290–299; 1987.
22. Pessin, M. S.; Kwan, E. S.; *et al.* Posterior cerebral artery stenosis. Ann. Neurol. 21:85–89; 1987.
23. Patterson, J. R.; Grabios, M. Locked in syndrome: a review of 139 cases. Stroke 17:758–764; 1986.
24. Bamford, J.; Sandercock, P.; *et al.* The natural

history of lacunar infarction: the Oxfordshire community stroke project. Stroke 18:545–551; 1987.

25. Tuszynski, M. M.; Petito, C. K.; *et al.* Risk factors and cervical manifestations of pathologically verified lacuna infarctions. Stroke 20:990–999; 1989.

26. Peterson, P.; Boysen, G.; *et al.* Placebo-controlled randomized trial of warfarin and aspirin for prevention of thromboembolitic complications in chronic atrial fibrillation. Lancet 1:175–179; 1989.

27. Rothrock, J. F.; Dietrich, H. C.; *et al.* Acute anticoagulation following corticoembolic stroke. Stroke 20:730–734; 1989.

28. Halsey, E. C., Jr.; Kassell, N. P.; *et al.* Failure of heparin to prevent progression in progressing ischemia infarction. Stroke 19:10–14; 1988.

29. Sinyor, D.; Amato, P. Post-stroke depression: relationship to functional impairment, coping strategies and rehabilitation outcome. Stroke 17:1102–1107; 1986.

30. Del Zoppo, G. J.; Ferbert, A.; *et al.* Local intra-arterial fibrinolytic therapy in acute carotid territory stroke. A pilot study. Stroke 19:307–313; 1988.

31. Hacke, W.; Zeumer, H.; *et al.* Intra-arterial thrombocytic therapy improves outcome in patients with acute vertebrobasilar occlusive disease. Stroke 19:1216–1222; 1988.

32. Gelmers, H. J.; Goster, K.; *et al.* A controlled trial of nimodipine in acute ischemic stroke. N. Engl. J. Med. 318:203–207; 1988.

33. Cummings, J. L.; Miller, B.; *et al.* Neuropsychiatric aspects of multi-infarct dementia and dementia of the Alzheimer's type. Arch. Neurol. 44:389–393; 1987.

34. Meyer, J. S.; Rogers, R. L.; *et al.* Cognition and cerebral blood flow fluctuate together in multi-infarct dementia. Stroke 19:163–169; 1988.

35. Kinkel, W. R.; Jacobs, L.; *et al.* Subcortical arteriosclerotic encephalopathy (Binswanger's disease) computed tomographic nuclear magnetic resonance and clinical correlations. Arch. Neurol. 42:951–959; 1985.

36. Jacobs, T. G. Cocaine abuse: neurovascular complications. Radiology 170:223–227; 1989.

37. Oppenheimer, S.; Hoffbrand, B. J. Optic neuritis and myelopathy in systemic lupus erythematosus. Can. J. Neurol. Sci. 13:129–132; 1986.

38. Yamamoto, M. Recurrent transverse myelitis associated with collagen disease. J. Neurol. 233:185–187; 1986.

39. Futrell, N.; Millikan, E. Frequency, etiology and prevention of stroke in patients with systemic lupus erythematosus. Stroke 20:583–591; 1989.

40. Solomon, S.; Cappa, K. G. The headache of temporal arteritis. J. Am. Geriatr. Soc. 35:163–165; 1987.

41. Wong, R. L.; Korn, J. H. Temporal arteritis with normal sedimentation rate. Am. J. Med. 80:959; 1986.

42. Koo, E. H.; Massey, E. W. Granulomatous angiitis of the central nervous system: protein manifestations and response to treatment. J. Neurol. Neurosurg. Psychiatry 51:1126–1133; 1988.

43. Miller, J. W.; Peterson, R. C.; *et al.* Transient global amnesia: clinical characteristics and prognosis. Neurology 37:733–737; 1987.

44. Guidotti, M. Transient global amnesia. J. Neurol. Neurosurg. Psychiatry 52:320–323; 1989.

45. Keane, J. R. Locked in syndrome after head and neck trauma. Neurology 36:80–82; 1986.

46. Levine, S. R.; Kieran, S.; *et al.* Cerebral venous thrombosis with lupus anticoagulant—Report of two cases. Stroke 18:801–804; 1987.

47. Bousser, M. G.; Chiras, J.; *et al.* Cerebral venous thrombosis—A review of 38 cases. Stroke 16:199–213; 1985.

48. Rothman, S. M.; Fulling, K. H.; *et al.* Sickle cell anemia and central nervous system infarction: a neuropathological study. Ann. Neurol. 20:684–690; 1986.

49. Broderick, J. P.; Swanson, J. W. Migraine-related strokes. Clinical profile and prognosis in 20 patients. Arch. Neurol. 44:868–871; 1987.

CHAPTER 9

SUBARACHNOID HEMORRHAGE

Subarachnoid hemorrhage is a syndrome in which there is bleeding into the subarachnoid space. It may be secondary to trauma or spontaneous. Spontaneous subarachnoid hemorrhage may result from an intracerebral hemorrhage that ruptures into the subarachnoid space or may follow primary subarachnoid hemorrhage. In primary subarachnoid hemorrhage spontaneous rupture of a blood vessel lying in the subarachnoid space results in bleeding into the subarachnoid space. Primary subarachnoid hemorrhage accounts for approximately 9 percent of acute cerebrovascular episodes. Rupture of a berry aneurysm or bleeding from an arteriovenous malformation are by far the commonest causes of primary subarachnoid hemorrhage. Table 9–1 lists less common etiologies of subarachnoid hemorrhage.

Berry Aneurysm

Berry aneurysms have been described in 1 to 18 percent of autopsied cases. This depends on the definition of an aneurysm by the pathologist. Aneurysms are usually single, but multiple aneurysms occur in about 15 percent of cases. Ninety percent of aneurysms occur in the anterior portion of the circle of Willis, and 10 percent occur in the vertebral basilar system. The commonest sites for berry aneurysm formation are at the terminal portion of the internal carotid artery, the junction of the anterior cerebral and anterior communicating arteries, or at the origin of the middle cerebral artery (see Figure 9–1). Subarachnoid hemorrhage due to ruptured aneurysm occurs in 26,000 people in the United States every year, an incidence of one in 10,000 people. Approximately 65 percent of cases die or experience severe disability (1).

Pathology. All berry aneurysms arise at the bifurcation of a cerebral artery. A number of theories have been advanced in an attempt to explain the development of cerebral aneurysms. These include:

1. *Aneurysms develop at the site of developmental defects in the cerebral vessels.* This theory proposes a lack of development of the internal elastic lamina at the bifurcation of a vessel in or near the circle of Willis. The vessels are crowded together in the embryonic state and the apposition of the vessel walls protects the potentially weak area. However, as the brain and the circle of Willis develop, the angle between the arteries increases, leaving a potentially weak area at the bifurcation of the two arteries. This area, lacking an internal elastic lamina, will become the site of an aneurysm if weakened by unusual stresses. These stresses may include chronic hypertension, atherosclerosis, or the hemodynamic effects of anomalous development of the circle of Willis.

2. *Aneurysms develop at the site of vestigial vessels.* There are numerous small vessels at the base of the embryonic brain, most of which disappear as the circle of Willis devel-

TABLE 9–1.   Subarachnoid Hemorrhage

A. Common Causes
   1. Traumatic subarachnoid hemorrhage
   2. Spontaneous subarachnoid hemorrhage
      a. Intracerebral hemorrhage with rupture into the subarachnoid space
      b. Primary subarachnoid hemorrhage
         1. Ruptured berry aneurysm
         2. Bleeding arteriovenous malformation
         3. Ruptured mycotic aneurysm

B. Rare Causes
   1. Developmental defects including pseudoxanthoma elasticum, Ehlers-Danlos syndrome, Sturge-Weber disease, hereditary hemorrhagic telangiectasia, telangiectasia pontis
   2. Infections. *Herpes simplex* encephalitis, acute hemorrhagic leukoencephalitis, brain abscess, tuberculous meningitis, syphilitic vasculitis
   3. Neoplasm. Primary or metastatic brain tumor. Hemangioblastoma of the cerebellum or brain stem
   4. Blood dyscrasias. Leukemia, Hodgkin's disease, thrombocytopenia, sickle cell anemia, hemophilia, aplastic anemia, pernicious anemia, anticoagulant therapy
   5. Vasculitis. Polyarteritis nodosa, anaphylactic purpura
   6 Arteriosclerosis. Rupture of an arteriosclerotic vessel
   7. Subdural hematoma

ops. This theory of aneurysm formation proposes that the lack of an internal elastic lamina occurs at the site of a vestigial vessel and that this region weakens and eventually becomes the site of an aneurysm.

3. *Aneurysms develop because of lack of intimal "cushions."* Examination of any circle of Willis reveals several areas that lack an internal elastic lamina, and it is probable that this is a common event. It is possible that these areas are protected by hypertrophy and hyperplasia of the intima with the formation of intimal "cushions," which prevent aneurysm formation. The failure of development of an intimal cushion exposes the weakened vessel to the stresses of chronic hypertension,

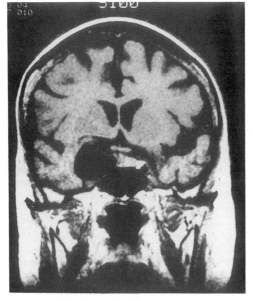
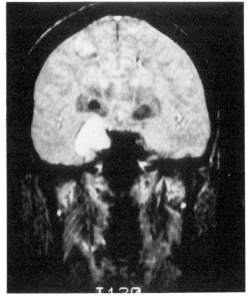

A   B

FIGURE 9–1.   MR scan coronal sections, T1(**A**) and T2 (**B**) weighted images, showing a large aneurysm of the terminal portion of the right internal carotid artery.

atherosclerosis, or abnormal flow in the circle of Willis, leading to the development of an aneurysm.

Pathologic changes following subarachnoid hemorrhage consist of staining of the subarachnoid space due to the presence of blood. The high-pressure jet of blood from a ruptured aneurysm frequently penetrates the brain parenchyma, forming an intracerebral hematoma. Occasionally, the blood tears through the dura into the subdural space, creating a subdural hematoma. The brain may show evidence of edema and ischemic infarction secondary to interruption of blood supply due to arterial spasm or compression of the circle of Willis by a hematoma.

Microscopic examination at the site of an aneurysm shows that the internal elastic lamina terminates on either side close to the aneurysm. The aneurysm has a very thin wall of fibrous tissue and is often lined by a laminated blood clot. Areas of calcification may occur in long-standing aneurysms.

Clinical Features. The signs and symptoms of subarachnoid hemorrhage due to rupture of an aneurysm depend on the site of the aneurysm (see Table 9–2).

Some patients have prodromal symptoms several days or weeks preceding rupture of an aneurysm. These include the sudden onset of a severe headache lasting a few hours to several days, then subsiding (sentinel headache). Intracavernous internal carotid aneurysms or aneurysms arising at the junction of the internal carotid and posterior communicating arteries may compress the third nerve in the lateral wall of the cavernous sinus, producing third nerve palsy with involvement of the pupil. Similarly, pressure on the ophthalmic or maxillary divisions of the fifth cranial

TABLE 9–2. **Signs and Symptoms of Aneurysms According to Site of Origin**

Origin of Aneurysm	Structure Involved	Signs and Symptoms
Internal carotid, cavernous portion	Compression of cranial nerves 3, 4, & 6; compression of ophthalmic division of cranial nerve 5; compression of pituitary; rupture into cavernous sinus producing an AV fistula	Mydriasis, diplopia, ptosis, trigeminal neuralgia, atypical facial pain, hypopituitarism, noise in the head
Internal carotid, supraclinoid portion	Compression of optic nerve, compression of optic chiasm, compression of cranial nerve 3	Visual failure, optic atrophy, visual field defects, mydriasis, diplopia, ptosis
Ophthalmic artery	Compression of optic nerve, compression of pituitary	Visual failure, optic atrophy, hypopituitarism
Middle cerebral artery	Irritation of the cortex	Usually causes few signs and symptoms before rupture, partial seizures
Anterior cerebral artery	Compression of optic chiasm, compression of olfactory tract	Visual field defects, unilateral anosmia
Posterior communicating artery	Compression of cranial nerve 3, compression of cranial nerve 6	Mydriasis, diplopia, ptosis, diplopia
Posterior cerebral artery	Compression of the midbrain	Usually causes few signs and symptoms before rupture, hydrocephalus, stupor, akinetic mutism
Basilar artery	Compression of cranial nerve 5, compression of cranial nerve 7, compression of midbrain	Trigeminal neuralgia, atypical facial pain, facial paralysis, hydrocephalus
Vertebral artery	Compression of cranial nerves 9 & 10, compression of brain stem	Paralysis of the palate, pharynx, dysphonia, dysphagia, vertigo, ataxia, vomiting

nerve in the lateral wall of the cavernous sinus may produce facial pain. Focal motor seizures or partial complex seizures (psychomotor seizures) are a rare complication of large aneurysms that irritate the cortical gray matter.

Rupture of an aneurysm usually occurs when a patient is active and alert. Many patients give a history of onset while working or engaged in other activities such as athletics or sports. Rupture of an aneurysm has been recorded during sexual intercourse, defecation, and immediately following micturition. Nevertheless, rupture can occur when the patient is asleep or quietly sitting and resting.

The onset of subarachnoid hemorrhage from a ruptured berry aneurysm is sudden in about 90 percent of cases, and there is rapid loss of consciousness in 20 percent. The majority of patients complain of severe generalized headache, with pain extending into the neck, and nausea and vomiting. Other symptoms include transient vertigo and a feeling of faintness or confusion. Seizures occur in 10 to 20 percent of cases (2). Patients occasionally report hearing loss, visual impairment, and diplopia. Many patients experience a brief loss of consciousness with gradual improvement, but a small number remain comatose from the onset of the illness. Onset with hemiparesis may mimic infarction. When first examined most patients show some impairment of consciousness and the presence of nuchal rigidity. Funduscopic examination may reveal the presence of a subhyaloid hemorrhage, and papilledema may develop within six hours of the onset of subarachnoid hemorrhage.

About 10 percent of patients with subarachnoid hemorrhage due to ruptured berry aneurysm have a more gradual onset with evolution of symptoms over a period ranging from several hours to several days. Although severe headache is a major complaint in the great majority of conscious patients, not all patients report headache, and approximately 2 percent of conscious patients are headache-free.

Complications.

1. Arterial spasm occurs in approximately 30 percent of cases of subarachnoid hemorrhage. The cause of the spasm is presumed to be due to the liberation of a vasospastic substance, including serotonin tryptophan, and prostaglandin $F_{2\alpha}$, by the disintegrating red cells in the subarachnoid space (3). This produces intense arterial vasospasm, which is often remote from the site of the aneurysm and is occasionally generalized. Arterial spasm usually develops within three days after the subarachnoid hemorrhage and lasts approximately 12 days.

The initial spasm may be followed by endothelial proliferation which maintains the narrowing of the vessel lumen, and the term vasospasm may be ultimately incorrect in the latter stages of arterial narrowing. The intense arterial constriction has the effect of producing delayed cerebral ischemia, multiple infarcts, and edema, and death may occur from brain swelling rather than the direct results of the subarachnoid hemorrhage (4).

2. Rebleeding following ruptured berry aneurysm is maximal in the first 24 hours with a cumulative risk of about 20 percent in the next 14 days. Rebleeding results in death in about 60 percent of affected cases.

3. Intracerebral hematoma can produce a dense contralateral homonymous hemianopia and hemiparesis.

4. A subdural hematoma may result from rupture of an aneurysm into the subdural space (5).

5. Acute hydrocephalus may result from the occlusion of the subarachnoid space by breakdown products of red cell disintegration and the inflammatory response. Hydrocephalus occurs in more than 50 percent of cases of subarachnoid hemorrhage within 30 days of the hemorrhage. Ventriculoperitoneal shunting may be required in those who show delayed neurologic deterioration and persistent ventricular enlargement (6).

6. Inappropriate secretion of antidiuretic hormone may occur in severe subarachnoid hemorrhage, or as a postoperative complication. Some patients develop hyponatremia due to inhibition of renal tubular sodium absorption rather than inappropriate secretion of antidiuretic hormone.

7. Pulmonary and urinary tract infections, dehydration, electrolyte disturbances, and the development of decubiti are not unusual in comatose patients.

Diagnostic Procedures. The diagnostic procedures are as follows:

1. Magnetic resonance imaging (MRI) or computed tomography (CT) scan. A scan will reveal blood in the basal cisterns in most patients with subarachnoid hemorrhage, and the extent of an intracerebral hematoma, cerebral infarction, cerebral edema, and acute hydrocephalus are readily demonstrated. Intraventricular and intracerebral bleeding and hydrocephalus have adverse effects on survival. Localized, thick, or diffuse collections

of subarachnoid blood are associated with a higher risk of vasospasm and a poorer prognosis (7–9). Aneurysms are occasionally seen in an enhanced CT scan (see Figure 9–2).

2. Lumbar puncture. Lumbar puncture reveals a bloody spinal fluid under increased pressure. The supernatant fluid is xanthochromic within six hours of subarachnoid hemorrhage. There is a polymorphonuclear pleocytosis within 24 hours and later appearance of mononuclear cells. Red blood cells usually disappear from the spinal fluid by five days; their persistence indicates that further hemorrhage has occurred. Xanthochromia usually lasts for approximately 28 days. An estimation of the date of onset of subarachnoid hemorrhage can be made by measuring the presence of oxyhemoglobin and bilirubin in the xanthochromic fluid by cerebrospinal fluid (CSF) spectrophotometry. Oxyhemoglobin appears at the onset of subarachnoid hemorrhage and gradually decreases; bilirubin appears after two or three days and increases in amount as oxyhemoglobin decreases. Recurrent hemorrhage is associated with a late rise in the presence of oxyhemoglobin (10).

3. Skull x-ray. X-ray of the skull occasionally shows the presence of calcification in the wall of an aneurysm. Erosion of the lateral wall of the sella or anterior clinoid processes may occur. Pineal shift occurs in the presence of a large hematoma. An ophthalmic aneurysm can cause enlargement of the optic foramen.

4. Arteriography. The presence of a berry aneurysm can be confirmed by arteriography in most cases.

Differential Diagnosis.

1. Migraine headache. The first "migraine headache" in a young individual may be confused with a subarachnoid hemorrhage. An MRI or CT scan and a lumbar puncture should be performed if the diagnosis is in doubt.

2. Systemic infection. Some systemic infections such as influenza can be associated with severe headache. Lumbar puncture will reveal a normal cerebrospinal fluid in such cases, and this procedure should always be performed if there is any doubt about the diagnosis.

3. Acute meningitis or encephalitis. The acute onset of severe headache and nuchal rigidity occurs in these acute inflammatory conditions and also occurs in subarachnoid hemorrhage. Lumbar puncture should be performed because of the presence of nuchal rigidity and will establish the correct diagnosis.

4. Hypertensive encephalopathy. Patients with severe hypertension may present with severe headache. Systemic evidence of hypertension, such as hypertensive retinopathy, cardiac enlargement, and proteinuria are usually present. There is no nuchal rigidity.

5. Cervical arthritis. This condition may be present in patients who develop acute headache from other causes such as migraine. The neck stiffness is present in all directions of head movement and is not of recent onset.

6. Cerebral infarction. The acute onset of hemiparesis may occasionally occur following forceful rupture of a berry aneurysm into the brain parenchyma or result from the development of vasospasm. Most cases with subarachnoid hemorrhage will have severe headache and nuchal rigidity. Magnetic resonance imaging or CT scan and lumbar puncture will establish the correct diagnosis in most cases, but arteriography may be necessary to differentiate between spontaneous intracerebral hemorrhage and ruptured berry aneurysm.

Treatment. See page 54, treatment of the comatose patient. In general, these measures apply to patients with subarachnoid hemor-

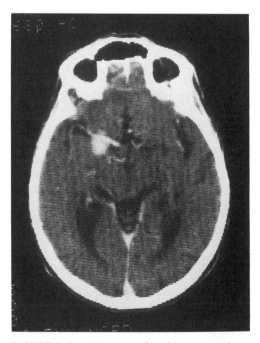

FIGURE 9–2. CT scan with enhancement showing a ruptured berry aneurysm of the middle cerebral artery.

rhage whether they are conscious or unconscious. Additional measures include:

1. At least three weeks of strict bed rest with adequate nursing care is a necessity.
2. Adequate use of narcotics in the conscious patient. Most patients will require meperedine (Demerol) 100 to 150 mg intramuscularly (IM) q4h p.r.n. for control of severe headache. Lesser doses are inadequate. Subarachnoid hemorrhage produces one of the most severe and distressing headaches known, and it is unfortunate that it is often inadequately treated.
3. In addition to narcotics, patients may require the regular administration of a phenothiazine or barbiturate to allay restlessness.
4. Hypertension should be controlled unless there are signs of increasing cerebral vasospasm.
5. Patients with progressive neurologic deficits due to cerebral vasospasm should be treated with volume expansion therapy. This entails the use of agents such as low molecular weight dextran to increase blood volume and elevate central venous pressure, and concomitant induction of hypertension. Since the areas of the brain affected by severe vasospasm and ischemia have lost autoregulation, blood flow through collateral should be increased by volume expansion and hypertension (11).
6. The calcium channel blocking agent nimodipine has been reported to improve neurological outcome in cases with neurologic deficits associated with vasospasm. A dose of 60 mg nimodipine every four hours for 21 days beginning within 96 hours of the subarachnoid hemorrhage is recommended (12).
7. Cerebral edema should be controlled with dexamethasone (Decadron) 12 mg initially followed by 4 mg q6h intravenously or mannitol 1g/kg in a 20 percent solution over 20 minutes followed by 0.25 g/kg IV q4h.
8. The use of antifibrinolytic agents has declined in popularity and remains controversial.
9. Continuous cardiac monitoring should be performed irrespective of early or delayed surgical treatment, because 90 percent of patients develop cardiac arrhythmias, of which 50 percent are serious and require prompt treatment (13).

Surgical Treatment of Berry Aneurysm. Immediate surgical treatment may be necessary as an emergency measure to relieve increased intracranial pressure, to evacuate an intracerebral hematoma or subdural hematoma, or to relieve acute hydrocephalus. Many surgeons still prefer to operate two weeks after rupture. This avoids operating in the presence of arterial spasm and development of arterial spasm in the postoperative period. All surgical procedures should be preceded by arteriography to be sure that no vasospasm is present. In addition, surgery should be performed only on good-risk patients who are conscious and easily aroused and who have minimal or mild neurologic deficits.

There is, however, a growing number of neurosurgeons who believe that patients with normal neurologic status or mild impairment of consciousness with focal neurologic deficits should receive early aneurysm surgery followed by volume expansion therapy. This approach, while technically more difficult than delayed surgery, has the advantage of eliminating the risk of rebleeding and frees the basal cisterns of blood clots which may reduce the risk of vasospasm (14).

Continuing medical treatment is indicated in all semicomatose or comatose patients, in those with severe neurologic deficit, and in those patients in whom arterial vasospasm persists. This latter group of patients may eventually receive surgery following relief of vasospasm. Finally, there are a number of patients who reject surgical treatment and will continue to require medical therapy.

When an unruptured aneurysm is identified, the risk of rupture is related to the size of the aneurysm. Aneurysms less than one centimeter in diameter have a very low probability of subsequent rupture. Aneurysms greater than one centimeter in diameter have a 50 percent chance of rupturing within two-and-a-half months and should be surgically managed whenever possible.

Prognosis. The outcome of subarachnoid hemorrhage following rupture of a berry aneurysm varies from center to center, but in general it can be said that 30 percent of patients die within 24 hours and 40 percent die within seven days. Of the survivors, 50 percent will have a second subarachnoid hemorrhage which carries a 40 percent mortality rate; 60 percent of patients with subarachnoid hemorrhage due to ruptured berry aneurysm die within six months of the initial bleed. The risk of rebleeding in survivors is low after six months, and approximately 1 percent of survivors eventually rebleed each year (15).

Arteriovenous Malformation

Definition. An arteriovenous malformation is a congenital, nonneoplastic mass composed of tortuous blood vessels which apparently result from agenesis of an interposing capillary system. The condition is occasionally inherited as an autosomal dominant trait (16).

Etiology and Pathology. The absence of an intervening capillary bed permits a greatly decreased vascular resistance, and the abnormal vessels undergo progressive dilatation. Most arteriovenous (AV) malformations (90 percent) are supratentorial and are located in the parietal cortex (see Figures 9–3 and 9–4). However, AV malformations can occur anywhere in the brain or spinal cord. They consist of thin-walled, dilated communications between arterial and venous systems. The surrounding brain shows staining, numerous small hemorrhages, and gliosis with disruption of surrounding neurons.

Clinical Features. Partial or generalized seizures occur in 18 percent of cases (2). Other patients report migraine-like headaches on the side of the malformation. The neurologic examination may reveal the presence of focal deficits including homonymous hemianopia, dysphasia, and hemiparesis. There is often a bruit, which can be heard on auscultation over the orbits or skull.

Approximately 50 percent of AV malformations bleed, causing subarachnoid hemorrhage. Subarachnoid hemorrhage from rupture of an arteriovenous malformation is often less dramatic than hemorrhage following rupture of an aneurysm since AV malformations are a low-pressure system. Formation of a hematoma at the site of the malformation is not unusual with a subsequent increase in focal neurologic signs. Repeated hemorrhage may lead to fibrosis and destruction of the subarachnoid space. This results in a normal pressure hydrocephalus and progressive dementia. There is an increased tendency toward subarachnoid hemorrhage from an AV malformation during the first three months of pregnancy due to an increase in circulating blood volume.

Diagnostic Procedures. As for berry aneurysm.

Treatment.

1. Seizures should be controlled with adequate anticonvulsant therapy with serial measurement of plasma anticonvulsant levels.

2. The medical treatment of subarachnoid hemorrhage from rupture of an AV malformation is the same as the treatment described under berry aneurysm. Surgical treatment with extirpation of the AV malformation should be carried out if it is possible to remove the malformation without producing serious neurologic deficit. Attempts at surgical removal may be preceded by embolization with small plastic beads or injection of a polymerizing glue, which reduces its size and renders the operation more feasible (see Figure 9–4).

Prognosis. The outlook following subarachnoid hemorrhage from an AV malformation is much better than that following hemorrhage from a ruptured berry aneurysm. Some patients suffer repeated subarachnoid hemorrhages with little residual neurologic abnormalities. Many AV malfor-

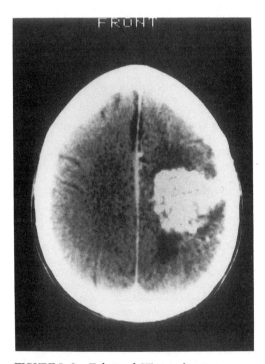

FIGURE 9–3 Enhanced CT scan showing an area of increased density in the left parietal area. A large arteriovenous malformation causing right sided partial motor seizures and occasional generalized seizures.

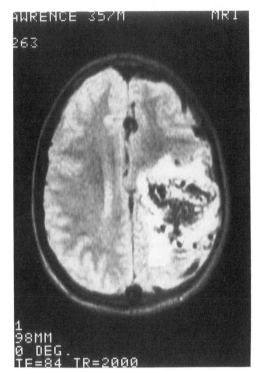

A

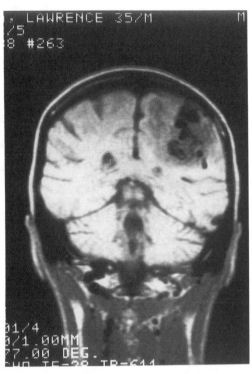

B

FIGURE 9–4. **A**, **B** and **C** MRI showing large arteriovenous malformation in the left parietal area. Dilated vessels can be seen at the periphery and within the substance of the malformation. Same patient as shown in Figure 9–3.

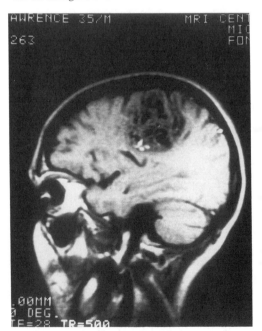

C

mations do not bleed and may be discovered in patients with seizures or incidentally during an evaluation for an unrelated problem (17).

Mycotic Aneurysm

Definition. A mycotic aneurysm is an aneurysm formation due to infection and subsequent weakening of the vessel wall.

Etiology and Pathology. The repeated introduction of bacterial organisms into the bloodstream by drug addicts who use contaminated syringes and needles results in subacute bacterial endocarditis and septic embolism. Septic emboli nearly always lodge in the middle cerebral artery, producing a low-grade infection of the arterial wall with formation of one or more mycotic aneurysms.

Clinical Features. Mycotic aneurysms of the middle cerebral artery were quite common at the turn of the century, but the incidence decreased with the declining incidence of rheumatic fever and subacute bacterial endocarditis. The condition became very rare after the introduction of antibiotics, but there has been an increase in identification of mycotic aneurysms in drug addicts in the last decade. Most cases of mycotic aneurysm remain undetected until the patient presents with subarachnoid hemorrhage. The symptoms have been described under ruptured berry aneurysm.

Diagnostic Procedures.

1. As for ruptured berry aneurysm.
2. The infecting organisms may be identified by repeated blood culture.

Treatment.

1. As for berry aneurysm.
2. Subacute bacterial endocarditis must be treated with the appropriate antibiotic therapy and many weeks of antibiotic treatment may be necessary.
3. Some aneurysms heal and disappear following antibiotic therapy. Persistent aneurysms can be treated surgically if they can be obliterated without occluding the vessel.

Prognosis. The prognosis of ruptured mycotic aneurysm is poor and most patients die once subarachnoid hemorrhage has occurred.

Subarachnoid Hemorrage—Cause Unknown

It is not possible to determine the cause of subarachnoid hemorrhage in about 10 percent of cases. The possibility of one of the rare causes should be considered (see Table 9-1), but investigation will not identify a cause in most cases when arteriography fails to reveal a berry aneurysm or an AV malformation. Since the false negative rate of 4-vessel arteriography is less than 2 percent, repeated studies are only recommended after rebleeding, which occurs in about 10 percent of cases. Subarachnoid hemorrhage of unknown etiology is a relatively benign disease with an early mortality of less than 5 percent, and a normal functioning capacity in about 90 percent of cases after many years of follow up (18).

Arteriosclerotic Aneurysms

An arteriosclerotic aneurysm is a dilatation of an arteriosclerotic cerebral vessel. Arteriosclerotic aneurysms usually occur in elderly patients. These aneurysms do not rupture and bleed but may exert pressure on surrounding structures. Arteriosclerotic aneurysms of the basilar artery can compress cranial nerves, particularly the fifth and seventh cranial

nerves, producing neurologic symptoms. Pressure from an arteriosclerotic aneurysm on the terminal portion of the internal carotid artery may cause optic atrophy on one side.

REFERENCES

1. Biller, J.; Godersky, J. C.; *et al.* Management of aneurysmal subarachnoid hemorrhage. Stroke 19:1300–1305; 1988.
2. Sundaram, M. B. H.; Chow, F. Seizures associated with spontaneous subarachnoid hemorrhage. Canad. J. Neurol. Sci. 13:229–231; 1986.
3. Chehrazi, B. B.; Giri, S.; *et al.* Prostaglandins and vasoactive aminos in cerebral vasospasm after aneurysmal subarachnoid hemorrhage. Stroke 20:217–224; 1989.
4. Hijdra, A.; Van Gijn, J.; *et al.* Delayed cerebral ischemia after aneurysmal subarachnoid hemorrhage. Clinico-anatomical correlations. Neurology 36:329–333; 1986.
5. Kotwicaz, Z.; Brzezinski, J. Chronic subdural hematoma presenting as spontaneous subarachnoid hemorrhage. J. Neurosurg. 63:691–692; 1985.
6. Black, P. McL. Hydrocephalus and vasospasm after subarachnoid hemorrhage from ruptured intracranial aneurysms. Neurosurgery 18:12–16; 1986.
7. Stober, T.; Emde, H.; *et al.* Blood distribution in computer cranial tomograms after subarachnoid hemorrhage with and without an aneurysm or angiography. Eur. Neurol. 24:319–323; 1985.
8. Sacco, R. L.; Wolf, P. A.; *et al.* Subarachnoid and intracerebral hemorrhage: natural history, prognosis, and precursive factors in the Framingham study. Neurology 34:847–854; 1984.
9. Adams, H. P. J.; Kassell, N. F.; Torner, J. C. Usefulness of computed tomography in predicting outcome after aneurysmal subarachnoid hemorrhage: a preliminary report of the Cooperative Aneurysm Study. Neurology 35:1263–1267; 1985.
10. Tsementzis, S. A.; Hitchcock, E. R.; *et al.* Comparative studies of the diagnostic value of cerebrospinal fluid spectrophotometry and computed tomographic scanning in subarachnoid hemorrhage. Neurosurgery 17:908–912; 1985.
11. Awad, I. A.; Carter, P.; *et al.* Clinical vasospasm after subarachnoid hemorrhage: response to hypervolemic, hemodilution and arterial hypertension. Stroke 18:365–372; 1987.
12. Ljunggren, B.; Brandt, L.; *et al.* Outcome in 60 consecutive patients treated with early aneurysmal operation and intravenous nimodipine. J. Neurosurg. 61:864–873; 1984.
13. Andreoli, A.; DePasquale, G.; *et al.* Subarachnoid hemorrhage: frequency and severity of cardiac arrhythmias. Stroke 18:558–564; 1987.
14. Solomon, R. A.; Fink, M. E. Current strategies for the management of aneurysmal subarach-

noid hemorrhage. Arch. Neurol. 44:769–774; 1987.

15. Nishioka, H.; Tarner, J. C.; *et al.* Cooperative study of intracranial aneurysms and subarachnoid hemorrhage: a long-term prognostic study. Arch. Neurol. 41:1142–1151; 1984.

16. Allard, J. C.; Hochberg, F. H.; *et al.* Magnetic resonance imaging in a family with hereditary cerebral arteriovenous malformations. Arch. Neurol. 46:184–187; 1989.

17. Crawford, P. M.; West, C. R.; *et al.* Arteriovenous malformations of the brain: natural history in unoperated patients. J. Neurol. Neurosurg. Psychiatry 49:1–10; 1986.

18. Ruelle, A.; Lasio, G.; *et al.* Long-term prognosis of subarachnoid hemorrhage of unknown etiology. J. Neurology 232:277–279; 1985.

CHAPTER 10

INTRACEREBRAL, PONTINE, AND INTRACEREBELLAR HEMORRHAGE

Although there has been a considerable decrease in the incidence of primary intracerebral hemorrhage in the past 20 years, the condition remains a dramatic event with high mortality, and there has been little improvement in therapy of cases with deeply situated hemorrhage. The decrease in incidence is probably related to improved control of hypertension in the population and is an indication of the success of antihypertensive therapy. This form of preventive medicine can be carried out by every practicing physician and is the keystone to the reduction in nearly all forms of cerebrovascular disease.

Primary Intracerebral Hemorrhage

Definition. Primary intracerebral hemorrhage is a syndrome characterized by spontaneous bleeding into the substance of the brain.

Etiology and Pathology.

1. Most cases of primary intracerebral hemorrhage occur in patients with chronic hypertension (1). This condition results in arteriosclerotic changes of small blood vessels, particularly in those branches of the middle cerebral artery that penetrate into the substance of the basal ganglia and internal capsule. These vessels show splitting and reduplication of the internal elastic lamina, hyalinization of the media, and the eventual formation of small aneurysms known as Charcot-Bou-

chard aneurysms. Similar changes probably occur in the penetrating vessels of the pons and cerebellum. Rupture of one of the weakened blood vessels results in hemorrhage into the substance of the brain.

2. Nontraumatic primary intracerebral hemorrhage in the normotensive and elderly is likely to be the result of cerebral amyloid angiopathy (2). This is an acellular thickening of the walls of small and medium sized arteries by amyloid. The affected vessels are weakened, undergo dilatation and microaneurysm formation and may rupture causing intracerebral hemorrhage (3).

3. An angiomatous malformation (arteriovenous malformation, cavernous angioma, venous angioma, or capillary telangiectasia) located at any site in the brain may rupture and produce an intracerebral hemorrhage of lobular type (4).

4. The abnormal vessels within high grade astrocytomas frequently rupture and may bleed extensively with the production of an intracerebral hemorrhage.

5. Rupture of a berry aneurysm can result in a massive intracerebral hemorrhage if the high pressure bleed is directed into the brain parenchyma.

6. Recreational amphetamine use can result in a vasculitis followed by arterial rupture and intracerebral hemorrhage (5).

7. Chronic cocaine use has been associated

169

with intracerebral hemorrhage. The mechanism has not been identified but the association is unequivocal (6, 7).

8. Anticoagulant therapy, particularly in the hypertensive individual treated for transient ischemic attacks (TIAs) or cerebral infarction, may result in intracerebral hemorrhage (8, 9).

9. Moya-moya disease, where there is an absence of the circle of Willis and a network of collateral vessels running into the brain parenchyma, has a high incidence of intracerebral hemorrhage.

10. Vasculitis—inflamed arteries with weakened walls found in granulomatous angiitis, may also result in intracerebral hemorrhage.

11. Leukemia with leukemic infiltration of the brain parenchyma can be followed by intracerebral hemorrhage.

12. Ingestion of phenylpropanolamine in dietary medications can result in intracerebral hemorrhage in some cases (10).

13. Sickle cell disease which produces a vasculopathy can be associated with arterial rupture or subarachnoid or intracerebral hemorrhage (11).

14. Idiopathic or acquired thrombocytopenia is a known cause of intracerebral hemorrhage.

15. Disseminated intravascular coagulopathy has been associated with intracerebral hemorrhage.

Risk factors identified in cases of intracerebral hemorrhage include hypertension, chronic alcoholism, hepatic disease, electrocardiographic abnormalities, prior cerebellar infarction or hemorrhage, and an abnormally high hematocrit (12, 13).

In the majority of cases hemorrhage occurs in the area of the thalamus (see Figure 10–1), internal capsule, or basal ganglia. However, the advent of computed tomography (CT) has demonstrated that focal hemorrhages situated in other areas of the cerebral hemisphere, such as the temporal lobe, are probably commoner than had been thought in the past (14).

An intracerebral hemorrhage produces direct destruction of tissue and compression of surrounding parenchyma. Deeply situated hemorrhages may rupture into the ventricular system (15) or, rarely, rupture through to the surface of the brain.

Clinical Features. In the majority of cases there is an acute onset of headache and rapid development of stupor followed by coma. Examination usually reveals systemic

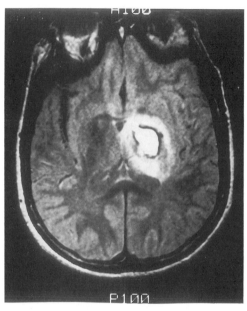

FIGURE 10–1. Left thalamic hemorrhage. MR scan showing presence of blood in the left thalamus and a surrounding halo of hemosiderin.

evidence of chronic hypertension. The signs and symptoms depend on the location of the hematoma, which acts like a mass lesion (see page 50). Uncal herniation with rostral-caudal loss of brain stem function may occur. Survivors gradually recover consciousness over a period of several days. Patients with temporal or frontal lobe hematomas may present with sudden onset of seizures followed by some degree of contralateral hemiparesis (16). Patients who recover from an intracerebral hemorrhage often have surprisingly good return of neurologic functioning (17).

Diagnostic Procedures.

1. Skull x-rays. X-rays of the skull may show a shift of the calcified pineal gland away from the side of the lesion.

2. Magnetic resonance (MR) or CT scanning readily reveals the presence of an intracerebral hematoma, shift of the midline, or intraventricular hemorrhage (see Figure 10–2).

3. Arteriography reveals a mass lesion (18).

Differential Diagnosis.

1. Other causes of acute coma (see page 49) and other causes of a mass lesion.

2. Cerebral infarction due to thrombosis or embolism. The acute onset and the pres-

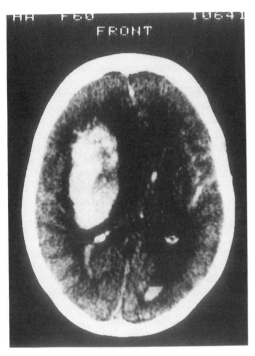

FIGURE 10–2. CT scan showing a large right intracerebral hemorrhage. There is a marked shift of midline structures to the left with blood in the left lateral ventricles which has gravitated to the occipital poles.

ence of blood in the cerebrospinal fluid will establish the diagnosis of intracerebral hemorrhage in the majority of cases. Small hematomas in the frontal or temporal lobes may be difficult to distinguish from cerebral infarction. The diagnosis will be established by MR or CT scan.

3. Ruptured berry aneurysm. This condition may occasionally present with severe headache, neck stiffness, and bloody spinal fluid without neurologic deficits. This rarely occurs in intracerebral hemorrhage. The two conditions are very difficult to differentiate when bleeding from an aneurysm has caused an intracerebral hematoma. The diagnosis can be established only by arteriography.

Treatment. See page 54, "treatment of the comatose patient." In general, these measures apply to patients with intraparenchymal hemorrhage. Additional measures include:

1. Careful control of hypertension; see page 146.
2. Cerebral edema should be reduced either with dexamethasone (Decadron) 12 mg

intravenously (IV) then 4 mg q6h or with mannitol when there is danger of herniation.

3. Surgical treatment may be lifesaving in selected cases with signs of rapidly increasing intracranial pressure. MR or CT scanning frequently reveals an acute hydrocephalus in these patients, apparently caused by an acute shift of the midline structures, which distorts and blocks the outflow of cerebrospinal fluid (CSF) from the ventricles. There may be dramatic improvement following emergency ventricular drainage, which should be maintained until the patient stabilizes. Patients with cerebral edema secondary to hematomas in the frontal or temporal lobes often improve following surgical evacuation of these hematomas. However, attempts to drain deeply situated hematomas are usually unsuccessful, and this form of treatment has been replaced by ventricular drainage in most centers.

Prognosis. The advent of MR and CT scanning has shown that intracerebral hemorrhage is not an inevitably fatal disease (see Figure 10–3). Nevertheless, mortality remains high, particularly when large hemorrhages involve the basal ganglia, internal capsule, and thalamus. A Glasgow Coma Scale score of less than 8, a wide pulse pressure, and a large hemorrhage indicate poor prognosis (19). Surviving patients usually have persistent neurologic deficits. Many function well, and every effort should be made to control those factors which lead to arteriosclerosis. In particular, hypertension must always be vigorously controlled.

Pontine Hemorrhage

Definition. A pontine hemorrhage is a hemorrhage into the pons. This condition is relatively rare and occurs in about 10 percent of cases with cerebral hemorrhage.

Etiology and Pathology. The most frequent cause of primary pontine hemorrhage is rupture of an arteriosclerotic vessel or rupture of a microaneurysm in a chronically hypertensive patient. Other possible causes include rupture of a small arteriovenous malformation.

The initial hemorrhage occurs either at the junction of the tegmentum and basilar portion of the pons or in the tegmentum at the midpontine level. When the hemorrhage involves the junction of the tegmentum and basilar pons, it may extend medially, ventrally, dorsally into the fourth ventricle, or

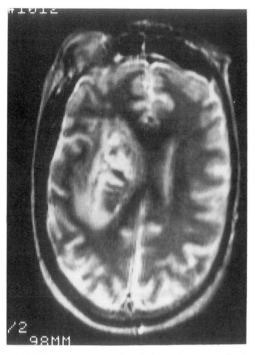

FIGURE 10–3. Large quadrilateral intracerebral hemorrhage. MR scan showing resolving hemorrhage involving basal ganglia internal and external capsules.

rostrally into the midbrain. When the hemorrhage is in the tegmentum at the midpontine level it tends to have limited extension.

Clinical Features. The onset is sudden with rapid loss of consciousness and coma in the majority of cases; a few patients present with stupor. Comatose patients are usually hypertensive with central neurogenic hyperventilation, and most exhibit decerebrate rigidity. There is extreme miosis in 50 percent of cases, and reflex conjugate eye movements are impaired in horizontal and vertical planes. Anisocoria, conjugate deviation of the eyes, or skew deviation are occasional occurrences. Most patients are quadriplegic or hemiplegic. The locked-in syndrome may occur (see page 155). Stuporous patients may show similar signs of eye involvement and motor deficits with additional hemisensory loss. Hyperpyrexia and gastrointestinal hemorrhage can occur in deeply comatose patients with extensive brain stem hemorrhages.

Diagnostic Procedures.

1. The MR or CT scan will demonstrate the hematoma (see Figures 10–4A and B).
2. Lumbar puncture usually reveals blood in the cerebrospinal fluid.
3. Arteriography reveals a mass in the area of the pons.

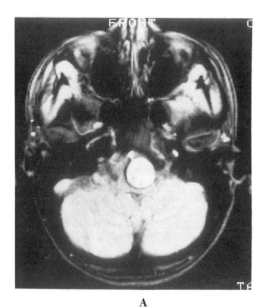

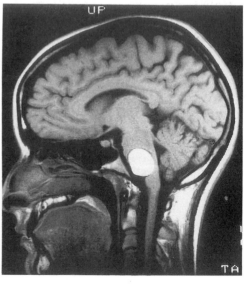

A   B

FIGURE 10–4. Pontine hemorrhage. A Axial and B lateral views of MR scan T1 weighted image showing well circumscribed area of increased signal in the pons.

Treatment. See page 146.

Prognosis. The prognosis is poor. When recovery does occur there are severe neurologic deficits.

Cerebellar Hemorrhage

Definition. A cerebellar hemorrhage is a hemorrhage originating within the substance of the cerebellum.

Etiology and Pathology. There are three major causes of cerebellar hemorrhage. These include:

1. Rupture of a penetrating artery, usually in the area of the dentate nucleus. In the chronic hypertensive patient penetrating arteries in the cerebellum undergo the same degenerative changes as the vessels of the cerebral hemispheres.
2. Rupture of an arteriovenous malformation.
3. Bleeding from a cerebellar hemangioblastoma (see page 241).

Hemorrhage is followed by hematoma formation within the substance of the cerebellum with dissection toward the subarachnoid space or toward the brain stem. The increasing volume of the hematoma produces distortion of the contents of the posterior fossa and pressure on the brain stem.

Clinical Features. There are three usual clinical presentations of cerebellar hemorrhage. The patient may present with:

1. Rapid onset with severe headache followed by clouding of consciousness and rapid progression. Sudden death may occur due to compression of the cardiorespiratory centers of the medulla. Since there are no localizing neurologic findings these cases are often diagnosed as intracerebral hemorrhage or subarachnoid hemorrhage.
2. Abrupt onset of occipital headache, severe vertigo, vomiting, and ataxia. There is progressive diminution of the level of consciousness followed by the appearance of central neurogenic hyperventilation indicating brain stem compression. These cases proceed to death within two to three days unless the hematoma is evacuated.
3. Approximately 20 percent of patients show slower progression following the development of occipital headache, vomiting, and vertigo. These patients are often conscious or obtunded and dysarthric. There are contralateral deviation of the eyes, ipsilateral cerebellar signs, contralateral hemiparesis, an extensor plantar response, and nuchal rigidity. The course is slowly progressive.

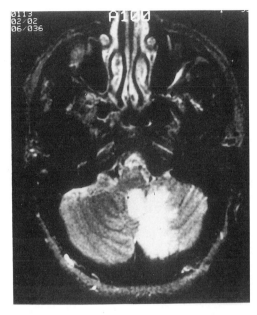

FIGURE 10–5. MR showing an intracerebellar hemorrhage with spread into the fourth ventricle and the subarachnoid space.

Diagnostic Procedures.

1. The MR or CT scan shows the presence of cerebellar hemorrhage with a circumscribed area of increased density lying within the substance of the cerebellum. The MR scan gives much better detail of the extent of the hemorrhage and proximity to or involvement of the brain stem (see Figure 10–5).
2. Arteriography reveals a posterior fossa mass.

Treatment. The hematoma should be evacuated as soon as the diagnosis is verified by CT scan.

Prognosis. The prognosis is good if evacuation occurs before there are signs of severe brain stem compression. There may be some residual signs of cerebellar ataxia, but these are often mild.

REFERENCES

1. Brott, T.; Thalinger, K.; *et al.* Hypertension as a risk factor for spontaneous intracerebral hemorrhage. Stroke 17:1078–1083; 1986.
2. Vinters, H. V. Cerebral amyloid angiopathy: a critical review. Stroke 18:311–324; 1987.
3. Kase, C. S. Intracerebral hemorrhage: non-hypertensive causes. Stroke 17:590–595; 1986.

4. Farmer, J. P.; Cosgrove, G. R.; *et al.* Intracranial cavernous angiomas. Neurology 38:1699–1704; 1988.
5. Toffol, G. J.; Biller, J.; *et al.* Nontraumatic intracerebral hemorrhage in young adults. Arch. Neurol. 44:483–485; 1987.
6. Wojate, J. G.; Flamm, E. S. Intracranial hemorrhage and cocaine use. Stroke 18:712–715; 1987.
7. Rowley, H. A.; Lowenstein, D. H.; *et al.* Thalamomesencephalic strokes after cocaine abuse. Neurology 39:428–430; 1989.
8. Levine, M.; Hirsch, J. Hemorrhagic complications of long-term anticoagulant therapy for ischemic vascular disease. Stroke 17:111–116; 1986.
9. Carlson, S. E.; Aldorich, M. S.; *et al.* Intracerebral hemorrhage complicating intravenous tissue plasminogen activator treatment. Arch. Neurol. 45:1070–1073, 1988.
10. Maher, L. M. Postpartum intracranial hemorrhage and phenylpropanolamine use. Neurology 37:1686; 1987.
11. Van Hoff, J.; Ritchey, A. K.; *et al.* Intracranial hemorrhage in children with sickle cell disease. Am. J. Dis. Child. 139:1120–1123; 1985.
12. Calandre, M. D.; Arnal, C.; *et al.* Risk factors for spontaneous cerebral hematomas. Case-control study. Stroke 17:1126–1128; 1986.
13. Bahemuka, M. Primary intracerebral hemorrhage and heart weight: a clinicopathological case-control review of 218 patients. Stroke 18:531–536; 1987.
14. Tanaka, Y.; Furuse, M.; *et al.* Lobar intracerebral hemorrhage: etiology and a long-term follow-up study of 32 patients. Stroke 17:51–57; 1986.
15. Gates, P. C.; Barnett, H. J. M.; *et al.* Primary intraventricular hemorrhage in adults. Stroke 17:872–877; 1986.
16. Berger, A. R.; Lipton, R. B.; *et al.* Early seizures following intracerebral hemorrhage. Neurology 38:1363–1365; 1988.
17. Verma, A. K.; Maheshwari, M. C. Hypesthetic-ataxic-hemiparesis in thalamic hemorrhage. Stroke 17:49–51; 1986.
18. Toffol, G. J.; Biller, J.; *et al.* The predicted value of angiography in non-traumatic intracerebral hemorrhage. Stroke 17:881–883; 1986.
19. Tuhrim, S.; Dambrosia, J. M.; *et al.* Prediction of intracerebral hemorrhage survival. Ann. Neurol. 24:258–263; 1988.

CHAPTER 11

STROKES IN CHILDREN AND YOUNG ADULTS

Strokes in children and young adults are encountered much less frequently than in the middle aged and elderly, but the result of a stroke in the younger age group is often devastating. Consequently, prevention, diagnosis, and treatment are extremely important in susceptible or afflicted individuals. There are many causes of stroke or stroke-like symptoms in young people (see Table 11–1) but many of these conditions are treatable. Consequently, appropriate treatment should reduce the risk of stroke or limit the neurologic deficit if the stroke has occurred.

Etiology. Hereditary conditions predisposing to stroke include sickle cell disease (1), sickle cell trait, hemoglobin S-C disease, homocystinuria, hyperlipidemia, and thrombocytosis. There is unfortunately as yet no adequate treatment for the hemoglobinopathies, but homocystinuria can be treated by diet and the hyperlipidemias will respond to diet or to lipid-reducing drugs if necessary. The identification and treatment of hyperlipidemia at an early age may slow the atherosclerotic process and reduce the risk of stroke or myocardial infarction which can be so crippling in the young adult (2).

Congenital conditions which predispose to stroke in the child or young adult include arteriovenous (AV) malformations and congenital heart disease which is a potent source of cerebral embolism and may cause cerebral thrombosis because of associated polycythemia. Right left shunt resulting in paradoxical embolism is probably underestimated as a cause of cerebral embolism (3). The septal defect may be very small and elude detection by standard investigative procedures unless the study is specifically directed to the detection of a right to left shunt (4). Embolism from a mitral valve prolapse is probably a rare cause of stroke and has been overemphasized in the past.

Intracerebral arteriovenous malformation is a potent cause of both seizures and stroke in young adults. The hemorrhage from a ruptured AV malformation can cause a large intracerebral hemorrhage and young females are at high risk during the first three months of pregnancy when there is a considerable increase in circulating blood volume.

Ruptured berry aneurysm carries a high mortality and morbidity (see page 159). The condition is rare in children but not uncommon in young adults. The neurologic deficits may be due to an intracerebral hematoma but are usually the result of arterial spasm which frequently accompanies subarachnoid hemorrhage.

Spontaneous arterial dissection involving the aorta or major vessels can occlude the lumen of the common carotid or vertebral arteries. Dissection is a feature of Marfan's syndrome or Ehlers Danlos syndrome but may also occur after trauma.

Trauma is a potent cause of childhood stroke and hemiparesis has been reported after closed head injury in children. Damage

TABLE 11–1.　Factors Known to Contribute to Stroke in Children and Young Adults

Hereditary:	Sickle cell disease, sickle cell trait, S-C disease, homocystinuria, hyperlipidemia, thrombocytosis
Congenital:	Mitral valve prolapse, arteriovenous malformation, congenital heart disease, paradoxical embolism, ruptured berry aneurysm, spontaneous arterial dissection
Traumatic:	Head trauma, subdural hematoma, subdural hygroma, brain contusion, traumatic intracerebral hemorrhage, direct trauma to carotid artery, accidental injection of carotid artery, traumatic dissection carotid artery, fat embolism
Infectious:	Infections in children: pneumonia, cervical adenitis, pharyngitis, retropharyngeal abscess, tonsillitis, sinusitis
	Cerebral venous thrombosis: infection of face, sinusitis, otitis media, mastoiditis
	Epidural abscess, cerebral abscess, encephalitis, viral arteritis, syphilitic arteritis, subacute bacterial endocarditis
Metabolic:	Hyperlipidemia, hypercholesterolemia, hyperuricemia, hypothyroidism, diabetes mellitus, smoking, obesity, pregnancy, acute alcoholic intoxication
Neoplastic:	Brain tumor, primary CNS tumor, lymphoma in AIDS
Blood dyscrasias:	Polycythemia, lupus anticoagulant, leukemia, homophilia, thrombocytopenia, thrombotic thrombocytopenic purpura, hemolytic uremic syndrome, postpartum state, "sticky platelets"
Toxic:	Alcohol abuse, heroin, cocaine (crack), IV sympathomimetic drugs
Cardiac:	Congenital heart disease, paradoxical embolism, subacute bacterial endocarditis, rheumatic heart disease, atrial fibrillation, paradoxical arrhythmias, mitral valve prolapse, ischemic heart disease, cardiac surgery
Vascular:	Hypertension, atherosclerosis, lupus erythematosus, polyarteritis nodosa, granulomatous giant cell arteritis, dermatomyositis, isolated intracranial arteritis, sarcoidosis, arteritis of herpes zoster
Degenerative:	Atherosclerosis
Miscellaneous:	Migraine, unilateral status epilepticus, dehydration

to the internal carotid artery following trauma to the neck may result in thrombosis and infarction. The internal carotid artery may also be damaged by trauma through the tonsillar fossa by a stick or pencil held in the mouth.

Injury to the carotid artery and stroke in young adults has been reported following a sudden blow to the neck by a ski when snow or water skiing. This results in damage to the intima followed by thrombosis and carotid occlusion or occlusion following traumatic dissection of the arterial wall.

Adolescents and young adults can suffer a major stroke following accidental injection of heroin into the carotid artery following an attempt to enter the jugular vein.

Fat embolism is an occasional cause of stroke in children.

A number of infectious conditions may be followed by a stroke. Infant and childhood hemiparesis has been associated with pneu-monia, cervical adenitis, pharyngitis, retropharyngeal abscess, tonsillitis, and sinusitis. The mechanism is presumed to be a local arteritis affecting the carotid artery with thrombosis and cerebral infarction. Cerebral venous thrombosis and venous sinus thrombosis can occur in the presence of infection of the face, paranasal sinuses, or middle ears.

The development of an epidural abscess or cerebral abscess is occasionally a rapid process producing a progressive hemiparesis and mimicking a stroke.

Viral encephalitis occasionally presents with a hemiparesis when the infection is predominantly in one hemisphere. Infection by the herpes zoster virus may be followed by an arteritis with vascular occlusion and stroke. The same mechanism occurs in syphilitic arteritis in young adults.

Subacute bacterial endocarditis causes stroke by embolism and vessel occlusion or rupture of a mycotic aneurysm and subarachnoid hemorrhage. Mycotic aneurysms usually occur in heroin addicts with bacterial endocarditis following numerous intravenous injections of bacteria which colonize dirty needles.

A number of metabolic abnormalities including diabetes mellitus, hyperlipidemia, hypercholesterolemia, hyperuricemia, and hypothyroidism predispose to cerebral infarction and stroke in young adults. The effect of these conditions may be accentuated by obesity, smoking, and frequent alcoholic intoxication. There is an increased incidence of stroke during pregnancy. The cause is probably multiple and includes metabolic changes, increased circulating blood volume, increased fibrinogen levels, and increased platelet activation.

Two types of brain tumor, a rapidly growing glioma and primary lymphoma in acquired immunodeficiency syndrome (AIDS), may mimic a stroke with a rapid development of hemiparesis.

Either primary or secondary polycythemia predisposes to stroke in children or young adults, while stroke has been reported to occur when the only abnormality is the presence of circulating lupus anticoagulant. Hemorrhagic infarction or intracerebral hemorrhage is a complication of leukemia, hemophilia, thrombocytopenia, thrombotic thrombocytopenia purpura, hemolytic uremic syndrome, and therapeutic anticoagulants.

Dehydration complicated by cerebral venous or venous sinus thrombosis may produce cerebral infarction in children. There is an increased risk of stroke due to cerebral venous thrombosis in the postpartum period in young adults.

A group of young adults with increased platelet hyperaggregability have been recognized. This has been called "sticky platelet syndrome" and results in both transient ischemic attacks and cerebral infarction in young adults.

Alcohol abuse increases the risk of stroke in young adults while heroin, cocaine, and "crack," a highly potent refined cocaine, can cause a cerebral arteritis resulting in a severe stroke in young adult drug addicts (5). Intravenous use of sympathomimetic drugs has also resulted in stroke.

Heart disease is a potent cause of stroke. Congenital heart disease may result in cerebral embolism because of periodic dysrhythmias or atrial fibrillation. Paradoxical embolism can occur when there is a right to left shunt (3); subacute bacterial endocarditis is an ever present risk in congenital heart disease.

Rheumatic heart disease has declined in the last several years but may cause stroke in young adults by embolism, subacute bacterial endocarditis, or paroxysmal fibrillation. As already indicated, mitral valve prolapse is an occasional but overestimated cause of cerebral embolism. Ischemic heart disease occasionally occurs in young adults and may be complicated by dysrhythmias, embolism, and stroke (6).

Cardiac surgery carries a not inconsiderable risk of cerebral infarction from embolism due to clots or entrance of particulate matter into the circulation, resulting in air embolism and hypoxia (7).

Severe hypertension predisposes to accelerated atherosclerosis and stroke, or may be complicated by intracerebral hemorrhage in young adults. Several arteritides such as those of lupus erythematosus, polyarteritis nodosa, granulomatous giant cell arteritis, dermatomyositis, isolated intracranial arteritis, sarcoidosis, syphilis, and herpes zoster can produce stroke in children and young adults.

A mild degree of atherosclerosis is not uncommon in young adults but marked development of atherosclerosis can occur even in children who are subject to prolonged action of predisposing factors such as hypertension and diabetes mellitus. Consequently, stroke in children or young adults may be the result of accelerated atherosclerosis in some cases (8).

Complex migraine is an occasional occurrence in children or young adults and may be accompanied by cerebral infarction and hemiplegia (9). Whether the infarction results from severe arterial spasm or damage to cortical neurons from another cause is open to debate.

The cause of hemiplegia following unilateral status epilepticus appears to be neuronal exhaustion and cell death. This process can occur as early as two hours after onset of seizure activity in children or young adults, indicating the urgent need for effective treatment of the seizures as soon as possible (see page 79).

Clinical Features. The majority of strokes affect the cerebral hemispheres, are of acute onset, and present with hemiparesis. Examination may show a homonymous visual field defect, dysphasia if the dominant hemisphere is involved, and hemisensory loss. Lesions such as AV malformations may be associated with contralateral involuntary movements.

Children and young adults with subarachnoid hemorrhage complain of headache and frequently have seizures and focal neurologic signs, including cranial nerve palsies and hemiparesis. Examination shows the presence of nuchal rigidity and occasionally subhyaloid hemorrhage.

Differential Diagnosis.

1. Trauma. All children who have suffered head trauma with neurologic deficit should be closely investigated for the possibility of epidural hematoma, subdural hematoma, cerebral contusion, or intracerebral hemorrhage.

2. Cerebral abscess. In this case the onset is usually gradual. There are headache, vomiting, and signs of increased intracranial pressure with the development of focal neurologic signs. The temperature is elevated and there may be signs of infection elsewhere or signs of congenital heart disease.

3. Encephalitis. The onset is usually acute with fever, headache, neck stiffness, and occasionally focal seizures followed by the development of focal neurologic signs. In some cases, however, the infection may develop without fever and only minimal headache with rather sudden development of hemiparesis. Such cases present some difficulty in diagnosis. If there is any doubt, obtain a head scan and follow up with a lumbar puncture. This will reveal an increase in pressure with pleocytosis, elevated protein content, and normal glucose content in viral encephalitis.

4. Bacterial meningitis. This may present with much the same symptoms of fever, headache, lethargy, seizures, and nuchal rigidity. In this case, however, the lumbar puncture will reveal a polymorphonuclear pleocytosis, elevated protein content, and decreased glucose content.

5. Uremia. The presence of hypertension associated with elevated blood urea nitrogen and anemia characterizes uremia.

6. Benign intracranial hypertension. The condition is quite common in children and young adults and there are no neurologic deficits. The patient complains of increasing headache and shows increasing lassitude. A history of excess vitamin A intake, recent ingestion of tetracyclines, withdrawal of corticosteroids, or laboratory tests suggesting hypoparathyroidism or Addison's disease contribute to the diagnosis. A number of cases are of unknown etiology and tend to occur in obese individuals. Other cases are associated with the menarche in adolescent girls.

7. Postictal (Todd's) paralysis. The acute onset of hemiparesis in a semicomatose child may indicate a postictal state following a seizure. In this case there will be rapid recovery of consciousness and resolution of the hemiparesis.

8. Migraine. The sudden onset of a neurologic deficit, usually hemiparesis, associated with a severe headache in a child with a history of previous headaches suggests hemiplegic migraine. Ophthalmoplegic migraine with third nerve palsy is rare in children but has been reported.

9. Lead encephalopathy. This condition may present acutely. There are signs of increased intracranial pressure with neurologic deficits. The diagnosis depends upon demonstration of elevated serum lead levels.

10. Tumor. Tumors can present with acute neurologic deficits, particularly following epileptic seizures. There may be signs of increased intracranial pressure, and the diagnosis can usually be established by magnetic resonance (MR) or computed tomography (CT) scan.

Diagnostic Procedures. Diagnostic procedures are outlined in Table 11–2.

Treatment.

A. In the acute situation:
   1. An airway should be established in an obtunded, semicomatose, or comatose patient.
   2. Adequate hydration should be maintained. Children become easily dehydrated. The requirement of fluids is 1,200 ml/sq m of body surface per day.
   3. Any electrolyte imbalance should be corrected.
   4. Any identified medical condition should be treated; for instance, patients with congenital heart disease may have dysrhythmia or heart failure and require appropriate treatment with digitalis and diuretics.
   5. Seizures should be controlled. If the patient is in status epilepticus, treat as status epilepticus (see page 79).
   6. In stroke due to cerebral embolism the patient should be heparinized (see page 148).
   7. In case of increased intracranial pressure patients should be admitted to an

TABLE 11–2. Strokes in Children and Young Adults: Diagnostic Procedures

An acute stroke in a child or young adult requires immediate investigation to rule out trauma, intracranial infection, intracranial mass lesion and congenital heart disease:

1. MR or CT scan should be obtained to rule out mass lesion including epidural and subdural hematoma, intracerebral hemorrhage, cerebral edema due to trauma, tumors, and cerebral abscess.

2. There should be x-rays of the mastoid air cells, paranasal sinuses, and chest to rule out infection.

3. Lumbar puncture should be performed, after the CT scan, in any case with fever and nuchal rigidity to rule out encephalitis and meningitis. The cerebrospinal fluid should be examined for cells and glucose and protein content. A smear should be stained by Gram's method and the fluid cultured aerobically and anaerobically.

4. Rule out congenital heart disease. Additional studies and consultation may be needed.

5. A blood sample should be drawn for complete blood count, platelet count, blood urea nitrogen, creatinine, sedimentation rate, and blood culture. Additional studies might include lupus anticoagulant, antinuclear antibody determination, sickle cell preparation, hemoglobin type, and aminoacid levels.

6. Arteriography will be required in all cases of nontraumatic subarachnoid hemorrhage of unknown etiology, to rule out the presence of a cerebral aneurysm or a small vascular malformation which has not been detected by MR or CT scanning. Arteriography is the definitive study for the diagnosis of cerebral arteritis in young adults (10).

intensive care unit and intracranial pressure monitoring carried out. Cerebral edema may be reduced by infusion of 20 percent mannitol in a dosage of 1.5 gm/Kg over a 20-minute period. It is then possible to titrate the requirements of mannitol by observing the intracranial pressure monitor readings. Dexamethasone is also helpful but is delayed in onset. An initial dose of 12 mg should be followed by 6 mg a day. The dosage can be gradually tapered over a period of 7 to 10 days. Acute neurosurgical procedures are indicated for epidural hematoma, subdural hematoma, and acute hydrocephalus secondary to intracerebral hematoma. Hydrocephalus can be relieved by ventricular drainage.

B. In the chronic situation:
1. Patients with residual neurologic deficits who are suffering from seizures should have adequate seizure control with appropriate anticonvulsants (see page 75). Frequent determinations of serum levels of anticonvulsants may be necessary to ensure control.
2. Patients with permanent neurologic problems require a planned multidisciplinary program to obtain optimum benefit. The emotional impact of the chronic illness on the child and the family should always be considered. A planned program of physical therapy extending over many months is useful. Speech therapy by a trained speech pathologist is indicated in patients with dysphasia. All children should receive full psychological evaluation, and the psychologist should be available for counseling if this is required by the child or family.

The psychological evaluation is useful in planning education for the impaired child or adolescent. In addition, the evaluation will detect and measure depression which is quite common following stroke in the young adult. Treatment with antidepressants and psychotherapy should be obtained if indicated. A social worker may also help in the counseling and in arranging for available community resources to be used in the rehabilitation process.

Prognosis. Although young children show much better recovery from motor and speech deficits following a stroke than adults, many children are left with obvious neurologic deficits following a stroke. One of the main problems is epilepsy, and almost all children with hemiplegia accompanied by seizures at onset have subsequent epileptic attacks. Many children with motor deficits also have intellectual impairment and hyperkinetic behavior. Language development is often delayed in children, or dysphasia is a problem in the young adult but recovery is often quite good over a period of the next two years. Permanent aphasia or severe dysphasia is rare if the neurologic deficit begins before the age of four years (11).

Some conditions producing stroke have a high risk of recurrence: homocystinuria, sickle cell disease, cerebral embolism from congenital heart disease, and particularly polyarteritis nodosa. The risk of cerebral embolism can be reduced by the use of long-term anticoagulants orally. Arteritis often responds to corticosteroids although immunosuppression will be required in some cases.

REFERENCES

1. Rothman, S. M.; Fulling, K. H.; *et al.* Sickle cell anemia and central nervous system infarction: a neuropathological study. Ann. Neurol. 20:684–690; 1986

2. Adams, H. P., Jr.; Butler, M. J.; *et al.* Nonhemorrhagic cerebral infarction in young adults. Arch. Neurol. 43:793–796; 1986.

3. Beller, J.; Adams, H. P., Jr.; *et al.* Paradoxical cerebral embolism: eight cases. Neurology 36:1356–1360; 1986.

4. Harvey, J. R.; Teague, S. M.; *et al.* Clinically silent atrial septal defects with evidence of cerebral embolization. Ann. Int. Med. 105:695–697; 1986.

5. Wojak, J. C.; Flamms, E. S. Intracranial hemorrhage and cocaine use. Stroke 18:712–715; 1987.

6. Flegel, K. M.; Shipley, M. J.; *et al.* Risk of stroke in non-rheumatic atrial fibrillation. Lancet 1:526–529; 1987.

7. Ferry, P. C. Neurological sequelae of cardiac surgery in children. Am. J. Dis. Child. 141:309–312; 1987.

8. Johnson, S. E.; Skre, H. Transient cerebral ischemia attacks in the young and middle aged. A population study. Stroke 17:662–666; 1986.

9. Poole, C. J. M.; Ross Russel, R. W.; *et al.* Amaurosis fugax under the age of forty years. J. Neurol. Neurosurg. Psychiatry 50:81–84, 1987.

10. Smoker, W. R. K.; Biller, J.; *et al.* Angiography of non-hemorrhage cerebral infarction in young adults. Stroke 18:708–711; 1987.

11. Bogousslavsky, J.; Regli, F. Ischemic stroke in adults younger than thirty years of age. Causes and prognosis. Arch. Neurol. 44:479–482; 1987.

CHAPTER 12

VASCULAR DISEASE OF THE SPINAL CORD

When compared to cerebrovascular disease, vascular disease of the spinal cord is uncommon, a fact that does not support the unsubstantiated claim that the spinal cord has a "poor blood supply." The blood supply to the spinal cord is adequate in a healthy individual with ample reserve and the capacity for development of substantial collateral circulation. There are many common factors in vascular disease of the brain and spinal cord (i.e., atherosclerosis). However, because of anatomic factors there are a number of additional factors that may produce vascular disease of the cord.

Anatomy of the Arterial Supply of the Spinal Cord

The anterior spinal artery runs the entire length of the spinal cord and is located in the anterior ventral sulcus of the cord. At the cranial end the anterior spinal artery arises from the fourth portion of the vertebral artery and descends over the ventral surface of the medulla toward the midline to join the anterior spinal artery from the opposite side. The two vessels are usually small but have the capacity for hypertrophy and are a potential source of collateral circulation to the medulla and spinal cord. The anterior spinal artery is reinforced by three anterior, anastomotic (medullary) arteries in the cervical area. These vessels take origin from the vertebral artery, the deep cervical artery, and the costocervical or ascending cervical artery and usually join the anterior spinal artery at the level of C_3, C_6 and C_8, respectively. The thoracic portion receives one or two anastomotic vessels, which arise from intercostal arteries. The commonest site is at T_4 or T_5. The thoracolumbar portion of the anterior spinal artery is joined by the great anterior anastomotic artery of Adamkiewicz, which arises anywhere between the levels of T_8 and L_4 on the left side in about 80 percent of cases. This vessel receives blood from the aorta via the lower intercostal or lumbar arteries. In its course over the cauda equina the anterior artery is joined by branches from the lumbar, iliolumbar, lateral, and medial sacral arteries.

The anterior spinal artery is not a continuous vessel but should be regarded as a series of anastomotic systems fed by anastomotic arteries such as the artery of Adamkiewicz. This physiologic concept suggests that the arterial system of the spinal cord is similar to the arterial systems of the brain and brain stem.

The branches of the anterior spinal artery are of two types.

1. Central arteries penetrate the median fissure and branch alternately to the right or to the left with an occasional bifurcating vessel. These branches extend to the anterior horn, where they divide into a rich capillary network and form a plexus involving the anterior horn cells, the gray commissure, the lateral horn, and the base of the posterior horn. The capillaries from this system also

181

penetrate the white matter and anastomose with branches of the centripetal system. There is also an additional anastomosis through intersegmental arterioles extending upward and downward in the cord which forms a connection between adjacent segmental arterial systems.

2. The centripetal system arises from the anterior spinal artery and extends around the periphery of the spinal cord as far as the posterior nerve root. These vessels give rise to numerous penetrating radial arteries, which enter the white matter and anastomose with the capillaries of the central system.

The posterior spinal arteries constitute an irregular system that traverses the length of the spinal cord immediately posterior to the entrance of the posterior nerve root. These vessels are reinforced by 12 to 16 small posterior anastomotic arteries. The posterior spinal system anastomoses superiorly with the vertebral arteries and inferiorly with the anterior spinal artery through many fine arterioles surrounding the terminal portion of the spinal cord and cauda equina. The posterior horns of the spinal cord and the posterior columns, which constitute the posterior third of the spinal cord, are supplied by penetrating vessels arising from numerous superficial anastomotic vessels joining the two posterior spinal arteries.

Anatomy of the Venous Drainage of the Spinal Cord

The intrinsic drainage of the spinal cord occurs through a central venous system and a radial group of veins.

The central veins of the spinal cord converge toward the anterior median fissure and enter the anterior median spinal vein. The radial veins pass to the surface of the cord, where a plexus is formed which drains into the anterior median spinal vein.

The posterior one-third of the spinal cord is also drained by a series of radial veins into a posterior plexus. Blood from the anterior median spinal vein and from the posterior plexus of veins enters a series of anastomotic veins, which penetrate the dura and enter the internal and external vertebral plexi. These systems extend throughout the length of the spinal canal and anastomose with the vena cava, the azygos, and the hemiazygos systems. It is possible that blood can be channeled into the pelvic plexus of veins and into the dural sinuses and cerebral veins at the level of the foramen magnum.

Spinal Cord Infarction

Definition. Spinal cord infarction results from inadequate blood supply to the spinal cord parenchyma.

Etiology and Pathology. The development of spinal cord infarction is influenced by a number of anatomic, physiologic, and pathologic factors. These factors include:

1. Site of occlusion. The farther from the cord the occlusion occurs, the better the chance of developing collateral circulation.
2. Anatomic variation. The greater the number of anastomotic vessels to the cord, the better the chance of avoiding infarction if an anastomotic vessel or its parent vessel should be occluded.
3. Onset of occlusion. Gradual occlusion permits the development of collateral circulation and is less likely to cause infarction than rapid occlusion of a vessel. A decrease in perfusion pressure in the anastomotic vessels produces spinal cord ischemia and increases the chance of infarction.
4. Systemic blood pressure. Hypotension decreases perfusion pressure and increases the chance of infarction.
5. Hypoxia. Chronic hypoxia results in lower arterial oxygen tension and increases the chance of infarction.
6. Atherosclerosis. Progressive atherosclerosis involving the anastomotic vessels or the spinal arteries reduces blood flow to the cord and increases the chance of infarction.
7. Inflammation. Arteritis of the anastomotic vessels or the anterior spinal artery and its branches will increase the chance of thrombosis and infarction.
8. Embolism. Emboli can arise from atherosclerotic plaques in the vertebral, intercostal, or lumbar arteries and enter the circulation of the spinal cord.
9. Trauma. The spinal arteries and anastomotic vessels are susceptible to trauma. Fracture dislocation, spondylosis, and disk protrusion may produce damage to the costal, lumbar, or anastomotic vessels.

The pathology of ischemia shows some variation according to the site of the involved vessel. When the aorta is involved, there may be occlusion at the origin of intercostal or lumbar arteries due to aneurysm, thrombosis, or surgical procedures of the aorta. The vertebral arteries are susceptible to thrombosis following cervical injury or chiropractic manipulation and from atherosclerosis. Intercostal and lumbar arteries are occasionally injured in thoracoplasty and resection of an aortic aneurysm. An anastomotic artery may be occluded following trauma to the spine or the development of primary or metastatic tumors of the spine. There may be involvement due to osteomyelitis of the spine or tuberculous osteomyelitis (Pott's disease). In addition, the vessels may be involved by an arteritis in syphilis or collagen diseases. Anterior and posterior spinal arteries may be occluded because of trauma with fracture dislocation of the spine or pressure from a herniated lumbar disk. The anterior spinal artery is particularly susceptible to compression in cervical spondylosis.

The pathologic changes in infarction of the spinal cord resemble those seen in ischemic infarction of the brain, with necrosis of the gray matter followed by astrocytic proliferation and the formation of a glial scar.

Clinical Features. All of the signs and symptoms of spinal cord infarction can be attributed to a lesion within the distribution of the occluded vessel.

Transient ischemic attacks of the spinal cord are difficult and probably impossible to recognize. It is possible that some "drop attacks" without loss or impairment of consciousness, which are attributed to sudden ischemia of the medulla, are caused by ischemia of the cervical cord.

When the anterior spinal artery is occluded, there are paresthesias and impaired pain and temperature sensation below the level of the infarction. There may be pain in a radicular distribution at the level of the infarction. Spinal shock with sudden loss of bladder control and flaccid paraparesis or paraplegia of the lower extremities is followed by a gradual development of lower limb spasticity as the signs of spinal shock resolve (1).

Occlusion of an anterior spinal cord ramus at the level of the medulla results in a sudden onset of contralateral hemiplegia with loss of contralateral vibration and position sense due to involvement of the medial lemniscus. Bilateral involvement of the spinal rami produces quadriparesis, and bilateral involvement of the medial lemniscus causes bilateral loss of vibration and position sense.

Occlusion of a cervical anastomotic branch of the anterior spinal artery produces a combination of upper and lower motor neuron abnormalities. There are weakness and wasting of the muscles in the upper limb supplied by the appropriate anterior horn cells at the level of the infarct with flaccid quadriparesis progressing gradually to spastic paraparesis and loss of pain and temperature sensation below the level of the lesion.

Infarction in the thoracic cord produces a flaccid paraplegia with gradual progression to spastic paraparesis. This is associated with a dissociated sensory loss and eventually with some return of bladder function.

Lesions of the lumbosacral cord tend to produce flaccid paraparesis because of destruction of the motor neurons of the anterior horn cells at this level. There are a dissociated sensory loss and incomplete improvement in bowel and bladder function.

It is not unusual to encounter incomplete infarction of the spinal cord. The effects of infarction are dependent upon the efficiency of the collateral circulation, and only small segments of the anterior two-thirds of the spinal cord may be irreversibly damaged following occlusion of the anterior spinal artery or its branches.

Posterior spinal artery occlusion is very rare. Syphilitic arteritis is believed to have been the major cause of this condition in the past. However, trauma, infection, or compression of the posterior spinal arteries may compromise the circulation sufficiently to produce infarction of the posterior one-third of the spinal cord. The clinical picture is tabetic-like with progressive ataxia and loss of vibration and position sense. Deep tendon reflexes are depressed or absent. There may be retention of urine with painless distention of the bladder. Spinal cord compression should be relieved and infection controlled by appropriate antibiotic therapy. Urinary retention or incomplete emptying can be managed with intermittent self-catheterization. Gait may be improved by physical therapy.

Diagnostic Procedures.

1. Lumbar puncture. The spinal fluid is normal in appearance, and there is little or no cellular response. The protein content may be elevated.
2. Arteriography. The occlusion may be demonstrated by arteriography.

Differential Diagnosis. See Table 12–1 (page 184).

Treatment. As for cerebral infarction (see page 146).

Prognosis. Many patients with spinal cord infarction show gratifying return of function in the lower limbs and considerable improvement in bowel and bladder function

TABLE 12–1. Differential Diagnosis: Cord Infarction, Transverse Myelopathy, Epidural Abscess

Infarction	Transverse Myelopathy	Epidural Abscess
Age		
Elderly, unless some unusual easily identifiable condition exists (e.g., syphilis)	Any age	Any age
Pain		
Acute onset, radicular distribution	Yes. Often interscapular with radiation into the abdomen and lower limbs	Yes. At site of abscess
Onset of Spasticity		
Acute onset, initially flaccid followed by development of spasticity	May be acute or insidious onset. May be prolonged flaccidity	Insidious onset, spastic lower extremities
Spinal Fluid		
Normal	Abnormal, Inflammatory cells and elevated protein content	Abnormal. Xanthochromic if complete block, polymorphonuclear leukocytosis, protein elevated, glucose normal
Peripheral Nerve Involvement		
None (except diabetic neuropathy)	Yes. Lesion may involve nerve roots	None (except diabetic neuropathy)
Dissociated sensory loss		
Yes	Unusual	No
X-ray spine		
Normal	Normal	Osteomyelitis in some cases
Myelogram		
Normal	Normal	Extradural compression, may be a complete block

over a period of several months. Prevention of further infarction depends upon the control of precipitating factors. Patients with atherosclerosis run a high risk of coronary artery disease and cerebral thrombosis.

Intermittent Claudication of the Spinal Cord

Intermittent ischemia of the spinal cord or cauda equina may result in transient pain, weakness, and numbness of one or both lower limbs during exercise. The disorder is believed to result from narrowing of the spinal canal, herniation of a lumbar disk, or lumbar spondylosis, which results in pressure on the spinal cord and/or cauda equina. Patients with this condition develop aching in one or both calves followed by paresthesias of one or both feet while walking. Continued walking may result in foot drop. Examination reveals that the circulation of both lower limbs is adequate. There is exaggeration of stretch reflexes if the spinal cord is involved. X-rays of the lumbosacral spine show the presence of osteoarthritis and narrowing of intervertebral disk spaces. Myelography will demonstrate multiple disk protrusions or lumbar stenosis. Surgical removal of herniated disks and decompression of spinal cord stenosis will result in improvement.

Chronic Ischemia of the Spinal Cord

It is quite likely that changes in the cervical cord in cervical spondylosis are due to a combination of compression of the cord and ischemia of the cord due to compression of the vasculature. This would account for the development of symptoms indicating damage to the cord above and below the site of the lesion.

Arteriovenous Malformation of the Spinal Cord

Definition. Most arteriovenous (AV) malformations involving the spinal cord are low flow conditions with a nidus located on the dura of the dorsal nerve root. Symptoms are probably the results of increased venous pressure and cord ischemia (2).

Clinical Features. Most patients with an AV malformation of the spinal cord experience pain at the level of the lesion or in the lower limbs. The pain may be constant or episodic and is often of an unpleasant burning quality. Some patients show progressive spastic paraparesis with or without evidence of a lower motor neuron lesion. Urgency, frequency, and incontinence are present in about two-thirds of patients. Sensory deficits occur below the level of the lesion and affect all sensory modalities. The neurologic deficits tend to progress in a stepwise fashion over a period of months or years. Sudden paraplegia from hemorrhage or infarction may occur at any time. Rupture of an AV malformation with spinal subarachnoid hemorrhage is unusual but has been reported (3).

Diagnostic Procedures.

1. Magnetic resonance (MR) scanning will demonstrate the site of the malformation and the presence of any hemorrhage.
2. Selective arteriography is needed to demonstrate the nidus.

Treatment. Direct removal of the dural nidus is curative. However, some malformations within the spinal cord cannot be totally excised without cord damage (4).

Venous Spinal Cord Infarction

Three types of venous infarction of the spinal cord have been recognized: embolic, hemorrhagic, and nonhemorrhagic. Embolic cases are associated with venous embolism elsewhere such as pulmonary embolism and produce sudden back pain with symmetric dysfunction and dissociate sensory loss. Hemorrhagic infarction is of equally sudden onset with back pain or radicular pain, progressive neurologic dysfunction, and a high mortality rate. Nonhemorrhagic infarction is more gradual and painless with neurologic signs evolving over several weeks (5).

Venous spinal cord infarction is often diag-nosed as a transverse myelitis. Arteriography may be helpful, and MR scanning will help to rule out hemorrhage. Nonhemorrhagic cases should be treated with anticoagulation.

Transverse Myelopathy (Myelitis)

Definition. Transverse myelopathy is a syndrome characterized by acute spinal cord dysfunction involving both halves of the cord in transverse section.

Eitiology and Pathology. The various etiologies of transverse myelopathy are outlined in Table 12–2. The condition may be a peri-infectious or postinfectious process and has been associated with many viral infections. In some cases there appears to be a direct viral involvement of the spinal cord by an inflammatory process. Transverse myelopathy has been associated with or has followed measles, varicella, mumps, rabies, typhoid, systemic lupus erythematosus (SLE), and a reaction to sulphonamides. Transverse myelopathy has also followed vaccination and immunization against rubella, diphtheria, and poliomyelitis. Vascular occlusion with softening of the cord may occur in syphilitic arteritis and in the arteritis associated with collagen diseases. Arterial occlusion due to dissecting aneurysm of the aorta, or following surgical resection of the aortic aneurysm, is another possible cause. Acute transverse myelopathy in heroin addicts is probably due to a focal arteritis. Transverse myelopathy may occur as an acute demyelinating process in multiple sclerosis, and a severe acute myelopathy has been described as a remote effect of carcinoma. The increasing survival of patients with treated neoplasms has led to the recognition of increasing numbers of cases of acute transverse myelopathy secondary to radiation therapy.

TABLE 12–2. **Etiologies of Transverse Myelopathy**

1. Congenital—vascular malformation
2. Infectious—viral infection
3. Autoimmune—periinfectious, postinfectious, or vaccinial myelitis
4. Multiple sclerosis
5. Neoplastic—paracarcinomatous necrosis
6. Toxic—secondary to heroin injections
7. Vascular—vascular insufficiency
8. Degenerative—irradiation
9. Idiopathic

Sudden bleeding from vascular malformations or capillary telangiectasia may produce a similar picture.

The pathologic changes vary. In most cases there is necrosis of the cord often involving several segments. The necrosis is maximal in the center of the cord, and even in severe cases there is always a thin rim of surviving tissue at the periphery. The posterior nerve roots and posterior root ganglia are occasionally involved in the process. In cases of vascular etiology, there is infarction of the spinal cord.

Clinical Features. A history of recent acute illness suggesting a viral or bacterial infection may be obtained in about one-third of the patients. The commonest complaint is a history of an upper respiratory tract infection or a "flulike" illness. Transverse myelopathy is occasionally preceded by a gastrointestinal illness. Patients with transverse myelopathy occurring as a paracarcinomatous condition have a history of preexisting neoplasia that is frequently metastatic. Radiation transverse myelopathy occurs several months to a year after radiation therapy.

Transverse myelopathy may present with the following:

1. Paresthesias, which are often described as numbness, tingling, or pins and needles. The paresthesias usually begin in the toes or the feet and extend up the lower limbs into the trunk with eventual involvement of the upper limbs.
2. Pain is of sudden onset, usually severe, and corresponds to the level of cord involvement. Consequently, the pain is often in the interscapular region.
3. Progressive leg weakness, often presenting with "stumbling or weakness of one lower limb."
4. Urinary retention occasionally occurs as the initial complaint and is usually followed by lower limb weakness in a short period of time.

The course of transverse myelopathy may vary. There may be:

1. A smooth progressive course, often beginning with involvement of the lower limbs followed by ascending paresthesias and weakness over a period of two weeks, at which time the condition stabilizes with paraplegia or quadriplegia and a well-defined sensory level.
2. A subacute progression, with symptoms appearing intermittently over a 10-day to 4-week period. During this time the illness may appear to stabilize only to be followed by the appearance of new symptoms after several days of apparent stabilization.
3. An acute catastrophic illness with all symptoms developing within 12 hours and sometimes in less than one hour after onset. This type of presentation is usually preceded by marked back pain. Recovery is slow and incomplete.

Examination of patients with transverse myelopathy usually reveals an area of sensory loss which is symmetric on the two sides and extends to the upper level of cord involvement. This site commonly lies between T_6 and T_{12}, but there may be extension into the cervical cord in some cases. The sensory loss is usually total, involving touch, pinprick, vibration, and proprioception, or the loss may be dissociated with loss of pinprick and preservation of posterior column functions. Bladder distention occurs early in the illness in the majority of patients and is followed by overflow incontinence. Fecal incontinence is less frequently encountered.

Diagnostic Procedures.

1. All cases should have an MR scan or myelography to rule out extradural abscess or tumor. The myelogram is usually negative in transverse myelopathy, but occasionally mild swelling of the cord may be demonstrated. There is no obstruction of the subarachnoid space.
2. Lumbar puncture. The cerebrospinal fluid may show a pleocytosis in about 50 percent of cases, which varies from a mild increase in leukocytes to a white count as high as 300 cells per cubic millimeter. The cells are predominantly monocytic. Protein content is elevated in about 40 percent of cases.

Differential Diagnosis. See Table 12–1.

Treatment. The patient should be placed on bedrest and turned every two hours to prevent the development of decubiti and also to promote drainage of the dependent portions of the lungs. The bladder should be catheterized and the urine cultured periodically to detect any infection. Appropriate antibiotics should be used if infection occurs. The bowels should be moved once every two days, and a diet with adequate bulk should be given as soon as possible to prevent fecal impaction. Physical therapy with passive movements of all joints should be performed twice a day. Application of foam rubber splints to the lower limbs helps to prevent contraction deformities. Patients with involvement of the upper limbs should have adequate splinting of the forearms, wrists, and hands.

As recovery occurs, efforts should be made to remove the bladder catheter as soon as possible, and urologic evaluation should be obtained to determine bladder function. Stimulants such as bethanechol chloride, a parasympathetic stimulant, 10 to 50 mg three or four times a day, may help to initiate micturition and empty the bladder in cases with persistent bladder paralysis.

Severe spasticity of the lower limbs can often be relieved by the use of baclofen (Lioresal) 10 mg q6h, increasing slowly to as high as 80 to 100 mg if necessary. The patient should be placed in a program of physical therapy as recovery occurs.

Prognosis. The majority of patients with transverse myelopathy show some degree of recovery, which varies from complete to minimal. More than 50 percent of patients with the idiopathic form of the disease regain the ability to walk within a year, although a number will be dependent upon orthopedic appliances. Twenty-five percent of patients show poor recovery, and the majority of these give a history of severe back pain preceding a rapid, catastrophic onset of transverse myelopathy.

Nontraumatic Subdural Hematoma of the Spinal Cord

Definition. Nontraumatic subdural hematoma of the spinal cord is a rare condition in which there is an accumulation of blood in the spinal subdural space.

Etiology and Pathology. The majority of cases of nontraumatic spinal subdural hematoma occur in patients with an underlying hematologic disorder such as hemophilia, leukemia, or thrombocytopenic purpura. Many cases have been reported following lumbar puncture and anticoagulant therapy. There is an accumulation of blood in the spinal subdural space with compression of the underlying spinal cord.

Clinical Features. The patient typically presents with a gradual onset of low back pain, followed by the development of progressive paraparesis over a period of several days.

Diagnostic Procedures. Myelography shows the presence of an extradural lesion with compression of the spinal cord.

Treatment.

1. Dexamethasone (Decadron) should be administered immediately, 12 mg IV and then 4 mg q6h.
2. The subdural hematoma should be surgically evacuated as soon as possible.

Prognosis. Patients who have surgical relief of a cord compression before the development of complete paraplegia may show considerable improvement in weakness of the lower limbs.

REFERENCES

1. Satran, R. Spinal cord infarction. Stroke 19:529–532; 1988.
2. Cahan, L. D.; Higashida, R. T.; *et al.* Variants of radiculomeningeal vascular malformations of the spine. J. Neurosurg. 66:333–337; 1987.
3. Gueguen, B.; Merland, J. J. Vascular malformations of the spinal cord: intrathecal perimedullary arteriovenous fistulas fed by medullaryarteries. Neurology 37:969–979; 1987.
4. Rosenblum, B.; Oldfield, E. H.; *et al.* Spinal arteriovenous malformations: a comparison of dural arteriovenous fistulas and intradural AVM's in 81 patients. J. Neurosurg. 67:795–802; 1987.
5. Kim, R. C. Nonhemorrhagic venous spinal cord infarction. Ann. Neurol. 15:379–385; 1984.

CHAPTER 13

SYNCOPE AND SLEEP DISORDERS

There are relatively few causes of sudden loss of consciousness. These are outlined in Table 13–1. There is a common misconception that conditions such as myocardial infarction and intracranial hemorrhage can produce a sudden loss of consciousness. This is incorrect and serves to emphasize the importance of obtaining an accurate history when faced with the problem of loss of consciousness.

SYNCOPE

Syncope is a loss of consciousness resulting from impairment of circulation to the brain. The classification of syncope is outlined in Table 13–2.

Adams-Stokes Attack

Definition. An Adams-Stokes attack is a syncopal episode which occurs secondary to sudden cardiac arrhythmia.

Clinical Features. The episodes are characteristically sudden in onset and brief in duration. Loss of consciousness occurs without warning, and the patient falls to the ground. On examination the patient appears pale and feels cold, the respirations are shallow, and the patient may be pulseless or have an irregular pulse. There is rapid recovery without confusion or other complaints.

Diagnostic Procedures. The diagnosis should be suspected in a patient with a history of sudden loss of consciousness and car-

diac disease. Cardiac monitoring will establish the diagnosis.

Treatment. The treatment is that of the cardiac disease.

Obstruction of Left Ventricular Blood Flow

The expulsion of blood from the left ventricle may be hampered by aortic stenosis, a left atrium atrial myxoma, or idiopathic hypertrophic subaortic stenosis. This can result in a sudden loss of consciousness that resembles an Adams-Stokes attack. The disorders may be differentiated by characteristic murmurs and cardiac evaluation. The treatment is that of the underlying cardiac disease.

Micturition Syncope

Definition. Micturition syncope is a sudden loss of consciousness that occurs immediately after completion of micturition in the male.

Etiology. Micturition syncope is believed to result from a combination of the following factors:

1. Autonomic overactivity producing bradycardia and peripheral vasodilation
2. Straining with the glottis closed, resulting in a Valsalva maneuver, which reduces venous return to the heart
3. Emptying a distended bladder, which results in the pooling of venous blood in the abdominal and pelvic organs

188

TABLE 13–1.   Causes of Sudden Loss of Consciousnes

1. Cardiac causes
   a. Arrhythmia (e.g., Adams-Stokes attack)
   b. Obstruction of left ventricular blood flow
      (1) Aortic stenosis
      (2) Atrial myxoma
      (3) Idiopathic hypertrophic subaortic stenosis
2. Reflex cardiac causes
   a. Carotid sinus sensitivity
   b. Deglutition syncope
   c. Micturition syncope
3. Cerebral causes
   a. Epilepsy (see page 67)
   b. Transient ischemic attacks (see page 134)
   c. Trauma—concussion

TABLE 13–2.   Causes of Syncope

1. Cardiovascular causes
   a. Impaired cardiac output
      (1) Arrhythmias (e.g., Adams-Stokes attack)
      (2) Extensive myocardial infarction
      (3) Obstruction of left ventricular blood flow
         (a) Aortic stenosis
         (b) Atrial myxoma—left atrium
         (c) Idiopathic hypertrophic subaortic stenosis
   b. Impaired venous return to the heart
      (1) Atrial myxoma—right atrium
      (2) Orthostatic hypotension
   c. Impaired blood flow to left side of heart
      (1) Pulmonary embolism
      (2) Pulmonic stenosis
   d. Reflex cardiac causes
      (1) Carotid sinus sensitivity
      (2) Cough syncope
      (3) Deglutition syncope
      (4) Vasovagal syncope
      (5) Micturition syncope
   e. Decreased oxygen supply in blood
      (1) Hypoxia
      (2) Anemia
2. Cerebral causes—transient ischemic attacks (see page 134)

Clinical Features. The condition occurs in middle-aged or elderly males who usually admit to a heavy alcohol intake prior to the syncopal episode. The patient arises to empty the bladder in the middle of the night and suddenly loses consciousness without warning immediately after emptying the bladder.

There may be a precipitous fall and injuries to the head. Recovery occurs in a few seconds.

Diagnostic Procedures. The diagnosis can be established by the characteristic history.

Treatment. The patient should avoid the precipitating factors of heavy alcohol intake, excessive straining, and standing while urinating.

Orthostatic Hypotension

Definition. Orthostatic hypotension is a condition characterized by increasing lightheadedness, blurring of vision, tinnitus, weakness, and ataxia, which is occasionally followed by syncope.

Etiology. There are many causes of orthostatic hypotension. The common causes are listed in Table 13–3.

Clinical Features. Patients with orthostatic hypotension experience symptoms on arising from a lying or sitting position. Progressive lightheadedness, blurring of vision, tinnitus, weakness, and ataxia occur and may culminate in syncope if the patient does not sit or assume a supine position. Examination reveals cold, clammy skin and a weak, shallow pulse. Orthostatic hypotension may result in the typical symptoms of a TIA in patients with a hemodynamically significant stenosis of the internal carotid artery (1).

TABLE 13–3.   Causes of Orthostatic Hypotension

1. Venous pooling in the lower extremities due to
   a. Prolonged standing
   b. Poor muscle and vascular tone
   c. Prolonged confinement to bed

2. Impairment of sympathetic vascular tone
   a. Postsympathectomy
   b. Peripheral and autonomic neuropathy (diabetic, alcoholic, postinfectious polyneuritis)
   c. Subacute combined degeneration of the spinal cord
   d. Syringomyelia
   e. Familial dysautonomia
   f. Shy-Drager syndrome

3. Drug use
   a. Antihypertensives, vasodilators
   b. Phenothiazines
   c. L-Dopa

4. Corticosteroid deficiency

5. Idiopathic orthostatic hypotension

Diagnostic Procedures. The diagnosis is established by demonstrating a drop in blood pressure and rise in pulse rate when the patient stands after lying or sitting for a few minutes. Patients with idiopathic orthostatic hypotension fail to show the expected rise in pulse rate on standing.

Treatment. The treatment of orthostatic hypotension should be directed toward the cause. Idiopathic orthostatic hypotension may be improved by the use of elastic hose, an abdominal binder, and/or drugs that increase the circulating blood volume, such as fludrohydrocortisone 0.1 mg q12h. A permanent cardiac pacemaker can be used when there is failure to respond to other forms of treatment.

Carotid Sinus Sensitivity

Carotid sinus sensitivity usually occurs in elderly patients with evidence of atherosclerosis but is occasionally seen in adolescence. Stimulation of the carotid sinus results in reflex bradycardia, a drop in arterial pressure, and syncope. The diagnosis can be established if the patient complains of "faintness" in association with a concomitant bradycardia on gentle pressure over the carotid sinus. The disorder can usually be controlled by use of anticholinergic drugs. Refractory cases may require a permanent cardiac pacemaker.

Cough Syncope

This condition can be easily diagnosed by history and observation. The attack begins with a prolonged period of deep coughing associated with increasing distress. There is a brief episode of lightheadedness followed by loss of consciousness and rapid recovery. The condition is probably caused by hypersensitivity of vagal mechanisms involved in the cough reflex with a "spillover" to produce cardiac standstill. An electrocardiogram (ECG) and electroencephalogram (EEG) should be performed and the patient instructed to cough. Slowing of the ECG will be followed almost immediately by slowing of the EEG.

Treatment. Some patients show a good response to the regular use of anticholinergic drugs, which reduce vagal hypersensitivity. Many cases require the insertion of a permanent cardiac pacemaker.

Deglutition Syncope

The condition is similar to cough syncope with the occurrence of a syncopal episode after swallowing. The mechanisms are probably much the same as cough syncope with vagal hypersensitivity. The diagnosis can be established as outlined under cough syncope. The treatment is the same.

Vasovagal Syncope

Definition. Vasovagal syncope is the most common cause of loss of consciousness. The condition occurs in all ages and is usually preceded by sudden, often unexpected, emotional stress.

Etiology. The vasovagal attack is frequently but not invariably preceded by an emotional stimulus that produces pain or discomfort. The attack seems to be generated by autonomic overactivity, which causes pooling of blood in the viscera and lower extremities, with reduction of venous return to the heart. Cardiac activity is not affected, but the heart receives decreasing volumes of venous blood resulting in a decrease in cardiac output and a sudden, precipitous hypotensive episode with loss of consciousness. There is immediate improvement in the venous return to the heart as soon as the patient assumes a horizontal position and recovery occurs.

Clinical Features. The patient experiences progressive lightheadedness, tinnitus, blurring of vision, increasing weakness, and ataxia, all of the well-known premonitory features associated with fainting. Recovery occurs as soon as the patient slumps to the ground and the venous return to the heart improves.

Diagnostic Procedures. The diagnosis can be established by history. No other procedures are necessary.

Treatment. Vasovagal syncope can be avoided by assuming a horizontal position. Patients should be instructed to lie down when premonitory symptoms occur or to avoid the precipitating emotional stress.

SLEEP DISORDERS

Narcolepsy

Definition. Narcolepsy is a condition characterized by excessive daytime fatigue and repetitive sleep attacks. It is often associated with cataplexy and less frequently with sleep paralysis, hypnagogic hallucinations, disrupted nighttime sleep, and automatic behavior.

Etiology. The etiology is unknown. Narcolepsy is believed to result from a disturbance of sleep-wake mechanisms probably resulting from a disturbance in the brain stem reticular activating system (2). The rare occurrence of narcolepsy and cataplexy following head injury (3) with probable damage to the brain stem, and the occasional narcolepsy in multiple sclerosis, supports the concept of involvement of the reticular activating system (4). There is some evidence that cataplexy may result from reduction of the bioavailability of 5 hyrdoxytryptamine (serotonin) in the brain (5).

Clinical Features. Narcolepsy is not uncommon and may affect as many as 200,000 people in the United States. Unfortunately, many cases are misdiagnosed as inattention in class, as most cases experience their first symptoms in their teens or 20s. Cataplexy usually develops later than the sleep attacks but may occasionally precede them.

The first symptom is usually excessive daytime sleeping, which develops over a period of years. The patient begins to fall asleep in situations of monotony such as a monotonous lecture, working alone at a repetitive task, or sitting in a warm room after a meal. The attacks gradually become more frequent and less appropriate until the individual falls asleep in an obviously inappropriate or hazardous situation, such as driving a car or working with machinery. In most cases the episodes are preceded by an intense feeling of fatigue and an irresistible urge to sleep. However, some patients fall asleep without any warning and at times do not realize that a short period of sleep has occurred. In most cases attacks last from a few seconds to about 30 minutes. The patient often awakens refreshed and alert, but some individuals complain of constant fatigue and the distress of attempting to suppress the urge to sleep.

A cataplectic attack is a brief sudden loss of voluntary muscle tone preceded by an emotional or stressful situation. The emotional stimulus is usually amusing, producing laughter, but an attack can be precipitated by other situations such as anger or fear.

Cataplexy is usually mild at the onset with no more than a sudden brief feeling of weakness. However, attacks often increase in frequency and severity until the patient falls to the ground. At this stage the mere thought of an amusing or stressful situation may provoke a cataplectic attack.

Patients with narcolepsy often experience sleep paralysis in which there are brief periods of inability to move and speak when falling asleep or immediately upon awakening. The narcoleptic may also experience vivid hypnagogic hallucinations, which can occur with or without sleep paralysis but always

occur at the beginning of sleep or occasionally on awakening in the morning. The experience often consists of an impression of a threatening intruder in the room and is accompanied by fear. The hallucination may involve a human figure, an animal, or a vague monstrous apparition.

Some patients with narcolepsy experience disrupted sleep and report that they usually awaken several times during the night. About 20 percent of men with narcolepsy have an associated sleep apnea. It is not unusual for a patient with narcolepsy to automatically perform repetitive tasks and have no recollection of the passage of time. Automatic behavior is occasionally inappropriate and the patient may interject comments that are completely out of context during a conversation.

Diagnostic Procedures. An EEG is recorded while the patient is given five opportunities to sleep (multiple sleep latency test) at 10 A.M., 12 noon, 2 P.M., 4 P.M., and 6 P.M. The occurrence of rapid eye movement (REM) and complete loss of muscle tone within 15 minutes of the onset of Stage I sleep occurring during two or more of the five test periods is highly suggestive of narcolepsy (6). However, about 15 percent of patients with clinical narcolepsy do not have rapid onset of REM when tested. This subgroup has been called idiopathic central nervous system (CNS) hypersomnia. Normal individuals do not develop REM sleep until 60 to 90 minutes after the onset of sleep.

Differential Diagnosis.

1. Inattention and inappropriate sleeping. The narcoleptic child may be reprimanded for inattention and subjected to unjustified punishment or restrictions for sleeping in class. Similarly, narcoleptic patients experience difficulty in retaining employment because of uncontrollable episodes of sleeping at work. The history, occurrence of other symptoms, and EEG will help to differentiate the narcoleptic from those who are sleeping excessively from other causes.

2. Partial complex seizures. The description of automatic behavior or frightening hallucinations may suggest the possibility of partial complex seizure activity. However, the history of excessive daytime sleeping and cataplexy helps to differentiate the narcoleptic patient.

3. Transient global amnesia. Episodes of automatic behavior are a feature of transient global amnesia, but this disorder is not associated with the other symptoms of narcolepsy.

4. Sleep apnea. This condition may lead to excessive daytime sleepiness suggesting narcolepsy.

Treatment.

1. Sleep attacks
   a. Methylphenidate (Ritalin) is the drug of choice. The initial dose of 10 mg in the morning and at noon may be increased to 80 to 100 mg per day. Methylphenidate can be used in combination with other drugs used in the treatment of cataplexy.
   b. Amphetamines are also useful and often very effective in treatment of excessive daytime sleeping but have a number of unpleasant side effects in some cases. These include progressive hypertension or personality changes ranging from emotional lability and mild depression to frank psychosis.
   c. Propranolol (Inderal) has recently been shown to be effective in reducing the number of sleep attacks in narcolepsy.
2. Cataplexy
   a. Imipramine (Tofranil) is widely used in the control of cataplexy. Imipramine is well tolerated in the majority of cases but may become less effective with the passage of time. This requires a gradual increase in dosage. An initial effective dose of 25 mg three times a day may rise to 50 mg three times a day over a two-year period. Imipramine may produce somnolence in some cases and has caused impotence and urinary retention.

Prognosis. Narcolepsy is a lifelong affliction that tends to increase slowly in severity until about the age of 50. Symptoms may become less disabling in older patients.

Sleep Apnea

Definition. There are two types of sleep apnea (7):
   a. Obstructive sleep apnea characterized by intermittent obstruction of the airway with cessation of breathing and interruption of sleep.
   b. Central sleep apnea due to loss of sensitivity of central respiratory control mechanism.

Obstructive Sleep Apnea

Etiology and Pathology. Obstructive sleep apnea results from narrowing of upper respiratory airways during sleep due to the loss of muscle tone in the uvulopalatopharyngeal muscles (8).

Clinical Features. Sufferers are known to snore loudly during sleep. This is interrupted by a sudden cessation of breathing followed by restlessness, gasping respiratory sounds, and interruption of sleep. The condition may occur many times during the night, and consequently patients with sleep apnea feel tired during the day and frequently sleep if inactive. The condition produces intermittent hypoxemia and hypercapnia, which increase the risk of systemic hypertension and cardiac arrhythmia. There is an association with narcolepsy.

Diagnostic Procedures.
   a. The diagnosis is established by polysonography, a sleep study which includes electroencephalography, electrocardiography, air flow, chest and abdominal movements, eye movements, electronystagmography, and oxygen saturation.
   b. Obstructive sleep apnea has been reported in some patients with cerebral infarction, brain stem infarction, syringobulbia, Shy-Drager syndrome, muscular dystrophy, poliomyelitis, multiple sclerosis, and achondroplasia (9).

Differential Diagnosis. Patients with sleep apnea sleep only when inactive and unlike narcoleptics, can avoid sleep by activity.

Treatment.

1. Many patients are obese. Weight reduction reduces upper respiratory obstruction and daytime hypersomnolence. Nocturnal oxygenation is important.
2. Alcohol and depressant hypnotic drugs increase upper airway obstruction and should be avoided.
3. Protriptylene, a tricyclic antidepressant, 10 to 20 mg h.s., reduces daytime hypersomnolence and may selectively stimulate upper respiratory muscles and reduce sleep apnea.
4. Continuous positive airway pressure applied to the nose through a mask will result in reversal of sleep apnea in the majority of cases (10).
5. The small number of cases that fail to respond to medical treatment may require uvulopalatopharyngoplasty or tracheotomy.

Central Sleep Apnea

This condition is not as common as obstructive sleep apnea and is believed to be due to a decreased sensitivity of central respiratory control and to changes in sensitivity of CO_2 chemoreceptors during sleep.

Central sleep apnea occurs in some cases at high altitudes. Others suffer from the obesity-hypoventilation hypersomnia (Pickwickian) syndrome. These latter cases often have a combination of obstructive and central sleep apnea (4). Olivopontocerebellar degeneration and other forms of spinocerebellar degeneration may be associated with central sleep apnea (11).

Diagnostic Procedures.

1. Pickwickian patients have a waking hypercapnia.
2. Hypothyroidism must be excluded.
3. Diagnosis is established by polysonography.

Treatment.

1. Acetazolamide 250 mg q.i.d. is effective in some cases of central sleep apnea.
2. Medroxyprogesterone acetate is effective in patients with the Pickwickian syndrome.
3. Trazodone 50 mg h.s. is also effective in central sleep apnea.

REFERENCES

1. Dobkin, B. H. Orthostatic hypotension as a risk factor for symptomatic cerebrovascular disease. Neurology 39:30–34; 1989.

2. Norman, M. E.; Dyer, J. A. Ophthalmic manifestations of narcolepsy. Am. J. Ophthalmol. 103:81–86; 1987.
3. Maccario, M.; Ruggles, K. H.; et al. Post-traumatic narcolepsy. Military Med. 152:370–371; 1987.
4. Poirer G.; Montplaisir, J.; et al. Clinical and sleep laboratory studies of narcoleptic symptoms in multiple sclerosis. Neurology 37:693–695; 1987.
5. Godbout, R.; Montplaisir, J. The effect of Zimelidine, a serotonin re-uptake blocker, on cataplexy and daytime sleepiness of narcoleptic patients. Clin. Neuropharmacol. 9:46–51; 1986.
6. Kales, A.; Bixler, E. O.; et al. Narcolepsy/cataplexy IV. Diagnostic value of daytime nap recordings. Acta Neurol. Scan. 75:223–230; 1987.
7. Guilleminault, C.; Quera-Salva, M.A.; et al. Central sleep apnea and partial obstruction of the upper airway. Ann. Neurol. 21:465–469; 1987.
8. Nahmias, J. S.; Karetzky, M. S. Current concepts in sleep apnea. N. J. Med, 84:475–479; 1987.
9. Manon-Espaillat, R.; Gothe, B.; et al. Familial 'sleep apnea plus' syndrome. Report of a family. Neurology 38:190–193; 1988.
10. Klonoff, H.; Fleetham, J.; et al. Treatment outcome of obstructive sleep apnea. Physiological and neuropsychological concomitants. J. Nerv. Ment. Dis. 175:208–217; 1987.
11. Salazar-Grueso, E. F.; Rosenberg, R. S.; et al. Sleep apnea in olivopantocerebellar degenerations: treatment with Trazodone. Ann. Neurol. 23:399–401; 1988.

CHAPTER 14

DEGENERATIVE DISEASES

Degenerative diseases of the central nervous system (CNS) can affect gray matter, white matter, or both. The involvement is often diffuse but usually affects one area or system more than another, which permits an anatomic classification of these conditions.

DISEASES OF THE GRAY MATTER

DISEASES OF THE CEREBRAL CORTEX: THE DEMENTIAS

Dementia may be defined as a progressive deterioration of intellectual capacity resulting from disease of the brain. Although Alzheimer's disease and multiinfarct dementia account for 80 percent of the dementias of old age, many neurologic diseases are associated with dementia. Any condition that damages the brain, including trauma, CNS infections, toxins, metabolic abnormalities, tumors, infarctions, or hemorrhages, may result in dementia. These conditions all have an identifiable and often treatable cause of dementia in contrast to a group of degenerative diseases of unknown etiology in which dementia is a predominant sign. This group of diseases includes Huntington's disease, Alzheimer's disease, Pick's disease, and normal pressure hydrocephalus. Such conditions constitute the majority of nonvascular cases with progressive dementia encountered in clinical practice.

Although dementia occurs predominantly in older people and is an increasing problem in our aging population, dementia should never be accepted as an inevitable concomitant of aging. There is an increasing recognition of the treatable causes of dementia, and each patient deserves full evaluation and correct diagnosis. This approach will obviate the use of such terms as "presenile dementia," "senile dementia," "senility," "organic brain syndrome," "getting old," and "hardening of the arteries" which implies failure to establish a diagnosis and consequently leads to delay in or lack of treatment. It is quite possible that some of the dementias are due to chronic (slow) virus infection. The evidence for this has evolved from studies of such neuronal diseases as kuru, Jakob-Creutzfeldt disease, and familial Alzheimer's disease. Studies involving kuru, a rare degenerative neurologic disease limited to an isolated community in Eastern New Guinea, showed that this disease was transmitted by cannibalism and that the viral agent was spread by the oral route. The virus of Jakob-Creutzfeldt disease has been passed through several generations of laboratory animals and has been accidentally transmitted from human to human. Familial Alzheimer's disease has also been passed from human material to laboratory animals.

At present about 20 percent of patients with dementia have a treatable condition.

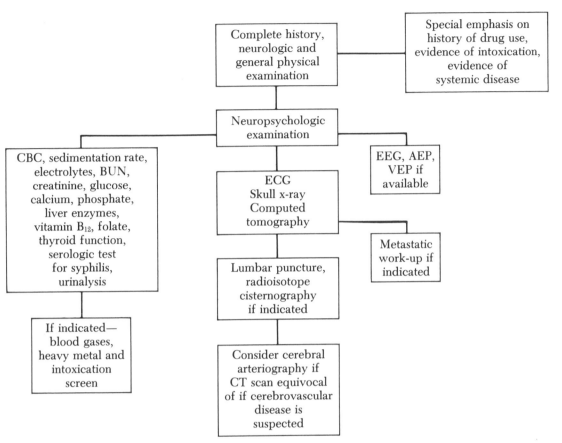

FIGURE 14–1. Evaluation of the patient with dementia.

Consequently it is incorrect to assume that a patient suffering from dementia is destined to a course of progressive intellectual deterioration. The suggested evaluation for the dementia patient is given in Figure 14–1, while Table 14–1 lists the more common causes of reversible or treatable dementia.

TABLE 14–1. **Treatable Dementia**

Therapeutic drug use: anticholinergics—atropine and related compounds; anticonvulsants—phenytoin, mephenytoin, barbiturates; antihypertensives—clonidine, methyldopa, propranolol; psychotropics—haloperidol, lithium carbonate, phenothiazines; miscellaneous—disulfiram, bromides, paraldehyde, quinidine

Metabolic–systemic disorders: electrolyte or acid-base disorders; hypo-, hyperglycemia; severe anemia; polycythemia vera; hyperlipidemia; hepatic failure; uremia; pulmonary insufficiency; hypopituitarism; thryoid, adrenal, or parathyroid dysfunction; cardiac dysfunction; hepatolenticular degeneration

Intracranial disorders: cerebrovascular insufficiency, chronic meningitis or encephalitis, neurosyphilis, epilepsy, tumor, abscess, subdural hematomas, multiple sclerosis, normal pressure hydrocephalus

Deficiency states: vitamin B_{12} deficiency, folate deficiency, pellagra (niacin)

Collagen-vascular disorders: systemic lupus erythematosus, temporal arteritis, sarcoidosis, Behçet's syndrome

Exogenous intoxication: alcohol, carbon monoxide, organophosphates, toluene, trichloroethylene, carbon disulfide, lead, mercury, arsenic, thallium, manganese, nitrobenzene, anilines, bromine hydrocarbons

Alzheimer's Disease

Definition. Alzheimer's disease is the commonest form of dementia and is due to neuronal degeneration.

Etiology and Pathology. The etiology of Alzheimer's disease is unknown. Reports of a viral etiology are speculative at this time. There is an accelerated loss of neurons in the CNS, possibly due to an abnormality in some essential intracellular enzymatic system, with decreased activity of enzymes involved in the biosynthesis of neurotransmitters. There are reports of reduction of enzymes involved in the synthesis of acetylcholine, giving rise to the concept that Alzheimer's disease is a cholinergic system failure (1,2). However, other systems including noradrenergic, serotonergic, dopaminergic, and GABAergic systems are also abnormal in Alzheimer's disease, giving rise to the concept that the disease is one of a symmetric multisystem involvement of the cerebral hemispheres (3–5).

Studies of Alzheimer's disease and Down's syndrome suggest the implication of genes or chromosome 21 in the genesis of the pathologic changes in Alzheimer's disease (6). However, other studies suggest that the rare Familial Alzheimer's disease may be inherited as an autosomal dominant trait (7,8).

The brain shows generalized atrophy with widening of the sulci and narrowing of the gyri. The atrophy involves both gray and white matter, and there is a compensatory diffuse ventricular dilatation (hydrocephalus *ex vacuo*). Microscopically, neuronal loss occurs in both cortical and subcortical gray matter bilaterally and symmetrically (9). Many surviving neurons show the presence of neurofibrillary tangles, which are degenerated neuronal filaments with an increased aluminum content. The gray matter contains numerous senile plaques consisting of amyloid surrounded by degenerated products of neurons and glia. The combination of neurofibrillary tangles and senile plaques is characteristic but not pathognomonic of Alzheimer's disease.

Clinical Features. There are probably 500,000 persons more than 65 years of age with Alzheimer's disease in the United States. It occurs in both sexes and can begin at any age after the early thirties.

Clinically, there is an early loss of operational judgment followed by failure of recent memory. The patient resorts to keeping written notes to circumvent the failure of recent memory. Loss of insight, inappropriate be-havior, uncritical statements, irritability, grandiosity, euphoria, depression, and any combination of these features may occur. The dominant symptom often reflects the premorbid personality of the patient. Focal signs, including dysphasia, dyscalculia, dyslexia, dysgraphia, and dyspraxia can develop at any time (10–12). Parkinsonian features are not uncommon. Olfaction is often impaired in Alzheimer's disease and eye movements are saccadic and occasionally show impersistence. Muscle tone may be increased with paratonia and resting or intention tremor is not uncommon. Patients may exhibit normal gait, a short-stepped bradykinetic gait, or apraxia of gait—an inability to initiate gait with the patient apparently "glued to the floor." The presence of apraxia of gait also creates a spurious impression of Parkinsonism; however, once the patient with Alzheimer's disease is able to initiate gait, it does not have the festinant quality of Parkinsonism. Seizures occur in a considerable number of patients with Alzheimer's disease. Sensory testing often reveals astereognosis or graphesthesia. More than 50 percent of patients have increased stretch reflexes or exhibit release signs such as the glabellar sign and snout, palmomental, and grasp reflexes (13).

Diagnostic Procedures. For the diagnostic procedures in the differential diagnosis of dementia, see Figure 14–1. More specifically:

1. The general physical examination, biochemical testing, and tests for infection are all negative.
2. The presence of the following criteria permit the diagnosis of Alzheimer's disease (14):
   A. Sustained deterioration in memory in an alert patient
   B. Plus impairment in three of the following:
      a) orientation
      b) judgment and problem solving
      c) function in community affairs
      d) function in home and hobbies
      e) function in personal care
   C. Gradual onset and progression
   D. Duration of six months or longer.
3. The electroencephalogram (EEG) shows progressive deterioration with loss of alpha activity and gradual development of generalized theta activity. The slowing may not be entirely symmetric, and focal slowing or focal seizure activity can occur.

4. Magnetic resonance (MR) or computed tomography (CT) scan of the brain shows the presence of diffuse atrophy with ventricular enlargement and enlarged cortical sulci. In the early stages there may be little evidence of cortical atrophy.
5. The development of testing to identify a protein marker in the cerebrospinal (CSF) fluid is likely in the near future (15).

Treatment.

1. Diet. Many patients with Alzheimer's disease develop the habit of taking a very restricted diet and may have an associated vitamin deficiency. It is important to ensure that the patient has an adequate diet with vitamin supplementation.
2. Adequate care. When the spouse of an elderly patient is infirm or incapable of providing care for the patient, a search should be made for aid through community resources. Most communities will provide aid to patients with chronic illnesses of all types. These resources should always be identified and the family made fully aware of their existence.
3. Planning with the family. It is important to discuss all aspects of the disease with the family and to indicate that there will be a progression of symptoms. The physician should be available to discuss the many problems of management with the family and to refer them to the appropriate agency when they decide to transfer the patient to a chronic care institution. The services of a social worker are invaluable at this time. When it is apparent that the patient is no longer competent to take care of his or her affairs, the family should be informed and advised that the patient should be declared mentally incompetent according to the laws of the state.
4. Sedation. Many patients with Alzheimer's disease require some form of sedation because of impulsive or combative behavior. Daytime sedation can be managed with a phenothiazine such as thioridazine (Mellaril). This should be given in small doses beginning with 25 mg q12h, followed by the addition of 25 to 50 mg every three days until there is a satisfactory change in the patient's behavior. This usually requires between 300 to 450 mg daily. When a family complains that the patient is unable to sleep at night, the physician should determine whether the patient is sleeping during the day. The correction of

this practice is often difficult but usually leads to restoration of a normal sleep pattern. However, if the patient remains restless at night, a simple sedative such as chloral hydrate 500 mg may be effective.
5. Depression. Signs and symptoms of depression may be treated with either fluoxetine hydrochloride (prozac) 20 mg q.d. or amitriptyline (Elavil) 75 to 300 mg in divided doses.
6. Drug therapy. Treatment with choline, lecithin, and intraventricular bethanicol has been without benefit in ameliorating the dementia of Alzheimer's disease (16). Physostigmine may improve memory and day-to-day functioning, but further studies are needed (17).

Prognosis. Patients with Alzheimer's disease have a mean survival time of 5 to 10 years after diagnosis and usually die of intercurrent infection.

Pick's Disease

Definition. Pick's disease is a rare type of dementia characterized by selective atrophy of the frontal and temporal lobes of the brain.

Etiology and Pathology. The cause of the neuronal degeneration is unknown. The brain shows a marked symmetric atrophy of the frontal and temporal lobes with compensatory dilatation of the lateral ventricles. The affected areas show loss of neurons, which is maximal in the outer three layers of the gray matter. Surviving neurons are small with argentophilic inclusions; because of their characteristic appearance these cells have been called Pick's cells. Senile plaques and neurofibrillary tangles are not a characteristic feature of Pick's disease.

Clinical Features. The clinical features are those of progressive dementia (see Alzheimer's disease, page 196). Pick's disease has occasionally been described as a familial disorder.

Diagnostic Procedures. MR or CT scanning shows dilatation of the frontal and temporal horns of the lateral ventricles. There is marked widening of the cortical sulci in the same areas, indicating maximal atrophic changes in the frontal and temporal lobes.

Positron emission tomography (PET) shows a marked decrease in metabolic rate for glucose in the frontal lobes, sufficiently distinctive to distinguish Pick's disease from Alzheimer's disease (18).

Treatment. The treatment is that of a progressive dementia.

Progressive Aphasia without Dementia

Definition. This is a rare condition often mistaken for Alzheimer's disease in which there is progressive failure of language without dementia.

Etiology and Pathology. The etiology is unknown. Autopsy studies have shown focal spongiform changes in the left inferior frontal gyrus without evidence of changes compatible with Alzheimer's disease, Pick's disease, or Jakob-Creutzfeldt's disease.

Clinical Features. The disease presents with anomic difficulties followed by nonfluent dysphasia with later addition of a receptive component to the dysphasia. Despite the profound involvement of language function, other cognitive and behavioral functions are relatively spared. This contrasts with cases of Alzheimer's disease which can present with dysphasia in that other signs of deterioration in judgment, insight, memory, cognition, and perception soon appear in Alzheimer's disease.

Treatment. There is no treatment for progressive aphasia without dementia but recognition of the condition is important since the patient can maintain independent living but may require help in developing alternative methods of communication.

Jakob-Creutzfelt's Disease

See page 290.

DISEASES OF THE BASAL GANGLIA

The majority of degenerative diseases that affect the basal ganglia are associated with involuntary movements and are discussed in Chapter 6.

Progressive Supranuclear Palsy

Definition. Progressive supranuclear palsy is a chronic degenerative disease involving the CNS that is characterized by early paralysis of eye movements.

Etiology and Pathology. The etiology is unknown, but the condition may be related to an antecedent viral infection.

The brain shows evidence of atrophy. There is decreased pigment in the substantia nigra and locus ceruleus and loss of neurons in the basal ganglia, brain stem, and cerebellum. Surviving neurons in these areas contain neurofibrillary tangles.

Clinical Features. The disease typically presents in the fifth decade with progressive loss of ability to move the eyes in a vertical plane. This is followed by loss of horizontal eye movements. Parkinsonian features including paucity of blinking, fixed facial expression, and generalized rigidity are prominent. Generalized spasticity, more apparent in lower than upper limbs, progressive dysarthria and dysphagia, increased reflexes, and extensor plantar responses are constant features. Torticollis, blepharospasm, and stuttering speech have been described. The dementia associated with supranuclear palsy is often mild and only slowly progressive (19). Eventually the patient becomes bedridden and dies from an intercurrent infection.

Diagnostic Procedures. The diagnosis depends largely on clinical presentation and the characteristic progression of the disease. Brain stem auditory evoked responses may be normal even in advanced stages of the disorder.

Treatment. The treatment is symptomatic. Antiparkinsonian agents (levodopa/carbidopa, trihexyphenidyl, amantadine, bromocriptine) and methysergide may reduce the severity of some of the disabling symptoms in this disease.

Prognosis. Median survival is about 10 years (20).

Shy-Drager Syndrome (Central Neurogenic Orthostatic Hypotension)

Definition. The Shy-Drager syndrome is a rare condition in which postural hypotension and other signs of autonomic dysfunction occur due to progressive neuronal degeneration.

Etiology and Pathology. The Shy-Drager syndrome is a neuronal degeneration of unknown etiology with involvement of central autonomic neurons.

Pathologic examination shows marked neuronal loss or chronic neuronal degeneration involving the cerebral cortex, basal ganglia, diencephalon, brain stem, cerebellum, anterior horn cells, and intermediolateral columns of the spinal cord and autonomic ganglia. Affected areas in the CNS show reactive gliosis. Surviving neurons show the presence of Lewy bodies in the locus ceruleus, substantia nigra, and sympathetic ganglia.

Clinical Features. This is a rare syndrome that is usually sporadic but has been described in families. The presenting symptoms consist of urinary hesitancy, xerostomia, constipation, impotence in the male, anhidrosis with heat intolerance, and postural hypotension manifested by lightheadedness and ataxia on change of posture and occasional syncope. The marked orthostatic hypotension is due to loss of sympathetic and parasympathetic reflexes and is reflected by impairment of cerebral autoregulation. Later developments include extraocular palsies associated with iris atrophy and laryngeal stridor due to cord abductor paralysis which may lead to severe obstructive sleep apnea (21). There is a change in muscle tone with the development of rigidity and/or spasticity. The patient shows loss of associated movements when walking, and some cases develop parkinsonian features or a cerebral tremor develops. Marked distal muscle wasting and fasciculations occur. The bladder is atonic, and there is loss of rectal sphincter tone. Advanced cases show impaired respiratory rhythm.

Diagnostic Procedures.

1. Electromyography shows the presence of fibrillations and fasciculations suggesting anterior horn cell involvement.
2. Slit lamp examination will reveal iris atrophy in some cases.
3. Urodynamic studies will demonstrate an atonic bladder.
4. Brain stem auditory evoked potentials are abnormal in contrast to the normal findings in Parkinson's disease (22).
5. MR imaging shows atrophy of the putamen (23).
6. Impaired release of antidiuretic hormone has been demonstrated in some cases.
7. There is a marked sensitivity to injection of small doses of pressor amine, such as 0.2 ml of 1:1,000 epinephrine solution subcutaneously, with severe tachycardia and elevation of blood pressure.

Treatment.

1. The patient should have a full cardiac evaluation, and efforts should be made to maintain the blood pressure, using fludrocortisone 0.1 mg q12h. This can be supplemented by the use of a leotard, which should extend as high as the upper thorax. Refractory cases may require a permanent cardiac pacemaker.
2. Tyramine combined with a monoamine oxidase inhibitor may relieve postural hypotension. Patients should be encouraged to eat food with high tyramine content, such as cheese and wine, on the assumption that this may lead to an increase in norepinephrine levels.
3. Oral   DL-Threo-3,4-dihydroxyphenylser-ine, a precursor amino acid of norepinephrine, improves hypotension in Shy-Drager syndrome (24).
4. Obstructive sleep apnea can be treated with trazodone. Alternative therapy includes a positive pressure face mask or, if this fails, either tracheotomy or crico-arytenoid pexis.
5. Bethanechol chloride may be titrated to relieve symptoms of anhidrosis, xerostomia, urinary hesitancy, and constipation.

DEGENERATIVE DISEASES OF THE CEREBELLUM AND SPINAL CORD—SPINOCEREBELLAR DEGENERATIONS AND MOTOR NEURON DISEASE

The spinocerebellar degenerations are a group of familial conditions identified more by a particular constellation of signs and symptoms than by specific pathologic changes within the CNS.

Friedreich's Ataxis

Definition. Friedreich's ataxia is a degenerative disease of adolescence and early adult life that primarily involves the long tracts of the spinal cord. This disease is inherited as an autosomal recessive trait and is the most common form of spinocerebellar degeneration.

Etiology and Pathology. The etiology is unknown. The relationship between Friedreich's ataxia and abnormalities in pyruvate, ketoglutarate, or the lipoamide moiety of dehydrogenase complexes remains uncertain at this time.

There is atrophy with demyelination involving the posterior columns and the spinocerebellar and corticospinal tracts of the spinal cord. The areas of degeneration show loss of axons and myelin with secondary gliosis. The degenerative changes begin in the neurons of the dorsal root ganglia and are followed by a dying back of axons of large myelinated fibers in peripheral nerve and in the posterior columns of the spinal cord (25). Similar neuronal changes eventually involve the nucleus gracilis and cuneatus with degenerative changes in the medial lemniscus. The dorsal and ventral spinocerebellar tracts are similarly involved. The corticospinal tracts show demyelination with increasing involvement in a caudal direction. Loss of Purkinje cells in the cerebellum and degeneration of the dentate nucleus with axonal loss and demyelination of the superior cerebellar peduncles also occur.

Cardiac hypertrophy and diffuse myocardial fibrosis with degeneration of cardiac muscle cells are an invariable finding.

Clinical Features. The first symptoms of ataxia begin in the early teens, and the majority of cases have well-established signs before the age of 20. The ataxia is progressive; it begins in the lower limbs with eventual involvement of the upper limbs. Tests of coordination show dysdiadochokinesia, dysmetria, nystagmus, and intention tremor bilaterally. The gait is wide-based due to a combination of spasticity and ataxia. Examination of the motor system reveals hypertonia and muscle weakness. Deep tendon reflexes are always absent in the lower limbs and depressed or absent in the upper limbs. There is a bilateral extensor plantar response. Examination of sensation shows that touch is usually intact, but there is impairment of temperature discrimination in the hands and feet. Vibration and position sense are always decreased in the lower limbs. The fully developed syndrome is characterized by a mild degree of dementia. Optic atrophy with visual failure is not unusual, and many patients have a progressive hearing loss. The speech is slow, staccato, and explosive in the more developed cases but many eventually become unintelligible in the later stages of the disease.

Deformity of the feet with pes cavus and extension of the metatarsophalangeal joints and flexion of the interphalangeal joints is present in about 90 percent of cases. Diabetes mellitus, cardiomyopathy, and deafness may also occur.

Diagnostic Procedures.

1. Clinical diabetes mellitus due to insulin resistant b cell deficiency, and type I diabetes is present in about 20 percent of cases (26).
2. Serum bilirubin levels are frequently elevated.
3. Pulmonary function tests show progressive impairment due to progressive kyphoscoliosis.
4. The electrocardiogram (ECG) is abnormal, and many patients have obstructive hypertrophic cardiomyopathy.
5. Electroencephalography shows mild nonspecific abnormalities in most cases.
6. Motor nerve conduction velocities are normal, but sensory conduction velocities are prolonged or absent in the lower limbs.
7. Somatosensory evoked potentials recorded following peroneal nerve stimulation are abnormal, indicating spinal cord involvement.

Differential Diagnosis.

1. Other forms of spinocerebellar degeneration. The characteristic findings, moderately rapid progression and cardiac involvement, differentiate Friedreich's ataxia from other spinocerebellar degenerations.
2. Congenital abnormalities. The Arnold-Chiari malformation, platybasia, and odontoid compression can be excluded by x-ray studies, computed tomography (CT), and myelography of the upper cervical spine and base of the skull.
3. Arteriovenous (AV) malformation of the spinal cord. Increased tone and hyperreflexia occur only below the level of the malformation. There are progressive urgency of micturition and a sensory level. The AV malformation can be demonstrated by MR or CT scanning, myelography, and arteriography.
4. Syphilis. Syphilitic pachymeningitis is rare. The condition is associated with a cerebrospinal fluid pleocytosis and increased protein content. The serologic test for syphilis is positive.
5. Subacute combined degeneration. This condition can cause confusion if it occurs before overt signs of pernicious anemia. Serum vitamin B_{12} levels are depressed.
6. Spinal cord tumor. Tumors tend to cause pain, particularly nerve root pain. There is progressive spasticity below the level of the lesion and progressive urgency of micturition. Examination shows a sensory level. The diagnosis can be established by MR or CT scanning and myelography.
7. Multiple sclerosis. Spinal cord forms of multiple sclerosis may cause some confusion with Friedreich's ataxia. There tends to be a relapsing and remitting course in multiple sclerosis, with bladder involvement and patchy sensory loss. Visual evoked potentials and auditory evoked potentials may be abnormal. The cerebrospinal fluid usually shows an elevated protein and gamma globulin content and increase in myelin basic protein. An MR scan of the brain is usually abnormal.
8. Vitamin E deficiency. A condition closely resembling Friedreich's ataxia can occur in severe vitamin E deficiency. Serum vitamin E levels are normal in Friedreich's ataxia (27).

Treatment. The treatment is symptomatic. Cardiac and pulmonary complications should receive prompt attention in advanced cases since they are frequently fatal.

Prognosis. The disease runs a progressive course, and most patients are unable to walk five years after the appearance of symptoms. Death occurs 10 to 20 years after onset from pulmonary or cardiac complications.

Olivopontocerebellar Degeneration

Definition. Olivopontocerebellar degeneration is form of spinocerebellar degeneration in which there is predominant involvement of the brain stem and cerebellum.

Etiology and Pathology. The disorder may be inherited as an autosomal dominant trait and is believed to be the result of a deficiency in the heat labile component of glutamate dehydrogenase (28).

Advanced cases show some degree of cerebral atrophy, but the striking features are the atrophic changes in the cerebellum and pons, which have a shrunken appearance. Microscopic examination shows loss of neurons in the medullary olives and pons and loss of Purkinje cells in the cerebellum.

Clinical Features. The notable characteristic of olivopontocerebellar degeneration is the wide variety of presenting symptoms. Affected members of the same family may present with a totally different clinical picture. Eventually, however, the affected members of the family will develop ataxia, nystagmus, intention tremor, and titubation of the head. There may be generalized rigidity and parkinsonian features in some cases. The speech becomes severely dysarthric. The tendon reflexes may be hyperactive or hypoactive, and there is a bilateral extensor plantar response. Some patients develop signs of dementia as a late feature of the disease, and there may be signs of autonomic disturbance due to involvement of autonomic neurons with incontinence and postural hypotension. Sleep disorders including hyposomnia, rapid eye movement (REM), sleep without atonia, and sleep apnea are present in some cases (29).

Diagnostic Procedures.

1. Magnetic resonance imaging and CT scanning. The scan shows atrophy of the brain stem and atrophy of the cerebellum with enlargement of the fourth ventricle and ambiens and prepontine cisterns.
2. Auditory evoked potentials indicate abnormality of the brain stem auditory pathways.
3. Lumbar puncture. There are no CSF abnormalities.

Treatment. Treatment is symptomatic. Sleep apnea may respond to trazodone 50 mg h.s.

Prognosis. There is typically a relentless progression of the disease with death occurring from intercurrent infection approximately 20 years after the development of the initial symptoms.

Vitamin E Deficiency and Spinocerebellar Degeneration

Etiology and Pathology. Chronic fat malabsorption in abetalipoproteinemia, cystic fibrosis, chronic cholestatic liver disease and acquired intestinal diseases can lead to chronic Vitamin E deficiency which is associated with a form of spinocerebellar degeneration. Vitamin E deficiency has occasionally occurred without fat malabsorption. Pathologic changes occur in the basal ganglia, substantia nigra and posterior columns of the spinal cord (30).

Clinical Features. The main features are ataxia, dysarthria, impaired vibration and position sense, areflexia and extensor plantar responses. Ophthalmoplegia, dystonic posturing of hands and feet, bradykinesis, fasciculations of the tongue and pigmentary degeneration of the retina have been described.

Diagnostic Procedures.

1. Serum vitamin E levels are depressed below 5 μg/ml.
2. Fecal fat may be increased.
3. Nerve conduction studies are abnormal.
4. Somatosensory evoked responses are abnormal indicating spinal cord involvement.
5. Peripheral neuropathy and myopathy can be demonstrated by biopsy.

Treatment. High doses of Vitamin E daily by mouth, up to 3500 units daily, may arrest the progression of this disease.

Hereditary Areflexic Dystasia (Roussy-Levy Syndrome)

Hereditary areflexic dystasia is a rare condition in which the patient has features of both Friedreich's ataxia and peroneal muscular atrophy. It is a very slowly progressive condition, characterized by the absence of nystagmus and deep tendon reflexes.

Hereditary Spastic Ataxia and Hereditary Spastic Paraparesis

Hereditary spastic ataxia and hereditary spastic paraparesis are probably forme frustes of other spinocerebellar degenerations in which the predominant feature is bilateral spasticity. It is important to rule out compressive conditions of the spinal cord, particularly cervical spondylosis, in all of these cases. These conditions are slowly progressive and in most cases are not associated with reduction of the normal life span.

Amyotrophic Lateral Sclerosis (Motor Neuron Disease)

Definition. Amyotrophic lateral sclerosis (ALS) is a chronic disease characterized by progressive degeneration of motor neurons in the spinal cord, brain stem, and cerebral cortex (31).

Etiology and Pathology. The etiology is unknown. While several conditions such as hexosamidase deficiency, glutamate dehydrogenase deficiency, hyperthyroidism, parathyroid disorders, macroglobulinemia, and heavy metal intoxication produce an ALS-like syndrome, they are clearly absent in amyotrophic lateral sclerosis. Nevertheless, a significant elevation of plasma glutamate has been demonstrated in amyotrophic lateral sclerosis, suggesting a defect in metabolism of glutamate in amyotrophic lateral sclerosis (32). Cerebral glucose utilization is reduced suggesting hypometabolism or nonfunction of cerebral neurons and a more complex and wide spread dysfunction of neurons beyond the motor pathway (33).

There are a progressive loss of motor neurons of the anterior horns of the spinal cord, loss of motor neurons of the brain stem, loss of the Betz cells of the cerebral cortex, and involvement of the corticospinal tracts.

Clinical Features. Amyotrophic lateral sclerosis is a rare disease with a prevalence of approximately 2 per 100,000, and a male-to-female ratio of 1.1:1. The median age of onset is 66 years.

Four types of amyotrophic lateral sclerosis are recognized:

1. Progressive muscular atrophy. In this condition there is a progressive loss of motor neurons in the anterior horns of the spinal cord, the condition often begins in the cervical area with progressive weakness, wasting, and fasciculations involving the small muscles of the hands. However, the loss may occur at any site in the spinal cord. There is no evidence of corticospinal tract involvement, and the sensory involvement is normal.

2. Progressive bulbar palsy. This condition involves the motor neurons of the cranial nerve nuclei and results in progressive weakness and wasting involving the pharyngeal muscles, the tongue, and the facial musculature. The patient develops progressive dysarthria and dysphagia. Fasciculations of the tongue are usually prominent and can be seen when the tongue is examined lying quietly on the floor of the mouth. The oculomotor nuclei are usually not involved.

3. Primary lateral sclerosis. In this type the motor neuronal loss occurs in the cortex and is associated with secondary degenerative changes involving the corticospinal tracts. The patient experiences progressive weakness and spasticity involving the limbs and truncal musculature. There is no atrophy, and fasciculations are not present. The stretch reflexes are increased, and there is a bilateral extensor plantar response. This form of amyotrophic lateral sclerosis is rather unusual.

4. Combined form. A combined form of ALS is the commonest form of the disease. The features of the three conditions described above are combined. The patient complains of increasing weakness, and examination reveals atrophy, fasciculations, and wasting of muscles in both upper and lower limbs associated with increased reflexes and extensor plantar responses. Eventually the brain stem nuclei are involved, resulting in dysphagia, dysarthria, and facial weakness. There are no sensory changes.

Diagnostic Procedures.

1. Electromyography shows the presence of fibrillations and fasciculations characteristic of denervation atrophy.
2. Muscle biopsy shows the typical appearance of denervation atrophy with atrophic fascicles coexisting with normal fascicles.
3. Muscle enzymes such as creatine phosphokinase (CPK) may be elevated in rapidly progressive cases.
4. Lumbar puncture. The cerebrospinal fluid is normal.
5. There are no myelographic abnormalities.

Differential Diagnosis.

1. Mass lesion impinging on the spinal cord (e.g., tumor, spondylosis, abscess). In these conditions the weakness, wasting, and fasciculations are confined to one or

more myotomes, and there is appropriate sensory loss in the affected dermatomes.

2. Benign fasciculations, myokymia. Benign fasciculations are not at all uncommon and are often diffuse. There are no other signs of neurologic involvement, and the general physical examination and neurologic examinations are perfectly normal. Follow-up examinations remain normal.

3. Chronic inflammation of meninges or spinal cord (e.g., adhesive arachnoiditis). In these conditions the CSF is abnormal. Myelography may be abnormal.

Treatment. There is no known method for arresting the course of this disease. Immunosuppressive therapy is not effective (34). Patients should be given full support and the family informed of the course of the disease. Community resources should be obtained through the help of a social worker, since the family requires increasing support as the patient becomes increasingly dependent. When dysphagia prevents normal feeding, feedings should be continued through a plastic nasogastric gastrostomy or jujenostomy tube using a pureed diet. The weakness and wasting often produces painful subluxation of the scapulohumeral joints, and the arms should be supported by hemiplegic slings. The patient should receive adequate analgesics for control of pain.

When respiratory failure occurs, the family should be assured that the patient will pass quietly into a carbon dioxide narcosis, coma, and death, and should be urged to avoid the use of a mechanical respirator. However, a number of patients develop respiratory failure in an early stage when there is still adequate function in the upper limbs. These individuals may lead a useful life of two or more years in some cases with portable mechanical respirator support. Death occurs from pulmonary infection as the patient becomes immobilized by muscle weakness.

The bulbar musculature tends to lose function at a slower rate than the muscles in the upper limbs (35), but bulbar involvement is more critical because of the dangers of aspiration.

Prognosis. The course is one of steady progression until death. Occasionally the process seems to be arrested for a period of several months before continuing the downhill course. Progressive muscular atrophy and primary lateral sclerosis have the best prognosis with survival beyond 15 years in some cases. Mean survival for all types is four years.

Spinal Muscular Atrophies

Definition. The spinal muscular atrophies are a group of diseases of unknown etiology that result from degeneration of the anterior horn cells of the spinal cord.

Etiology and Pathology. The etiology is unknown. In most cases the condition is inherited as an autosomal recessive trait, although unusual pedigree patterns are occasionally reported (35).

The primary pathologic process appears to be degeneration and atrophy of the anterior horn cells. However, chromatolytic changes with enhanced mitochondrial and oxidative activity in surviving neurons suggest that the primary change may be distal in the axons.

The muscle shows evidence of denervation atrophy with atrophic motor units surrounded by normal-appearing muscle fibers. However, histochemical studies show that the surrounding fibers are all of one histochemical fiber type because of reinnervation of denervated fibers by sprouting collaterals from axons of surviving anterior horn cells. Other helpful findings include the presence of angular fibers and target or targetoid fibers.

Clinical Features. There are four clinical forms based on age at onset of signs and symptoms. These include:

Infantile Form (Werdnig-Hoffman). The condition is present at birth, and the mother frequently reports diminution of the child's movements in utero in the latter weeks of pregnancy. The infant is weak at birth and shows progressive muscular weakness and hypotonia (floppy infant). This produces a characteristic "frog" position when the baby is prone. The arm is abducted at the shoulder and flexed at the elbow, and the lower limbs are abducted and externally rotated at the hips and flexed at the knees. There is progressive weakness of respiratory muscles, paradoxical respirations leading to respiratory insufficiency and pneumonia and death within 12 to 18 months.

Late Infantile Forms. These children have normal movements at birth but develop progressive muscle weakness and hypotonia within two months. The lower limbs are weaker than the upper limbs, and the child is never able to stand or crawl. Fasciculations of the tongue occur in about 50 percent of cases. Death usually occurs within two years, but some children survive for several years.

Childhood Form. Children with this form of spinal muscular atrophy develop normally up to or beyond the first birthday and are able to stand and crawl. Many are able to walk for a short period of time, but progressive weakness, wasting, hypotonia, and hyporeflexia with proximal or distal preponderance impose increasing restriction of activities. Fasciculations are unusual in limb muscles but may be present in the tongue. Focal or even diffuse muscle hypertrophy can occur due to hypertrophy of surviving motor units. There may be a fine asynchronous tremor of the outstretched hands due to the firing of large motor units; this results from reinnervation of denervated muscles by surviving nerve fibers. Voluntary contraction fasciculations, which disappear on relaxation, may be present. Palpation of the contracting muscle may yield a vibration-like sensation. Auscultation may reveal a low-pitched rumbling. Late changes include joint contractures and scoliosis. Severe scoliosis may lead to spinal cord compression and result in hyperreflexia and extensor plantar responses. The combination of scoliosis and respiratory muscle involvement can produce severe respiratory insufficiency.

Adolescent Form (Familial Spinal Muscular Atrophy—Kugelberg-Welander Syndrome). This is a more benign form of spinal muscular atrophy that is inherited as an autosomal dominant or autosomal recessive trait and begins at about two years of age. Wasting and weakness may be confined to the proximal limb-girdle musculature. There may be fasciculations in the limb-girdle muscles, and the tongue, and some hypertrophy of muscle can occur. Both hypo- and hyperreflexia are reported. The disease is often confused with the limb-girdle type of muscular dystrophy but can be distinguished by muscle biopsy. This is the most benign form of generalized spinal muscular atrophy. The patient survives into adult life, at which time there is slowing or apparent arrest of the muscle weakness.

Focal forms of the disease present with:

1. Scapulohumeral distribution which is usually benign but may present as a rapidly progressive disease in adults with death from respiratory failure within three years (36).
2. Scapuloperoneal distribution. This form also occurs in adolescents and adults. The atrophy involves muscles of the scapula and periscapular region and the anterior compartment of the legs.
3. Ocular and facial muscle involvement. This form occurs in children and adults and constitutes one of the conditions in the syndrome of "ocular myopathy."
4. Bulbar involvement (Fazio-Londe dis-

ease). This is a rapidly progressive form of muscular atrophy involving bulbar motor neurons and begins in early childhood. The atrophy is most marked in the bulbar musculature, with weakness and wasting of the extraocular, facial, and pharyngeal muscles. Death occurs from respiratory insufficiency and pneumonia.

Diagnostic Procedures.

1. It is possible to produce fasciculations in suspected cases by injecting 1 mg of prostigmine IM.
2. Electromyography may show the presence of fasciculations and fibrillations.
3. Muscle biopsy with histochemistry is abnormal. The findings are outlined above under "Etiology and Pathology."

Treatment. The infantile form of spinal muscular atrophy runs a rapid course with death from respiratory failure 6 to 18 months after birth. Patients with the more chronic forms of the disease should receive:

1. Treatment directed toward maintaining ambulation as long as possible. This includes physical therapy, orthopedic consultation, bracing, and surgical procedures (37).
2. Prompt treatment of all upper respiratory tract infections that may lead to pneumonia, pulmonary insufficiency, and death.
3. A normal education, since the intelligence is not affected.

Prognosis. The life span is reduced in all forms of generalized spinal muscular atrophy, but a normal span is possible in some cases with focal forms of the disease.

DISEASES OF THE WHITE MATTER— INBORN ERRORS OF METABOLISM CAUSING DEGENERATION

THE LEUKODYSTROPHIES

The leukodystrophies are a rare group of genetically determined conditions characterized by metabolic defects in formation or breakdown of myelin (see Table 14–2). Metachromatic leukodystrophy is the most frequently encountered of these rare metabolic disorders.

Metachromatic Leukodystrophy

Definition. Metachromatic leukodystrophy is an autosomal recessive disorder characterized by degeneration of myelin in the

TABLE 14–2. Disorders of Sphingomyelin Metabolism

Disease	Inheritance	Enzyme Deficiency	Metabolite Which Accumulates
Metachromatic leukodystrophy	Autosomal recessive	Sulfatidase	Sulfatide
Globoid cell leukodystrophy (Krabbe)	Autosomal recessive	Galactocerebroside-β-galactosidase	Galactocerebroside
GM$_1$ Gangliosidoses (generalized)	Autosomal recessive	Ganglioside GM$_1$-β-galactosidase	Ganglioside GM$_1$
Tay-Sachs disease (infantile)	Autosomal recessive	Hexosaminidase A	Ganglioside GM$_2$
Tay-Sachs disease (juvenile)	Autosomal recessive	Hexosaminidase B	Ganglioside GM$_2$
Tay-Sachs disease (Sandhoff-Jatzkewitz)	Autosomal recessive	Hexosaminidase A, B	Ganglioside GM$_2$
Fabry's disease	X-linked recessive	Ceramidetrihexoside-α-galactosidase	Ceramidetrihexoside
Gaucher's disease	Autosomal recessive	Glycocerebroside-β-galactosidase	Glucocerebroside
Niemann-Pick's disease	Autosomal recessive	Sphingomyelinase	Sphingomyelin

central and peripheral nervous system due to the lack of activity of the enzyme cerebroside sulfate sulfitase (38).

Etiology and Pathology. There is disturbance of sphingolipid metabolism in which galactosyl-3-sulfate ceramide (sulfatide) is metabolized by sulfitase. The decreased activity of the enzyme in metachromatic leukodystrophy leads to accumulation of the sulfatide in the central and peripheral nervous system.

The brain is normal in size and weight. The white matter is firm and brownish in appearance with occasional cavitation. Microscopic abnormalities include loss of myelin sheaths, axonal degeneration, loss of oligodendrocytes, and accumulation of lipid lying free or within macrophages and neurons. The peripheral nerves show myelin degeneration and axonal loss with accumulation of lipid. Lipid deposits are also present in the Kupffer cells of the liver and the renal tubules. The ganglion cells of the retina are heavily involved.

Clinical Features. There are three clinical forms of metachromatic leukodystrophy:

Late Infantile Form. This form has its onset at 12 to 18 months of age with progressive weakness of the lower limbs. The gait is abnormal due to hypotonia, spasticity, or ataxia. Gradual visual loss develops, followed

by optic atrophy. Occasionally macular degeneration and a "cherry red spot" appearance occurs. Progressive dementia, loss of speech, ataxia, spasticity, and tremors are seen. Seizures occur in about 50 percent of cases. The condition progresses to severe dementia, blindness, and spastic tetraplegia with decerebration in the terminal stages. Death occurs 2 to 10 years after onset.

Juvenile Form. In this form symptoms do not appear until 5 to 10 years of age. The child develops progressive dementia and ataxia with a somewhat slower progression than in the infantile form of the disease.

Adult Form. Early symptoms often suggest a psychiatric illness with emotional abnormalities and abnormal behavior. This is followed by progressive dementia and death after several years of illness (39).

Diagnostic Procedures.

1. Metachromatic bodies can be seen in frozen sections of the sural nerve following biopsy.
2. Metachromatic bodies or abnormal urinary lipids can be demonstrated in the urine.
3. A deficiency of arylsulfatase A (which parallels levels of sulfitase) can be demonstrated in the urine, in leukocytes, and in cultured skin fibroblasts.

4. Peripheral nerve conduction velocities are prolonged.
5. Magnetic resonance imaging shows cortical atrophy, ventricular enlargement and abnormal increased T2 tissue densities in the periventricular white matter. Computed tomography scans show scattered areas of decreased density in the central white matter or decreased white matter attenuation near the frontal and occipital horns (40).
6. The cerebrospinal fluid protein is elevated in some cases.
7. Prenatal diagnosis is possible by demonstrating lack of arylsulfatase A in the amniotic fluid.

Treatment. Treatment is symptomatic.

Globoid Cell Leukodystrophy (Krabbe)
Definition. Globoid cell leukodystrophy is a disorder characterized by degeneration of myelin due to a deficiency of galactocerebroside-β-galactosidase and is inherited as an autosomal recessive trait.
Etiology and Pathology. There is an abnormality of the enzyme cereboside-β-galactosidase, which is necessary for sphingolipid metabolism; see Table 14–2.

The brain is small, and there is a diffuse loss of myelin. Microscopic examination shows the presence of multinucleated histiocytic (globoid) cells in the white matter, which contain galactocerebroside. The cortex remains remarkably normal in appearance despite isolation from subcortical centers and loss of interhemispheric connections.
Clinical Features. Globoid cell leukodystrophy occurs only in an infantile form. Symptoms begin in infancy with loss of ability to sit, hold up the head, and reach other developmental milestones. Hyperirritability, hyperesthesia, and episodic fever occur. There are gradual development of optic atrophy, deafness, and progression to hypotonic or spastic quadriparesis. Seizures may occur. Terminal decerebration and death occur within one year of onset.
Diagnostic Procedures.

1. There is diminished activity of galactocerebroside-β-galactosidase in leukocytes or cultured fibroblasts.
2. CT scanning shows areas of low density in the white matter of the cerebral hemispheres and cerebellum and occasionally symmetric high density areas in the thalami, posterior limbs of the internal capsule and corona radiata (39).

3. MRI shows plaque like lesions with high T1 and T2 values in the white matter of the central semiovale with diffuse reduction in gray matter and white matter mass (41).
4. Nerve conduction velocities are slowed.
5. The cerebrospinal fluid protein may be elevated.
6. Antenatal diagnosis can be made by amniocentesis and demonstration of deficient galactocerebroside-β-galactosidase in cultured amniotic fluid cells (42).

Treatment. Treatment is symptomatic.

Adrenoleukodystrophy
Definition. Adrenoleukodystrophy is a sex-linked recessive disorder characterized by degeneration of myelin and adrenal insufficiency.
Etiology and Pathology. The etiology is unknown but the disease is characterized by the accumulation of very long chain fatty acids, particularly hexacosanoate in the tissues. There is symmetric demyelination of the cerebrum, brain stem, cerebellum, and spinal cord. Microscopic examination shows sudanophilic lipids within macrophages lying in the perivascular spaces of the white matter. The adrenal glands are atrophic and contain ballooned cells with eccentric nuclei.
Clinical Features. The disease begins in young males ages four to eight. There is progressive failure of academic achievement in school followed by progressive deterioration of vision. Ataxia and spasticity develop, and seizures may occur. There is deterioration to decorticate and decerebrate states. Death occurs one to four years after onset.

Heterozygous females are usually asymptomatic but may develop a chronic spinal cord degeneration (43).
Diagnostic Procedures.

1. Magnetic resonance imaging shows diffuse areas of increased signal density in the white matter of the cerebrum. These areas appear as symmetrical areas of decreased density in the CT scan.
2. The electroencephalogram shows symmetric slowing, which increases as the disease progresses.
3. The ACTH infusion test is abnormal indicating primary adrenal insufficiency.
4. The cerebrospinal fluid protein content may be elevated.
5. Adrenal cortical biopsy will reveal the characteristic ballooned cells and establish the diagnosis.

6. Auditory evoked potentials. Waves VI and VII may be absent on auditory evoked potentials.

Treatment. A diet enriched in oleic acid with restricted hexacosanoate may be of value (44).

Palizaeus-Merzbacher Disease

Definition. Palizaeus-Merzbacher disease is a rare sex-linked recessive disorder characterized by degeneration of myelin.

Etiology and Pathology. The etiology is unknown. The disorder has been considered a dysgenesis of myelin or a degeneration of already formed myelin.

There is a severe degree of atrophy of the brain, which shows irregular areas of demyelination in the cerebral hemispheres, cerebellum, and brain stem, giving a so-called tigroid appearance. The cerebellum shows loss of Purkinje cells and granular cells in addition to demyelination. Subcortical U-fibers are frequently spared.

Clinical Features. The condition is apparent shortly after birth with failure to attain expected developmental milestones. Progressive spasticity, cerebellar ataxia, coarse nystagmus, choreoathetosis, optic atrophy, and mental retardation occur. Death occurs from intercurrent infection after several years. A few cases show slower progression and survive to adolescence. A rare adult form of the disease has been described (45).

Diagnostic Procedures.

1. Computed tomography shows irregular areas of decreased density in the white matter of the cerebrum and cerebellum compatible with demyelination.
2. Serial EEG's show progressive symmetric slowing as the disease progresses.
3. Auditory, visual, and somatosensory evoked potentials are all prolonged.
4. In early cases a lower than normal percentage of REM sleep has been reported.

Leukodystrophy with Diffuse Rosenthal Fiber Formation (Alexander)

Definition. Leukodystrophy with diffuse Rosenthal fiber formation is a sex-linked recessive disorder characterized by demyelination and progressive deterioration.

Etiology and Pathology. The etiology is unknown but is believed to be a metabolic defect of astrocytes (46).

The brain is normal in size or enlarged. There is diffuse demyelination with proliferation of astrocytes and primitive oligodendroglial cells. The proliferating cells degenerate and are converted into refractile Rosenthal fibers.

Clinical Features. There are three clinical forms of presentation of this disorder. These are as follows:

Infantile Onset. This form occurs in males and is characterized by progressive psychomotor retardation, spasticity, megaloencephaly, and seizures at approximately six months of age. Death occurs by age three.

Juvenile Onset. This form of the disorder occurs equally in males and females; begins in late childhood and is characterized by progressive paresis, bulbar signs, and hyperreflexia. The patient succumbs in the late teens.

Adult Onset. The adult onset form may resemble multiple sclerosis. There may be a remittent course with ataxia, nystagmus, and spastic paraparesis or quadriparesis.

Sensory symptoms are not singificant in any of the clinical presentations.

Diagnostic Procedures. The diagnosis is established by brain biopsy with demonstration of refractile Rosenthal fibers in relation to astrocytes.

Treatment. Treatment is symptomatic.

Spongy Degeneration (Canavan)

Spongy degeneration is a sex-linked recessive disorder that occurs predominantly in Jewish families and is characterized by demyelination and progressive deterioration. The etiology is unknown. There is progressive megalencephaly, spasticity, and developmental delay. The CT scan is reported to show symmetric decrease in white matter density.

THE LIPIDOSES (LIPID STORAGE DISEASE)

The lipidoses are a group of genetically determined storage diseases characterized by accumulation of a catabolite. Sphingomyelin is usually stored within cellular lysosomes. The specific enzyme deficiencies have been identified in the majority of cases but are as yet untreatable. Although they are traditionally listed under disorders of white matter, some of these disorders, such as gangliosidoses, types II and III; Gaucher's disease; and the neuronal ceroid lipofuscinoses also affect the gray matter.

Sphingomyelin is a structural molecule of cell membranes in the central nervous system. The metabolism of sphingomyelin is represented schematically in Table 14–2.

GM₁ Gangliosidoses (Generalized)

GM₁ gangliosidoses are autosomal recessive, degenerative disorders characterized by a deficiency of the enzyme ganglioside GM₁-β-galactosidase (see Table 14–2). GM₁ ganglioside accumulates in the nervous system, liver, spleen, and bone marrow. There are two clinical variants of GM₁ gangliosidoses. In the infantile form the patient presents with coarse facial features, bony abnormalities, hepatosplenomegaly, seizures, an exaggerated startle reflex, and progressive visual, motor, and intellectual deterioration. The patient usually succumbs by the age of three years. A cherry red spot is seen in the area of the fovea due to retinal degeneration. This is caused by accumulation of GM₁ ganglioside in the ganglion cells of the retina producing a grayish appearance. Since the fovea is devoid of ganglion cells, it appears as a dark red area. Patients with juvenile onset GM₁ gangliosidoses are normal at birth and develop ataxia and progressive motor and intellectual deterioration late in childhood. Cherry red spots, visual disturbance, hepatosplenomegaly, and bony abnormalities are not seen in the juvenile form. The diagnosis is established by the demonstration of a deficiency of ganglioside GM₁-β-galactosidase in cultured white cells or skin fibroblasts. Prenatal diagnosis is possible, and the treatment is symptomatic.

Tay-Sachs Disease

Definition. Tay-Sachs disease is an autosomal recessive disturbance of sphingomyelin metabolism in which the enzyme N-acetylhexosaminidase A is deficient (see Table 14–2).

Etiology and Pathology. There are two forms of the enzyme hexosaminidase. Hexosaminidase A is lacking in Tay-Sachs disease (infantile onset GM₂ gangliosidoses). Hexosaminidase A is also absent in the juvenile variant of GM₂ gangliosidoses. Both A and B hexosaminidase are decreased in the Sandhoff variant. Deficiency has also been identified in infants, children, and adults with cerebellar ataxia, spinal muscular atrophy, dementia, and basal ganglia deficits (47).

Pathologic changes in the central nervous system consist of diffuse demyelination, astrocytosis, and accumulation of GM₂ ganglioside within the neurons of the brain and spinal cord. The optic nerves show marked demyelination.

Clinical Features. The disorder occurs predominantly in patients of Ashkenazi Jewish descent. There are two clinical forms of the disease based on age of onset. In the infantile form, the patient develops loss of interest in surroundings and progressive visual impairment beginning at approximately six months of age. There are progressive weakness, spasticity, intellectual impairment, seizures, and death occurs in early childhood. Examination of the fundus reveals the presence of a cherry red spot. The juvenile form of the disorder is rather rare and begins at three to four years of age. It is also characterized by progressive deterioration, but the cherry red spot is absent. Early onset, rapid progression, and a severe seizure disorder characterize the Sandhoff-Jatzkewitz form of Tay-Sachs disease.

Diagnostic Procedures.

1. The diagnosis depends on demonstration of decreased hexosaminidase activity in serum or cultured fibroblasts. Amniocentesis allows identification of an affected fetus when therapeutic abortion is still possible.
2. MR or CT scan reveal cortical atrophy and ventricular dilatation.
3. Brain biopsy or rectal biopsy reveals neurons distended with lipid.

Treatment. Intrathecal injections of hexosaminidase A have been attempted but have not proved beneficial at this time.

Fabry's Disease

Fabry's disease is an X-linked recessive disorder of sphingomyelin metabolism characterized by deficiency of ceramidetrihexoside-α-galactosidase with accumulation of ceramidetrihexose (CTH) in the tissues (see Table 14–2). The majority of the neurologic manifestations are caused by arterial thrombi, which result from deposition of CTH in blood vessel walls (48). The diagnosis should be considered when dermatologic abnormalities consisting of elevated, brownish-red zones, are associated with excruciating, burning pains in the extremities; inability to sweat, disturbances of renal and cardiac function (49); corneal and lens opacities; vascular lesions of the retina; and ischemic CNS signs and symptoms (hemiplegia, asphasia, etc.). The diagnosis is established by demonstration of deficient -α-galactosidase. Prenatal diagnosis has been made by demonstration of -α-galactosidase deficiency in chorionic villi and amniotic fluid cells. Treatment is asymptomatic. The patient usually dies of renal disease. Heterozygous females may show corneal opacities and electrocardiographic abnormalities (48).

Gaucher's Disease (Cerebroside Lipidoses)

Gaucher's disease is an autosomal recessive disorder of sphingomyelin metabolism in which the enzyme glucocerebroside-β-glucosidase is deficient and glucocerebroside accumulates in various tissues (50) including neurons (51). There are three types of clinical presentation. In type I Gaucher's disease (the adult form) the liver, spleen, lungs, and bones are affected and the central nervous system is spared. The patient, typically a young adult, presents with hepatosplenomegaly, aseptic necrosis of the bones, and a hemorrhagic diathesis. In addition to systemic features, the CNS is affected in the type II and III forms of the disease; seizures, myoclonus, ataxia, and intellectual and motor function deterioration may occur. Type II patients (the infantile form) develop symptoms by age three months and typically succumb in two years. Type III patients (the juvenile form) have a course similar to type I patients but later develop neurologic abnormalities. Patients who appear to have the type I form of the disease but actually have type III may be distinguished by EEG. These patients are more likely to have EEG abnormalities and eventually may develop characteristic 6 to 10/second, multiple, rhythmic, spike and wave discharges, which are more prominent over the posterior head region. The diagnosis depends on demonstration of deficient glucocerebrosidase. Prenatal diagnosis is possible. MR scanning is useful in demonstrating bone marrow involvement and joint abnormalities in Gaucher's disease (52).

Niemann-Pick's Disease

Niemann-Pick's disease is an autosomal recessive disorder of sphingomyelin metabolism in which the enzyme sphingomyelinase is reduced in activity or absent (see Table 14–2). This result in accumulation of sphingomyelin and cholesterol, which appear as large foam cells, particularly in the cerebellum, liver, spleen, lymphoid tissue, and bone marrow. In the (Type A) severe infantile form, onset of anorexia and hepatosplenomegaly occurs by six months of age followed by progressive visual loss, intellectual deterioration, and hypotonia. The type B form is characterized by visceral involvement with sparing of the central nervous system. The childhood form (type C) is similar to the infantile form except that the symptoms occur

in late childhood or in the teens. The type D form of the disease is characterized by a clinical presentation similar to A and C but the patients are from the Nova Scotia area. Diagnosis depends on the demonstration of a deficiency of sphingomyelinase. Prenatal diagnosis is possible. Successful treatment by implantation of human amniotic membrane cells in a subcutaneous pouch has been reported (53).

Neuronal Ceroid Lipofuscinoses

The neuronal ceroid lipofuscinoses are rare, genetically determined disorders of cellular metabolism characterized by accumulation of autofluorescent lipopigments. There is believed to be a lack of an enzyme, or decreased activity, which results in excessive peroxidation and accumulation of insoluble lipopigments in the central and peripheral nervous system, skeletal muscle, various visceral organs, and circulating lymphocytes. The disorders are usually inherited as autosomal recessive traits and present in three forms: The infantile onset form (Bielschowsky-Jansky) is characterized by onset at two to four years of age and progressive visual loss, seizures, and intellectual and motor function deterioration. In the juvenile onset form (Batten, Vogt-Spielmeyer, or Spielmeyer-Sjogran) the patient develops visual loss at four to eight years of age followed by more gradual development of intellectual and motor function deterioration. Macular degeneration, retinitis pigmentosa, and seizures may be present. Adult onset disease (Kufs) begins after age 20 and is characterized by intellectual deterioration, ataxia, spasticity, and seizures. Visual loss is not characteristic. Serious, often fatal infections may occur during the course of all three forms. The diagnosis is established by demonstration of the characteristic inclusions (54). The treatment is asymptomatic.

Cerebrotendinous Xanthomatosis

Cerebrotendinous xanthomatosis is a rare, degenerative disorder of deranged cholesterol metabolism that is inherited as an autosomal dominant trait. Pathologically the disease is associated with a defect in the blood brain barrier and the accumulation of cholesterol and cholestanol in the central nervous system, particularly the brain stem and cerebellum (55). The cornea, lungs, tendons and peripheral nerves (56) are also involved. The disorder presents as a progressive visual loss in the second to third decade, enlarged Achilles tendons, progressive cerebellar ataxia, and dementia beginning in the sixth decade. The diagnosis depends upon the demonstration of cholesterol and cholestanol in biopsied material. Treatment with chenodeoxycholic acid reduces cholestanol synthesis and plasma cholestanol levels (55).

AMINOACIDURIAS

Phenylketonuria

Definition. Phenylketonuria is a heterogeneous group of conditions characterized by the development of hyperphenylalaninemia in response to a normal diet.

Etiology and Pathology. Phenylketonuria is inherited as an autosomal recessive trait and is an inborn error of metabolism in which a mutant allele is expressed in an environment containing an abundance of the amino acid L-phenylalanine. There are three biochemical phenotypes including absent or reduced phenylalanine hydroxylase (PH—), absent or reduced dihydropteridin reductase (DHPR—), and deficient biopterin synthetase (BH_2). The BH_2—phenotype also involves hydroxylation of tryptophan and tyrosine. In each phenotype there is an increase in phenylalanine concentration in the brain resulting in brain damage. The exact metabolic abnormalities leading to brain damage are not clearly understood at this time.

In untreated cases the brain is underweight and shows diffuse demyelination with some reactive gliosis.

Clinical Features. There is progressive delay in development beginning shortly after birth with failure to achieve expected normal developmental milestones. Seizures occur in about one-third of the cases, and two-thirds become severe retarded. Examination shows an irritable, hyperactive, retarded child. Eczema occurs in 30 percent of cases.

Diagnostic Procedures.

1. A filter paper sample of capillary blood should be analyzed for phenylalanine content by fluorometric or microbiologic techniques. The sample should be obtained in full-term infants at least 24 hours after milk feeding has begun or from the premature infant between the fifth and seventh day of life.
2. Infants with elevated phenylalanine levels should be tested to determine the biochemical phenotype of phenylketonuria.

Treatment. The classic form of phenylketonuria (PH—) should be treated with a low-phenylalanine diet. Diet should be adjusted to maintain blood phenylalanine levels within the normal range. Dietary treatment should be maintained as long as possible but may be relaxed although still restricted in older children and adults (55). The BH_2—phenotype requires a low-phenylalanine diet and additional treatment with L-dopa, 5-hydroxytryptophan, and a dopa decarboxylase inhibitor.

Prognosis. The dietary treatment of phenylketonuria has produced a remarkable change in prognosis in this disease. Early treatment prevents mental retardation and allows normal mental development (57). Most patients with phenylketonuria now lead a normal life.

Pregnant women with phenylketonuria should be given phenylalanine restricted diets to prevent fetal microcephaly and mental retardation (58).

DISEASES INVOLVING THE TRICARBOXYLIC ACID CYCLE

Subacute Necrotizing Encephalopathy (Leigh)

Definition. Subacute necrotizing encephalopathy is a rare disease characterized by symmetric areas of necrosis in the neuropile of the brain stem with lesser involvement of the cerebral hemispheres and cerebellum.

Etiology and Pathology. Subacute necrotizing encephalopathy (SNE) is believed to be caused by more than biochemical defect. Pyruvate dehydrogenase deficiency has been established in some cases, while other patients have demonstrated an abnormality in mitochondrial metabolism with cytochrome C oxidase deficiency (59).

The pathologic changes are similar in both types of Leigh's disease and resemble those seen in Wernicke's encephalopathy. However, the pattern of distribution is different and the mammillary bodies are usually spared. The brain is normal in appearance, but the brain stem shows the presence of widespread symmetric necrosis involving the periaqueductal gray, inferior colliculi, cranial nerve nuclei, inferior olives, superior olives, and nuclei gracilis and cuneatus. Microscopic examination shows vacuolization of the white matter with loss of myelin and preservation of neuronal cell bodies. There are capillary proliferation and a reactive gliosis.

Clinical Features. The disease may run a rapidly fatal course in children under five years of age but has a more chronic course extending over a period of many years in older children and adults. The acute onset in infants and children is characterized by progressive cerebellar ataxia, cranial nerve palsies, hemiparesis, pseudobulbar palsy, quadriplegia, and death within a few weeks from respiratory failure. The more chronic form presents with mental deterioration, involuntary movements, ataxia, seizures, and a slow progression to quadriparesis and death from intercurrent infection.

Diagnostic Procedures. Most cases have been diagnosed at autopsy. If the diagnosis is suspected it may be confirmed by the demonstration of an inhibitor to the enzyme adenosine triphosphate-thiamine dysphosphate phosphotansferase in the blood, urine, or cerebrospinal fluid. Pyruvate and lactic acidemia are present. In the early stages of the illness the MR scan shows increased signal density surrounding the aqueduct and involving the tectum of the midbrain. Serial MR scans show the lesions extending symmetrically into the substantia nigra, globus pallidus putamen and caudate nucleus (60).

DISEASES OF PURINE METABOLISM

Lesch-Nyhan Syndrome

The Lesch-Nyhan syndrome is a sex-linked recessive disorder of purine metabolism characterized by self-mutilation. The enzyme hypoxanthineguanine phosphoriboxyltransferase (HGPRT) is deficient, resulting in build-up of the purine base hypoxanthine. Thickening of blood vessel walls, perivascular demyelination, and marked degeneration of cerebellar granular cells occur. The disorder presents in infancy with progressive intellectual deterioration and spasticity. Self-mutilation occurs. Serum uric acid is elevated, and there is a marked deficiency of the enzyme HGPRT. Treatment is oriented toward decreasing serum uric acid via allopurinol 10 mg/kg/day. Some patients improve with carbidopa-levodopa, others with tetrabenazine therapy (61).

NEUROECTODERMAL DEGENERATIONS— PHAKOMATOSES

The neuroectodermal degenerations are hereditary diseases characterized by lesions involving the skin and nervous system. They include:

1. Neurofibromatosis (von Recklinhausen's disease)
2. Tuberous sclerosis (Bourneville's disease)
3. Sturge-Weber disease (encephalotrigeminal vascular syndrome)
4. Von Hippell-Lindau disease (retinocerebellar angiomatosis)
5. Ataxis telangiectasia (Louis-Bar syndrome).

Neurofibromatosis (von Recklinhausen's Disease)

Definition. Neurofibromatosis is a neuroectodermal degeneration characterized by localized overgrowths of both mesodermal and ectodermal elements in the skin and nervous system. Neurofibromatosis is inherited as an autosomal dominant trait, the gene responsible located on chromosome 17 in the common NF-1 type of the disease (62). The gene responsible for the rarer central NF-2 type of the disease is located on chromosome 22.

Pathology. The condition consists of hyperpigmented lesions (cafe-au-lait patches) and multiple neurofibromas involving the skin and deeper structures. The tumors are usually multiple. There is an increased incidence of central nervous system tumors, including gliomas, meningiomas, and acoustic neurilemomas, in patients with neurofibromatosis.

Clinical Features. There are two forms of neurifibromatosis, the common peripheral NF-1 type and the rare central NF-2 type. The NF-1 type is characterized by multiple cafe-au-lait spots and subcutaneous neurofibromatosis and can be associated with the development of more deeply located neurofibromata. The NF-2 type consists of bilateral acoustic neurilemomas, the presence of one or more cafe-au-lait spots, and subcutaneous neurofibromas (63).

In the NF-1 type of the disease the cutaneous lesions include pigmentary nevi, cafe-au-lait spots, and sessile or pedunculated neurofibromas. The cafe-au-lait spots are brown in color, greater than five in number, and usually located on the trunk. Neurofibromas are of two types, smooth tumors which can be palpated along the course of peripheral nerves and pedunculated neurofibromas scattered over the trunk, head, and extremities. These tumors may produce pain and muscle weakness by compression of the brachial plexus or lumbosacral plexus and by pressure on individual nerves or nerve roots. A neurofibroma developing on the spinal nerve root may extend through the intervertebral foramen in dumbbell fashion to compress the spinal cord. These tumors may attain considerable size in the posterior mediastinum or retroperitoneal space.

The majority of patients with neurofibromatosis show the presence of Lisch nodules (pigmented iris hamartomas). Other occasional features include macrocephaly, short statue, pseudoarthrosis, kyposcoliosis, intellectual decline, speech impediments, headache, seizures, syringomyelia, learning disabilities, attention deficit disorders, intracranial tumors, spinal cord tumors, ganglioneuromas and pheochromocytomas. An increased incidence of stroke, often the result of internal carotid artery occlusion, has been reported.

The NF-2 type of the disease presents with the development of a neurilemoma on the eighth cranial nerve, although other cranial nerves are occasionally involved. The tumors may be bilateral or multiple, and there are signs of cutaneous neurofibromatosis.

A number of congenital malformations may be associated with neurofibromatosis. These include bony malformations of the spine, syringomyelia, aqueductal stenosis, cortical dysplasias, and heterotopias.

Diagnostic Procedures. The diagnostic criteria for the NF-1 type of neurofibromatosis are met when an individual shows two or more of the following conditions (64).

1. Six or more cafe-au-lait macules more than 5 mm in greatest diameter in prepubital individuals and over 15 mm in diameter in postpubital individuals.
2. Two or more neurofibromas of any type or one plexiform neurofibroma.
3. Freckling in the axillary or inguinal regions.
4. Optic glioma.
5. Two or more Lisch nodules (iris hamartomas).
6. A distinctive osseous lesion such as a sphenoid dysplasia or thinning of long bone cortex with or without pseudoarthrosis.
7. A first-degree relative (parent, sibling or offspring) with NF-1 by the above criteria.

The criteria for NF-2 neurofibromatosis are met by an individual who has

1. Bilateral eighth nerve masses seen by appropriate imaging techniques (CT or MR scan).
2. A first degree relative with NF-2 and either unilateral eighth nerve mass or two of the following: neurofibroma, meningioma, glioma, schwannoma, or juvenile posterior subcapsular lenticular opacity.

Treatment. The majority of patients with neurofibromatosis do not suffer any serious complications. Neurofibromas producing peripheral nerve or spinal cord compression require surgical removal. This is often incomplete, and symptoms may recur years later. The treatment of acoustic neurilemomas is discussed on page 239.

Tuberous Sclerosis (Epiloia, Bourneville's Disease)

Definition. Tuberous sclerosis is a neuroectodermal degeneration characterized by epileptic seizures, mental retardation, and adenoma sebaceum. It is inherited as an autosomal dominant or recessive trait or may occur sporadically. The gene for tuberous sclerosis is believed to be located on the distal long arm of chromosome 9 (65).

Pathology. The brain is normal in size and may show the presence of tubers on the cortical and ventricular surfaces. Microscopically the cortex shows a diffuse disturbance of structure with gliosis and atypical monster or giant cell forms. Nodules composed of masses of subependymal glial cells with incorporation of distorted neurons or giant glial cells protrude into the ventricles. Calcification may occur.

Adenoma sebaceum is a cutaneous disorder in which hyperplasia of connective and vascular tissue results in small, approximately 2 mm, pinkish-yellow, wartlike lesions. Other skin changes include cafe-au-lait spots and shagreen patches of thick yellowish skin over the lower trunk.

There are an increased incidence of glial tumors; rhabdomyomas of the skeletal muscle and heart; endocrine tumors; cyst formation in the kidneys, pancreas, and liver; and a honeycomb appearance of the lung in tuberous sclerosis.

Clinical Features. Patients with tuberous sclerosis present with a progressive mental deterioration and seizures, usually beginning in childhood. The seizures may be partial or generalized and are often difficult to control. Focal neurologic deficits may occur, resulting from the local growth of tubers in the brain. Dystonia and athetosis may develop in some cases.

Adenoma sebaceum typically occurs in a butterfly distribution over the bridge of the nose and cheeks. Some cases may present with only a few lesions in the nasolabial folds. These patients often have subungual fibromas beneath the fingernail. Ophthalmoscopic examination may reveal the presence of white nodules (phakomata) in the retina.

There is an increased incidence of hydrocephalus, spina bifida, and other congenital abnormalities in tuberous sclerosis.

Diagnostic Procedures. The diagnosis may be established by the typical clinical appearance and the occurrence of periventricular calcifications on skull x-ray or by MR imaging or CT scan (see Figure 14-2).

Treatment. Treatment is symptomatic.

Prognosis. Some cases show a slow progression, and death occurs in adolescence or early adult life. Incomplete or abortive forms of tuberous sclerosis may have a better prognosis, and there is a tendency for seizures to decrease with age.

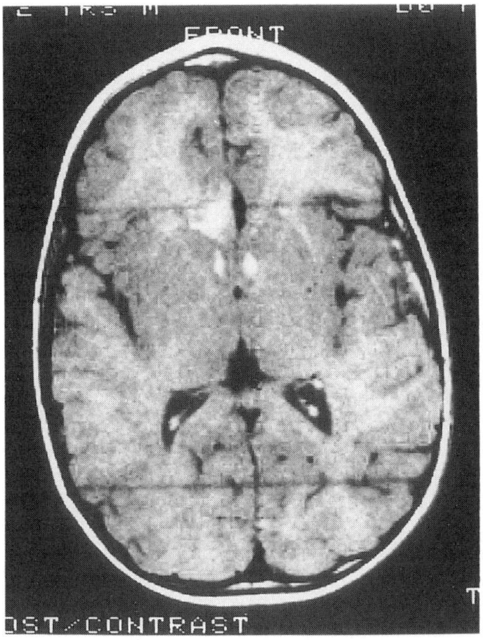

Sturge-Weber Disease (Encephalotrigeminal Vascular Syndrome)

Definition. Sturge-Weber disease is a neuroectodermal degeneration characterized by a unilateral cavernous or capillary cutaneous hemangioma in the distribution of the ophthalmic division of the trigeminal nerve, a venous hemangioma of the meninges, and gliosis and calcification of the underlying cortex.

Pathology. The changes consist of a hemangiomatous malformation involving the ophthalmic division of the trigeminal nerve. The hemangioma may spread to involve other divisions of the trigeminal nerve in some cases. When the ophthalmic division is involved, the occipital lobes are usually the site of the venous hemangioma and cortical degeneration. The brain on the side of the lesion is atrophied with a venous hemangioma in the parieto-occipital region and calcification in the second and third layers of the cortex.

Clinical Features. The condition is associated with seizures, which usually begin in infancy or early childhood. There is some degree of mental retardation and a contralateral hemiparesis in severe cases. The eye on the side of the lesion is often involved, with protrusion (buphthalmos) and later development of glaucoma and blindness. Megencephaly has been reported (66).

Diagnostic Procedures. The diagnosis is established by the typical clinical appearance and the occurrence of cortical calcifications on skull x-ray and computed tomography. On skull x-ray the calcifications appear as parallel lines, "railroad tracks." MR scanning may show accelerated myelination in the affected hemisphere in the early stages of Sturge-Weber disease (67).

Treatment. Seizures can be controlled by administration of adequate doses of anticonvulsant drugs and monitoring plasma anticonvulsant levels (see page 71).

Von-Hippell-Lindau Syndrome (Retinocerebellar Angiomatosis)

Definition. Von-Hippell-Lindau syndrome is a rare neuroectodermal degeneration characterized by the presence of a hemangiomatous malformation of the retina associated with a hemangioblastoma of the cerebellum; angiomas and cysts of the liver, pancreas, and kidneys; and with tumors of the kidney, epididymis, or adrenals (see page 241). The condition is inherited as an autosomal dominant trait but may occur sporadically.

Pathology. There is a combination of vascular tumors and/or malformations involving the retina and a hemangioblastoma of the cerebellum, spinal cord, brain stem or adrenals (68). Angiomas and cysts of other organs including the liver, pancreas, and kidneys and adenomas of the liver, epididymis and adrenals, and renal carcinoma are present in some cases. Additional lesions including meningeal, hemangioblastomas, lung and ovarian cysts, angiomas of bone, epididymis and skin, pheochromocytoma and islet cell tumors have been reported (69).

Clinical Features. Symptoms do not usually occur until late adolescence or adult life. The cerebellar hemangioblastoma may pre-

FIGURE 14-2. MRI. T2 weighted image showing multiple areas of increased signal in both gray and white matter in tuberous sclerosis.

sent with signs of progressive cerebellar ataxia or increased intracranial pressure, while the retinal lesion produces progressive loss of vision. The condition has been associated with syringomyelia.

Diagnostic Procedures. The diagnostic procedures for cerebellar hemangioblastoma are outlined on page 241. The condition may have a coexistent polycythemia.

Treatment.

1. The hemangioblastoma of the cerebellum should be removed surgically if possible.
2. The retinal lesion may be treated by photocoagulation.
3. Patients with Von-Hippell-Lindau disease and their at risk relatives should be screened with annual indirect ophthalmoscopy from age five years. Urine VA and metadrenaline estimation should be introduced at 10 years of age. Biannual MR or CT scans of the abdomen to visualize kidneys, adrenals and the pancreas should be performed from the age of 20 years (70).

Ataxia Telangiectasia (Louis-Bar Syndrome)

Definition. Ataxia telangiectasia is a neuroectodermal degeneration characterized by telangiectasia of the bulbar conjunctivae and skin associated with mental retardation and cerebellar degeneration. The condition is inherited as an autosomal recessive trait.

Pathology. There are an extensive loss of Purkinje cells in the cerebellar cortex and degeneration of neurons in the cerebral cortex, basal ganglia, brain stem, and anterior horns of the spinal cord.

Clinical Features. The condition presents in childhood with progressive cerebellar ataxia often labeled "clumsiness" by the parents. Other stigmata of the disease may be absent at the time but gradually develop as the neurologic condition deteriorates. The child is noted to have a characteristic facial appearance, which has been described as "sad." Many affected children have strabismus. Telangiectasia first appear in the conjunctiva with later development on the cheeks and across the bridge of the nose in a butterfly distribution. The eyelids and pinnae may also be involved. Many children have repeated attacks of sinusitis and pneumonia because of altered resistance to infection leading to chronic bronchitis and bronchiectasis. There is an increased incidence of cancer, particularly lymphomas and lymphocytic leukemia, and to a lesser degree carcinomas of stomach, liver, ovary, salivary glands, mouth, breast and pancreas in patients with ataxia telangiectasia, and heterozygous carriers (71). Endocrine disturbances including insulin-resistant diabetes, hypogonadism, and delayed development of secondary sex characteristics have been described. Most children show some degree of mental retardation, usually of mild degree, and progressive cerebellar ataxia with impaired coordination, dysmetria, intention tremor, truncal ataxia, and ataxia of gait. Speech becomes progressively dysarthric, and there may be excessive drooling. Choreoathetosis appears in adolescence. There is generalized hypotonia with depression of stretch reflexes.

Diagnostic Procedures.

1. Depression of IgA and IgE. This indicates an alteration in the normal immune system with increased susceptibility to infection.
2. Serum alpha fetoprotein levels are elevated indicating impairment of liver function.
3. Skull x-rays frequently show the presence of chronic sinusitis.
4. X-ray of the chest may show the presence of pneumonia or increased markings associated with chronic bronchitis and bronchiectasis.
5. MR or CT scanning shows the presence of cerebellar atrophy in older children and adolescents.

Treatment.

1. Infections should be controlled with appropriate antibiotic therapy.
2. Most children require special schooling because of mental retardation and the associated ataxia.
3. An ongoing program of physical therapy will help to keep children ambulatory, although the majority will be confined to a wheelchair by the time they reach adolescence.

Prognosis. The majority of children with ataxia telangiectasia die from intercurrent infection in late childhood or early adolescence.

DISEASES OF THE OPTIC NERVE AND RETINA

Leber's Optic Atrophy

Definition. Leber's optic atrophy is a form of hereditary optic atrophy associated with degenerative changes in the central nerous system, which develop later in the course of the disease.

Etiology and Pathology. It is postulated that Leber's optic atrophy is due to a hereditary failure of cyanide metabolism and one of the enzymes, thiosulphate sulphurtransferase (rhondanase), used in the detoxication of cyanide, is deficient in this disease (72).

Pathologic changes consist of loss of ganglion cells in the retina with secondary demyelination of the optic nerve. After an interval of several years some neuronal loss and patchy demyelination develop in the central nervous system.

Clinical Features. Leber's optic atrophy is inherited as an autosomal dominant trait, though sporadic cases have been reported. The onset is usually in adolescence or early adult life with progressive visual failure. This often proceeds rapidly to severe impairment of vision or complete blindness with optic atrophy. However, a number of patients show some visual improvement in one or both eyes.

Symptoms of progressive dementia, cerebellar ataxia, spastic paraparesis, impairment of sphincter control, and signs of bulbar involvement appear in some cases in later life.

Diagnostic Procedures.

1. Serial visual evoked potential tests are useful in assessing the progression of the optic atrophy.
2. All patients should be thoroughly investigated to exclude the possibility of a pituitary or parapituitary tumor producing pressure on the optic chiasm.

Differential Diagnosis.

1. Mass lesion with pressure on the optic chiasm. Compressive lesions of the optic chiasm typically produce bitemporal hemianopsia, whereas Leber's optic atrophy presents with large bilateral central scotomas in the early stages.
2. Multiple sclerosis. The onset with rapidly progressive optic atrophy followed by signs and symptoms of patchy involvement of the central nervous system in later life may mimic multiple sclerosis.

Treatment.

1. Those conditions which might increase serum cyanide levels should be avoided. These include:
   a. Tobacco smoking.
   b. Certain bacterial infections, particularly urinary tract infections by *Escherichia coli* and *Pseudomonas aerugi-*

nosa, which increase serum cyanide levels (Infections by these organisms should be treated promptly with appropriate antibiotics.)
2. Large doses of vitamin B_{12}, hydroxycobalamin, are said to be helpful since this vitamin has cyanide-binding properties.

Melas Syndrome

Definition. A familial disease characterized by mitochondrial encephalomyopathy, lactic acidosis and stroke (MELAS). The mode of inheritance is uncertain.

Etiology and Pathology. The condition is probably the result of a defect in any one of several enzymes in the respiratory chain.

Clinical Features. Both childhood and adult forms of the disease are recognized (73). The patient often exhibits short stature and sensorineural hearing loss. There is a gradual decline in intellectual functioning and memory associated with seizures, episodic confusion, persistent headache, nausea, vomiting and recurrent cerebral infarction.

Diagnostic Procedures.

1. The serum and cerebrospinal fluid lactate is persistently elevated.
2. MR or CT scanning shows bilateral basal ganglia calcifications.
3. Muscle biopsy is positive for mitochondrial myopathy with ragged red fibers on trichrome acid or red O staining.

Treatment. A combination of methylprednisolone and chlorpromazine may produce clinical improvement. Seizures respond to anticonvulsant medication.

DISORDERS OF CEREBROSPINAL FLUID CIRCULATION

Hydrocephalus

Hydrocephalus is an excessive accumulation of cerebrospinal fluid within the cranial cavity. Cerebrospinal fluid (CSF) is secreted by the cells of the choroid plexus of the lateral, third, and fourth ventricles and flows through the ventricular system and the foramina of Luschka and Magendie into the subarachnoid space. The fluid then flows up and over the cerebral convexities and is absorbed principally through the arachnoid granulations along the superior sagittal sinus. Part of the fluid passes into the central canal of the spinal cord and is absorbed into the general circulation. Transependymal and transmeningeal flow has also been demonstrated. There is approximately 150 ml of CSF in the adult, 30 ml of which is in the ventricular system.

Hydrocephalus may occur under the following conditions:

1. Cerebral malformation. A failure or arrest in development of a part of the brain is associated with accumulation of CSF in the area of the abnormality. These defects vary from failure of development of the cerebral hemispheres (anencephaly) to minor developmental abnormalities.
2. Increased production of CSF. This rare condition occurs with papilloma of the choroid plexus and responds to excision of the tumor.
3. Obstruction of CSF circulation. Obstruction may occur within the ventricular system (internal, obstructive or noncommunicating hydrocephalus).
4. Reduced absorption of CSF. The absorptive capacity of the arachnoid granulations may be damaged following meningitis or subarachnoid hemorrhage. A thrombosis of the major venous sinuses may also decrease CSF absorption.
5. Compensation for cerebral atrophy. Loss of brain substance leads to accumulation of increasing amounts of CSF in the ventricular system and over the surface of the brain. This is termed hydrocephalus ex vacuo.

Infantile Hydrocephalus

Definition. Infantile hydrocephalus is a progressive hydrocephalus that develops in infants and children.

Etiology and Pathology. The most common cause of infantile hydrocephalus is obstruction of the sylvian aqueduct at the level of the midbrain. The aqueduct may show the presence of stenosis with or without gliosis, "forking," in which the aqueduct is replaced by a number of small, inefficient channels; or septum formation.

A number of malformations are associated with infantile hydrocephalus. These include the Arnold-Chiari malformation (see pages 58–59) and the Dandy-Walker syndrome, in which atresia of the foramen of Magendie is associated with failure of development of the vermis of the cerebellum.

Other causes of infantile hydrocephalus include meningitis, in which the inflammation exudate and subsequent fibrosis block the sylvian aqueduct, the foramen of Luschka or Magendie, or the subarachnoid space at the base of the brain. Subarachnoid hemorrhage, which usually results from trauma in children, produces the same effect. Posterior fossa tumors are a rare but potent cause of hydrocephalus in children.

Infantile hydrocephalus is characterized by marked dilatation of the ventricular system and compression of the brain. The width of tissue between the dilated ventricle and the surface of the brain may be less than 2 cm in some cases. The increased intracranial pressure results in enlargement of the skull and separation of the cranial structures.

Clinical Features. Hydrocephalus is unusual at birth but can cause difficult labor, which may require cesarean section. The great majority of hydrocephalic children appear normal at birth, and signs and symptoms do not appear until later in infancy or early childhood. There is a gradual enlargement of the head, and the normal proportions of the cranial cavity are distorted. The face has abnormal appearance, but there may be some degree of exophthalmos and prominence of sclera due to anterior displacement of orbital contents. The children are often surprisingly alert but eventually fall behind in developmental milestones. Examination reveals an enlarged head, prominent scalp veins, and enlarged fontanelles. There may be progressive visual loss and optic atrophy with a poor pupillary reaction to light, failure of upward gaze, impairment of lateral gaze, strabismus, nystagmus, paralysis or spasm of convergence, and absence of visual fixation. Percussion of the skull produces a typical "cracked-pot" sound. In advanced cases the head may be so enlarged that the child is unable to lift the head from the pillow. Increased intraventricular pressure results in damage to the corticospinal tracts with increased stretch reflexes and a bilateral extensor plantar response.

Untreated cases eventually develop necrosis of the scalp with leakage of cerebrospinal fluid, infection, and death. A minority of cases used to survive before shunting procedures were available, and the child with arrested hydrocephalus would show enlargement of the head, some degree of mental retardation, spasticity of the limbs, and impairment of bladder function.

Diagnostic Procedures.

1. The skull should be measured at each visit to record the progression of the hydrocephalus.
2. The fundi should be examined for the development of optic atrophy. The presence

of papilledema is unusual. All infants should receive transillumination to exclude hydranencephaly and subdural hygroma.

3. X-rays of the skull will show enlargement with separation of sutures and increased intracranial markings as a feature of increased intracranial pressure.

4. MR or CT scan will clearly define the extent of the hydrocephalus and the presence or absence of any cerebral malformations.

Treatment. All cases of infantile hydrocephalus should have a ventriculoatrial or ventriculoperitoneal shunting procedure. The procedure is not without complications which include shunt occlusion, infection of the valve, subdural hematoma, low pressure headaches and thromboembolism (75).

Prognosis. More than 80 percent of children with infantile hydrocephalus will benefit from a shunting procedure. Irreversible damage from previous meningitis or subarachnoid hemorrhage may produce permanent neurologic deficits. Shunting should be performed as soon as possible to avoid the development of permanent neurologic deficits such as visual impairment and mental retardation. The results of shunt procedures for hydrocephalus by fetal surgery are under review (74).

Normal Pressure Hydrocephalus

Definition. Normal pressure hydrocephalus is a chronic hydrocephalus that occurs in adults and is associated with a delay in circulation or absorption of CSF and progressive neurologic deficit.

Etiology and Pathology. In the majority of cases the etiology cannot be determined. Obstruction of the subarachnoid space may occur months or years after subarachnoid hemorrhage or chronic meningoencephalitis. It is possible that some cases are due to aqueductal stenosis, which slowly decompensates as the patient ages. Other causes include obstruction of the third ventricle by slowly growing tumor or cyst or by an elongated basilar artery. It has been postulated that the condition is initiated by intermittent elevation of CSF pressure. Once the ventricles begin to dilate, the dilatation continues in a chronic fashion despite the presence of normal CSF pressure.

Pathologic changes consist of dilatation of all of the ventricles without cortical atrophy.

Clinical Features. The syndrome presents with increasing clumsiness of gait. The gait disturbance is followed by urgency of micturition and eventual incontinence. After a period of several months or a year or two, there is definite evidence of dementia. The patient shows progressive unsteadiness and frequent falls due to a mixture of ataxia, spasticity and dyspraxia of gait. There is a general slowing of function with complaints of weakness and fatigue. The patient may develop dysesthesias of the feet and lower legs. Patients who become ill, undergo surgical procedures, or are injured show poor recuperation.

Diagnostic Procedures.

1. MR or CT scanning shows the presence of ventricular dilatation with enlargement of the third, fourth, and lateral ventricles. Cortical atrophy is often absent, but the presence of cortical atrophy does not rule out the diagnosis of normal pressure hydrocephalus.

2. The cerebrospinal fluid is under normal pressures. The appearance, cell count and chemical composition are normal. Improvement in gait after removal of 50 ml of fluid correlates with a good outcome following a shunting procedure.

3. Radioactive cisternography, which is performed by injecting a radiopharmaceutical into the lumbar subarachnoid space, shows prolonged retention of the radioactive material within the ventricular system and impaired movement of radioactive material over the cerebral convexities.

Treatment.

1. There may be transient improvement in the early stages by repeated lumbar puncture with removal of 15 to 20 ml cerebrospinal fluid.

2. A ventriculoatrial or ventriculoperitoneal shunt may produce dramatic improvement in some cases. Improvement in postoperative cognitive functioning is more likely if there was a known cause, hypertension, short history, small sulci and periventricular hypodensity by CT scan (76).

Syringomyelia, Syringobulbia

Definition. Syringomyelia is a cavitation of the spinal cord. It is a rare and destructive condition involving the cord and occasionally the brain stem (syringobulbia).

Etiology and Pathology. The etiology of syringomyelia is unknown. There are several theories as to why the cavity formation occurs. These include:

1. Cavity formation occurs because of obstruction of the outflow of cerebrospinal fluid from the fourth ventricle. This leads to an increased pressure of the spinal fluid, which is transmitted to the central canal of the spinal cord leading to cavity formation. This theory is supported by the fact that syringomyelia is often associated with other congenital abnormalities such as spina bifida, hydrocephalus, the Arnold-Chiari malformation, and the Klippel-Feil syndrome.
2. Syringomyelia represents a degeneration of a low-grade glioma of the spinal cord. This theory is supported by the demonstration of glial elements in the wall of the syrinx.
3. Syringomyelia represents the effects of proliferation and subsequent degeneration of cell rests, which are incorporated into the spinal cord during embryogenesis.

The syrinx usually occurs in the cervical or upper thoracic spinal cord. Extension into the medulla is not uncommon. Syringobulbia has been described with extension rostrally into the thalamus. The spinal cord is enlarged at the site of the syrinx and the cavity is usually irregular and may be slitlike or involve most of the spinal cord parenchyma. The syrinx is usually anterior to the central canal either to the right or the left of the midline. The cavity is lined by degenerating glial tissue, which includes Rosenthal fibers.

Clinical Features. Syringomyelia occurs most commonly in the cervical area of the cord, and the clinical features can be explained by the anatomic location of the tracts of the spinal cord (see Figure 14–3).

Extension of the cavity in an anterolateral direction produces pressure on and destruction of the anterior horn cells, resulting in weakness and wasting of the small muscles of the hand. Fasciculations may be seen. Expansion laterally exerts pressure on the corticospinal tract producing spasticity, increased reflexes below the level of the lesion, and extensor plantar responses. Lateral extension involves the lateral spinothalamic tract with subsequent loss of pain and temperature sensation on the opposite side of the body. When the cavity expands anteriorly it interrupts the decussating fibers of the lateral spinothalamic

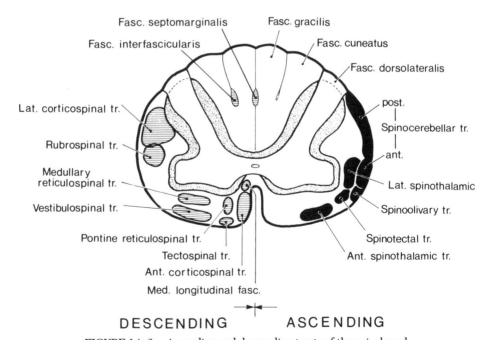

FIGURE 14–3. Ascending and descending tracts of the spinal cord.

tracts and results in bilateral loss of pain and temperature sensation. Loss of pain sensation results in undetected injury of the affected areas of the hands and fingers. Infection and joint deformities may result. The presence of Charcot joints in the shoulders is nearly always due to syringomyelia and only occasionally occurs in other conditions such as chronic, diabetic peripheral neuropathy. Involvement of descending sympathetic fibers may result in an ipsilateral Horner's syndrome.

In syringobulbia the patient usually presents with weakness and wasting of the tongue and/or dysphagia and dysarthria due to involvement of the vagal complex. Lateral extension may involve the spinal tract of the trigeminal nerve producing loss of pain and temperature sensation of the ipsilateral face. If the decussating fibers of the medial lemniscus are involved, ipsilateral loss of touch, vibration, and proprioception may result. Involvement of the medial longitudinal fasciculus may result in nystagmus or internuclear ophthalmoplegia. With more rostral extension diplopia and ptosis may occur.

Diagnostic Procedures.

1. X-rays of the cervical spine may reveal widening of the spinal canal.
2. Computed tomography. Computed tomography scanning may reveal widening of the spinal cord and canal.
3. MR scanning will usually demonstrate the presence of the syrinx within the spinal cord and the extent of the abnormality on saggital sections (see Figure 14–4).
4. Electrophysiological studies show reduction of hypothenar compound muscle action potentials in the presence of a cervical syrinx with fibrillations and reduced motor potentials in the small muscles of the hand. Ulnar and median somatosensory evoked potentials are normal in the presence of dissociated sensory loss but abnormal when all sensory modalities are impaired. The tibial nerve somatosensory evoked potentials are usually abnormal (77).

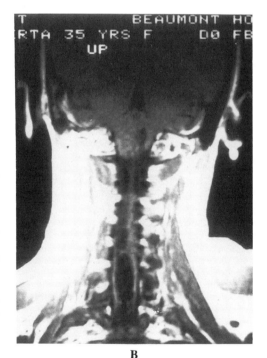

A   B

FIGURE 14–4. (**A.**) Syringomyelia. MR scan showing widening of cervical portion spinal cord containing an irregular cavity.

FIGURE 14–4. (**B.**) Syringomyelia. MR scan showing widening of cervical portion spinal cord containing an irregular cavity.

Differential Diagnosis.

1. Hematomyelia. In hematomyelia there is a sudden onset with pain in the involved area and a history of trauma.
2. Intramedullary tumor. An intramedullary tumor tends to have a more rapid course, and CSF protein is elevated.
3. Extramedullary tumor. An extramedullary tumor is more likely to present with root pain and obstruction or block of the subarachnoid space. CSF protein is elevated.
4. Amyotrophic lateral sclerosis. There is no sensory abnormality, and there are generalized increased reflexes in ALS.
5. Cervical spondylosis. The sensory loss is confined to involved nerve roots in cervical spondylosis.

Treatment. A small syrinx with very slow deterioration does not require treatment. In cases with increasing neurologic deficit the syrinx should be drained.

Pain that fails to respond to simple analgesics may respond to carbamazepine or transcutaneous nerve stimulation.

Prognosis. Syringomyelia and syringobulbia are usually slowly progressive diseases but can eventually prove to be severely disabling. Some patients show remission with no further deterioration for many years.

REFERENCES

1. Hansen, L. A.; DeTeresa, R.,; *et al.* Neurocortical morphometry. Lesion counts and choline acetyltransferase levels in the age spectrum of Alzheimer's disease. Neurology 38:48–54; 1988.
2. Zubenko, G. S.; Moosey, J.; *et al.* Bilateral symmetry of cholinergic deficits in Alzheimer's disease. Arch. Neurol. 45: 254–259; 1988.
3. Chu, D. C. M.; Penney, J. B.; *et al.* Cortical GABA$_B$ and GABA$_A$ receptors in Alzheimer's disease. A quantitative autoradiographic study. Neurology 37:1454–1459; 1987.
4. Saper, C. B.; German, D. C. Hypothalamic pathology in Alzheimer's disease. Neuroscience Letters 74:364–370; 1987.
5. Mann, D. M. A.; Yates, P. O.; *et al.* Dopaminergic neurotransmitter systems in Alzheimer's disease and in Down's syndrome at middle age. J. Neurol. Neurosurg. Psychiatry 50:341–344; 1987.
6. Goate, A. M.; Owen, M. J.; *et al.* Predisposing lows for Alzheimer's disease on chromosome 21. Lancet 1:352–355; 1989.
7. Huff, F. J.; Auerbach, J.; *et al.* Risk of dementia in relatives of patients with Alzheimer's disease. Neurology 38:786–790; 1988.
8. Fitch, N.; Becker, R.; *et al.* The inheritance of Alzheimer's disease: A new interpretation. Ann. Neurol. 23:14–19; 1988.
9. Moosey, J.; Zubenko, G. S.; *et al.* Bilateral symmetry of morphologic lesions in Alzheimer's disease. Arch. Neurol. 45:251–253; 1988.
10. Huff, F. J.; Boller, F.; *et al.* The neurologic examination in patients with probable Alzheimer's disease. Arch. Neurol. 44:929–932; 1987.
11. Horner, J.; Heyman, A.; *et al.* The relationship of agraphia to the severity of dementia in Alzheimer's disease. Arch. Neurol. 45:760–763; 1988.
12. Faber-Langendoen, K.; Morris, J. C.; *et al.* Aphasia in senile dementia of the Alzheimer type. Ann. Neurol. 23:365–370; 1988.
13. Tierney, M. C.; Fisher, R. H.; *et al.* The NINCDS-ADRNA work group criteria for the clinical diagnosis of probable Alzheimer's disease: A clinicopathologic study of 57 cases. Neurology 38:359–364; 1988.
14. Morris, J. C.; McKeel, D. W.; *et al.* Validation of clinical diagnostic criteria for Alzheimer's disease. Ann. Neurol. 24:17–22; 1988.
15. Townsend, L. E.; Gilroy, J.; *et al.* Comparison of methods for analysis of CSF proteins in patients with Alzheimer's disease. Neurochem. Pathol. 6:213–229; 1987.
16. Penn, R. D.; Martin, E. M.; *et al.* Intraventricular bethanecol infusion for Alzheimer's disease. Neurology 38:219–222; 1988.
17. Thal, L. J.; Masur, D. M.; *et al.* Chronic oral physostigmine without lecithin improves memory in Alzheimer's disease. J. Amer. Geriatr. Soc. 37:42–48; 1989.
18. Kamo, H.; McGee, P. L.; *et al.* Positron emission tomography and histopathology in Pick's disease. Neurology 37:434–445; 1987.
19. Dubois, B.; Pillon, B.; *et al.* Slowing of cognitive processing in progressive supranuclear palsy: A comparison with Parkinson's disease. Arch. Neurol. 45:1194–1199; 1988.
20. Golbi, L. I.; Davis, P. H. The prevalence and history of progressive supranuclear palsy. Neurology 38:1031–1034; 1988.
21. DeReunk Van Lendegem, W. The posterior craco-arytenoid muscle in two cases of Shy-Drager syndrome with laryngeal strider. J. Neurol. 234:187–190; 1987.
22. Prasher, D.; Bannister, R.: Brain stem auditory evoked potentials in patients with multiple system atrophy with progressive autonomic failure (Shy-Drager Syndrome). J. Neurol. Neurosurg. Psychiatry 49:278–289; 1986.
23. Pastakia, B.; Polinsky, R.; *et al.* Multiple system atrophy (Shy-Drager Syndrome): MR imaging. Radiology 159:499–502; 1986.
24. Sakoda, S.; Suzuki, T.; *et al.* Treatment of orthostatic hypotension in Shy-Drager Syndrome with DL-Threo-3,4-dihydroxyphenylserine: A case report. Eur. Neurol. 24:330–334; 1985.
25. Said, G.; Marion, M.-H.; *et al.* Hypotrophic and dying back nerve fibers in Friedreich's ataxia. Neurology 36:1292–1299; 1986.

26. Finocchiaro, G.; Baio, G.; *et al.* Glucose metabolism alterations in Friedreich's ataxia. Neurology 38:1292–1296; 1988.

27. Miller, D. P. R.; Mathews, S.; *et al.* Serum vitamin E concentrations are normal in Freidreich's ataxia. J Neurol Neurosurg Psychiatry, 50:625–627; 1987.

28. Konagaya, Y.; Konagaya, M.; *et al.* Glutamate dehydrogenase and its izoenzyme activity in olivopontocerebellar atrophy. J. Neurol. 74:231–236; 1986.

29. Salazar-Gruesco, E. F.; Rosenberg, R. S. Sleep apnea in olivopontocerebellar degeneration: Treatment with Trazodone. Ann. Neurol. 23:399–401; 1988.

30. Krendel, D. A.; Gilchrist, J. M.; *et al.* Isolated deficiency with Vitamin E with progressive neurologic deficit. Neurology 37:538–540; 1987.

31. Amyotrophic lateral sclerosis. Brooks, B. R., ed. Neurologic Clinics 5:1–195; 1987.

32. Plaitakis, A.; Caroscio, J. T. Abnormal glutamate metabolism in amyotrophic lateral sclerosis. Ann. Neurol. 22:575–579; 1987.

33. Dalakas, M. C.; Hatazawa, J.; *et al.* Lowered cerebral glucose utilization in amyotrophic lateral sclerosis. Ann. Neurol. 22:580–586; 1987.

34. Appel, S. H.; Stewart, S. S.; *et al.* A double-blind study of the effectiveness of cyclosporin in amyotrophic lateral sclerosis. Arch. Neurol. 45:381–386; 1988.

35. Munsat, T. L.; Andres, P. L.; *et al.* The natural history of motorneuron loss in amyotrophic lateral sclerosis. Neurology 38:409–413; 1988.

36. Jansen, P. H. P.; Joosten, E. M. G.; *et al.* A rapidly progressive autosomal dominant scapulohumeral form of spinal muscular atrophy. Ann. Neurol. 20:538–540; 1986.

37. Granata, C.; Cornelio, F.; *et al.* Promotion of ambulation of patients with spinal muscular atrophy by early fitting of knee-ankle-foot orthoses. Dev. Med. Clin. Neurol. 29:221–224; 1986.

38. Morell, P.; Wiesmann, U. A correlative synopsis of the leukodystrophies. Neuropediatrics Suppl. 15:62–65; 1984.

39. Alves, D.; Peres, M. M.; *et al.* Four cases of late onset metachromatic leukodystrophy in a family. Clinical, biochemical and neuropathological studies. J. Neurol. Neurosurg. Psychiatry 49:1417–1422; 1986.

40. Waltz, G.; Harch, S. I.; *et al.* Adult metachromatic leukodystrophy. Value of computed tomographic scanning and magnetic resonance imaging of the brain. Arch. Neurol. 44:225–227; 1987.

41. Baram, T. Z.; Goldman, A. M.; *et al.* Krabbe Disease: Specific MRI and CT findings. Neurology 36:111–115; 1986.

42. Giles, L.; Cooper, A.; *et al.* Krabbe's Disease: First trimester diagnosis confirmed on cultured amniotic fluid cells and fetal tissue. Prenat. Diagnosis 7:329–332; 1987.

43. Noetgel, M. J.; Landau, W. M.; *et al.* Adrenoleukodystrophy carrier state presenting as a chronic nonprogressive spinal cord disorder. Arch. Neurol. 44:566–567; 1987.

44. Rizzo, W. B.; Phillip, M. W.; *et al.* Adrenoleukodystrophy: Dietary oleic acid lowers hexacosanoate levels. Ann. Neurol. 21:232–239; 1987.

45. Pamphlett, P.; Silberstein, P. Pelizaeus-Merzbacher Disease in a brother and sister. Acta. Neuropathol. (Berl.) 69:343–346; 1986.

46. Borrett, D.; Becker, L. E. Alexander's disease, a disease of astrocytes. Brain 108:367–385; 1985.

47. Adams, C.; Green, J. Late onset hexosamidase A and Hexosamidase B deficiency—Family study and review. Devel. Med. Child. Neurol. 28:236–243; 1986.

48. Yokoyama, A.; Yamazoe, M.; *et al.* A case of heterozygous Fabry's disease with a short P-R interval and giant negative T waves. Brit. Heart J. 57:296–299; 1987.

49. Kaye, E. M.; Kolodny, E. H.; *et al.* Nervous system involvement in Fabry's disease: Clinicopathological and biochemical correlation. Ann. Neurol. 23:508–509; 1988.

50. Beaulet, A. L. Gaucher's disease—Editorial. N. Engl. J. Med. 316:619–621; 1987.

51. Grafe, M.; Thomas, C.; *et al.* Infantile Gaucher's disease: A case with neuronal storage. Ann. Neurol. 23:300–303; 1988.

52. Kerr, R. Gaucher's disease. Orthopedics 10:204–210; 1987.

53. Scaggiante, B.; Pineschi, A.; *et al.* Successful therapy of Niemann-Pick disease by implantation of human amniotic membrane. Transplantation 44:59–61; 1987.

54. Isetic, E.; Amano, N.; *et al.* A case of adult neuronal ceroid-lipofuscinosis with the appearance of membranous cytoplasmic bodies localized in the spinal anterior horn. Acta. Neuropathol. (Berl.) 72:362–368; 1987.

55. Salem, G.; Berginer, V. Increased concentration of cholestanol and apolipoprotein B in the cerebrospinal fluid of patients with cerebrotendinosus xanthomatosis. N. Engl. J. Med. 316:1233–1236; 1987.

56. Argov, Z.; Soffer, D.; *et al.* Chronic demyelinating peripheral neuropathy in cerebrotendinous xanthomatosis. Ann. Neurol. 20:89–91; 1986.

57. Fishler, K.; Azen, C. G.; *et al.* Psychoeducational findings among children treated for phenylketonuria. Am. J. Mental Def. 92:65–73; 1987.

58. Rohr, F. J.; Doherty, L. B.; *et al.* New England Maternal PKU Project: Prospective study of untreated and treated pregnancies and their outcome. J. Pediatr. 110:391–398; 1987.

59. DeMauro, S.; Servidei, S.; *et al.* Cytochromic oxidase deficiency in Leigh Syndrome. Ann. Neurol. 22:498–506; 1987.

60. Kissel, J. T.; Kolkins, J.; *et al.* Magnetic resonance imaging in a case of autopsy-proved

adult subacute necrotizing encephalomyelopathy (Leigh's disease). Arch. Neurol. 44:563–566; 1987.

61. Jankovic, J.; Caskey, T. C.; *et al.* Lesch-Nylan syndrome: A study of motor behavior and cerebrospinal fluid neurotransmitters. Ann. Neurol. 23:466–469; 1988.

62. Barker, D.; Wright, E.; *et al.* Gene for von Recklinhousen neurofibromatosis is in the pericentromeric region of chromasome 17. Science 236:1100–1102; 1987.

63. Gillespie, S. M.; Shaywitz, B. A. Neurological manifestations of neurofibromatosis. Conn. Med. 51:215–219; 1987.

64. Neurofibromatosis Conference Statement. National Institutes of Health Consensus Development Conference. Arch. Neurol. 45:575–578; 1988.

65. Fayer, A. E.; Chalmers, A.; *et al.* Evidence that the gene for tuberous sclerosis in on chromosome 9. Lancet 1:659–662; 1987.

66. Fishman, M. A.; Baram, T. Z. Megalencephaly due to impaired cerebral venous return in a Sturge-Weber variant syndrome. J. Child. Neurol. 1:115–118; 1986.

67. Jacoby, C. G.; Yuh, W. T. C.; *et al.* Accelerated myelination in early Sturge-Weber syndrome demonstrated by MR imaging. J. Comput. Ass. Tomogr. 11:226–231; 1987.

68. Burns, C.; Levine, P. H.; *et al.* Case Report: Adrenal hemangioblastoma in Von Hippel-Lindau disease as a cause of secondary erythocytosis. Am. J. Med. Sci. 293:119–121; 1987.

69. Seitz, M. L.; Shenker, I. R.; *et al.* Von-Hippel-Lindau disease in an adolescent. Pediatrics 79:632–637; 1987.

70. Huson, S. M.; Harper, P. S.; *et al.* Cerebellar haemangioblastoma and Von-Hippel-Lindau disease. Brain 104:1297–1310; 1986.

71. Swift, M.; Reitnauer, P. M.; *et al.* Breast and other cancers in families with ataxictelangiectasia. N. Engl. J. Med. 316:1269–1294; 1987.

72. Poole, C. J. M.; Kind, P. R. N. Deficiency of thiosulphate sulphurtransferase (rhondanese) in Leber's hereditary optic atrophy. Br. Med. J. 292:1229–1230; 1986.

73. Driscoll, P. F.; Larsen, P. D.; *et al.* MELAS syndrome involving a mother and two children. Arch. Neurol. 44:971–973; 1987.

74. Manning, F. A.; Harrison, M. R.; *et al.* Catheter shunts for fetal hydronephrosis and hydrocephalus. Report of the International Fetal Surgery Registry. N. Engl. J. Med. 315:336–340; 1986.

75. Sainte-Rose, C.; Hooven, M. D.; *et al.* A new approach in the treatment of hydrocephalus. J. Neurosurg. 66:213–226; 1987.

76. Graff-Radford, N. R.; Godersky, J. C. Idiopathic normal pressure hydrocephalus and hypertension. Neurology 37:868–871; 1987.

77. Veilleux, M.; Stevens, J. C. Syringomyelia: Electrophysiologic aspects. Muscle Nerve 10:449–458; 1987.

CHAPTER 15

TUMORS

Neoplasia can affect the central nervous system in three ways: Primary tumors may develop in the brain, spinal cord, or surrounding structures; metastatic tumors may spread to the central nervous system from primary cancer elsewhere; or the brain and spinal cord may be damaged indirectly by the presence of a tumor elsewhere in the body. This latter condition is discussed under the remote effects of cancer (see page 314).

Tumors arising within the central nervous system or from surrounding structures, including the meninges, blood vessels, embryonic cell rests, and bone, constitute approximately 10 percent of all tumors and account for 1.7 percent of deaths from cancerous tumors.

The types of tumors and their relative frequency are listed in Table 15–1. This indicates that 80 percent of all tumors are primary tumors, while 20 percent are metastatic. The gliomas are the most common tumor type with astrocytomas and glioblastoma multiforme exceeding the oligodendrogliomas and ependymomas in frequency. Nongliomatous tumors consist of meningiomas (10 percent), pituitary adenomas (10 percent), and neurilemomas (5 percent), with a large group of miscellaneous tumors making up another 5 percent. There is some difference in the frequency and distribution of tumors affecting the brain and spinal cord. The gliomas are the most common brain tumors,

followed by meningiomas and pituitary adenomas. In contrast, the neurilemomas are the most common tumors affecting the spinal cord, followed by meningiomas and gliomas.

In general, tumors that arise from embryonic tissue such as the medulloblastoma tend to occur early in life, but identification may be delayed until adolescence or adult life in some cases. Gliomas occur at all ages with increasing frequency up to 65 years of age. Metastatic tumors are usually seen among older patients with a steady increase in incidence after the age of 50.

Etiology

It is not possible to identify etiologic factors in the great majority of brain tumors. Heredity plays a relatively minor role, although there are occasional reports of gliomas, meningiomas, and medulloblastomas in siblings. There is an increased incidence of brain tumors in neurofibromatosis and tuberous sclerosis, but these conditions are relatively uncommon. Congenital abnormalities, particularly incorporation of embryonic tissue in the developing brain or cranial cavity, are believed to be responsible for craniopharyngiomas, chordomas, colloid cysts of the third ventricle, and some pineal tumors. Inclusion of dermal elements may be followed by the development of dermoid and epidermoid tumors. The effects of trauma, infection,

223

TABLE 15–1. Neoplasms Affecting the Central Nervous System

Adult	Neoplasms	Child
Primary Tumors		
45% gliomas	Astrocytomas, glioblastoma multiforme Oligodendroglioma	30%
	Ependymoma	10%
5%	Medulloblastoma Pinealoma	30%
10%	Pituitary adenomas	
10%	Meningiomas	
5%	Neurilemoma	
5% miscellaneous	Craniopharyngioma	10%
	Vascular tumors and malformations Colloid cyst Dermoid and epidermoid cyst Germinoma Teratoma Miscellaneous— fibroma, maglignant lymphoma, lipoma, melanoma Neoplasma of the skull and spine— osteomas, sarcomas, chondromas, myelomas	
Secondary Tumors		
20%	Metastatic lesions, meningeal carcinomatosis	

and carcinogenic viruses or agents are unclear, and there is little evidence that they play a major role in the development of brain tumors. Radiation treatment for scalp ringworm in children is, however, associated with an increased rate of developing brain tumors late in life (1).

Classification

There is no generally accepted classification of neoplasms of the central nervous system at this time. Consequently the description here will follow the outline given in Table 15–1.

Astrocytoma

Definition. Astrocytomas are benign neoplasms of astrocytic origin and are the most common type of intracranial tumors in children. The malignant counterpart of the astrocytoma is the glioblastoma multiforme, which is discussed separately. There have been several attempts to classify astrocytomas based on the histologic subtypes of the astrocyte that normally exist. However, some astrocytomas cannot be categorized in this fashion since they contain not only several histologic subtypes of astrocytes but also other glial cells. It is probably better, therefore, to base the description of astrocytomas on their location within the central nervous system.

Cerebral Astrocytoma (Astrocytoma Grades 1–2). Pathology. This tumor presents as a solid, gray mass with indistinct boundaries. Microscopic examination shows the presence of fibrillary astrocytes with a glassy eosinophilic cytoplasm and cell processes. Cells with unusually plump cytoplasm are occasionally encountered and are termed gemistocytes. There is a spectrum of differentiation from well-differentiated (grade 1) tumors to more anaplastic (grade 2) tumors. Astrocytomas may undergo a malignant transformation to glioblastoma multiforme at any time.

Clinical Features. The peak incidence of cerebral astrocytomas occurs during the third and fourth decades of life, but astrocytomas can also develop in childhood, in which case they are usually well-differentiated tumors. The frontal lobes are the most common site for astrocytomas followed by the temporal lobes, parietal lobes, basal ganglia, and occipital lobes in decreasing order of frequency. Thalamic astrocytomas are occasionally seen in children.

The patient often complains of unilateral or focal headache that becomes generalized with the development of increased intracranial pressure. Some cases present with focal or generalized seizures (2). Other signs depend upon the location of the tumor (see Figures 15–1, 15–2, 15–3, and 15–4; Table 15–2).

Diagnostic Procedures.

1. Skull x-rays. Intracranial calcification is not unusual in slowly growing tumors. There may be displacement of a calcified pineal gland. Signs of increased intracranial pressure may be present and include decalcification of the posterior clinoid

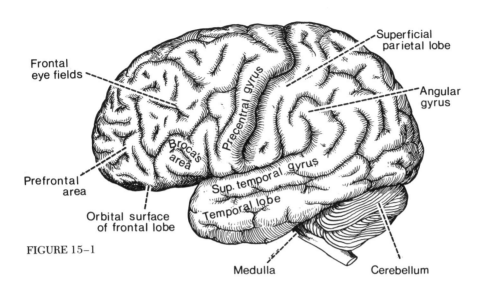

FIGURE 15–1

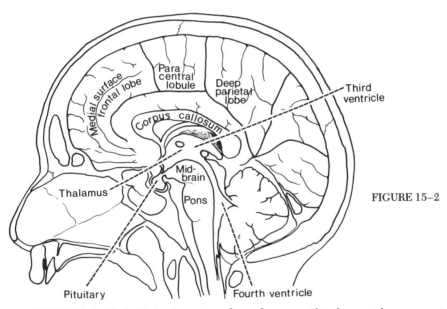

FIGURE 15–2

FIGURE 15–1, 15–2, 15–3.   Locations of specific areas within the central nervous system.

processes and floor of the dorsum sellae, increased digital markings in the skull, and separation of the cranial sutures in children.

2. Magnetic resonance and computed tomography scanning: MR scanning with demonstration of the tumor in axial, coronal and sagittal planes is the method of choice in cases of suspected astrocytoma. MR gives a more accurate delineation of tumor boundaries than CT, and regular MR scans can be obtained in follow-up without risk to the patient (see Figure 15–5). With CT scanning astrocytomas usually present as areas of increased density that show enhancement after infusion of iodine. There are displacement of midline structures and effacement of the wall of the lateral ventricle on the side of the tumor.

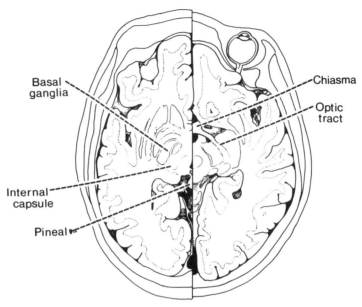

Basal ganglia

Chiasma

Optic tract

Internal capsule

Pineal

FIGURE 15–3

3. Arteriography. There is displacement of both arteries and veins by the relatively avascular tumor mass.

Treatment. Astrocytomas should be surgically excised whenever possible. Radiation therapy is advised when total excision cannot be accomplished or when there is recurrence of the tumor.

The pathology of deep nonresectable tumors can be established using an MR or CT guided stereotactic biopsy instrument before radiation therapy (3).

Recent developments in treatment including the use of MR or CT guided laser probes are encouraging. Other new techniques include brachytherapy—the temporary stereotactic implantation of a high energy radiation source—and the use of chemotherapy and radiation therapy.

Prognosis. Approximately 40 percent of adults with astrocytoma grade I are alive 10 years following total excision of the tumor. Children have a survival rate of 85 percent 10 years after surgery. Patients with poorly differentiated grade 2 astrocytomas have a postoperative five-year survival rate of 20 to 40 percent.

Cerebellar Astrocytoma. Pathology. These tumors are often cystic and usually well circumscribed. In some cases a large cyst is associated with a small mural nodule of tumor. On microscopic examination the tumor is usually composed of protoplasmic and pilocytic astrocytes. These tumors are histologically and biologically benign.

Clinical Features. The cerebellar astrocytoma is the most common infratentorial tumor of childhood. It is commoner in males and usually occurs during the first two decades of life. The tumor can develop in the cerebellar hemispheres or the vermis. The presenting symptoms are usually unilateral cerebellar ataxia involving the limbs and trunk followed by signs of increased intracranial pressure.

Diagnostic Procedures.

1. MR or CT scanning will reveal a cystic cerebellar mass (see Figure 15–6). The much greater detail of the MR scan is an advantage in delineating the boundaries of the cystic mass and the mural nodule which may appear in the CT scan only after constrast enhancement. The use of gadolinium DTPA enhanced MRI provides even better definition of tumors and their anatomical relationships (4).

2. Arteriography may reveal an avascular mass in the posterior fossa and will reveal the location of the mural nodule.

Treatment and Prognosis. The tumor should be excised whenever possible since virtually 100 percent of patients are alive 10 years following total removal.

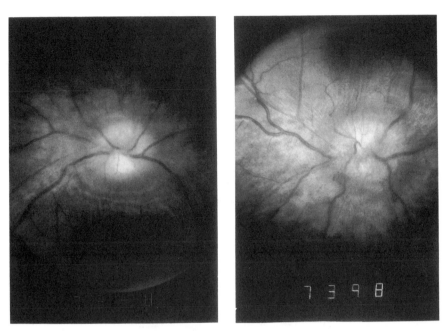

FIGURE 15–4.   **A** Bilateral papilledema in a 17 year old male with an astrocytoma in the posterior third ventricle obstructing outflow of cerebrospinal fluid.

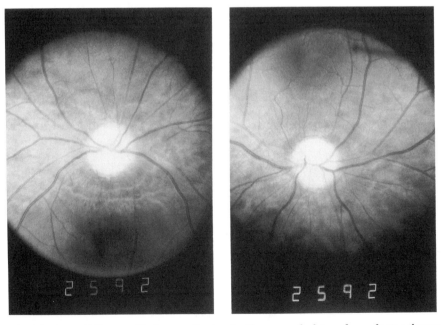

FIGURE 15–4.   **B** Post papilledema optic atrophy three months later after radiation theapy.

TABLE 15–2. Signs Associated with Localized Lesions (see Figs. 15–1 to 15–3)

Location of Lesion	Associated Signs
Prefrontal area	Loss of judgment, failure of memory, inappropriate behavior, apathy, poor attention span, easily distractible, release phenomena
Frontal eye fields	Failure to sustain gaze to opposite size, saccadic eye movements, impersistence, seizures with forced deviation of the eyes to the opposite side
Precentral gyrus	Partial motor seizures, jacksonian seizures, generalized seizures, hemiparesis
Superficial parietal lobe	Partial sensory seizures, loss of cortical sensation including two-point discrimination, tactile localization, stereognosis and graphism
Angular gyrus	Agraphia, acalculia, finger agnosia, allochiria (right-left confusion) (Gerstmann's syndrome)
Broca's area	Motor dysphasia
Superior temporal gyrus	Receptive dysphasia
Midbrain	Early hydrocephalus; loss of upward gaze; pupillary abnormalities; third nerve involvement—ptosis, external strabismus, diplopia; ipsilateral cerebellar signs; contralateral hemiparesis; parkinsonism; akinetic mutism
Cerebellar hemisphere	Ipsilateral cerebellar ataxia with hypotonia, dysmetria, intention tremor, nystagmus to side of lesion.
Pons	Sixth nerve involvement—diplopia, internal strabismus; seventh nerve involvement—ipsilateral facial paralysis; contralateral hemiparesis; contralateral hemisensory loss; ipsilateral cerebellar ataxia; locked-in syndrome
Medial surface of frontal lobe	Apraxia of gait, urinary incontinence
Corpus callosum	Left-hand apraxia and agraphia, generalized tonic-clonic seizures
Thalamus	Contralateral "thalamic pain," contralateral hemisensory loss
Temporal lobe	Partial complex seizures, contralateral homonymous upper quadrant-anopsia
Paracentral lobule	Progressive spastic paraparesis, urgency of micturition, incontinence
Deep parietal lobe	Autotopagnosia, anosognosia, contralateral homonymous lower quadrantanopsia
Third ventricle	Paroxysmal headache, hydrocephalus
Fourth ventricle	Hydrocephalus, progressive cerebellar ataxia, progressive spastic hemiparesis or quadriparesis
Cerebellopontine angle	Hearing loss, tinnitus, cerebellar ataxis, facial pain, facial weakness, dysphagia, dysarthria
Olfactory groove	Ipsilateral anosmia, ipsilateral optic atrophy, contralateral papilledema (Foster-Kennedy syndrome)
Optic chiasm	Incongruous bitemporal field defects, bitemporal hemianopsia, optic atrophy
Orbital surface frontal lobe	Partial complex seizures, paroxysmal atrial tachycardia
Optic nerve	Visual failure of one eye, optic atrophy
Uncus	Partial complex seizures with olfactory hallucinations (uncinate fits)
Basal ganglia	Contralacteral choreoathetosis, contralateral dystonia
Internal capsule	Contralateral hemiplegia, hemisensory loss, and homonymous hemianopsia

TABLE 15–2. **Continued**

Location of Lesion	Associated Signs
Pineal gland	Loss of upward gaze (Parinaud's syndrome), early hydrocephalus, lid retraction, pupillary abnormalities
Occipital lobe	Partial seizures with elementary visual phenomena, homonymous hemianopsia with macular sparing
Hypothalamus/pituitary	Precocious puberty (children), impotence, amenorrhea, galactorrhea, hypothyroidism, hypopituitarism, diabetes insipidus, cachexia, diencephalic autonomic seizures

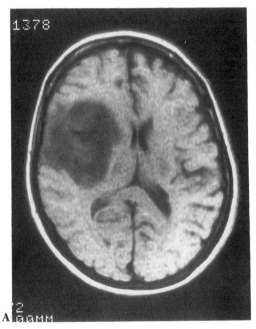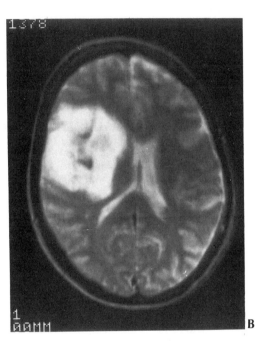

FIGURE 15–5. MR scan T1 weighted image (**A**) and T2 weighted image (**B**) showing an abnormality in the right cerebral hemisphere, compatible with a low grade astrocytoma or an oligodendroglioma. The patient has been asymptomatic for many years apart from occasional left-side focal seizure activity.

Glioblastoma Multiforme (Astrocytoma-Grade 3, 4: Spongioblastoma Multiforme)

Definition. Glioblastoma multiforme is the most common intracranial neoplasm of the adult.

Etiology and Pathology. The brain is swollen and the neoplasm appears as a pinkish-gray, well-demarcated mass with scattered areas of hemorrhage within its substance. There may be areas of cystic degeneration and a central area of creamy necrosis. Microscopically, the tumor is characterized by hypercellularity and pleomorphism, and the cells show hyperchromatic nuclei and occasional mitoses. Multinucleated giant cells are a feature of the more anaplastic tumors; there are few normal astrocytes. The numerous blood vessels show endothelial proliferation. Despite the presence of a well-demarcated border the tumor infiltrates the surrounding brain and is associated with considerable edema.

Clinical Features. Glioblastoma multiforme occurs most commonly in the fifth and sixth decades and is somewhat commoner in males. The tumor is found most frequently in one frontal lobe and may spread through the corpus callosum to the opposite side. Glio-

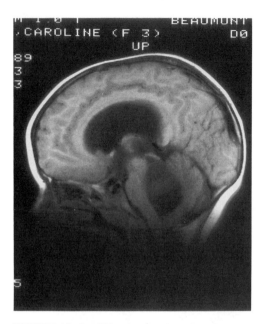

FIGURE 15-6. CT scan showing a cystic astro-cytoma in the cerebellum compressing the fourth ventricle and hydrocephalus.

blastomas also occur in the temporal, parietal, and occipital lobes, and in the basal ganglia and thalamus. This tumor is the most common glioma of the pons.

There is usually a rapid progression of signs and symptoms. The patient may present with unilateral headache over the site of the tumor, but this is rapidly followed by generalized headache, indicating an increase in intracranial pressure due to tumor mass edema or hydrocephalus (see Figure 15-7). Onset with focal or generalized seizures or the development of seizures early in the course of the illness is not unusual. Additional signs and symptoms depend on the location of the neoplasm (see Table 15-2).

Diagnostic Procedures.

1. MR scanning is the most sensitive imaging technique in the detection of glioblastoma multiforme and in the delineation of the boundaries of the tumor (see Figure 15-8). The volume of the tumor is usually greater than that identified by the CT scan.
2. CT scanning shows a mass with irregular margins containing areas of high and low density. There are usually significant mass effect and marked surrounding edema.

There is usually a homogeneous, irregular, or ring pattern of enhancement following infusion of contrast material. Calcification occurs in about 15 percent of cases, and they may be areas of cystic, necrotic, or hemorrhagic change within the tumor substance.

3. Arteriography. Arteriography shows displacement of arteries and veins which are draped over the tumor mass. There may be abnormal vessels and a "tumor blush" indicating a high degree of vascularity in the tumor.

Treatment.

1. The malignant nature, invasiveness, and rapid progression of the neoplasm precludes excision in most cases. Nevertheless patients who have a total resection of the tumor have a significantly longer survival time than those who have a partial resection (5,6). Surgical decompression, radiation, and chemotherapy are associated with a median survival of 11.5 months. Poorly differentiated tumors are associated with a shorter survival time.
2. Dexamethasone (Decadron) 4 mg q6h reduces cerebral edema and produces symptomatic improvement in most cases without prolonging life.
3. Chemotherapy with BCNU may prolong survival of patients with a glioblastoma if given following radiation therapy (7). While CCNU is beneficial, CCNU plus misonidazole provides a longer survival (8). Intravenous VP-16 (etoposide) is also effective in some cases.

Oligodendrogliomas

Definition. Oligodendrogliomas constitute approximately 5 percent of all gliomas. These tumors usually occur in adults and are located predominantly in the cerebral hemispheres. Oligodendrogliomas are rarely curable by excision but are often associated with a reasonably long life expectancy.

Pathology. The neoplasm presents as a gray-pink to red cystic area in the brain. Microscopic examination reveals a honeycomb appearance at low power due to the presence of a fibrovascular stroma. On higher power the cells have a uniform appearance with a central nucleus surrounded by clear cytoplasm. The presence of some mitoses is not unusual. Approximately 70 percent of these tumors show some evidence of calcification. The neoplasm expands toward the cortex,

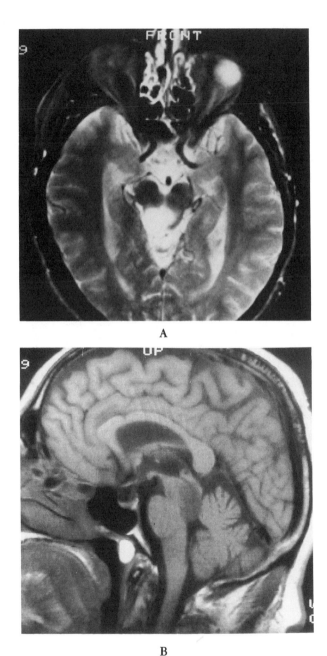

A

B

FIGURE 15–7.   Axial (**A**) and sagittal (**B**) MR scans showing a glioma of the midbrain with compression of the aqueduct.

may spread through it and eventually may attach to the dura.

Clinical Features. Oligodendrogliomas are commoner during the third and fourth decades and usually occur in the frontal lobes. Chronic headaches and partial or generalized seizures may be the only complaints for several years. Additional signs and symptoms depend on the location of the tumor (see p. 228).

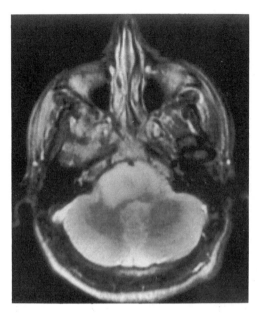

FIGURE 15–8. Pontine glioma. MR scan, T2 weighted image, showing enlargement of the pons by an astrocytoma.

Diagnostic Procedures.

1. Skull x-rays often show evidence of increased intracranial pressure and calcification in the area of the neoplasm; 40 to 50 percent of the tumors show some calcification on plain skull x-rays.
2. MR and CT scanning. The MR scan will clearly define the oligodendroglioma and its boundaries. The nonenhanced CT scan shows clusters of dense calcification lying within an area of decreased density. There are some surrounding edema and ventricular displacement. There may be little change on contrast enhancement or slight enhancement of the surrounding area.
3. Arteriography reveals an avascular mass with displacement and draping of surrounding arteries and the occasional presence of early draining veins.
4. Tissue diagnosis may be established by stereotactic tumor biopsy.

Treatment. Since the boundaries of the tumor can often be defined by MR scanning in three planes, resection may be possible by laser probe using MR scans to control the extent of the operative procedure.

Prognosis. In the standard procedure of partial resection followed by radiation therapy, the mean postoperative survival is be-

tween five and seven years. Cases with complete resection have survived beyond 10 years (see Figure 15–9).

Ependymoma

Definition. Ependymomas are neoplasms derived from the ependymal cell lining of the ventricular system and the central canal of the spinal cord. These tumors are commoner in childhood and have a 50 percent five-year survival rate.

Pathology. Ependymomas are usually reddish, lobulated, and well-circumscribed tumors, said to resemble a cauliflower in shape. There are two histologic types. Epithelial ependymomas contain ependymal cells, which form true rosettes. This histologic type is most common in tumors involving the cerebral hemispheres and posterior fossa. Papillary ependymomas consist of ependymal cells which resemble simple epithelium or glial fibrillary stroma arranged in papillary configuration. This type is most common in the spinal cord and filum terminale. There may be cystic areas and calcification within the tumor. The tumor is usually benign but 10 to 20 percent are malignant with a tendency toward local extension and spread throughout the subarachnoid space.

Clinical Features. Ependymomas are the third most frequent posterior fossa neoplasm of childhood. Supratentorial ependymomas are usually found in the parietooccipital area and are more aggressive tumors. Spinal cord ependymomas commonly involve the lumbosacral area and filum terminale and are often relatively benign.

The signs and symptoms of this neoplasm depend on the location. Ependymomas involving the fourth ventricle are likely to be detected at an early stage because of signs and symptoms of increased intracranial pressure including headache, nausea, vomiting, and papilledema. However, supratentorial ependymomas often grow to a considerable size before detection.

Diagnostic Procedures. MR and CT scanning shows displacement, distortion or obliteration of the fourth ventricle by a midline mass which may show cystic areas and foci of calcification (see Figure 15–10). However, the boundaries of the mass are shown in much greater detail by the MR scan (9). Supratentorial ependymomas have features similar to those of the glioblastoma multiforme.

Treatment. The treatment of choice is partial resection with removal of as much of the tumor as possible followed by radiation

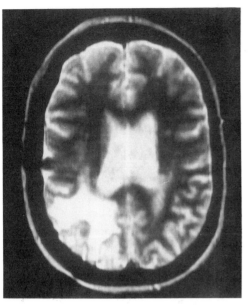
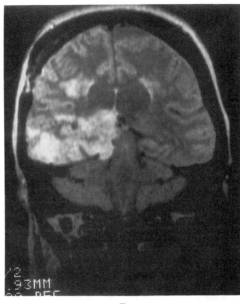

A   B

FIGURE 15-9.   Axial (A) and Coronal (B) MR scans. Recurrent glioma multiforme in the right posterior temporal parietal and occipital areas. The abnormal signal identified within the white matter may represent radiation changes.

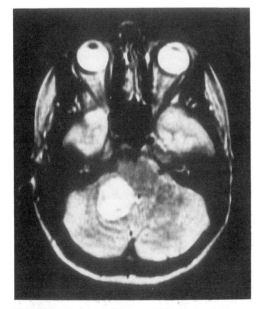

FIGURE 15-10.   MR scan T2 weighted image. Tumor mass within the right cerebellar hemisphere pressing upon and displacing the fourth ventricle and brain stem to the left.

therapy. Hydrocephalus should be treated by a ventricular shunting procedure.

Prognosis.   There is a mean survival rate of 55 percent five years postoperatively for ependymomas of the fourth ventricle. Supratentorial ependymomas carry a poor prognosis.

Choroid Plexus Papilloma

The choroid plexus papilloma is a low-grade neoplasm of the choroid plexus which bears a close structural resemblance to normal choroid plexus. This is a rare neoplasm and is usually found in children where it is often associated with overproduction of cerebrospinal fluid and hydrocephalus. The hydrocephalus and the tumor can be demonstrated by MR or CT scan (see Figure 15-11).

The papilloma can usually be completely removed with subsequent resolution of the hydrocephalus.

Medulloblastoma

Definition.   Medulloblastomas are the second most common posterior fossa tumors of childhood. Medulloblastomas are highly malignant and usually develop in the vermis of the cerebellum.

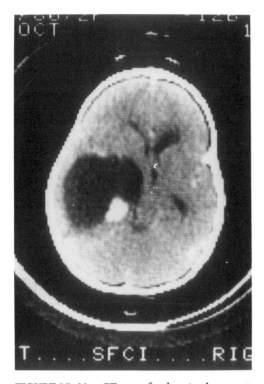

FIGURE 15-11. CT scan of a choreic plexus papilloma associated with a large cyst containing cerebrospinal fluid. There is marked lateral displacement of the ventricular system.

Pathology. Medulloblastomas present as well-circumscribed, soft, reddish-gray tumors. Microscopic examination reveals closely packed cells with deeply staining nuclei and scant cytoplasm. The cells occur in random formation but occasionally form pseudorosettes or appear in rows. The tumor is highly vascular and contains numerous small blood vessels. It has a tendency to seed into the subarachnoid space, and there is a high rate of recurrence.

Clinical Features. Medulloblastomas are commoner in males with a male-to-female ratio of 2–3:1. The tumors usually develop in the cerebellar vermis and are more aggressive in younger children. The presence of tumor close to the fourth ventricle results in the early development of hydrocephalus with signs of increased intracranial pressure (see Figure 15–12). This is often accompanied by signs of cerebellar dysfunction, usually presenting as truncal ataxia.

Diagnostic Procedures.

1. Skull x-rays, in children, often show separation of the sutures indicating increased intracranial pressure.
2. The MR scan is clearly superior to CT scanning in demonstrating the posterior fossa mass with distortion and compression of the fourth ventricle (see Figure 15–13).

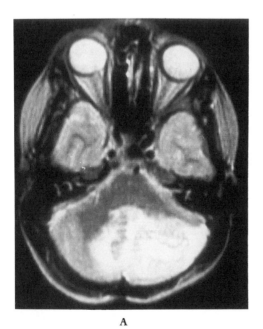

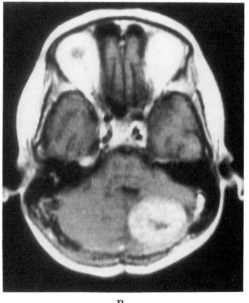

A   B

FIGURE 15–12. Medulloblastoma left cerebellar hemisphere. MR scan pre-gadolinium (A) and post-gadolinium (B).

Treatment.

1. High dosage corticosteroid therapy should be started at the time of diagnosis to reduce edema around the tumor.
2. Emergency ventricular drainage may be necessary to relieve the symptoms of acute intracranial pressure.
3. An attempt should be made to resect as much tumor as possible before radiation therapy. Tumor resection may be facilitated by ultrasonic aspirators which emulsify tumor tissue, or by the use of laser to vaporize tumor fragments.
4. Craniospinal radiation therapy should follow resection.
5. The tumor tends to recur in the posterior fossa or in the subarachnoid space and chemotherapy with vincristine, BCNU, and methotrexate will produce temporary improvement in some cases with recurrence. Edema can be reduced by the use of dexamethasone (Decadron); see page 54.

Prognosis. The postoperative survival is 6 to 12 months for patients treated by surgery alone. Combined surgery and radiation therapy has a 10-year survival rate of 40 to 50 percent. Deficiencies of growth hormone and and thyrotropin induced by chemotherapy should be corrected by replacement therapy (10).

Pinealoma

Definition. Pinealomas are a heterogeneous group of tumors found in the area of the pineal gland. True neoplasms of the pineal gland constitute less than 1 percent of all intracranial tumors.

Pathology. Neoplasms arising in the pineal area include pineal parenchymal tumors (pineocytoma, pineoblastoma), germ cell tumors (germinoma teratoma, teratocarcinoma, embryonic carcinoma, yoke-sac tumor and choriocarcinoma), glial tumors and cysts.

Pinealomas are soft masses that replace the pineal gland and are often the site of necrosis, hemorrhage, or cyst formation. Pineocytomas consist of cells resembling normal pineal tissue. Pinealoblastomas have an appearance similar to medulloblastomas. Teratomas contain mixtures of hair, bone, cartilage, and muscle.

Germinomas have the microscopic appearance of germinomas of the testes (11).

Clinical Features. Pineal tumors produce symptoms due to pressure on the midbrain at the level of the quadrigeminal plate. Symptoms of increased intracranial pressure, including occipital headache, nausea, and vom-

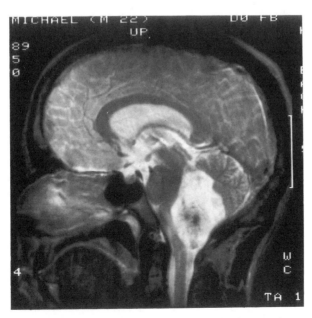

FIGURE 15–13.   Medulloblastoma. MR scan T2 weighted image showing involvement of the anterior cerebellum and brain stem and compression of the fourth ventricle and hydrocephalus.

iting appear at an early stage because of distortion of the cerebral aqueduct and resultant hydrocephalus. Examination frequently shows the loss of vertical upward gaze (Parinaud's syndrome) due to pressure on the superior colliculi. Other signs include lid retraction and pupillary abnormalities such as poor reaction to light or Argyll-Robertson pupils when there is pretectal involvement. More severe compression of the midbrain causes ataxia and nystagmus. There may be bilateral signs of corticospinal tract involvement caused by forward displacement of the midbrain with compression of the cerebral peduncles.

Diagnostic Procedures.

1. Skull x-ray. Pinealomas produce increased calcification in the area of the pineal gland in the adult. The presence of calcification in the pineal gland in a child younger than 10 years of age who has hydrocephalus is suggestive of pinealoma.
2. MR scanning shows the presence of a pineal tumor in multiple planes and demonstrates the precise anatomical relations of the tumor including vascular structures such as the internal cerebral veins, vein of Galen and straight sinus. The presence of fat within the tumor, shown by MR or CT scan, suggests the presence of a teratoma, epidermoid or dermoid tumor and excludes germinoma (12).
3. Arteriography. With the demonstration of vascular structures by MR scanning, arteriography is only necessary if it is believed that the mass is a vascular tumor.

Treatment. The hydrocephalus requires immediate treatment with a ventriculoperitoneal shunt. Germinomas, pinealocytomas and pinealoblastomas are treated by radiation therapy. Dermoids, epidermoids and teratomas require surgical resection. Teratocarcinomas, embryonic carcinomas, yolk-sac tumors and choriocarcinomas are more malignant and should be treated with subtotal resection, radiation therapy and chemotherapy.

Prognosis. Shunting and radiation therapy is associated with a 60 to 70 percent five-year survival rate for germinomas.

Pituitary Adenoma

Definition. Pituitary adenomas are tumors derived from cells of the anterior portion of the pituitary gland and represent approximately 10 percent of all intracranial tumors.

Pathology. The current classification of pituitary adenomas has replaced the previous categories of eosinophilic, basophilic, and chromophobe adenoma, which depended upon the identification of the predominant cell type by light microscopy. The introduction of histochemical techniques, electron microscopy, and immunochemical techniques now permits classification of adenomas according to those that possess secretory capability—including somatotroph, prolactin, melanocorticotroph, and thyrotroph adenomas—and those adenomas without secretory capability. It is likely that additional refinements of histopathologic techniques will result in further change in the categorization of these tumors in the future.

Clinical Features. Pituitary adenomas are usually found in middle-aged or older individuals. The tumors may develop from cellular adenoplasia of the pituitary gland which has been reported in approximately 25 percent of all autopsies.

The clinical signs and symptoms of pituitary adenomas are caused by secretion of hormones, by compression of the normally functioning pituitary producing hypopituitarism, or by extension beyond the sella to involve the optic chiasm, frontal lobes, or hypothalamus.

Thyrotroph adenomas secrete thyrotrophic hormone and may produce primary hyperthyroidism or hypothyroidism.

Melanocorticotroph adenomas secrete adrenocorticotrophic hormone (ACTH), which produces Cushing's disease. This condition is characterized by hypertension, facial and truncal obesity, osteoporosis, abnormal carbohydrate metabolism, muscle weakness, menstrual abnormalities, and female hirsutism.

Somatotroph adenomas secrete growth hormone, which results in gigantism in children and adolescents prior to fusion of the bony epiphyses, and acromegaly in the adult. Acromegaly is characterized by hypertrophy of bone and connective tissue, producing progressive enlargement of the hands, feet, thorax, skull, and jaw, leading to "coarsening" of the features.

Prolactin-secreting adenomas are more common in women and result in secondary amenorrhea and galactorrhea. The same tumors cause impotence, infertility, and hypogonadism in the male.

Patients who are found to have a pituitary adenoma should be investigated for the multiendocrine adenoma (MEA) Type I syndrome in which there is a positive family history of parathyroid and pancreatic dysfunction.

Diagnostic Procedures

1. MR or CT scanning in the axial, coronal and sagittal planes will reveal even the smallest of microadenomas and display the relationship of the tumor to the surrounding structures–cavernous sinus, optic chiasm, carotid arteries and the hypothalamus (13) (see Figure 15–14).
2. Immunochemical techniques are useful in the measurement of increased hormone levels in the serum and urine. Excess levels of prolactin (<100 ng/ml) growth hormone (<5 mg/ml), or thyroid-stimulating hormone may be demonstrated in some cases. Increase in the 24-hr urine excretion of free cortisol or 17-hydroxycorticosteroids associated with nonsuppression of ACTH and cortisol by dexamethasone are indicative of pituitary dysfunction.

Treatment. Microneurosurgical techniques and the transphenoidal approach to the sella have improved the prognosis and cure rates of pituitary tumors. Radiation therapy is advised when surgical removal is incomplete or there is recurrence.

Total hypophysectomy may be required in seriously ill patients with Cushing's disease. This can be followed by radiation therapy to the sella and blocking corticosteroid produc-tion by metyrapone if ACTH levels remain elevated. However, transsphenoidal adenomectomy is effective in most cases of Cushing's disease (14).

The dopamine receptor agonist bromocriptine has been successful in reversing symptoms of hormonal overactivity in prolactin-secreting tumors prior to surgery or when symptoms persist after surgery. Bromocriptine is also reported to be effective in the control of hormone secretion in growth hormone-secreting tumors. Preoperative treatment of acromegaly with the long-acting somatostatin analogue SMS 201-295 produced decreases in tumor size and growth hormone levels fell to normal. This facilitates transsphenoidal resection of the pituitary adenoma and improves prognosis (15).

Meningioma

Definition. Meningiomas are benign, slow-growing tumors that are believed to be derived from the cells and vascular elements of the meninges.

Pathology. The majority of meningiomas are of four basic types. Meningothelial meningiomas are derived from arachnoid cap cells and composed of sheets of cells with large vesicular nuclei. Fibrous meningiomas are derived from connective tissue elements of the arachnoid and consist of strands of interlacing spindle cells with long fibrils. Psam-

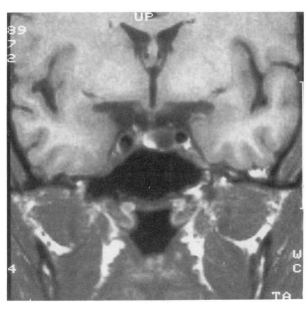

FIGURE 15–14.   MR scan showing a pituitary tumor with suprasellar extension. The elevated carotid arteries are clearly demonstrated.

momatous meningiomas consist of whirls of spindle cells with a central area that degenerates, calcifies, and forms a concretion or psammoma body. Angiomatous meningiomas contain numerous vascular spaces lined by endothelial cells. Many meningiomas undergo secondary xanthomatous or myxomatous change, while others calcify or contain melanin, bone, or cartilage. Most meningiomas grow as well-encapsulated tumors, but others develop in relatively thin sheets along the dura; the latter type of tumor has been termed "meningioma en plaque."

Clinical Features. Meningiomas constitute 10 percent of intracranial tumors. They are most common in the later years of life and are more frequent in women, particularly in those who have had breast cancer. Meningiomas can be found wherever arachnoic cap cells or connective tissue portions of arachnoid are located. These areas include the convexities of the cerebral hemispheres, the basal skull areas, sphenoid ridge, olfactory groove, sellar and parasellar areas, posterior fossa, choroid plexus, and rarely in the spinal canal.

Since meningiomas are slow-growing tumors producing compression of the brain, abnormal signs and symptoms may evolve over a period of many years. Neurologic abnormalities depend upon the location of the tumor (see p. 228).

Diagnostic Procedures.

1. Skull x-rays. Changes in the skull are not infrequent due to the proximity of the tumor to the inner table of the skull. X-ray abnormalities consist of thinning or thickening of bone and widening of vascular bone shadows. The tumor may contain calcifications in 30 to 60 percent of cases.
2. MR and CT scanning. The tumor usually appears as a dense, sharply demarcated homogeneous mass located near the bone or in close relationship to the falx or tentorium cerebelli. About 30 percent present as low-density areas and there is dense enhancement following infusion of contrast material (see Figure 15–15A and B).
3. Angiography. Angiographic findings are compatible with an extracerebral mass with a dense "tumor" stain. There may be hypertrophy of the arteries supplying the dura.

Treatment. Meningiomas should be excised. Complete removal offers the greatest likelihood of cure.

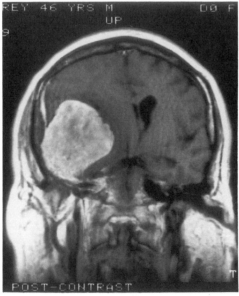
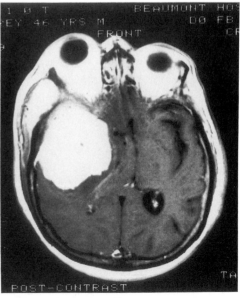

A   B

FIGURE 15–15. **A** and **B** CT scan showing a meningioma right middle cranial fossa with pressure on the right temporal lobe. There is marked right to left shift of the ventricular system.

Prognosis. Complete removal is usually followed by resolution of neurologic deficits and permanent recovery. Tumor recurrence is not unusual following incomplete excision, and a second operation may be necessary several years later. Radiation therapy prevents or delays recurrence of the tumor in most cases (16).

Neurilemomas (Neurinoma, Schwannoma)

Definition. Neurilemomas are slow-growing, benign tumors that originate from Schwann cells and most commonly develop on the vestibular portion of the eighth cranial nerve (acoustic neurinoma).

Pathology. Grossly the tumor is thickly encapsulated and lobulated. Microscopic examination shows that it consists of spindle-shaped cells with rod-shaped nuclei, which often lie in parallel rows. The tumor is often highly vascular and may contain areas of cystic granulation or loose reticular tissue. Axons are found only in the capsule of this tumor in contrast to the neurofibroma where axons are often contained in the substance of the tumor.

Clinical Features. The acoustic neurilemoma is the most common cerebellopontine angle tumor. It typically presents with tinnitus, progressive hearing loss, and episodic vertigo. As the tumor grows, it involves other

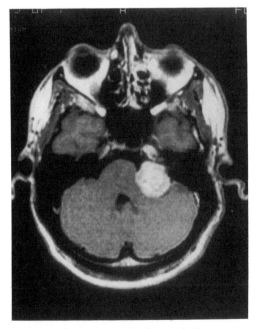

FIGURE 15–16. Large right cerebellar pontine mass extending into the internal auditory canal. Gadolinium enhanced MR scan.

cranial nerves, beginning with the trigeminal and facial nerves. This involvement produces loss of the corneal reflex, unilateral facial hypalgesia, and mild facial paralysis of the peripheral type. Pressure on the cerebellum results in ipsilateral cerebellar ataxia, while extension over the ventral surface of the medulla involves the glossopharyngeal and vagus nerves producing dysphonia, dysarthria, and dysphagia. Deformity and obstruction of the fourth ventricle result in hydrocephalus with headache, vomiting, and other signs and symptoms of increased intracranial pressure.

Neurilemomas are often found attached to other cranial nerves and to nerve roots of the spinal nerves, usually in the thoracic area, where they are subdural in location and involve the dorsal sensory nerve root. These tumors may grow out of the intervertebral foramen into the mediastinum, in so-called dumbbell fashion.

Bilateral acoustic neurinomas are occasionally encountered in patients with the subcutaneous nodules and *café-au-lait* lesions of neurofibromatosis.

Diagnostic Procedures.

1. Audiologic testing shows a high tone hearing loss and impaired speech discrimination.
2. Impedance audiometry is abnormal with absence of acoustic reflex in the affected side.
3. Brain stem auditory evoked potentials are abnormal with absence of wave 1 or prolongation of all absolute latencies.
4. Caloric testing shows reduced or absent response on the affected side.
5. MR scans clearly outline even the smallest tumor in axial, coronal and sagittal planes (17). MRI is particularly useful for the diagnosis of intracanalicular tumors (18) (see Figure 15–16).
6. Polytomes of the skull may reveal enlargement of the internal auditory meatus. Polytomes of the thoracic vertebrae may reveal enlargement of the intervertebral foramina in cases of a neurilemoma developing on a spinal nerve root.
7. CT scanning with enhancement reveals a sharply marginated, homogeneous, dense mass in the cerebellopontine angle. Hydrocephalus is often present in longstanding cases.

Treatment. Surgical removal is the treatment of choice. The tumor has a tendency to recur unless there has been complete removal.

Craniopharyngioma

Definition. The craniopharyngioma is a tumor of congenital origin that is histologically benign and occurs most commonly in the suprasellar region in children and adults.

Etiology and Pathology. The neoplasm is believed to develop from the squamous cell remnants of Rathke's pouch. The tumor is yellow-brown in color, encapsulated, nodular in appearance, and frequently cystic. Microscopically it is characterized by interlacing trabeculae of squamous epithelial cells with a peripheral layer of palisading, columnar epithelial cells. Keratinization results in formation of squamous "horny pearls," which frequently calcify. Cystic components are lined by stratified squamous epithelium, and the contents are oily brown in consistency and contain cholesterol crystals. There is an intense gliosis in the surrounding brain.

Clinical Features. The craniopharyngioma is the most common supratentorial tumor of childhood. The tumor accounts for 2 to 3 percent of all intracranial tumors and is usually detected during the first three decades of life. It occurs predominantly in males, with a 3:2 male-to-female ratio. Clinically the tumor can present with a variety of signs and symptoms. These include increased intracranial pressure, visual disorders, neuroendocrine disorders, hypothalmic involvement, cranial nerve palsies, hydrocephalus, and progressive dementia. There may be evidence of recurrent, aseptic, chemical meningitis if the cystic contents are discharged into the subarachnoid space. Diabetes insipidus may precede the appearance of other symptoms for some years in children with occult craniopharyngiomas, pituitary tumors or hypothalamic tumors (19).

Diagnostic Procedures.

1. Skull x-rays may reveal thickening, erosion, or enlargement of the sella. There may be evidence of bony invasion. Suprasellar calcifications are present in 80 percent of children with craniopharyngiomas but only in 40 to 50 percent of adult patients with this tumor.
2. MR scanning will clearly delineate the tumor in axial, coronal and sagittal planes (see Figure 15–17).
3. CT scanning is characterized by the presence of a calcified high-density mass or an isodense lesion in the case of intrasellar craniopharyngiomas. Cystic tumors show a well-defined capsule containing high-density areas of calcification surrounding a low-density core. The capsule often shows dense contrast enhancement. Hydrocephalus may be present if the tumor extends into the area of the third ventricle.

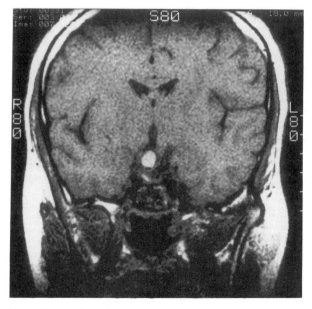

FIGURE 15–17. MR scan showing a craniopharyngioma with upward extension into the hypothalamus and third ventricle.

4. Endocrine studies should be obtained to establish the function of the pituitary and hypothalamus. A moderate hyperprolactinemia is not uncommon. Levels greater than 3000 mU/L (150 ng/ml) suggest the presence of an associated pituitary microadenoma (20).

5. Arteriography is useful in the preoperative period to delineate the blood supply to the tumor.

6. Lumbar puncture is indicated in cases with clinical evidence of meningeal involvement. The cerebrospinal fluid shows a polymorphonuclear leukocytosis. There are normal or slightly decreased glucose content and elevated protein content.

Treatment. The treatment of choice is surgical removal of all neoplastic tissue. However, total removal is not always feasible because of adherence to vital structures such as the optic chiasm, hypothalamus, and circle of Willis. In these cases as much tumor as possible is removed, the cystic contents are aspirated, and the patient is treated with postoperative radiotherapy. Some cases may require repeated stereotactic percutaneous drainage of cysts. Others may be treated by insertion of an Ommaya reservoir for intermittent aspiration of cysts.

Prognosis. The overall 10-year survival rate is approximately 60 percent. The rate is higher in the pediatric population than in adults. Hormonal deficiencies may be permanent and must be corrected by appropriate substitution therapy.

Hemangioblastoma

Definition. The hemangioblastoma is believed to be a tumor of capillary endothelial origin commonly located in the cerebellum.

Etiology and Pathology. The tumor is most frequently located in the cerebellar hemisphere or vermis. It may also develop in the brain stem or in the spinal cord where it may be associated with syrinx formation or supratentorially where it frequently attaches to the dura. The association of a cerebellar hemangioblastoma with angiomas and cysts of the liver, pancreas, and kidneys and with tumors of the kidney, epididymis, or adrenals has been termed Lindau's syndrome. The association of a retinal angioma and Lindau's syndrome is often referred to as the Von-Hippel-Lindau syndrome.

Hemangioblastomas are yellowish-red in color, well circumscribed, lobulated, and cystic in appearance. Small mural nodules of tumor may be located on the cyst walls. Microscopically the tumor is composed of an endothelial cell portion and a stromal portion, which is frequently distended with lipid. Reticular fibers separate the two portions. Some tumors have the apparent capacity to stimulate erythropoiesis.

Clinical Features. Hemangioblastomas usually develop during the third or fourth decade in men and frequently present as a posterior fossa mass with evidence of increased intracranial pressure and signs of cerebellar dysfunction. Brain stem involvement produces cranial nerve palsies and long tract signs (21). Polycythemia, or evidence of the Lindau or Von Hippel-Lindau syndrome may be present. Cerebellar tonsillar herniation may cause sudden death.

Diagnostic Procedures. The diagnostic procedures include:

1. MR and CT scanning reveals a well-circumscribed solid and/or cystic mass in the posterior fossa, which may contain calcifications (see Figure 15–18). Solid tumors show enhancement following injection of contrast material.

2. Arteriography. Arteriography usually shows the presence of the abnormal blood

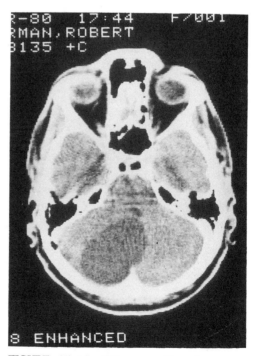

FIGURE 15–18. CT scan with enhancement showing a cystic cerebellar hemangioma.

supply and the vascular nodule in cystic tumors.

Treatment. In the case of cystic hemangioblastoma the cyst and mural nodule should be removed since this is usually curative. Solid tumors that can only be partially resected, multiple tumors, or inaccessible tumors may benefit from radiotherapy.

Colloid Cysts of the Third Ventricle

A colloid cyst is a rare congenital lesion derived from an outpouching of the ependyma at the site of the paraphysis. The cyst enlarges and contains a clear gelatinous substance. Symptoms occur when the cyst causes intermittent obstruction of the flow of cerebrospinal fluid through the third ventricle. The patient experiences intermittent headache, which is relieved by change in posture. Sudden death may occur.

An MR or CT scan will show the presence of a midline cystic lesion in the third ventricle with associated hydrocephalus (see Figure 15–19). The treatment of choice is total surgical removal. If this is not possible, the cyst may be drained stereotaxically or a bilateral ventricular shunting procedure may be necessary.

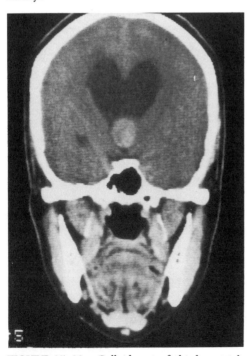

FIGURE 15–19. Colloid cyst of third ventricle CT scan with enhancement.

Dermoids and Epidermoid Cysts (Pearly Tumors)

Dermoids and epidermoid cysts are believed to result from incorporation of a portion of the ectoderm in the developing neural tube. The cysts have a thin capsule of epidermis or dermis and enlarge when desquamation occurs. Dermoid cysts may contain hair or sebaceous glands and are often calcified. They are usually associated with a dermal sinus or an occipital bone defect. The cysts are typically midline in the posterior fossa, cerebellopontine angle, intra- and suprasellar region, or the lumbosacral region. Dermoid cysts occasionally develop in the temporal lobe of the brain. These tumors present as a slowly growing intracranial mass producing partial or generalized seizures and increased intracranial pressure. Cerebellopontine angle cysts present with symptoms suggesting an acoustic neurilemoma (see p. 239). Intra- and suprasellar dermoid cysts may compress the pituitary gland and cause hypopituitarism. An MR scan is the procedure of choice while CT shows a cystic lesion often with negative density values. There may be peripheral calcification. Dermoid and epidermoid cysts should be excised with care, since contamination of the subarachnoid space may result in a severe chemical meningitis, which may be fatal.

Chordoma

Definition. A chordoma is a congenital neoplasm that may arise wherever notochordal tissue is present during embryonic development.

Etiology and Pathology. The chordoma is believed to arise from remnants of notochordal tissue and is most commonly located in the sacrococcygeal area or in the vicinity of the clivus. The tumor appears as a whitish or reddish-brown, lobulated structure containing gelatinous material. In some areas the cells are grossly distorted by vacuolation and have indistinct boundaries. These have been termed physaliphorous cells. This tumor has locally invasive tendencies.

Clinical Features. The chordoma is most frequently encountered in the third to seventh decades and is twice as common in males. Signs and symptoms depend on the site of the tumor. When the tumor is in the area of the clivus, it may extend forward to the suprasellar region to involve the optic chiasm or laterally into the middle fossa. There may be progressive cranial nerve involvement, usually beginning with the sixth cranial nerve and followed by hemiparesis or quadriparesis (22).

Diagnostic Procedures.

1. Skull x-ray may reveal sellar enlargement, bony erosion or calcification in the area of the tumor. Separation of the cranial sutures and enlargement of the skull can occur in children.
2. MR scanning is the diagnostic procedure of choice. The MR scan gives a clear definition of the extent of the tumor and the degree of destruction of the clivus.
3. A CT scan reveals a density at the base of the skull, which occasionally shows enhancement following infusion of iodine.

Treatment. Most tumors cannot be resected and should be treated by radiation therapy in an attempt to slow tumor growth. Partial resection by the transpharyngeal route, combined with retromastoid craniotomy may be possible in selected cases. This should be followed by radiation therapy. Combined treatment produces an average survival of five years (23).

Arachnoid Cysts

Definition. Arachnoid cysts are encapsulated cysts containing cerebrospinal fluid lying within the arachnoid space. The cysts may cause compression of the brain or spinal cord.

Etiology and Pathology. The majority of arachnoid cysts are of developmental origin and result from failure of fusion of the two layers of the arachnoid in early fetal life, followed by accumulation of cerebrospinal fluid and cyst formation. Between 20 and 30 percent of arachnoid cysts are associated with other congenital abnormalities, including aqueductal stenosis, agenesis of the corpus callosum, and hamartomas. A number of cases follow head trauma with herniation of the arachnoid between the two layers of the dura resulting in cyst formation. It is also possible that arachnoid cysts develop after subarachnoid inflammation and the formation of arachnoid adhesions.

Arachnoid cysts are thin-walled structures bounded by arachnoid. The cyst compresses the brain or spinal cord producing deformity and atrophy.

Clinical Features. Arachnoid cysts are commoner in infants and young children and may present with a local bulging of the skull. The cysts may occur in any part of the cranial cavity but are somewhat commoner in the posterior fossa. Older children and adults usually complain of increasing headache and other symptoms suggesting an expanding intracranial mass lesion.

Arachnoid cysts of the spinal canal are usually located posteriorly and produce progressive paraparesis without pain. Examination shows a well-demarcated sensory level at the site of compression.

Diagnostic Procedures.

1. X-ray of the skull may reveal asymmetry and local bulging and thinning of the bone.
2. MR and CT scanning reveals a lucent area with the density of cerebrospinal fluid and a clearly defined border (24) (see Figure 15–20).
3. Arachnoid cysts may be demonstrated by ultrasound in infants.

Treatment. Treatment consists of cyst peritoneal shunting when cyst compression is present. Many cases require a ventriculoperitoneal shunting procedure because of associated hydrocephalus (25).

Metastatic Neoplasms

Definition. Metastatic tumors comprise approximately 20 percent of all intracranial neoplasms. The most common primary site is the lung, and 10 percent of bronchial carcinomas present with neurologic symptoms before there is any evidence of lung involvement. Metastatic brain tumors are most

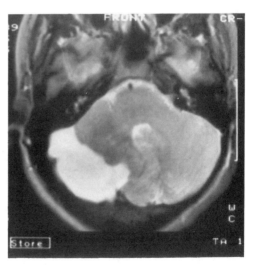

FIGURE 15–20. Arachnoid cyst. MR scan T2 weighted image showing a large cyst compressing the right cerebellar hemisphere.

frequently reported between the fourth and seventh decade.

Etiology and Pathology. The great majority of metastases reach the central nervous system through the arterial system. A smaller number arise by direct extension from extracranial sites such as the pharynx, neck, or paranasal sinuses. There is a theoretical pathway from the pelvis through the vertebral venous plexus, but it is doubtful that metastases in the brain originate in this manner. Most metastatic tumors develop in the cerebral hemispheres in the distribution of the middle cerebral artery at the junction of the gray and white matter. Approximately 35 percent of metastatic brain tumors arise from a primary lung tumor, 20 percent are associated with carcinoma of the breast, 10 percent from melanomatous tumors of the skin, 10 percent from gastrointestinal carcinomas, 5 percent from carcinoma of the kidney, and the remainder from the genitourinary system and the endocrine glands. Most metastases present as multiple, spherical, gray-pink tumors with sharply defined margins but without encapsulation and are typically associated with large areas of edema in the surrounding brain. It is not unusual to see a small tumor measuring 1 cm in diameter associated with massive cerebral edema. This edema is believed to arise in response to the presence of lipids released by tumor necrosis. Massive hemorrhage into tumors is rare and usually occurs with melanoma.

It is not always possible to determine the location of the primary lesion from the study of histologic characteristics of a metastatic tumor.

Clinical Features. Most metastatic tumors present with headache and partial or generalized seizures. Other signs and symptoms depend on the location and the rapidity of development of the tumor (see p. 228).

Diagnostic Procedures.

1. MR scanning is the procedure of choice in metastatic disease (see Figure 15–21). MR scanning is more sensitive than CT scanning and will often reveal multiple metastases which have escaped detection by CT scanning (see Figure 15–22).
2. CT scanning should be performed with both nonenhanced and contrast enhanced studies. If only one scan can be performed a contrast-enhanced study is recommended, although it is not possible to differentiate between hemorrhage or tumor enhancement in a contrast-enhanced scan.

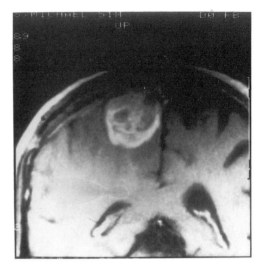

FIGURE 15–21.   MR scan with gadolinium showing a well-defined metastatic tumor in the left parietal area.

Metastatic tumors most often appear as high-density nodular or spherical mass often surrounded by frondlike areas of lucency, representing edema. There is increased density on contrast enhancement often appearing as a ring-shaped area.

3. Chest x-rays. X-ray of the chest will reveal one or more lesions indicating the presence of primary or metastatic tumors in the lung in most cases.
4. Arteriography. Arteriography shows displacement of arteries and veins by a mass lesion with marked neovascularity within the tumor mass.
5. The presence of carcinoembryonic antigen (CEA) in the cerebrospinal fluid in a patient with a solitary mass lesion in the brain suggests that the tumor is metastatic in origin (26).

Treatment.

1. Edema can be controlled by corticosteroids such as dexamethasone (Decadron) 12 mg initially followed by 4 mg q6h. A more rapid reduction of intracranial pressure using intravenous mannitol is indicated when there is a marked shift of the midline structures with the possibility of herniation.
2. Solitary metastasis should be excised when the primary lesion can be successfully treated or when the symptoms produced by the lesion are incapacitating.

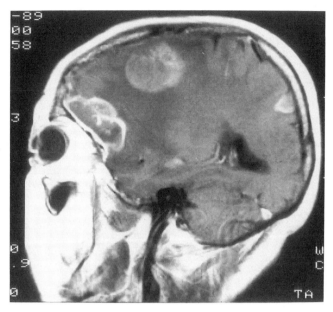

FIGURE 15–22.   MR scan with gadolinium showing multiple metastatic tumors.

3. Radiation therapy is the treatment of choice for multiple metastases since many are sensitive to radiation. There is usually improvement in symptoms following radiation therapy and some increase in months of survival.

Meningeal Carcinomatosis

Definition. Meningeal carcinomatosis is the least common form of intracranial metastatic disease and is usually associated with a well-differentiated primary carcinoma of the breast or lung.

Etiology and Pathology. Most cases of meningeal carcinomatosis occur as a complication of primary adenocarcinoma of the breast. The remaining cases are usually associated with carcinoma of the lung, stomach, and pancreas and malignant melanoma.

The meninges appear dull, gray, and hazy and show the presence of numerous tumor cells and an inflammatory reaction.

Clinical Features. The disorder is uncommon but not rare. Symptoms include headache, changes in mentation, signs of meningeal irritation, and cranial nerve palsies, particularly paralysis of the oculomotor and facial nerves. Spinal cord involvement with radicular pain or paresthesias is an occasional presentation.

Diagnostic Procedures.

1. Lumbar puncture usually reveals a clear cerebrospinal fluid under increased pressure with a slight lymphocytic pleocytosis, moderately elevated protein content, and a marked reduction in glucose content. The presence of tumor cells can be demonstrated by the millipore filter technique. There is an elevated carcinoembryonic antigen (CEA) level in CSF in patients with meningeal carcinomatosis due to cancer of the breast, lung, alimentary tract and genitourinary tract. The CEA level may be of value in monitoring response to treatment and relapse.

2. Cerebrospinal fluid lactate dehydrogenase levels often show marked elevation in meningeal carcinomatosis. Similar elevations can occur in bacterial meningitis but the test may be useful in suspected cases of meningeal carcinomatosis (27).

3. MR and CT scanning are usually normal in meningeal carcinomatosis but may reveal the presence of unsuspected metastatic lesions elsewhere in the neuraxis.

Differential Diagnosis. Meningeal carcinomatosis must be differentiated from all forms of chronic meningitis, including tuberculous meningitis, fungal meningitis, syphilis, or sarcoidosis involving the central nervous system.

Treatment. Irradiation and intrathecal methotrexate are the only available means of treating meningeal carcinomatosis. Most cases show progressive deterioration, but adequate treatment may provide a period of useful remission. Corticosteroids may provide some symptomatic improvement.

Brain Tumors in Children

Brain tumors in children are usually located in the posterior fossa although the incidence of astrocytomas may be 50 percent above and below the tentorium cerebelli. The most frequently encountered tumors in children are the astrocytomas, medulloblastoma, ependymoma and the brain stem glioma (28).

Clinical Features. Tumors involving the cerebral aqueduct or the fourth ventricle, such as an ependymoma or medulloblastoma, produce hydrocephalus with headache, nausea, and vomiting at an early stage. The brain stem glioma, a slowly growing tumor, does not produce hydrocephalus until late in the course of the disease (29).

Progressive cranial nerve palsies involving the cranial nerves, arising in the pons and medulla are a feature of brain stem glioma.

Cerebellar ataxia occurs in cases of cerebellar astrocytoma and follows hydrocephalus in patients with ependymoma and medulloblastoma.

1. The MR scan will give a detailed outline of the brain stem or cerebellar tumor in axial, coronal or sagittal planes.
2. The CT scan is adequate in cerebral tumors but often fails to detect the early stages of brain stem or fourth ventricular tumors.
3. Lumbar puncture is contraindicated in posterior fossa tumors because of the risk of downward herniation of the swollen cerebellar tonsils into the foramen magnum and fatal brain stem compression.

Treatment.

1. High dosage dexamethasone is indicated as soon as the diagnosis is made to reduce edema around the tumor.
2. Emergency ventricular drainage is required in some cases with symptoms of acute hydrocephalus.
3. Complete resection of cystic astrocytomas of the cerebellum is usually possible.

4. Postoperative radiation therapy is indicated for medulloblastomas and may increase survival in brain stem ependymomas and gliomas.
5. Chemotherapy does not appear to benefit brain stem or posterior fossa tumors in children (30).

Tumors of the Spinal Cord and Spinal Canal

Tumors of the spinal cord and spinal canal are uncommon with an annual incidence of between 0.9 to 2.5 per 100,000 population. The commonest tumor is the neurilemoma followed by the meningioma, glioma, and arteriovenous malformation. Approximately 25 percent of tumors arise in the area of the cervical canal; 55 percent originating in the area of the thoracic canal and 20 percent in the lumbosacral area. Twenty percent are extradural, 50 percent are extradural and intradural, and 30 percent are intradural. Tumors occur at all ages, but congenital tumors tend to occur with increasing frequency in infants and children.

Clinical Features.

1. Pain. Most cases of spinal cord tumor present with pain due to nerve root irritation. This is particularly common in extradural tumors and is frequently misdiagnosed as cervical spondylosis or herniated intervertebral disk. The pain is frequently exacerbated by coughing, sneezing, or straining. Root pains are less common with intramedullary tumors but have been reported. The association of root pain with asymmetry of reflexes and an insidious onset is strongly suggestive of spinal cord tumor.

2. Motor weakness. Root pain may be followed by the development of weakness and wasting of the muscles supplied by the affected nerve root. Extension of an extramedullary tumor may produce pressure on anterior horn cells at several segments in the spinal cord with gradual increase in muscle involvement. Compression of the corticospinal tracts produces weakness and spasticity below the level of the lesion. This usually takes the form of a progressive spastic paraparesis.

3. Sensory change. Many patients experience a dysesthesia in the limbs below the level of the lesion. This is often described as a feeling of temperature change, particularly a feeling of cold. Examination shows a dissociated sensory loss in about one-third of cases. This type of sensory loss is likely to

occur in intramedullary tumors but is not confined to this type and can be seen with extramedullary tumors.

4. Sphincter disturbances. Tumors affecting the cervical, thoracic, and upper lumbar spinal cord produce early symptoms of sphincter dysfunction with increasing frequency and urgency of micturition. Rectal disturbances tend to occur somewhat later in most cases. Tumors of the lower lumbar cord and the conus medullaris destroy the parasympathetic neurons responsible for bladder control. This results in retention of urine with overflow incontinence. The development of sphincter disturbances is frequently followed by impotence in men.

5. Syringomyelia-like symptoms. Some intramedullary tumors produce destruction of the decussating lateral spinothalamic fibers in the center of the spinal cord with loss of pain and temperature sensation below the level of the lesion on one or both sides of the body. This is often coupled with pressure on the descending corticospinal tracts and progressive spastic paraparesis. Anterior extension of the tumor involves the anterior horn cells at the level of the lesion and results in muscle weakness, wasting, and fasciculations in the muscles supplied by the anterior horn cells.

6. Brown-Sequard–like symptoms. Involvement of one-half of the spinal cord produces a characteristic constellation of symptoms known as the Brown-Sequard syndrome. This consists of progressive weakness, increased tone, clonus, increased reflexes, and an extensor plantar response on the same side below the level of the lesion. There is a dissociated sensory loss on the contralateral side with impairment of pain and temperature sensations. Posterior column involvement produces ipsilateral loss of vibration and position sense. The Brown-Sequard syndrome is much commoner in extramedullary tumors, which are usually benign and operable.

7. Papilledema. Some cases of spinal cord tumor are associated with papilledema. The reason for this development is not clear. It has been postulated that the high protein content of the CSF stimulates increased production of CSF, resulting in papilledema, but this cannot be the sole explanation for this phenomenon. Papilledema is more likely to occur in spinal cord ependymomas but has been described with both intramedullary and extramedullary tumors of other types. The occurrence of papilledema is much more common with tumors of the thoracic and lumbosacral regions.

8. Subarachnoid hemorrhage. Most cases of spinal subarachnoid hemorrhage are due to rupture of an arteriovenous malformation of the cord, and spinal cord tumors rarely cause subarachnoid hemorrhage.

9. Presence of a bruit. It is occasionally possible to detect the presence of a murmur over an arteriovenous malformation with careful auscultation.

The clinical features of spinal cord tumors at different levels include:

1. Upper cervical cord. There is usually involvement of the lower cranial nerves if the tumor extends up through the foramen magnum. A progressive spastic quadriparesis and a positive Lhermitte's sign may be seen. Nystagmus is not unusual due to involvement of the medial longitudinal fasciculus, which descends from the medulla into the upper cervical cord. Pressure on the vertebral arteries as they ascend over the ventral surface of the medulla may lead to intermittent symptoms of vertebrobasilar insufficiency. Patients may experience pain and stiffness of the neck with an abnormal posture of the head. Obstruction of the flow of the CSF at the level of the foramen magnum may lead to hydrocephalus and raised intracranial pressure with papilledema.

2. The lower cervical cord. Atrophy of the small muscles of the head may be caused by an anteriorly placed meningioma but has been reported in tumors at the level of the foramen magnum due to pressure on the anterior spinal artery with ischemia of the anterior horn cells in the lower cervical cord. Intramedullary and extramedullary tumors of the lower cervical area produce weakness and increased tone below the level of the tumor, often presenting with progressive spastic paraparesis, associated with increasing sphincter disturbances. Sensory examination may show the presence of abnormal sensation up to the level of the tumor on both sides of the body. Extramedullary tumors tend to produce a Brown-Sequard syndrome and unilateral Horner's syndrome due to involvement of the sympathetic outflow from the lower cervical and upper thoracic cord.

3. Thoracic cord lesions. Most thoracic tumors produce severe root pain, which radiates in a girdle fashion around the chest or upper abdomen. This is associated with progressive spastic paraparesis and bladder dysfunction. Examination may show a sensory

level, and Horner's syndrome may occur with lesions of the upper thoracic cord.

4. Lumbosacral tumors. Tumors in this area usually present with severe root pain followed by sphincter disturbances of the bladder and rectum. There is impotence in the male. Examination shows the presence of flaccid paralysis in the lower extremities with loss of stretch reflexes. There may be a sensory loss in the "saddle" area. Tumors in the lumbosacral area may mimic a herniated lumbar disk with the production of typical sciatic pain. This occurs with neurilemomas, meningiomas, and gliomas of the lower lumbosacral cord. Intramedullary lesions of the lumbar portion of the cord may produce flaccid paralysis on one side and evidence of spasticity with increased deep tendon reflexes and an extensor plantar response on the opposite side.

Diagnostic Procedures.

1. MR scanning is the method of choice in the diagnosis of tumors involving the spinal cord and spinal canal. The extraordinary detail obtained in sagittal axial or coronal sections of the spinal canal and spinal cord has replaced other procedures or relegated them to second choice (31) (see Figure 15–23).

2. X-rays of the cervical spine. The presence of a spinal cord tumor may lead to widening of the spinal canal and extramedullary

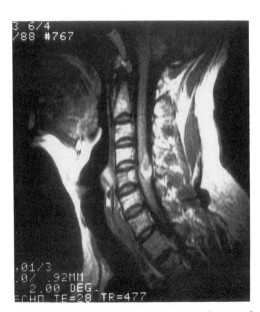

FIGURE 15–23. MR scan showing widening of the spinal cord at the fifth cervical segment with increased signal due to glioma.

tumors may produce erosion of the posterior aspect of the vertebral bodies. Neurilemomas may produce unilateral enlargement of the intervertebral foramina while neurilemomas, meningiomas, and metastatic tumors frequently produce erosion of the pedicles and laminae. Congenital tumors in children are frequently accompanied by abnormal curvature of the spine. Calcification is unusual but occasionally occurs in some spinal tumors. Malignant extradural tumors frequently produce bone destruction, and more benign tumors such as a meningioma may be associated with new bone formation.

3. Myelography. In most cases a myelogram will locate a spinal cord tumor and differentiate between an intramedullary and an extramedullary tumor. The combination of computed tomography and myelography using a water-soluble contrast material is particularly helpful in the diagnosis of spinal cord tumors.

4. Electromyography. Extramedullary tumors tend to be associated with unilateral denervation, which can be detected by electromyography. Bilateral denervation at the same level suggests the presence of an intramedullary tumor.

5. Angiography. Selective angiography of the spinal arteries is particularly useful in the diagnosis of arteriovenous malformations. Arteriography is not usually required for the diagnosis of other tumors.

6. Lumbar puncture. This procedure has become redundant in most cases because of MR scanning, but is utilized for the introduction of contrast material for myelography when the following observations can be made. Extramedullary and intramedullary tumors are likely to produce some change in pressure dynamics ranging from a slow rise in pressure following insertion of the needle to a failure to register any increase in pressure and a positive Queckenstedt test (see p. 252), indicating a block in the spinal subarachnoid space. In these cases the fluid is likely to be xanthochromic and the protein content markedly elevated. It is usual, however, to find some increase in the protein content of the spinal fluid even when there is no obstruction of the spinal subarachnoid space.

Differential Diagnosis. There are no clinical signs exclusively found with intramedullary tumors rather than extramedullary tumors. The presence of root pain and an ascending, segmental sensory loss occurs more often with extramedullary tumors than with intramedullary tumors. Fasciculations and descending, dissociated sensory loss are more characteristic of an intramedullary tumor.

The association of root pain with hypesthesia to pinprick and weakness of muscles supplied by the same nerve root is strongly suggestive of a neurilemoma. Meningiomas tend to produce bilateral root pain and paresthesias followed by unilateral then bilateral motor disturbances.

Treatment. Extramedullary tumors should be surgically removed. Intramedullary tumors producing cord compression are treated by surgical decompression followed by irradiation.

Prognosis. The prognosis of spinal cord tumors varies according to the histologic type and the degree of malignancy. If all spinal cord tumors are considered, approximately 66 percent of the patients survive five years following diagnosis and treatment. Most neurilemomas and meningiomas can be excised successfully with complete cure. Ependymomas have a 50 percent survival rate of more than five years' duration, while astrocytomas carry a poor prognosis. Congenital tumors in children, including dermoids, epidermoids, lipomas, and teratomas, have a good prognosis, although residual neurologic deficits including muscle wasting and weakness of the lower limbs and urinary incontinence persist.

REFERENCES

1. Ron, E. Tumors of the brain and nervous system after radiotherapy in childhood. N. Engl. J. Med. 319:1033–1039; 1988.
2. Goldring, S.; Rich, K. M.; *et al.* Experience with gliomas in patients presenting with a chronic seizure disorder. Clin. Neurosurg. 33:15–42; 1986.
3. Walker, M. O. CT scans, stereotactic equipment and localization of a tumor biopsy. J. Neuro. Oncol. 4:315–316; 1987.
4. Cohen, B. H.; Bury, E.; *et al.* Gadolinium-DTPA-enhanced magnetic resonance imaging in childhood brain tumors. Neurology 39:1178–1183; 1989.
5. Ammerati, M.; Vick, N.; *et al.* Effect of the extent of surgical resection on survival and quality of life in patients with supratentorial glioblastomas and anaplastic astrocytomas. Neurosurgery 21:201–206; 1987.
6. Fadul, C.; Wood, J.; *et al.* Morbidity and mortality of craniotomy for excision of supratentorial gliomas. Neurology 38:1374–1379; 1988.
7. Chemotherapy for malignant gliomas? Committee on health care issues. American Neurological Association. Ann. Neurol. 25:88–89; 1989.
8. Fulton, D. S.; Urtasum, R. C.; *et al.* Misonidazole and CCNU chemotherapy for recurrent primary brain tumor. J. Neuro. Oncol. 4:383–388; 1987.
9. Houang, M. T. W.; Coffey, G. L.; *et al.* Diagnosis of a posterior fossa tumor by magnetic resonance imaging. Med. J. Aust. 146:97–99; 1987.
10. Pasqualini, T.; Diez, B.; *et al.* Long-term endocrine sequelae after surgery, radiotherapy and chemotherapy in children with medulloblastoma. Cancer 59:801–806; 1987.
11. Graziano, S. L.; Paolozzi, F. P.; *et al.* Mixed germ-cell tumor of the pineal region. Case report. J. Neurosurg. 66:300–304; 1987.
12. Hudgins, R. J.; Rhyner, P. A.; *et al.* Magnetic resonance imaging and management of a pineal region dermoid. Surg. Neurol. 27:558–562; 1987.
13. Davis, P. C.; Hoffman, J. C., Jr.; *et al.* MR imaging of pituitary adenoma: CT, clinical and surgical correlation. AJR 148:797–802; 1987.
14. Mampalam, T. J.; Tyrrell, J. B.; *et al.* Transsphenoidal microsurgery for Cushing disease. A report of 216 cases. Ann. Intern. Med. 109:487–493; 1988.
15. Bartean, A. L.; Lloyd, R. V.; *et al.* Pre-operative treatment of acromegaly with long acting somatostation analo SMS 201-995: Shrinkage of invasive pituitary macroadenomas and improves surgical remission rate. J. Clin. Endocrinol. Metab. 67:1040–1048; 1988.
16. Barbaro, N. M.; Gutin, P. H.; *et al.* Radiation therapy in the treatment of partially resected meningiomas. Neurosurgery 20:525–528; 1987.
17. Gentry, L. R.; Jacoby, C. G.; *et al.* Cerebellopontine angle—petromastoid mass lesions: Comparative study of diagnosis with MR imaging and CT. Radiology 162:513–520; 1987.
18. Daniels, D. R.; Millen, S. J.; *et al.* MR detection of tumor in the internal auditory canal. AJR 148:1219–1222; 1987.
19. Sherwood, M. C.; Stanhope, R.; *et al.* Diabetes insipidus and occult intracranial tumors. Arch. Dis. Child. 61:1222–1224; 1986.
20. Wheatley, T.; Clark, J. D. A.; *et al.* Craniopharyngioma with hyperprolactinemia due to prolactinoma. J. Neurol. Neurosurg. Psychiatry 49:1305–1307; 1986.
21. Togretti, F.; Galassi, E.; *et al.* Haemangioblastomas of the brainstem. Neurochirurgia 29:230–234; 1986.
22. Handi, J.; Suzuki, F.; *et al.* Clivus chordoma in childhood. Surg. Neurol. 28:58–62; 1987.
23. Raffel, C.; Wright, D. C.; *et al.* Cranial chordomas: Clinical presentation and results of operative and radiation therapy in twenty-six patients. Neurosurgery 17:703–710; 1985.
24. Chuang, S.; Harwood-Nash, D. Tumors and cysts. Neuroradiology 28:463–475; 1986.
25. Gandy, S. E.; Heier, L. A. Clinical and magnetic resonance features of primary intracra-

nial arachnoid cysts. Ann. Neurol. 21:342–348; 1987.

26. Jacobi, C.; Reiber, H.; *et al.* The clinical relevance of locally produced carcinoembryogenic antigen in cerebrospinal fluid. J. Neurol. 233:358–361; 1986.

27. Van Zanten, A. P.; Twiznstra, A.; *et al.* Cerebrospinal fluid lactate dehydrogenase activities in patients with central nervous system metastases. Clinica. Chemica. Acta. 161:259–268; 1986.

28. Mori, K.; Kunsaka, M. Brain tumors in childhood: Statistical analyses of cases from benign tumor registry in Japan. Child's Nerv. Syst. 2:233–237; 1986.

29. Stroink, A. R.; Hoffman, H. J.; *et al.* Diagnosis and management of pediatric brainstem gliomas. J. Neurosurg. 65:745–750; 1986.

30. Jenkins, R. D.; Boesel, C.; *et al.* Brain-stem tumors in childhood: a prospective randomized trial of irradiation with and without adjuvant CCNU, VCR and Prednisone. A report of the Children's Cancer Study Group. J. Neurosurg. 66:227–223; 1987.

31. Talcemato, K.; Matsumaru, Y.; *et al.* MR imaging of intraspinal tumors. Capability in histological differentiation and compartmentalization of extramedullary tumors. Neuroradiology 30:303–309; 1988.

CHAPTER 16

INFECTIOUS DISEASE

Infectious diseases of the nervous system may result from a wide variety of agents. These include bacterial organisms, rickettsial organisms, fungi, protozoan organisms, viruses, and slow viruses. Early recognition of infection and identification of the source are necessary for effective management. The lumbar puncture and analysis of cerebrospinal fluid are the most objective means of identifying the etiologic agent.

Lumbar Puncture—Indications, Contraindications, Technique, and Complications

Indications. Lumbar puncture is indicated

1. To confirm a diagnosis
2. To identify the organism
3. To test for antibiotic sensitivity
4. To establish the need for treatment of children who are contacts in the case of meningococcal or hemophilus meningitis.

Contraindications. Lumbar puncture is contraindicated when there is suspicion of increased intracranial pressure due to an intracranial mass lesion, when there is serious cardiorespiratory disease, or when the area through which the spinal needle must pass is infected.

If available a magnetic resonance (MR) or computed tomography (CT) scan should always be obtained prior to lumbar puncture. Contraindications to lumbar puncture be-cause of increased risk of herniation include lateral shift of the midline structures, loss of suprachiasmatic and basilar cisterns, obliteration of the fourth ventricle or obliteration of the superior cerebellar and quadrigeminal cisterns with sparing of the ambient cisterns (1,2).

Treatment without lumbar puncture can be considered in cases where there is an unequivocal diagnosis of meningitis in a seriously ill individual with a positive blood culture who has impaired consciousness, raised intracranial pressure and signs of brain stem involvement by uncal herniation or central pressure.

Technique. The patient should be near the edge of the bed in the lateral decubitus position with neck, trunk, hips, and knees flexed (see Figure 16–1). The shoulders and hips must be perpendicular to the bed, and it may be necessary to place a small pillow beneath the head and/or trunk. The site of puncture is most commonly the L_4–L_5 interspace, which is located at the level of an imaginary line drawn between the highest points of the iliac crests.

The area should be cleansed with povidone-iodine solution and then wiped with alcohol. The puncture site should be located and the patient draped. It is necessary to change gloves to avoid contaminating the lumbar puncture needle with povidone-iodine. The lumbar puncture site is infiltrated with 1

251

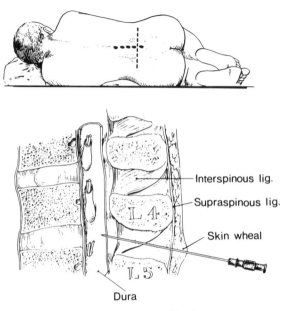

FIGURE 16–1.   Technique of lumbar puncture.

percent lidocaine hydrochloride for local anesthesia. The needle is then inserted at an angle of 10 to 20 degrees cephalad with the bevel of the needle parallel to the long axis of the spine. The needle should be advanced until a "pop" is felt indicating penetration of the meninges. When the needle has been advanced to the appropriate depth without the sensation of a "give" or "pop," the stylet should be removed every 2 to 3 mm as the needle is advanced to check for cerebrospinal fluid (CSF) return. If the needle fails to enter the subarachnoid space, it may be necessary to try again at a different interspace.

Once the needle is in place the manometer should be attached using a three-way stopcock and the patient's lower limbs extended before recording the opening pressure. Approximately 1 ml of CSF is collected into each of four tubes, and the closing pressure is measured. The manometer is then detached, the stylet replaced, and the needle removed. Blood should be drawn for glucose determination to allow comparison with the CSF glucose level. Table 16–1 lists the normal CSF indices. Table 16–2 compares CSF findings in various central nervous system disorders.

If there is suspicion of a spinal subarachnoid block, the Queckenstedt test may be performed after the opening pressure is recorded. To perform the test the jugular veins are compressed, usually manually, with enough force to occlude the veins but without interfering with carotid flow or respiration. Compression should be followed by a prompt rise in recorded pressure on the manometer followed by a fall to original pressure. If compression with enough force to occlude the jugular veins does not result in a rise in recorded pressure, the Queckenstedt test is termed positive, and it is presumed

TABLE 16–1.   **Normal CSF Indices**

Appearance: clear, colorless, does not clot in tube

Opening pressure: 70–200 mm H_2O

Cells: 0–5/mm^3 (mononuclear)

Na^+: 142–150 mEq/L; K^+: 2.2–3.3 mEq/L; CL: 120–130 mEq/L

CO_2: 25 mEq/L; pH: 7.35–7.40

Glucose: 45–80 mg%

Protein: 5–15 mg% (ventricular), 10–25 mg% (cisternal), 15–45 mg% (lumbar)

Gamma globulin: 5–12% of total protein

Transaminase (GOT): 7–49 U; LDH: 15–71 U; CPK: 0–3 IU

BUN: 5–25 mg%; bilirubin: 0

Amino acids: 30% of blood level

Lactic acid 0.8 to 2.8 mmol/L

TABLE 16–2. Cerebrospinal Fluid Findings in Various Central Nervous System Disorders

	Pressure	Appearance	Glucose	Protein	Cells
Viral encephalitis	Normal or mildly increased	Clear, colorless	Normal	Mildly increased	Increased lymphocytes
Aseptic meningitis	Normal	Usually clear, colorless	Normal	Mildly increased	Mildly increased lymphocytes
Acute pyogenic meningitis	Increased	Cloudy	Decreased	Increased	Increased polymorphonuclears
Tuberculous meningitis, syphilis	Increased	Usually clear, may be cloudy	Decreased	Increased	Increased lymphocytes
Fungal infections	Increased	Varies with organism	Varies with organism	Increased	Increased lymphocytes
Abscess	Increased	Clear, colorless	Normal	Increased	Increased polymorphonuclears
Cerebral infarction	Normal or mildly increased	Clear, colorless	Normal	Normal or mildly increased	Normal or very mild increase in polymorphonuclear cells <50 cu mm
Subarachnoid hemorrhage	Increased	Bloody, does not clot, supernatant— xanthochromic	Normal	Increased	Red cells maximal at onset decreasing and disappearing in about 5 days; mild to moderate polymorphonuclear and later lymphocytic pleocytosis occur as fluid clears
Traumatic LP	Normal	Bloody, clots spontaneously, supernatant— not xanthochromic	Normal	4 mg/dl increase per 5,000 RBC	Same as peripheral blood; fewer red cells last specimen than first specimen
Spinal cord tumor	Decreased	Cloudy, may be xanthochromic	Normal	Increased, may clot spontaneously (Froin syndrome)	May be mildly increased lymphocytes
Frequent seizures	Normal	Clear, colorless	Normal	Normal	<80/cu mm mostly polymorphonuclear

that a spinal subarachnoid block is present. This test should never be performed if there is increased intracranial pressure or suspicion of a mass lesion above the level of the foramen magnum.

Complications.

1. Headache. Postlumbar puncture headache is probably due to continued leakage of CSF through the needle tract. This causes a reduction in intracranial pressure and traction on the intracerebral dura. Headache can be avoided by maintaining the patient's hydration, using a small-gauge needle (20 gauge), and by removing the smallest volume of CSF necessary for chemical and bacteriologic studies.

2. Backache. Postlumbar puncture backache is usually the result of multiple unsuccessful attempts to place the needle in the subarachnoid space. The resultant muscle spasm produces pain. This may be avoided by improved technique.

3. Intracranial subdural hematoma. A subdural hematoma may result in patients with brain atrophy and tension on the perforating veins crossing the subdural space. A sudden decrease in pressure produces further traction and rupture of the veins. This complication should always be considered in elderly patients who become less responsive or develop hemiplegia following lumbar puncture.

4. Infection. Infection, including meningitis or subdural empyema, may result from a break in sterile technique during lumbar puncture.

5. Herniation. Uncal herniation is the most devasting complication of lumbar puncture and is due to a sudden change in intracranial pressure. A lumbar puncture should not be performed in the presence of an intracranial mass lesion with increased intracranial pressure.

6. Traumatic tap. A traumatic tap results from the laceration of vessels in the venous plexus of the spinal canal. Bleeding can be avoided by keeping the needle in the midline and not penetrating to the anterior wall of the spinal canal.

BACTERIAL INFECTIONS

Acute Pyogenic Meningitis

Definition. Acute pyogenic meningitis is an inflammatory response to bacterial infection involving the pia and arachnoid membranes covering the brain and spinal cord. Many microorganisms can produce pyogenic meningitis, which is classified according to the specific etiologic agent.

Etiology and Pathology. The three most common organisms causing acute pyogenic meningitis are *Diplococcus pneumoniae, Neisseria meningitidis,* and *Haemophilus influenzae.* (See Table 16–3) for distinguishing characteristics of the etiologic agents.) There is a considerable change in the incidence of bacterial types, with age (see Table 16–4).

Bacteria may reach the subarachnoid space via the blood stream; by extension from an adjacent area such as the ear, sinuses, or scalp; via direct implantation following trauma; or, rarely, following neurosurgical procedures or lumbar puncture. Once the organisms have crossed the blood-brain barrier they flourish in the CSF. There is a typical inflammatory response with an outpouring of polymorphonuclear cells into the cerebrospinal fluid, which becomes cloudy or milky in appearance. The inflammatory reaction is particularly intense in the basal cisterns and over the convexities of the brain. The pia and arachnoid become congested and opaque and the exudate rapidly becomes fibrinopurulent. The inflammation extends into layers 1 and 2 of the cortex and involves cortical veins producing cortical thrombophlebitis with thrombosis and infarction. The acute inflammatory response may be followed by thickening and fibrosis, and adhesions occur between the meninges and the brain, impairing the circulation of CSF and forming a scar around the cranial nerves at the base of the brain.

Clinical Features. The incidence of acute pyogenic meningitis is approximately 5 per 100,000. The condition occurs equally in both sexes, and the majority of cases occur in the winter months. Children aged six months to one year are at greatest risk, and children under 15 years of age comprise 75 percent of all cases. There are many predisposing factors, including infection of the lungs, middle ear, sinuses, skull bones, throat, nasopharynx, or mastoids; a history of recent head trauma, neurosurgery, or spinal anesthesia; contact with a patient who has a meningococcal infection; and debilitating conditions such as sickle cell anemia, alcoholism, leukemia, AIDS, or chronic immunosuppressive therapy.

The cardinal signs of meningitis include a stiff and painful neck, positive Kernig and Brudzinski signs, high fever, and a clouded sensorium. A positive Kernig's sign is indicated by the presence of pain in the lumbar area and the posterior aspects of the thigh on attempting to extend the patient's leg when the hip is flexed. Brudzinski's sign is positive if flexion of the patient's neck produces flexion of both legs and thighs. Other signs include stupor and coma, cranial nerve palsies, opisthotonus, and convulsions (especially in children less than 18 months of age). Papilledema is rare in meningitis and suggests the presence of brain abscess, subdural empyema, or venous sinus thrombosis (3).

Course. The disease may run a fulminant course in which the patient's condition reaches maximal severity within 24 hours. In other cases there is an insidious progression of symptoms over several days to weeks. In general, cases with rapid progression of symptoms carry a poorer prognosis. Once proper treatment is begun, the fever should diminish and the CSF should contain a preponderance of mononuclear cells within 72 hours. The most common residual deficit following acute pyogenic meningitis is deafness.

Complications. The most common causes of fever after seven days of proper antibiotic therapy are listed in Table 16–5.

1. Inappropriate secretion of antidiuretic hormone (SIADH). The syndrome of inappropriate secretion of ADH is a common complication of bacterial meningitis and occurs in approximately 80 percent of cases. It is characterized by a serum sodium concentration less that 130 mEq/L, elevated urine sodium, elevated urine osmolarity, and a normal or low blood urea nitrogen. It is managed by fluid restriction.

2. Subdural effusion. Subdural effusion occurs in as many as 32 percent of infants and children with bacterial meningitis. It should be suspected if there is recurrent vomiting, fever, failure to improve, bulging of the fontanelle, increasing head circumference, or convulsions. The diagnosis is made by transillumination of the skull, computed tomography, and tapping of the effusion. If the protein content of the fluid is less than 100 mg percent, it is not a subdural effusion. Repeated taps are not usually necessary.

3. Abscess. Failure to improve associated with progressive signs of focal neurologic deficit or evidence of increased intracranial pressure suggests the presence of a brain abscess (see p. 259).

4. Disseminated intravascular coagulation (DIC). Disseminated intravascular coagulation is most commonly associated with meningococcal and gram-negative meningitis and is characterized by petechiae, purpura, and hypotension. The diagnosis is established if fibrinogen levels are low, the prothrombin time is prolonged, and the platelet count is reduced. The condition is treated with heparin.

5. Hydrocephalus. Adhesions between the meninges and brain may block the circulation of CSF and result in hydrocephalus or a subarachnoid cyst. This should be considered if the CSF glucose remains depressed and the head continues to enlarge in infants and young children. Hydrocephalus may resolve as the infection is controlled. Refractory cases require placement of a ventricular shunt.

6. Subdural empyema. The spread of the inflammatory process and infection to the subdural space can result in the development of a subdural empyema. This is a rare complication and can be diagnosed by MR or CT scanning.

7. Ventriculitis. Ventriculitis should be considered in the pediatric patient who does not promptly respond to appropriate antibiotic therapy. It occurs most often in the neonatal age group with gram-negative meningitis, and the diagnosis is made by tapping the ventricles. Treatment requires intraventricular administration of antibiotics.

Differential Diagnosis. There are usually three considerations in the differential diagnosis of meningitis. These are bacterial, viral, and tuberculous or fungal infections. Table 16–6 illustrates the distinguishing characteristics of these conditions. There is always a possibility that bacterial meningitis not due to *H. influenzae, N. meningitidis,* or *D. pneumoniae* may be secondary to a ruptured brain abscess.

Diagnostic Procedures.

1. Lumbar puncture. Lumbar puncture is the only absolute means of substantiating a diagnosis of meningitis. In acute pyogenic meningitis the opening pressure is elevated, usually greater than 180 mm of water, with a mean of 300 mm of water. The CSF is cloudy and organisms are present on a direct smear in 40 percent of cases. There is a marked pleocytosis with a preponderance of polymorphonuclear cells in the early stages followed by a gradual increase of mononuclear cells. The CSF glucose is usually less than 40 mg percent and less than 50 percent of the level in a blood sample taken at the time of lumbar puncture. The CSF protein is elevated and varies from 100 to 2,000 mg percent. The CSF should be sent for culture.

2. Blood culture. Blood cultures are positive in more than 50 percent of cases.

3. Counterimmunoelectrophoresis (CIE). CIE is useful in determining the bacterial species and serotype of encapsulated bacteria.

4. X-rays. Chest, skull, mastoid, and paranasal x-rays should be taken to rule out fracture, sinusitis, or mastoiditis which may be a focus of infection.

5. CSF enzymes. Elevated CSF lactic acid dehydrogenase isoenzymes 4 and 5, and elevated glutamic-oxaloacetic transaminase have been reported in bacterial meningitis. C reactive protein is present in the CSF in acute bacterial and tuberculous meningitis but is reported to be absent in viral (aseptic) meningitis.

6. MR or CT scanning may reveal evidence of a subdural empyema, brain abscess, or infarction. MR scanning may show areas of high signal intensity on T2 weighted images of the brain stem when that structure is involved.

TABLE 16–3. Distinguishing Characteristics of Etiologic Agents Producing Acute Pyogenic Meningitis

Etiologic Agent	Microbiologic Characteristics	Distinguishing Epidemiologic Characteristics	Distinguishing Clinical Features	Mortality	Complications	Therapeutic Drug of Choice	Alternative Therapy
Diplococcus pneumoniae (Pneumococcus)	Gram positive, lancet-shaped diplococcus, encapsulated	Adult, head trauma, sickle cell disease, anemic or alcoholic	Cough, positive blood culture (56%)	20–60% depends on population	May be recurrent, subdural effusions, endocarditis,	Penicillin G	Cephatoxime
Neisseria meningitidis serotypes A, B, C, D, Y (5)	Gram negative, kidney-shaped diplococcus, intracellular, encapsulated	Youth (6 yr–20 yr), epidemics, occurs in early spring or winter	Sore throat, petechiae, and purpura	6–7%	Disseminated intravascular coagulation, endocarditis, adrenal hemorrhage (rare)	Penicillin G	Chloramphenicol
Haemophilus influenzae serotype B (5, 6)	Gram negative, pleomorphic rod, encapsulated	Child (2 mo–6 yr), occurs in late fall or winter	Earache, positive blood culture (79%)	7–8%	Subdural effusions, hydrocephalus	Cephatoxime	Ampicillin + Chloramphenicol
Streptococcus group B	Gram positive, cocci in chains	Neonates, premature rupture of membranes		1–2-day-old: 80%; 7–14-day-old: 40–50%	Endocarditis	Penicillin G	Chloramphenicol

Organism	Gram stain	Patient population	Clinical features		Associated condition	Treatment	
Escherichia coli	Gram negative rod	Neonates, head trauma or neurosurgery	Urinary tract infection 40%	50%	Endocarditis	Cephatoxime	
Klebsiella pneumoniae	Gram negative, encapsulated rod	Immunosuppressed or alcoholic patients				Cephatoxime	Vancomycin + gentamicin
Pseudomonas aeruginosa	Gram negative rod, motile	Head trauma, immunosuppressed, neurosurgery	Greenish CSF			Cephazidime	nafcillin + gentamicin
Staphylococcus species	Gram positive, cocci in clusters	Neonates, elderly; head trauma or neurosurgery				nafcillin	Vancomycin + gentamicin
Listeria monocytogenes	Gram positive rod, often mistaken for diphtheroids	Renal transplant patient or neonate	Absence of nuchal rigidity			Ampicillin + cephatoxime	Ampicillin + gentamicin
Neisseria gonorrhoeae	Gram negative, kidney-shaped diplococcus, intracellular	Pregnant	Gonorrhea joint involvement		Endocarditis	Penicillin G	Chloramphenicol
Clostridium perfringens (7)	Gram positive rods	Recent head trauma or neurosurgery		33%		Penicillin G	Cefatoxime or Vancomycin

257

TABLE 16–4. Age Relationship to Etiology of
Acute Pyogenic Meningitis

Age	Microorganism
Neonate (0–2 mo.)	Streptococcus, group B E. coli—coliforms Staph. aureus Enterobacter Pseudomonas
Child	Haemophilus influenzae N. meningitidis D. pneumoniae
Youth (6–20 yr)	N. meningitidis D. pneumoniae H. influenzae
Adult (>20 yr)	D. pneumoniae N. meningitidis Streptococcus Staphylococcus

TABLE 16–5. Causes of Fever After 7 Days of
Proper Antibiotic Therapy

1. Phlebitis due to intravenous (IV) administration of antibiotics
2. Intercurrent, hospital-acquired infection or persistence of particular foci of infection (e.g., otitis media)
3. Developing cerebral abscess
4. Drug fever
5. Subdural effusion
6. Subdural empyema
7. Ventriculitis

should receive dexamethasone (Decadron) and mannitol (see p. 54).

5. Seizures can be controlled with intravenous diazepam (Valium) 5 to 10 mg and intravenous phenytoin (Dilantin) (see p. 79). Seizures usually resolve as the infection is controlled, and a protracted course of anticonvulsants is unnecessary.

Prognosis. More than 90 percent of patients with bacterial meningitis died in the preantibiotic era. Currently, 10 to 20 percent of patients succumb to the infection or its complications. The majority are in the neonatal age group. There is a poorer prognosis for those who are very young or very old, when there is delayed or inadequate therapy, or if the patient has an associated systemic illness. Absence of marked leukocytosis (less than 15,000 polymorphonuclear leukocytes/cu mm), marked hyperpyrexia (greater than 40° C rectally), hypotension (blood pressure less than 100 mmHg systolic—adult, less than 70 mmHg systolic—child), seizures, coma, and thrombocytopenia are also associated with a poorer outcome. During outbreaks of meningococcal meningitis, carriers detected by positive swabs should be treated with rifampicin 10 mg/kg b.i.d. for 48 hours. (4).

Treatment.
1. Patients with acute meningitis require complete bed rest with noise and other extraneous stimuli kept to a minimum. Known or suspected meningococcal disease requires isolation until the patient has received several days of appropriate antibiotic therapy.
2. Fluid balance and electrolytes must be carefully monitored because of the possibility of inappropriate secretion of antidiuretic hormone and shock. A central venous pressure line aids in maintaining adequate hydration.
3. Antibiotic therapy as outlined in Tables 16–3, 16–7 and 16–8 should be administered. A minimum of two weeks of therapy is recommended. The CSF should be reexamined if there is any doubt regarding clinical improvement. The CSF should always be evaluated when antibiotics are discontinued.
4. Cerebral edema. If there is papilledema or evidence of herniation, the patient

TABLE 16–6. Differential Diagnosis of Meningitis

Type of Meningitis	Cells	Glucose	Protein	Smear	CSF Lactic Acid
Bacterial	Thousands of polymorphonuclear leukocytes	<$\frac{1}{2}$ blood glucose	>45 mg%	Organisms	>35 mg/dl
Viral	Hundreds of mononuclear cells	Normal	Mild increase	No organisms	<35 mg/dl
Tuberculous, fungal	Hundreds of mononuclear cells	Moderate or marked decrease	Marked increase	+, −	>35 mg/dl

TABLE 16–7. Suggested Dosages of Antibiotics in Treatment of Meningitis

Antibiotic	Infant	Child	Adult
Penicillin G	200,000 units/kg/ day in 6 doses q4h IV	250,000 units/kg/ day in 6 doses q4h IV	20 million U/day in 6 doses q4h IV
Ampicillin	200 mg/kg/day in 3 doses q8h IV	300–400 mg/kg per day in 4 doses q6h IV	18 g/day in 6 doses q4h IV
Nafcillin	200 mg/kg/day in 3 doses q8h IV	100 mg/kg/day in 4 doses q6h IV	18 g/day in 6 doses q4h IV
Chloramphenicol	50 mg/kg/day in 2 doses q12h IV	100 mg/kg/day in 4 doses q6h IV	4 g/day in 4 doses q6h IV
Cephatoxime	100 mg/kg/day in 2 doses q12h IV	200 mg/kg/day in 3 doses q8h IV	12 g/day in 6 doses q4h IV
Cephazidime	60 mg/kg/day in 2 doses q12h IV	150 mg/kg/day in 3 doses q8h IV	6 g/day in 3 doses q8h IV
Vancomycin	30 mg/kg/day in 2 doses q12h IV	50 mg/kg/day in 4 doses q6h IV	2 g/day in 4 doses q6h IV
Gentamicin	7.5 mg/kg/day in 3 doses q8h IM	5 mg/kg/day in 3 doses q8h IV	5 mg/kg/day in 3 doses q8h IV

TABLE 16–8. Initial Antibiotic Therapy Before Results of Culture Are Available

Type of Patient	Drug of Choice
Neonatal	Ampicillin and gentamicin ± intrathecal (IT), intramuscular (IM)
Children	Ampicillin and chloramphenicol
Adult	Ampicillin or penicillin G
Postneurosurgical	Cephazidime
Immunosuppressed or *Pseudomonas* suspect	Ampicillin and gentamicin ± (IT)

Brain Abscess

Definition. A brain abscess is a circumscribed collection of pyogenic material located within the brain parenchyma.

Etiology and Pathology. Brain abscesses are due to pyogenic bacteria, which gain access to the central nervous system by hematogenous spread from a distant septic focus, by direct extension from an adjacent infected area, such as frontal sinusitis induced by snorting cocaine (8), following trauma or neurosurgery, or as a rare complication of pyogenic meningitis. Most cases of brain abscess are the result of direct extension of infection from otitis media or sinusitis. Table 16–9 lists the most common etiologic factors, their distinguishing characteristics, and the type of organism usually encountered.

A brain abscess begins as an area of focal cerebritis. Once fully developed, a brain abscess resembles an abscess found anywhere else in the body with a central cavity containing debris and polymorphonuclear cells surrounded by a capsule of granulation tissue and a compact fibrotic, gliotic outer layer. There is usually marked cerebral edema in the surrounding tissues. Abscesses that arise by hematogenous spread usually develop at the junction of gray and white matter and extend into the white matter.

Clinical Features. Brain abscesses occur in all age groups. The overall incidence is approximately 1/100,000, and brain abscess is twice as likely to occur in males as in females. The frontal, parietal, and temporal lobes are most frequently involved and, 9 percent of cases have multiple abscesses.

The patient with a brain abscess usually presents with fever, chills, headache, and progressive focal neurologic signs. However, evidence of infection may be absent, and the patient may present with symptoms suggesting brain tumor, including increased intracranial pressure, nausea and vomiting, papilledema, bradycardia, and focal signs such as hemiparesis or homonymous hemianopia (see

TABLE 16–9. Epidemiologic Characteristics in Brain Abscess

Common Etiologic Factors in Descending Frequency	Distinguishing Characteristics	Microorganisms Typically Involved	
		Aerobes	Anaerobes
Middle ear, paranasal sinus, or mastoid infection	Ear infection: temporal lobe abscess. Sinus infection: frontal lobe abscess. Mastoid infection: cerebellar abscess	Aerobic Streptococci *Staph. aureus*	Anaerobic streptococci *Bacterioides*
Metastatic emboli from lung, pulmonary abscess, bronchiectasis, or chronic empyema	Multiple abscesses	*Staph. aureus* *Klebsiella* *D. pneumoniae*	Anaerobic streptococci Fusobacteria
Head trauma or neurosurgery	Gunshot wounds are most common head trauma associated with abscess	*Staph. aureus* *Pseudomonas*	Anaerobic streptococci
Endocarditis	Drug abuser	*Staph. aureus*	————
Rare Causes: Dental procedures Metastatic emboli from abdominal infections or pelvic inflammatory disease Osteomyelitis of skull	————	————	————

p. 228). A history of predisposing factors should lead to consideration of brain abscess in such cases.

The neurologic examination may reveal papilledema and focal neurologic signs, depending on the localization of the abscess. Patients with multiple cerebral abscesses have a more rapid increase in intracranial pressure with headache, drowsiness progressing to stupor, and increasing signs of neurologic dysfunction.

Course. The patient with a brain abscess may follow one of several courses. The abscess may behave like a low-grade astrocytoma or meningioma with a slow progression of symptoms. Others present with a more rapid course and deteriorate over a relatively short period of time. An untreated abscess will continue to extend with increasing edema, leading to herniation and secondary brain stem compression and death. Rupture of a cerebral abscess into the subarachnoid space or ventricles is a rare occurrence.

Complications. The complications of brain abscess include herniation, seizures, and rupture of the abscess into the subarachnoid space or into a ventricle. Herniation can be recognized by progressive brain stem compression (see p. 50). This condition re-

quires emergency treatment with mannitol and dexamethasone (Decadron), and immediate surgery. Rupture of the abscess is followed by development of acute pyogenic meningitis due to contamination of the subarachnoid space. Rupture of an abscess into a ventricle is rapidly fatal.

Differential Diagnosis.

1. Intracranial tumor. A brain abscess may resemble a tumor in that both show progression and focal neurologic signs. However, a history of infection and the appearance on computed tomography will usually differentiate the two conditions.

2. Meningitis. An early brain infection producing focal cerebritis may resemble meningitis with fever, headache, and meningismus, but a fully developed abscess usually presents as a mass lesion with focal signs and papilledema.

3. Chronic subdural hematoma. The history of trauma, lack of infection, and the appearance on MR or CT scans establish the diagnosis of subdural hematoma.

4. Subdural empyema. A subdural empyema may closely resemble a cerebral abscess. MR or CT scanning will distinguish the two conditions.

5. Cerebral infarction. Infarction is more

sudden in onset, and the triangular, wedge-shaped appearance on computed tomography differs from the typical "ring" appearance of an abscess.

6. Tuberculoma. The history of tuberculosis and the appearance on computed tomography help to differentiate abscess and tuberculoma.

Diagnostic Procedures.

1. There is evidence of infection with an elevated white blood cell count and an elevated sedimentation rate.

2. A lumbar puncture should not be performed in suspected cases of cerebral abscess. The procedure rarely adds any significant information and has been associated with herniation in a significant number of cases. Patients with suspected meningitis and focal neurologic signs should have an MR or CT scan.

3. The MR scan shows an area of increased signal density in the T2 weighted image which is homogeneous and represents the area of both abscess and surrounding edema. There is improved definition in a gad-olinium enhanced MR scan (see Figure 16–2A and B).

4. The CT scan is the procedure of choice in the diagnosis of brain abscess (9). An abscess has a central area of low density surrounded by a ring of increased density, which shows marked enhancement following injection of intravenous contrast material. The CT scan is the superior procedure in the delineation of multiloculated, interconnecting and multiple abscesses.

5. Bacterial culture. Bacterial culture should be obtained from any site which may have served as a focus of infection, although antibiotic coverage should not be based entirely on the results of these cultures.

6. Skull x-rays. Skull x-rays should be obtained since they may reveal changes indicating chronic increased intracranial pressure, pineal displacement, gas in the abscess cavity, or abnormalities compatible with infection of the mastoid air cells or paranasal sinuses.

Treatment. A brain abscess should be treated with antibiotic therapy and surgical excision or drainage. The patient should be

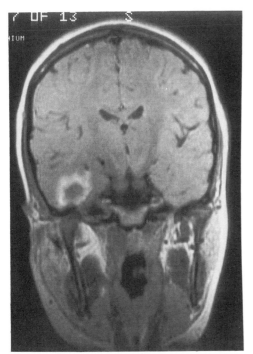

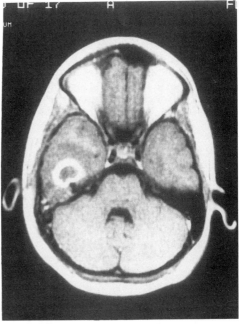

A   B

FIGURE 16–2.   (A) and (B) Temporal lobe abscess. Gadolinium enhanced MR scan showing a temporal lobe abscess secondary to pseudomonas infection in an individual with a chronic ear infection.

TABLE 16–10. Choice of Antibiotics Based on Suspected Etiology

Suspected Etiology	First Choice	Second Choice
Sinus infection	Penicillin G + Metronidazole	Chloramphenicol
Ear infection	Penicillin G + Metronidazole + Cefatoxime	Penicillin G + Chloramphenicol
Trauma	Ceftazidime + nafcillin + Gentamicin	Vancomycin + Gentamicin

placed on the appropriate antibiotic (see Table 16–10) to reduce infection, and dexamethasone (Decadron) to reduce edema. Some abscesses will resolve totally without surgical treatment but others require total excision when the abscess is sterile and has a well formed capsule. However, when the patient is debilitated or when the abscess has a thin capsule, treatment by repeated aspiration or fractional drainage is preferable. Antibiotics should be continued for at least two to three weeks after surgery. Focal epilepsy can be controlled with adequate anticonvulsant therapy (see pp. 76–77).

Prognosis. The mortality of brain abscess has remained at approximately 40 percent since World War II. The mortality is increased in multiple abscesses and in those located in the brain stem or occipital lobes. Coma, deeply located abscesses, ruptured abscesses, and the presence of anaerobic streptococci are also poor prognostic factors.

Cranial Subdural Empyema
Definition. A collection of purulent material in the subdural space.
Etiology and Pathology. Spread of infection from the paranasal sinuses or the mastoid air cells is the commonest etiological factor (10).
Clinical Features. There is a history of otitis media or infection involving the paranasal sinuses followed by focal neurologic signs such as focal seizures, hemiparesis, dysphasia and visual field defects. Empyema of the falx may cause bilateral lower limb weakness. Signs of increased intracranial pressure, including headache, vomiting, and papilledema, may be followed by rapid deterioration, signs of progressive brain stem dysfunction and death.

Diagnostic Procedures.
1. X-rays of the skull will demonstrate infection of the mastoid or paranasal sinuses.
2. Magnetic resonance or CT scanning will demonstrate an elliptical area of abnormality adjacent to the inner table of the skull. There is better detection of subdural empyema by MRI as compared with CT (11).

Treatment. Pus should be aspirated through bur holes and appropriate and aggressive chemotherapy instituted. (12).

Cranial Epidural Abscess
Definition. A collection of purulent material in the cranial epidural space.
Etiology and Pathology. As for cranial subdural empyema.
Clinical Features. Cranial epidural abscess has many of the features of cranial subdural empyema. Fever and headache are common but focal neurologic signs are infrequent because of the limited space available due to the close apposition of the dura to the inner table of the cranium.
Treatment. See cranial epidural empyema, above.

Spinal Epidural Abscess
Definition. A spinal epidural abscess is a collection of purulent material in the spinal epidural space.
Etiology and Pathology. Most cases of spinal epidural abscess occur in patients with diabetes mellitus. There may be a history of associated infection elsewhere such as furunculosis, a dental abscess, or a decubitus ulcer. Minor back trauma or intravenous drug abuse are also predisposing factors.
The infection begins as an osteomyelitis involving the vertebral body, lamina, or pedicle and spreads into the spinal epidural space. The inflammation and subsequent pus formation spread posteriorly over several segments.
Clinical Features. The patient with a spinal epidural abscess presents with severe pain in the spine. There is marked limitation of movement and spasm of the erector spinae muscles with tenderness to palpation over the affected area. The back pain is followed by the development of root pain on the side of the abscess and progressive cord compression with rapid onset of paraparesis progressing to paraplegia. Bladder function is paralyzed, there is a sensory loss below the level of the lesion, stretch reflexes are increased in the

lower limbs, and there is a bilateral extensor plantar response.

Differential Diagnosis.

1. Acute transverse myelitis. This condition may be easily confused but is usually associated with less pain.

2. Postinfectious polyneuritis (Guillain-Barré syndrome). This presents as an ascending flaccid paralysis with an ill-defined sensory loss.

3. Poliomyelitis. In this case the paralysis is usually asymmetric and flaccid, and there is no sensory involvement.

4. Cord compression from other causes, including tumor, hematoma, and disk herniation.

Diagnostic Procedures.

1. Spinal x-rays. X-rays of the spine may reveal osteomyelitis of the vertebrae.

2. An MR scan of the spine or a myelogram followed by computed tomography of the area reveals complete obstruction of the spinal subarachnoid space (13).

3. Lumbar puncture. If lumbar puncture is performed, the needle may enter the abscess with aspiration of pus. If the needle enters the subarachnoid space, the CSF is often xanthochromic with a polymorphonuclear pleocytosis and elevated protein content. The opening pressure is often low, and the Queckenstedt test indicates the presence of a spinal block.

Treatment

1. The abscess should be drained or excised as soon as possible to relieve cord compression.

2. An appropriate antibiotic should be administered. Penicillin G (30 million units) or methicillin (1 g q3h IM) may be given until the culture and sensitivity studies are available.

Prognosis. Paraparesis secondary to cord compression is a surgical emergency, and the compression must be relieved before paraplegia occurs. There is little chance of recovery of function once the patient is paraplegic (14).

Chronic Spinal Epidural Abscess

Chronic spinal epidural abscesses are usually secondary to tuberculous osteomyelitis of the vertebral body. A "cold" abscess develops and spreads to involve the spinal epidural space. Other causes of infection of the spinal epidural space include syphilis, which can produce granulomatous inflammation and thickening of the meninges (pachymeningitis

cervicalis hypertrophica), coccidioidomycosis, brucellosis, and cryptococcosis. A tuberculous abscess usually occurs in the upper or midthoracic region. The abscesses may extend around the thoracic or abdominal wall, external to the pleura or peritoneum, and present anteriorly, as a fluctuating mass, or extend through the psoas sheath and present in the inguinal area as a psoas abscess. Cord damage may be due to direct pressure from the cold abscess, pressure on spinal arteries producing cord ischemia, arteritis of the spinal arteries passing through the area of the abscess, or angulation of the spinal canal due to collapse of diseased vertebral bodies.

The condition usually presents with root pains radiating in segmental fashion around the chest or abdomen. This is followed by slowly progressive spastic paraparesis, hyperreflexia and bilateral extensor plantar responses, urgency of micturition followed by incontinence, and development of a sensory level. Spinal deformity is a late complication. The diagnostic procedures are discussed under spinal epidural abscess. Tuberculous infections require prolonged treatment with antituberculous drugs (see p. 273). Cases with syphilitic pachymeningitis may respond to penicillin. The compression must be relieved before paraplegia occurs.

Spinal Subdural Abscess

A spinal subdural abscess is a rare condition in which abscess formation occurs in the spinal subdural space. The etiology and pathology, clinical features, diagnostic procedures, and treatment have been described under spinal epidural abscess.

Acute Intramedullary Abscess of the Spinal Cord

Definition. An acute abscess of the spinal cord is a rare condition in which abscess formation occurs within the spinal cord substance.

Etiology and Pathology. Abscess formation usually follows septicemia in patients who are debilitated or have a chronic disease such as diabetes mellitus or alcoholism. An intramedullary abscess is occasionally associated with an epidural or subdural abscess. The infection is occasionally introduced by a stab wound.

The spinal cord is swollen and the abscess is surrounded by considerable edema.

Clinical Features. The patient is often severely debilitated and septic with signs of progressive spinal cord compression.

Diagnostic Procedures.

1. There is evidence of severe systemic infection.
2. The intramedullary abscess can be demonstrated by MR scanning or myelography followed by computed tomography of the area. This demonstrates a complete or partial block of the subarachnoid space and swelling of the spinal cord.

Treatment

1. The patient should be treated with high doses of broad-spectrum antibiotics pending results of cultures and sensitivities.
2. The cord compression should be relieved as rapidly as possible.

Chronic Spinal Subdural and Intramedullary Abscess

Most chronic subdural and intramedullary abscesses are due to tuberculous infection. Syphilis, schistosomiasis, fungi, and yeast infections may occasionally give rise to chronic abscesses. Rarely, a chronic abscess may complicate acute pyogenic meningitis.

The clinical course suggests the presence of a slowly expanding lesion of the spinal cord with progressive paraparesis and impairment of bladder function. The diagnosis is established by myelography combined with computed tomography. The condition should be treated by appropriate antibiotic therapy and surgical relief of cord compression if this is indicated by progression of the paraparesis.

Tetanus

Definition. Tetanus is an acute toxemia caused by the elaboration of neurotoxin from the infectious bacillus *Clostridium tetani.* The disorder is characterized by periodic, severe muscle spasms.

Etiology and Pathology. Clostridium tetani is a gram-positive, spore-forming bacillus. The most important factor in pathogenesis of tetanus is the necessity of an anaerobic environment, since the organism is an obligate anaerobe. Under suitable conditions spores germinate and the organism elaborates an extremely toxic neurotoxin, tetanospasmin. All of the characteristic clinical symptoms are due to this toxin. It binds to peripheral nerve terminals and is believed to gain access to the central nervous system, either by retrograde transport up the peripheral nerve axons or via the blood or lymph circulation. The toxin selectively disturbs motor neuron function by blocking synaptic inhibition of motor neurons and by damaging cell bodies.

Clinical Features. The occurrence of tetanus is sporadic and worldwide because of the ubiquitous nature of the organism. The condition favoring development of tetanus is a deep puncture wound with introduction of infected soil. However, tetanus has been reported after trivial scratches, insect bites, and vaccinations. In some cases there is no evidence of any kind of wound.

The incubation period is usually 4 to 10 days after infection, but symptoms have been recorded hours to weeks after injury. Initially the patient may complain of chills, fever, and pain and swelling of the wound site. In a few rare cases, the disease may remain in a localized form with pain and rigidity restricted to muscles close to the wound. More commonly the generalized form occurs following dissemination of toxin throughout the central nervous system. Tetanospasmin has a specific affinity for motor neurons supplying the face and jaw, and this results in the early signs of lockjaw (trismus) and risus sardonicus (sardonic smile). Eventually more and more muscle groups become involved, and spasmodic contortion of the body is determined by the contraction of the strongest muscles affected. The spasms are usually of brief duration but are intensely painful and tend to increase in frequency. They may be precipitated by a sudden noise or by touching the patient or may occur spontaneously. The disease may continue for several weeks.

Complications.

1. The spasms may be of sufficient strength and duration to fracture bones.
2. Asphyxia may occur if the diaphragm, intercostal muscles, and/or glottis are involved.

Diagnostic Procedures. The diagnosis of tetanus is based on the clinical picture, since a positive culture of *C. tetani* can be obtained in the absence of the disease and tetanus may occur without evidence of a recent wound.

Treatment.

1. Human tetanus immune globulin should be administered in a dosage of 100 U/kg IM or IV to neutralize all unbound toxin.
2. Puncture wounds should be opened, cleansed, debrided, and dressed.
3. Procaine penicillin G should be administered, 1.2 million units q6h for 10 days IM

or IV. Tetracycline 2 g/qd is the alternative antibiotic of choice for those allergic to penicillin.

4. The patient should be adequately sedated and kept in a quiet, dark room. Care should be taken to keep all stimuli to a minimum. Good nursing care is essential.

5. In severe cases, neuromuscular blocking agents should be administered, a tracheostomy performed, and respirations maintained with a mechanical respirator.

6. Pronounced autonomic nervous system instability with release of large amounts of catecholamine can be controlled by heavy sedation and infusion of magnesium sulphate 2 to 3 g per hour (15).

7. All patients who recover should be immunized, 0.5 ml of tetanus toxoid each month for three doses beginning six to eight weeks after the last antitoxin dose, since the disease does not confer immunity.

8. All children should be immunized. Children six weeks to six years of age should be given one dose of diphtheria, pertussis, tetanus toxoid on four occasions. Persons older than seven years of age should receive three doses of diphtheria, tetanus toxoid with a booster dose every 10 years.

Prognosis. The prognosis is poor when the incubation period is short, the initial wound is near the head, there is a rapid evolution of the disease, or the spasms are frequent and severe. Death tends to occur early in tetanus; the longer the survival the better the prognosis. The mortality rate is still approximately 15 percent in the best medical centers.

Botulism

Definition. Botulism is an acute, potentially fatal toxemia that results from the ingestion of botulinum neurotoxin and is characterized by symmetric cranial neuropathies followed by a descending symmetric muscle weakness and paralysis.

Etiology and Pathology. *Clostridium botulinum* is a strictly anaerobic, gram-positive, spore-forming bacillus which is the source of the most potent toxin known. Botulinum toxin is released upon death and autolysis of organisms that have survived in improperly home-canned foods. Following ingestion the toxin is absorbed through the gastrointestinal tract and disseminated throughout the body. The toxin prevents acetylcholine release from presynaptic nerve terminals. Cholinergic function is unaffected in the central nervous system.

Clinical Features. There are eight known strains of *C. botulinum* (A–G), but only types A, B, E, and F affect man. Types A and B account for the majority of outbreaks, with type A occurring most commonly in the Pacific Coast states, the Rocky Mountains, and the Northeastern United States, and type B predominating in the Mississippi River Valley area, the Great Lakes area, and the Southeastern United States. Type E has been reported in the Great Lakes area, and type F is occasionally reported along the Pacific Coast. Home-canned green beans are the most commonly incriminated source of botulism poisoning.

There is usually a history of ingestion of home-canned foods, and it is rare that a traumatic wound is the source of contamination. Sinus infection with *C. botulinum* can occur in cases of acute sinusitis due to inhalation of contaminated cocaine (16). Early symptoms occur 12 hours to 10 days after ingestion and usually consist of diplopia, ptosis, blurred vision, and photophobia. More caudal cranial nerves may become involved resulting in dysphonia, dysphagia, and dysarthria. A descending flaccid, symmetric paralysis that threatens respiratory function may develop quite rapidly. Parasympathetic autonomic dysfunction may be manifested by constipation, dry mouth and eyes, and urinary retention. The patient remains alert, oriented, and afebrile, and sensation is intact.

Differential Diagnosis. Guillain-Barré syndrome, myasthenia gravis, brain stem infarction, familial periodic paralysis, diphtheria, tick paralysis, poliomyelitis, and psychiatric disorders may be confused with early or atypical cases of botulism. The history, the development of similar symptoms in others, a normal cerebrospinal fluid, and the progression of the disorder will differentiate botulism from other conditions. (17).

Diagnostic Procedures.

1. The patient's serum, feces, gastric washings, and suspect food are potential sources of toxin, which can be identified by mouse innoculation, culture, and immunofluorescence. The Centers for Disease Control in Atlanta, Georgia, should be notified [phone by day, (404)329-3311].

2. Electrodiagnostic studies should include rapid repetitive stimulation of nerves

which will elicit an incremental response in most cases and is a more sensitive test than nerve stimulation at low frequencies which may fail to elicit a decremental (myasthenic) response in some cases.

Treatment.

1. The patient should receive a skin test before administration of equine trivalent antitoxin, since 20 percent of patients are allergic to the preparation and may require desensitization before treatment. However, the antitoxin should be administered as soon as possible.
2. If ileus is not present, cathartics and enemas should be administered to remove excess toxin from the intestinal tract.
3. Respiratory care is critical. An adequate airway must be maintained by suctioning. Intubation, tracheostomy, and mechanical ventilation may be necessary.
4. Fluid and electrolyte balance and the nutritional state must be carefully monitored.
5. Guanidine 15 mg/kg/day in divided doses increasing to 50 mg/kg is reported to increase the amount of acetylcholine released at nerve terminals. The benefit of guanidine therapy is not established.

Prognosis. While many outbreaks of botulism are mild Type A, Type A botulism toxemia has a reported mortality of 50 to 70 percent, followed by type E (30 percent) and type B (20 percent). Recovery occurs slowly, and the patient may be left with residual ocular paralysis.

Cerebral Brucellosis

Brucella infection by the organisms *Brucella abortus, melitensis*, and *suis* may affect the nervous system. The infection is usually acquired by contact with infected farm animals or ingestion of infected milk. The patient presents with an acute febrile illness with severe headache, myalgia, and weakness. Meningomyelitis, mycotic aneurysms, peripheral neuritis, or spondylitis may develop. Meningoencephalitis can result in cranial nerve palsies, hemiplegia, paraplegia, and transient parkinsonism (18).

Untreated infections or those that relapse following therapy may progress to the chronic form of the disease, which may mimic multiple sclerosis (19). Serologic tests are the most reliable means of identifying the organism. The patient with acute brucelosis should be given tetracycline 2 g daily for 28 days

alone or in combination with streptomycin. Doxycycline (Vibramycin) is also effective. Chloramphenicol or trimethoprim/sulphamethoxadole may be substituted for tetracycline in children under eight years of age.

Psittacosis (Chlamydiosis)

Psittacosis is an infection by the organism *Chlamydia psittaci*, which may be acquired by contact with infected wild or domestic birds. Meningitis or encephalitis may occur. The infection responds to tetracycline.

Lyme Meningoencephalitis

Definition. Lyme disease is an epidemic multisystem disease caused by a spirochete *Borrelia burgdorferi* which is transmitted by the bite of *Ixodes dammini* ticks.

Clinical Features. The acute illness is characterized by fever, fatigue, arthralgias of large joints and a unique skin rash, erythema chronicum migrans. This is often followed by persistent fatigue, migratory joint pains and brief recurrent attacks of joint swelling in larger joints, particularly the knees. Myocarditis, pericarditis, and cardiac conduction defects have been reported. Neurologic manifestations consist of aseptic meningitis, meningoencephalitis with headache, and personality change. Cranial nerve abnormalities, particularly facial nerve paresis, brachial neuritis or painful polyradiculoneuropathies may occur. Peripheral neuropathy with prominent limb paresthesias is common in late lyme disease (20). Guillain-Barré-like syndrome has been described.

Diagnostic Procedures. Serological tests using an enzyme linked immunosorbent assay (ELISA) or direct immunofluorescence assay (IFA) are available but are subject to false-positive and false-negative reactions (21).

Treatment. The infection responds to IV Penicillin G 24 million units daily for 10 days or cephtrioxone 2 g b.i.d. for 14 days (22).

GRANULOMATOUS INFLAMMATIONS

Syphilis

Infection with *Treponema pallidum* may result in syphilitic meningitis, chronic basal meningitis, syphilitic arteritis, gumma formation, general paresis, syphilitic optic atrophy, congenital neurosyphilis, syphilis of the spinal cord, and tabes dorsalis.

Prevention of neurosyphilis depends upon adequate screening of persons at risk even though recommended treatment for persons with syphilis has been given. In addition to cerebrospinal fluid examination, tests for pupillary abnormalities, abnormal pursuit movements, and brain stem auditory evoked potentials may be useful (23).

Syphilitic Meningitis. A mild meningeal reaction has been described during the primary stage of syphilis when the *T. pallidum* organism is disseminated throughout the body. Acute syphilitic meningitis is an occasional feature of the secondary and tertiary stages of syphilis.

Pathology. The presence of the *T. pallidum* leads to an inflammatory response involving the meninges and the superficial areas of the brain and spinal cord. Marked lymphocytic infiltration of the meninges and perivascular cuffing of the blood vessels occur in the superficial areas of the central nervous system. These vessels are also the site of an endarteritis.

Clinical Features. The patient presents with typical signs of acute meningitis, including headache, fever, nuchal rigidity, nausea, vomiting, and cranial nerve palsies.

Diagnostic Procedures.

1. The spinal fluid is under increased pressure and is clear, cloudy, or occasionally xanthochromic. Examination shows a pleocytosis with the presence of 50 to 2,000 lymphocytes per cubic millimeter. The protein content is increased, and the glucose occasionally depressed.
2. There is a positive serologic test for syphilis in the blood and CSF.

Treatment. See page 271.

Chronic Basal Meningitis. Chronic basal meningitis is a chronic granulomatous change of the meninges at the base of the brain that occurs in tertiary syphilis.

Pathology. The meninges show thickening due to the presence of granulomatous inflammation, particularly around the base of the brain and brain stem. This inflammatory process involves the circle of Willis, the basilar artery, and the upper cranial nerves. There is an extension onto the floor of the fourth ventricle, and obstruction of the foramina of the fourth ventricle may lead to hydrocephalus. Microscopic examination shows the presence of diffuse fibrosis with infiltration of lymphocytes and plasma cells.

Clinical Features. The condition usually presents with progressive involvement of the cranial nerves beginning with paralysis of the third and sixth cranial nerves. Extension of

this process may lead to involvement of the optic nerves and optic atrophy (24).

Diagnostic Procedures.

1. There is a lymphocytic pleocytosis in the cerebrospinal fluid with elevated protein and a marked increase in gamma globulin.
2. Serologic tests for syphilis are positive in the blood and spinal fluid.

Treatment. See page 271. Hydrocephalus may persist despite adequate treatment and may require placement of a ventricular shunt.

Syphilitic Arteritis. Syphilitic arteritis is a panarteritis secondary to syphilitic infection involving the cerebral blood vessels.

Pathology. Blood vessels in the brain stem and spinal cord show the presence of chronic inflammation with lymphocytes and plasma cells in all layers of the vessel wall. The internal lamina is preserved but shows reduplication. Endothelial proliferation produces narrowing of the lumen of the vessels with an increasing tendency to thrombosis. The penetrating vessels of the brain show a marked perivascular inflammatory response, and there is involvement of the meninges at the base of the brain with granulomatous inflammatory change.

Clinical Features. Syphilitic arteritis usually produces symptoms of transient ischemia or cerebral infarction in younger individuals. The commonest syndrome is syphilitic hemiplegia due to infarction in the distribution of the middle cerebral artey. Brain stem infarction is probably second in frequency; vertebrobasilar insufficiency also occurs. Involvement of the penetrating vessels of the frontal lobes may produce acute personality change followed by clouding of consciousness, delirium, delusions, and hallucinations. There is a progressive dementia, which can be arrested by adequate treatment. Arteritis involving the vessels supplying the brain stem and basal ganglia may result in parkinsonism, dystonia, or ballism.

Diagnostic Procedures.

1. Serologic tests for syphilis are positive in blood and cerebrospinal fluid.
2. The cerebrospinal fluid shows the presence of excess lymphocytes with increased protein and gamma globulin contents.
3. The arteritis can be demonstrated by arteriography, which shows an irregular involvement of the blood vessels and vascular occlusion.

Treatment. See page 271. Although the process is promptly arrested by adequate antibiotic treatment, residual neurologic deficits due to infarction are often severe.

Syphilitic Gumma. A syphilitic gumma is a tumorlike mass of granulation tissue occurring in the meninges or brain parenchyma of a patient with tertiary syphilis.

Pathology. A gumma is a solitary mass of granulation tissue consisting of epithelioid cells, plasma cells, and giant cells surrounding a central area of necrosis.

Clinical Features. Gummas of the central nervous system are extremely rare and behave as expanding mass lesions.

Diagnostic Procedures.

1. Serologic tests for syphilis are positive in the blood and cerebrospinal fluid.
2. The cerebrospinal fluid shows the presence of a lymphocyte pleocytosis, elevated protein content, and elevated gamma globulin.
3. There are focal changes on the electroencephalogram compatible with a focal structural lesion.
4. Diagnosis of a mass lesion can be made by MR or CT scan.
5. Arteriographic changes are compatible with the presence of a mass lesion.

Treatment. See page 271. Gummas presenting as an expanding intracranial mass are often excised, and the diagnosis is established postoperatively by histologic examination.

General Paresis. General paresis is a chronic syphilitic encephalitis caused by the presence of *T. pallidum* in the brain.

Pathology. In advanced cases the brain shows diffuse cortical atrophy and ventricular dilatation. The ependymal lining of the ventricles is thickened and has a granular appearance. The condition is termed "granular ependymitis." Histologic examination shows thickening of the meninges, which are infiltrated with plasma cells and lymphocytes. The gray matter of the brain shows loss of neurons and proliferation of astrocytes and microglia. The microglia have a typical rod-shaped appearance often oriented in a perpendicular fashion to the surface of the brain. Blood vessels show the presence of a diffuse syphilitic arteritis. There is marked perivascular cuffing of the vessels penetrating the surface of the brain. Numerous spirochetes may be demonstrated by special staining techniques.

Clinical Features. The patient shows progressive intellectual deterioration beginning with loss of operational judgment followed by impairment of insight, gradual loss of acceptable social behavior, impairment of recent memory, and personality change. With the passage of time the affect becomes flat and the patient becomes severely demented and apathetic.

The examination of the patient with established general paresis shows the presence of Argyll-Robertson pupils in all cases. There is a tremor involving the eyelids, lips, tongue, and fingers. The voice is tremulous, and rapid alternating movements are impaired because of dyspraxia. Deep tendon reflexes are symmetric but diffusely increased. There may be extensor plantar responses.

Diagnostic Procedures.

1. Serologic tests for syphilis are positive in blood and cerebrospinal fluid.
2. Cerebrospinal fluid shows the presence of a lymphocytic pleocytosis, increased protein content, and increased gamma globulin.
3. Serial electroencephalography will show gradual deterioration in the records with loss of alpha activity and replacement with theta activity and eventual appearance of delta activity. The activity is symmetric over both hemispheres.
4. Diffuse cortical atrophy and ventricular dilatation can be demonstrated by MR or CT scan of the brain.

Treatment. See page 271. Adequate treatment of general paresis in the early stages can arrest the disease prior to the development of severe dementia. Relapse is rare and will require a second course of treatment.

Syphilitic Optic Atrophy. Syphilitic optic atrophy is optic atrophy caused by or related to infection by *T. pallidum.*

Etiology and Pathology. There are two forms of neurosyphilitic optic atrophy. In primary optic atrophy the condition is a consequence of an inflammatory reaction of the optic nerve. Secondary syphilitic atrophy is caused by pressure on the optic nerve due to chronic basal meningitis or increased intracranial pressure resulting from hydrocephalus secondary to syphilitic meningitis.

In primary optic atrophy the optic nerve shows the presence of an inflammatory reaction surrounding the blood vessels that penetrate the nerve (vasa nervorum). This reaction is followed by loss of nerve fibers and demyelination beginning peripherally and gradually involving the center of the optic nerve. Optic atrophy eventually results.

Clinical Features. Syphilitic optic atrophy is characterized by progressive restriction of the visual fields beginning peripherally and extending toward the center. The visual loss is usually eccentric, and visual loss is total within a 10-year period. Examination shows marked pallor of the optic disks.

Diagnostic Procedures. The blood serologic test for syphilis is positive in most cases but may be negative in patients with optic atrophy and tabes dorsalis.

Treatment. See page 271. Syphilitic optic atrophy is often progressive despite adequate penicillin therapy, and repeated courses of treatment may not prevent the development of blindness.

Congenital Neurosyphilis. Congenital neurosyphilis results when there is transplacental infection of the fetus by the *T. pallidum.*

Pathology. The developing fetus is infected during the fourth month of pregnancy; adequate treatment of the mother with active syphilis before the fourth month of pregnancy prevents fetal infection. The pathologic changes are those of syphilis in its early stages.

Clinical Features. The child may be stillborn or show signs of congenital syphilis at birth. All untreated cases with congenital syphilis may develop all of the signs of neurosyphilis at a later stage. The conditions include syphilitic meningitis, chronic basal meningitis, syphilitic arteritis, and juvenile general paresis. General paresis presents during the second decade as a rapidly progressive dementia. Tabes dorsalis has rarely been described in congenital syphilis.

Diagnostic Procedures.

1. The blood serologic test for syphilis is positive.
2. The cerebrospinal fluid will show the presence of a lymphocytic pleocytosis with elevated protein content. The serologic test for syphilis is positive.

Treatment. See page 271.

Syphilis of the Spinal Cord. Syphilitic involvement of the spinal cord is rare and has been virtually eliminated with penicillin ther-

apy. Acute syphilitic transverse myelitis may occur and is due to an acute infarction of the spinal cord secondary to syphilitic arteritis of the anterior spinal artery or its branches.

Syphilitic meningomyelitis, which is a diffuse granulomatous meningitis involving the spinal cord, may produce progressive paraparesis. Pachymeningitis cervicalis hypertrophica is a condition in which marked thickening of the meninges over the cervical area of the spinal cord occurs. This condition is also associated with a progressive paraparesis. In addition, involvement of the motor nerve roots in the cervical area produces wasting of the muscles of the hands and upper limb girdles. Syphilitic amyotrophy resembles amyotrophic lateral sclerosis and is caused by progressive loss of anterior horn cells secondary to ischemia due to an arteritis involving the penetrating branches from the anterior spinal artery. Spinal gummas may rarely occur and present as a spinal cord tumor.

Diagnostic Procedures.

1. The blood serologic test for syphilis will be positive in all cases.
2. Lumbar puncture may show evidence of occlusion of the subarachnoid space with low opening pressure, positive Queckenstedt test, xanthochromic spinal fluid, lymphocytic pleocytosis, and elevated protein content. The serologic test for syphilis will be positive in the spinal fluid.
3. Areas of spinal cord compression can be demonstrated by MR scan or myelography.

Treatment. Most cases respond to adequate penicillin therapy. Cord pressure may be relieved surgically by removal of a gumma or excision of thickened meninges.

Tabes Dorsalis. Tabes dorsalis, a slowly progressive degenerative condition, is a late manifestation of syphilis and results from involvement of the dorsal nerve roots and posterior columns of the spinal cord.

Etiology and Pathology. Tabes dorsalis is known to be associated with late syphilis. It is extremely difficult to demonstrate the presence of *T. pallidum* organisms in tabes dorsalis, but the pathologic changes are believed to be due to the activity of the spirochetes. Pathologic changes begin in the posterior nerve root at the site of penetration of the pia just before the nerve root enters the spinal cord. The degenerative changes in the nerve root spread into the posterior column with progressive loss of axons and myelin. The end result is almost total bilateral destruction of the posterior columns.

Clinical Features. Patients with tabes dorsalis experience paroxysmal lancinating pains in the lower limbs for many years before the appearance of neurologic signs. These "lightning pains" are often termed "rheumatic pains" by the patients and may occasionally spread beyond the lower limbs to involve the abdomen, thorax, and occasionally the face. After several years of lightning pains, the patient develops a progressive ataxia beginning in the lower limbs. The gait becomes wide-based, and the feet are elevated abnormally when walking, producing a loud slapping sound. The loss of proprioception is severe and, the patient depends upon visual cues in order to maintain balance. This results in falling in poorly lighted or dark surroundings or, in extreme cases, when the patient closes the eyes. Patients with established ataxia experience loss of sensation in the feet, often described as "walking on cotton." Paresthesias of the limbs, trunk, and perioral area of the face are not uncommon. There may be an unpleasant hyperesthesia produced by contact with clothing, shoes, or bedcovers.

Loss of bladder sensation leads to painless distention of the bladder and retention of urine with overflow. The bladder may be extremely distended and contain several liters of urine. Impairment of sensation in the genital area and interference with the nerves supplying reflex activity lead to loss of libido in both men and women.

Paroxysmal episodes of abdominal pain (gastric crisis), pelvic pain (bladder crisis), rectal pain (rectal crisis), genital pain (genital crisis), and paroxysmal coughing (laryngeal crisis) can occur in established tabes dorsalis. The commonest form of this complication is gastric crisis in which the patient experiences paroxysmal upper abdominal pain associated with vomiting. Examination shows a distressed patient with boardlike rigidity of the abdomen, and the condition is often misdiagnosed as a perforated peptic ulcer. However, the patient shows the presence of Argyll-Robertson pupils and other signs of tabes dorsalis. There is hyperesthesia of the abdominal wall, which is not seen with ruptured abdominal viscera.

The loss of joint sensation results in accelerated degenerative changes in the joints of the lower limbs (Charcot joints), which become swollen and distorted. There is often hypermobility without pain, and the joints show the presence of marked effusion. Syphilitic optic atrophy is not uncommon in tabes dorsalis and may lead to total blindness. Loss of cutaneous sensation leads to the development of trophic ulcers over areas subjected to pressure. There is often ulceration of the soles of the feet, over the heads of the first metatarsal bone, or over the heels.

Clinical examination of the patient with tabes dorsalis shows the presence of Argyll-Robertson pupils (see p. 22). Some cases show the presence of syphilitic optic atrophy with disk pallor and constricted visual fields. There is a rather typical facial appearance with bilateral ptosis and prominent nasolabial folds, and cranial nerve palsies secondary to an associated syphilitic basal meningitis may be present. Examination of the motor system shows generalized hypotonia, and the gait is wide-based and ataxic. The Romberg test is positive. Sensation shows a loss of vibration and position sense in the lower limbs, later extending to involve the upper limbs. Patchy loss of appreciation of pinprick over the face, trunk, and limbs may occur. There may be trophic ulcers over the feet, the presence of Charcot joints, and a distended bladder.

Diagnostic Procedures.

1. The blood serologic test for syphilis is positive in about 50 percent of cases of tabes dorsalis.
2. Cerebrospinal fluid examination reveals clear fluid under normal pressure. There may be a slight increase in lymphocyte content with normal or slightly elevated protein content and increased gamma globulin. The serologic test for syphilis is abnormal in the early stages of tabes dorsalis but is often normal in the later stages of the disease.

Treatment. The treatment of tabes dorsalis is outlined under syphilis of more than one year's duration in Table 16–11. Lightning pains respond to the use of carbamazepine (Tegretol) in some cases; phenytoin (Dilantin) also may be effective. Gastric crisis requires intravenous fluids and sedation. Charcot joints may require bracing or orthopedic fusion. Patients with bladder involvement should employ self-catheterization. Some males may benefit from transurethral resection of the prostate. Trophic ulcers of the feet should be treated with extra care to avoid infection, which leads to bony necrosis.

TABLE 16–11. Current Treatment of Syphilis

A tabular summary of the current recommended treatment schedules from the Centers for Disease Control follows:°

Early Syphilis (Less than 1 year's duration)	Syphilis of More than 1 Year's Duration (Latent syphilis of indeterminate or more than 1 yr's duration, cardiovascular, late benign, neurosyphilis)	Syphilis in Pregnancy	Congenital Syphilis
(1) Benzanthine penicillin G 2.4 million units IM at a single session OR (2) Aqueous procaine penicillin G 4.8 million units Total: 600,000 units IM daily for 8 days. *If Allergic to Penicillin* (1) Tetracycline HCl 500 mg q.i.d. (PO) for 15 days *Note:* Other tetracyclines are not more effective. Avoid food, milk, iron preparations, and antacids with tetracycline as they impair absorption OR (2) Erythromycin 500 mg q.i.d. (PO) for 15 days	(1) Benzathine penicillin G 7.2 million units Total: 2.4 million units IM weekly for 3 successive weeks OR (2) Aqueous procaine penicillin G 9.0 million units Total: 600,000 units IM daily for 15 days *If Allergic to Penicillin* (1) Tetracycline HCl 500 mg q.i.d. (PO) for 30 days OR (2) Erythromycin 500 mg q.i.d. (PO) for 30 days	(1) Penicillin in dosage schedules appropriate for the stage of syphilis as recommended for nonpregnant patients *If Allergic to Penicillin* (1) Erythromycin in dosage schedule appropriate for the stage of syphilis recommended for nonpregnant patients *Note:* Erythromycin estolate and tetracycline are not recommended for syphilitic infections in pregnant women because of potential adverse effects on mother and fetus	Infants with abnormal CSF: (1) Aqueous crystalline penicillin G: 50,000 units/kg IM or IV daily in 2 divided doses for 10 days minimum OR (2) Aqueous procaine penicillin G: 50,000 units/kg IM daily for 10 day minimum Infants with normal CSF: (1) Benzathine penicillin G: 50,000 units/kg IM × 1 dose

° NOTE: All cases of early syphilis with human immunodeficiency virus (HIV) infection (acquired immunodeficiency syndrome—AIDS) should be treated as syphilis of more than one year's duration (25).

Tuberculous Meningitis

Definition. Tuberculous (TB) meningitis is an infection of the meninges caused by the acid-fast bacillus *Mycobacterium tuberculosis.*

Etiology and Pathology. The bacilli usually enter the body by inhalation. Transmission through the skin or by ingestion are rare causes of infection. Once introduced the organisms undergo multiplication and hematogenous dissemination; it is during this stage that the meninges are most likely to become involved. The subarachnoid space is infected by the rupture of a meningeal tubercle. Rup-ture of an intracerebral tuberculoma or direct extension from an adjacent focus (e.g., from the spine or nasal sinuses) into the subarachnoid space is rare.

The presence of the bacilli in the subarachnoid space is followed by an intense granulomatous inflammation of the leptomeninges and subjacent cortex. A thick, heavy, fibrous, and necrotic exudate is produced, which tends to collect at the base of the brain.

The arteries at the base of the brain are involved, and there is inflammation of the adventitia and media with narrowing and thrombosis of the lumen. Cranial nerves two and three, and occasionally seven and eight, are subjected to compression by the heavy exudate.

Clinical Features. Although the incidence of TB meningitis has decreased in the United States, the condition carries a high mortality in other parts of the world. The disease occurs at all ages, but the incidence is higher in infants, young children, and the aged. It is more common among the undernourished and in those areas of the world characterized by poor hygiene and overcrowding.

There is a history of contact with an infected individual or a history of previously active tuberculosis in 30 to 50 percent of patients. In the early stages of the disease the patient experiences anorexia, intermittent headache, lethargy, aching muscles, and low-grade fever. Irritability and poor feeding may be the only evidence of the illness in infants. Some two weeks after the initial febrile illness, the patient may begin to complain of persistent headache and a stiff neck. This is associated with other signs of meningeal irritation, increased intracranial pressure, and focal neurologic deficits including cranial nerve palsies or hemiparesis. Infants may have a tense, bulging fontanelle. There is a slow progression over a period of weeks to months with increasing drowsiness, evidence of progressive neurologic dysfunction, and terminal coma and eventual death. In some cases the infection is confined to the spinal cord and presents as a radiculomyelopathy. The course of the illness depends on the extent of the meningeal involvement, the immune response of the host, the virulence of the organism, and the stage at which treatment is administered.

Complications.

1. Infarction. Arteritis may be followed by thrombosis of a major artery resulting in cerebral infarction.

2. Hydrocephalus. The granulomatous exudate or an arachnoiditis may block the aqueduct of Sylvius, the foramina of Luschka and Magendie, or the subarachnoid space, impeding the flow of cerebrospinal fluid and causing hydrocephalus.

3. Seizures. Seizures may occur at any time during the illness and are most common in children less than two years of age.

Differential Diagnosis. The differential diagnosis of TB meningitis includes viral encephalitis, partially treated pyogenic meningitis, fungal infection, and other inflammatory disorders, which produce progressive neurologic dysfunction. The presence of active tuberculosis elsewhere and the results of cerebrospinal fluid examination are usually sufficient to establish the diagnosis.

Diagnostic Procedures.

1. Lumbar puncture (LP). This is the only definitive procedure in the diagnosis of TB meningitis. The cerebrospinal fluid is under increased pressure, is clear or slightly cloudy, and contains a predominance of mononuclears (usually >400/cu mm), increased protein (100–400 mg percent), and a decreased glucose content. It is usually difficult to identify the bacilli in the CSF; examination of the fibrin clot after centrifugation and careful staining by the Ziehl-Neelsen method is necessary. Fluorescent antibody staining may also be helpful. Bacterial culture and guinea pig inoculation require four to six weeks incubation before examination for tubercle bacilli. The LP should be repeated at weekly intervals in cases with clinical signs of tuberculous meningitis until the diagnosis is established.

1. Cerebrospinal fluid protein levels greater than 1,000 mg percent and a decreasing opening pressure on serial LP's suggest a spinal block. The Queckenstedt test usually reveals lack of communication through the subarachnoid space. A myelogram should be performed to confirm the presence of arachnoiditis.

2. Skull x-rays. Skull x-rays may reveal tuberculous osteomyelitis or evidence of increased intracranial pressure.

3. Evidence of systemic disease. More than 50 percent of patients will have an elevated sedimentation rate, a positive tuberculin skin test, or a positive chest x-ray.

4. Computed tomography. The CT scan may reveal enhancement of the basal cisterns. Tuberculomas appear as modular or ring enhanced masses. The target sign, a central area of calcification and peripheral ring enhancement is highly suggestive of tuberculoma. Serial CT scans are useful in identifying incipient complications such as hydrocephalus.

5. Magnetic resonance scans may be more sensitive than CT in detecting tuberculomas. The development of a tuberculoma during treatment for tuberculous meningitis does not necessarily indicate treatment failure.

6. Arteriography. Arteriography may show the presence of arteritis of the circle of Willis or its major branches. Affected vessels show irregular areas of narrowing and occlusion.

Treatment.

1. Tuberculous meningitis should be treated with a combination of antituberculous drugs. The regimen listed in Table 16–12 is recommended until culture and sensitivity results are obtained. At that time it may be necessary to substitute more toxic drugs such as ethambutol, cycloserine, pyrazinamide, or ethionamide, which require careful observation for the development of side effects. Pyridoxine must be administered in a dosage of 50 mg daily to avoid the development of isoniazid-(INH)-induced neuropathy, encephalopathy, and/or seizures. Intrathecal streptomycin therapy may be necessary in cases with fulminating meningitis or in those with impending occlusion of the spinal subarachnoid space.

2. Spinal arachnoiditis, arteritis, and hydrocephalus can be treated with intrathecal or intracisternal hydrocortisone 50 mg twice a week for six weeks.

3. Seizures should be adequately controlled with anticonvulsants. The dosage of phenytoin (Dilantin) may require careful adjustment with frequent monitoring of plasma phenytoin levels since INH inhibits the metabolism of phenytoin.

4. Ventriculoperitoneal shunting may be necessary in the treatment of hydrocephalus.

Prognosis. The mortality of TB meningitis is still between 10 and 20 percent. The prognosis is poor in infants and the elderly, when treatment is delayed, and in patients with poor nutrition or debilitation from other chronic diseases.

Tuberculoma

A tuberculoma is a granulomatous mass resulting from enlargement of a caseous tubercle. Tuberculoma formation is a rare indication of tuberculous infection in the United States and is more commonly encountered in Great Britain, Asia, and Africa. Tuberculomas vary in size and are usually supratentorial and multiple. Most are located in the parietal lobes and may be attached to the dura and predominantly extracerebral or located deep within the brain parenchyma. Signs and symptoms depend primarily on the location of the mass, but most cases present with headache, vomiting, and seizures. The diagnosis is usually considered if there is evidence of systemic tuberculosis. Computed tomography or MR scanning will identify a space-occupying mass, but there are no pathognomonic signs in these studies. Tuberculomas that produce neurologic dysfunction are usually excised, and diagnosis is established by microscopic examination of the specimen.

Tuberculosis of the Spine

Single or multiple vertebral involvement by tuberculosis is frequently followed by spinal cord compression due to the development of a cold abscess in the epidural space.

The condition presents with pain in the back followed by signs of spinal cord involvement including spastic paraparesis, urinary frequency and incontinence and loss of sensation below the level of the cord compression. The site of compression can be localized by MR scanning.

Treatment consists of antituberculous therapy and surgical decompression using an anterior spinal decompression and fusion (26).

Sarcoidosis

Definition. Sarcoidosis is an idiopathic noncaseating granulomatous disease that may involve any organ.

Etiology and Pathology. The etiology is unknown. Lesions of sarcoidosis are closely related to blood vessels and consist of nodular collections of epithelioid cells without necrosis and caseation. The nervous system may be involved at the following sites:

1. The meninges around the base of the brain

TABLE 16–12. Suggested Treatment of Tuberculous Meningitis (24)

		Dosage	
	Drugs	Child	Adult
Initial Treatment (two months)	IM streptomycin	10 mg/kg/day	1 g/day
	oral isoniazid (INH)	20 mg/kg/day	500 mg/day
	oral rifampin	15 mg/kg/day	600 mg/day
	oral pyrazinamide	20 mg/kg/day	20 mg/kg/day
Continued Treatment (to nine months)	oral isoniazid (INH) oral rifampin		

2. The infundibulum and floor of the third ventricle
3. The optic nerves and chiasm
4. Granulomatous involvement of the brain or spinal cord
5. Mononeuropathy or polymononeuropathy of any cranial or peripheral nerves.

Clinical Features. Sarcoidosis of the nervous system probably occurs in about 5 percent of cases of sarcoidosis. The disease occurs in both sexes and is commonest in the 20-to-40 age group.

Signs of systemic sarcoidosis are usually present in patients with involvement of the nervous system and include hilar lymphadenopathy, pulmonary infiltration, parotitis, uveitis, chorioretinitis, papilledema, proximal muscle weakness due to myopathy, and polyarthritis often preceded by bilateral heel pain (27).

Sarcoidosis can damage any cranial nerve, but the facial and optic nerves are most commonly involved. Changes in personality and dementia can occur because of space-occupying granulomas, hydrocephalus due to basal meningitis, or metabolic changes secondary to hypothalamic and pituitary involvement. Metabolic encephalopathy may result from hypercalcemia, pulmonary insufficiency and carbon dioxide narcosis, uremia secondary to kidney involvement, or hepatic encephalopathy in severe liver involvement. Meningeal sarcoidosis may present as a chronic meningitis with CSF pleocytosis, normal or reduced glucose, and elevated protein content. Generalized or partial seizures of all types have been described in sarcoidosis. Choreiform movements, parkinsonism, and ballism are rare complications. Sarcoid granulomas may occasionally mimic brain tumors and produce focal signs of brain involvement and increased intracranial pressure. Hypothalamic and pituitary involvement is probably the commonest sign of intracranial sarcoidosis. Diabetes insipidus occurs in about one-third of patients with neurologic sarcoidosis. Signs of endocrine deficiency can be demonstrated in many cases. Signs of brain stem and cerebellar dysfunction are not unusual in cases with multiple cranial nerve involvement. Myelopathy is rare, but granulomas may occur in the spinal meninges, in the nerve roots, and in the parenchyma of the spinal cord. Transient ischemic attacks may be the only clinical manifestation of intracranial sarcoidosis, and cerebral or brain stem ischemia can result from granulomatous involvement of blood vessels. Mononeuropathies and polymononeuropathies result in paresthesias, numbness, pain, muscle weakness and wasting.

Diagnostic Procedures.
1. Skull and chest x-ray. Sarcoidosis rarely produces radiolucent areas on the skull x-ray. Hilar lymphadenopathy is common, and changes in the lung parenchyma are not unusual in this disease.
2. Blood tests. The sedimentation rate is often elevated; serum calcium and alkaline phosphatase levels are increased. Serum proteins are elevated with increase in the globulin fraction.
3. Electroencephalography. The EEG may show focal slowing, seizure activity, or generalized slowing.
4. Visual evoked potentials. Optic nerve and optic chiasm involvement is not uncommon, producing abnormal visual evoked responses.
5. Magnetic resonance and CT scans are usually abnormal in intracranial sarcoidosis with demonstration of granulomatous lesions at the base of the brain, over the convexities, or intrahemisphericly and occasionally periventricularly (see Figure 16–3). Hydrocephalus may be present (28).
6. Lumbar puncture. The CSF shows a lymphocyte pleocytosis and elevated protein content. Glucose content is occasionally reduced. Cultures are negative.
7. Arteriography. The arteriogram may show the presence of an arteritis.
8. Nerve conduction studies. Nerve conduction studies will demonstrate a peripheral neuropathy.
9. Biopsy. Histologic confirmation of sarcoidosis may be obtained with biopsy of muscle, nerve, liver, or scalene lymph node.
10. Endocrine studies. Endocrine studies are indicated in all cases with intracranial involvement because of the high risk of hypothalamic and pituitary involvement.
11. Skin tests. The tuberculin test is usually negative. The Kveim test (intracutaneous inoculation of a suspension of sarcoid tissue) produces a granulomatous papule in about six weeks in 80 percent of cases.

Treatment.
1. The effect of corticosteroids in neurologic sarcoidosis has not been firmly established, but some patients show dramatic improvement when treated with these drugs. Dexamethasone (Decadron) 12 mg daily or methylprednisolone (Medrol) 80 mg daily can be reduced to a minimal effective dose once symptoms resolve and can be continued for many months. In some cases short courses

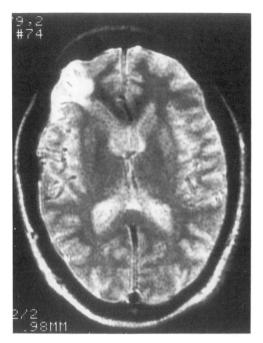

FIGURE 16–3. MR scan. T2 weighted image showing an area of increased signal right frontal lobe in a patient with cerebral sarcoidosis.

of corticosteroids can be used and discontinued when symptoms abate. This method tends to delay the development of side effects (29).

2. Increased intracranial pressure and hydrocephalus can be relieved by a ventriculoperitoneal shunt procedure.

3. Diabetes insipidus and other endocrine deficiencies should be treated with appropriate substitution therapy.

4. Seizures respond to therapeutic doses of anticonvulsants.

5. Occasionally large intracranial granulomatous masses can be removed surgically.

Prognosis. Many cases show spontaneous regression and apparent recovery, while others have a chronic relapsing-remitting course. The condition can be fatal. The prognosis is better in patients with involvement of only the peripheral nervous system.

Cat Scratch Disease

Definition. A rare infection caused by a gram negative bacterium transmitted by cat scratch.

The infection usually results in a benign lymphadenitis draining the lymph nodes draining the area of the cat scratch. Occa-

sional cases of encephalitis or cerebral arteritis have been reported.

Diagnosis depends upon demonstration of a rising titer of antibodies against the cultured bacteria (30).

Rickettsial Infections

The central nervous system is frequently affected during epidemic typhus *(Rickettsia prowazekii)*, murine typhus *(Rickettsia mooseri)*, scrub typhus *(Rickettsia tsutsugamushi)*, and Rocky Mountain spotted fever *(Rickettsia rickettsii)*.

Etiology and Pathology. The rickettsial infections are transmitted to man by insect vectors, including fleas, lice, ticks, and mites.

Pathologic changes include swelling of blood vessel endothelial linings and thrombosis. This is followed by a perivascular leukocytosis and formation of a typhus nodule. Eventually astrocytosis forms a glial scar.

Clinical Features. Typhus is rare in the United States, but Rocky Mountain spotted fever is increasing in frequency.

Typhus presents as a severe encephalitis often associated with seizures and focal neurologic deficits. In Rocky Mountain spotted fever nausea, vomiting, headache, and fever are followed by the development of a maculopapular rash on the ankles and wrists, which spreads distally and then proximally. There may be signs of meningeal irritation, seizures, and focal deficits including hemiplegia or hemiparesis.

Diagnostic Procedures.

1. There is a progressive rise in serum antibodies to rickettsiae.

2. The Weil-Felix reaction is positive.

Treatment.

1. Persons who reside in an endemic area should be immunized against the rickettsiae.

2. Typhus and Rocky Mountain spotted fever respond to chloramphenicol or tetracycline. Steroid therapy is indicated when there are signs of cerebral edema.

Fungal Infections

Definition. The systemic fungal infections discussed in this section have the capacity to invade the central nervous system either directly or through the bloodstream, producing a serious, often fatal, disorder that is exceedingly difficult to treat.

Etiology and Pathology. There are approximately twenty genera of fungi capable of producing central nervous system disease. Table 16–13 lists 12 of the most common

TABLE 16–13. Fungal Characteristics

Fungus	Characteristics	Portal of Entry	Epidemiology	Persons at Risk	Pathology
Cryptococcus neoformans (35)	Yeastlike, budding Large gelatinous capsule Predilection for CNS	Respiratory	Worldwide Found in soil and pigeon droppings	Those who have leukemia, renal transplants, lymphoma, AIDS, or who have undergone chronic corticosteroid therapy	Perivascular cyst formation
Coccidioides immitis	Nonbudding, thick-walled Spherules filled with endospores	Respiratory or skin	Southwestern U.S. Dust-borne	Those who live in an endemic area	
Candida albicans	Yeastlike, budding Small, oval Stains gram positive	Endocarditis GI, urinary respiratory	Worldwide Skin, GI, mucous membrane flora	Drug addicts The elderly Those who are immunosuppressed or have AIDS	Abscess formation
Aspergillus fumigatus	Septate branching, hyphae with small green spores Common laboratory contaminant	Respiratory or skin	Worldwide Soil, water, air Warm, humid climate		Inflammatory granulomas Abscess formation Thrombus formation
Phycomycetes mucor and *rhizopus*	Large broad nonseptate hyphae Common laboratory contaminant	Nasal sinus or orbit	Worldwide Nasal and throat flora Soil and decaying matter	Diabetics in ketoacidosis Immunosuppressed persons Heroin addicts	Hyphae have affinity for vasculature

276

Organism	Morphology	Portal / Clinical	Source / Geography	Risk group	Complications
Histoplasm capsulatum	Yeastlike, budding Small, oval Predilection for reticuloendothelial system	Respiratory	Central U.S. Soil, bird droppings, bats	Those who live in an endemic area	Inflammatory granulomas
Blastomyces	Yeastlike, single or budding Round, doubly refractile wall	Respiratory or skin	Midwest U.S. Soil	Those who live in an endemic area	Abscess formation
Paracoccidio idomyces brasiliensis	Yeastlike Multiple, budding	Oral cavity	South America Central America	Those who live in an endemic area	
Sporothrix schenckii (36)	Budding Round to oval Stains gram positive	Skin	GI flora		
Cladosporium bantianum	Septate, branching, brown hyphae	Respiratory			Abscess formation
Nocardia asteroides	Anaerobic Stains gram positive, acid-fast	Respiratory	Soil, water, grass	Those who are immunosuppressed	Abscess formation, multiloculated, multiple abscesses
Actinomyces	Actinomycotic "granules"—clumps of tangled filaments with radiating terminal "clubs"	Dental abscess Tooth extraction Poor dentition Chronic otitis Chronic sinusitis	Worldwide	Those with poor dentition	Cerebral abscess Subdural empyema Meningitis Actinomycoma

species, the tissue characteristics of these fungi, their usual portal of entry to the body, and characteristic pathology.

The majority of fungi gain access to the central nervous system via hematogenous dissemination from a distant source. Some (e.g., Phycomycetes [mucor]) may spread directly from an infected orbit or sinus (31, 32). The fungi spread through the subarachnoid space and produce a chronic basal meningitis with granulomatous lesions composed of epithelioid cells, giant cells, lymphocytes, and plasma cells. Some of the fungi also have the capacity to invade the brain parenchyma, and tissue destruction is followed by abscess or cyst formation. Involvement of cerebral vessels may result in thrombosis and ischemic infarction. *Candida* species are the most frequently identified cause of central nervous system infection.

Clinical Features. See Table 16–13. There has been a steady increase in the number of cases of fungal disease of the central nervous system due to increasing numbers of susceptible patients, greater physician awareness, and improved diagnostic capability.

The majority of patients present with a history of chronic or subacute, relapsing illness. Factors predisposing to fungal infection may be present and include broad-spectrum antibiotic therapy, drug-induced immunosuppression, malignancy, the presence of debilitating diseases such as diabetes mellitus or alcoholism, trauma, a ventriculoperitoneal shunt, narcotic addiction, residence in an endemic area, or prior history of fungal disease. The initial symptoms of neurologic involvement are often nonspecific and consist of headache, anorexia, nausea, vomiting, and insomnia. This may be followed by signs of meningeal irritation and papilledema or focal signs of cranial nerve involvement or hemiparesis. At the same time there may be evidence of involvement of other organs, including the liver, spleen, and kidney.

Patients who present with chronic sinusitis followed by sudden blindness in one eye, proptosis, a reddish-black nasal discharge, and involvement of the third, fourth, and/or sixth cranial nerves are usually infected by the genera Phycomycetes (mucormycosis).

Course. Most fungal diseases have a subacute or chronic course, although Phycomycetes is often rapidly fatal (33). The mortality approaches 100 percent in untreated fungal disease involving the central nervous system. Death results from a terminal meningitis, brain herniation, or systemic involvement.

Complications. The course of disease may be complicated by hydrocephalus, vertebral involvement with spinal cord compression, the development of fungal mycotic aneurysms, or a relapsing course despite adequate chemotherapy.

Diagnostic Procedures.

1. Lumbar puncture is the definitive procedure in the diagnosis and determination of the etiology of fungal disease. The CSF is either clear, turbid, or xanthochromic and is usually under elevated pressure. The fluid has monocytic pleocytosis, an elevated protein content, a decreased glucose content, and elevated lactic acid levels (34). Occasionally there are organisms in the centrifuged specimen stained with 10 percent potassium hydroxide. India ink is a useful stain in cases of suspected cryptococcosis. A large volume (20–50 ml) of CSF may be required to isolate the organism by culture. Cisternal puncture is strongly recommended when there is a high level of suspicion of fungal infection with repeatedly negative cultures following lumbar puncture.

2. Skin tests, complement fixation tests, fluorescent antibody tests, and serum Ag and Ab titers are available for the majority of fungi listed in Table 16–13.

3. The presence of a leukocytosis or abnormal chest x-ray may be evidence of infection elsewhere in the body. Cultures and smears of sputum and skin lesions may be positive for fungi. Bone marrow biopsy and culture are usually positive in disseminated histoplasmosis.

4. Either MR or CT scans may show the presence of an abscess, granuloma, or hydrocephalus.

5. Skull x-rays may reveal osteomyelitis.

Differential Diagnosis. The presence of tuberculous meningitis, bacterial meningitis, brain abscess, or neoplasm should be considered when evidence of fungal infection is lacking.

Treatment.

1. Amphotericin B is the treatment of choice in all fungal infections of the central nervous system except actinomycosis and nocardiosis.

The initial IV dosage of amphotericin B is 0.1–0.25 mg/kg/day. The maximum daily dose is 1.0 mg/kg. A combination of amphotericin B and oral 5-fluorocytocine 150 mg/kg/q6h is recommended for aspergillus candida and cryptococcal infections (37). Full blood counts, electrolytes, renal function, and 5-fluorocytocine levels must be monitored regularly. Intrathecal amphotericin B should be reserved for patients who fail to respond to IV amphotericin B, for those who relapse and the very ill. Intrathecal therapy can be given by intralumbar or intracisternal injections or through an Ommaya reservoir. Intrathecal (IT) therapy should be given on alternate days with an initial dose of 0.25 mg followed by an increase of 0.025 mg q.o.d. When the IT dose reaches 0.1 mg the amount is increased by 0.1 mg q.o.d. to 0.5 mg IT twice per week. A minimum course of six weeks is recommended. Unfortunately, amphotericin B is a toxic drug with a high incidence of side effects. It regularly produces headache, fever, nausea, vomiting, and hypotension. Higher doses result in disturbance of renal function with azotemia and hyperkalemia; the bone marrow is suppressed, producing anemia; and phlebitis occurs at the infusion site.

Penicillin G is the preferred antibiotic for the treatment of actinomycoses infections (38). Nocardial infections respond to treatment with sulphonamides or trimethoprim/sulphamethoxazole (39).

2. Symptomatic treatment is necessary for seizures, hydrocephalus, increased intracranial pressure, and the toxic effects of amphotericin.

3. Miconazole has been reported to be effective in the treatment of mycotic disease, particularly *Cryptococcus, Histoplasma,* and *Candida,* and is, fortunately, less toxic than amphotericin B. The intravenous dosage is 30 mg/kg/day. Intrathecal therapy is usually required; 20 mg may be slowly injected. Side effects include nausea, anemia, phlebitis, confusion, tremor, dizziness, and seizures.

Protozoan Diseases

Toxoplasmosis, amebiasis, and malaria are protozoan organisms that occasionally produce infection in the central nervous system.

Toxoplasmosis

Definition. Toxoplasma gondii usually produces an asymptomatic infection in adults but can cause a severe and potentially fatal encephalitis in immunosuppressed persons, particularly following organ transplantation or complicating AIDS. Toxoplasmosis can cause severe brain damage when transmitted transplacentally to a developing fetus.

Etiology and Pathology. The natural host of *Toxoplasma gondii* is the cat, but other animals may serve as hosts. Humans are infected by ingesting poorly cooked meat containing encysted trophozoites or, more commonly, by ingesting the oocyst excreted in cat feces. A parasitemia results, and the organisms are distributed throughout the body. The encysted organism is walled off by the body, and a granuloma results, which may eventually calcify.

Clinical Features. Infection of the adult is usually asymptomatic. However, an encephalitis can occur in immunosuppressed persons, particularly those with AIDS. Presenting symptoms consist of headache, disorientation, seizures, and hemiparesis.

Congenital infection with toxoplasmosis results in hepatosplenomegaly, jaundice, hydrocephalus, and encephalitis. Surviving children are often microcephalic, with chorioretinitis, seizures, and mental retardation.

Diagnostic Procedures.

1. Lumbar puncture. Cerebrospinal fluid analysis reveals a lymphocytic pleocytosis, xanthochromia, and an elevated protein content.
2. Skull x-rays. Skull x-rays may reveal intracranial calcifications or evidence of increased intracranial pressure.
3. Either MR or CT scans may reveal intracranial calcifications and hydrocephalus.
4. Brain biopsy is necessary for diagnosis of encephalitis in most cases.
5. Serologic tests. Serum antibody titers exceeding 1:32 indicate recent infection.
6. A positive Sabin-Feldman dye test, with titers exceeding 1:1,000, may be seen in congenital toxoplasmosis.

Differential Diagnosis. The differential diagnosis of congenital toxoplasmosis includes congenital rubella encephalitis and cytomegalic inclusion disease (see Table 16–14).

Treatment.

1. Immunocompromised persons should be treated with high dose pyrimethamine 50 to 100 mg/day combined with sulphadiazine 2 to 6 g/day and folinic acid 5 to 50 mg/day IM for two months. Treatment should be repeated if relapse occurs. Toxicity as a result of pyrimethamine and sulphonamide therapy consisting of leukopenia, thrombocytopenia and a rash occurs in about 6 percent of cases. Intravenous clindamycin should be used in those circumstances (40).
2. Pyramethamine and sulphonamides will eradicate the trophozoids and prevent

TABLE 16–14. Differential Diagnosis of Congenital Rubella, Cytomegalic Inclusion Disease, and Toxoplasmosis

Toxoplasmosis	CMV	Rubella
Hepatosplenomegaly, jaundice		
+	+	+
Premature growth failure, microcephaly		
+	+	+
Intracranial calcifications		
Throughout brain	Periventricular	+ −
Abnormal CSF		
Xanthochromic, +++ elevated protein	+ Elevated protein	+ Elevated protein
Hearing deficit		
+	−	+++
Cerebral palsy, minimal brain damage		
+	+	+
Cardiac abnormalities		
Very rare	Very rare	+ Patient ductus
Ocular abnormalities		
Chorioretinitis	Chorioretinitis	Cataract, salt and pepper retinopathy

further deterioration in infants. The parents should be reassured that subsequent infants will not be affected because the mother is immune to further infection.

Amebiasis

Primary amebic meningoencephalitis is an acute, severe meningoencephalitis that results from infection by free-living amebae of the genera *Naegleria*. The infection affects children and young adults and is acquired through the nasal passages while swimming in infected water. There are an acute onset of fever, nausea, and vomiting, severe headache, and meningeal irritation rapidly followed by stupor, seizures, and coma. Lumbar puncture reveals cloudy CSF under increased pressure. There is a polymorphonuclear pleocytosis with a decreased glucose and elevated protein content. Motile amebas may be evident on wet preparations. Treatment must be administered early and consists of amphoter-icin B and rifampin (Rifadin, Rimactane). The mortality approaches 100 percent.

Malaria

The central nervous system is involved in approximately 1 to 2 percent of infections with *Plasmodium falciparum*. This rare, potentially fatal complication results in a vasculitis, which aggravates existing anemia and shock. There is an abrupt onset of confusion and clouding of consciousness with progression to stupor and coma. Partial or generalized seizures, dysphasia, hemianopia, or hemiparesis may occur. Examination of peripheral blood smears will reveal the presence of the malarial parasites.

Treatment. The patient should be given a loading dose of quinine or quinidine intravenously with continuous electrocardiographic monitoring. This can be followed by oral quinine sulphate 600 mg q8h for six days and tetracycline 500 g q6h for seven days (41). Cerebral edema may be reduced with mannitol or dexamethasone (Decadron) (see p. 54).

Cysticercosis

Definition. *Cysticercus cellulosae* is the larval stage of development of the cestode *Taenia solium* (pork tapeworm).

Etiology and Pathology. Cysticercosis is acquired by the ingestion of the eggs from a gravid adult worm. The covering is dissolved in the stomach and the larvae traverse the mucosal lining of the stomach, enter the bloodstream, and are disseminated throughout the body, including the brain. When mature, the larval stage is known as a cysticercus. It is found in three forms within the central nervous system: a cystic form involving the ventricles and brain parenchyma, a racemose form involving the meninges, and a miliary form, which is commoner in children. The presence of the parasite results in an intense tissue reaction and the formation of a capsule. The cyst contents and capsule calcify after the larva dies.

Clinical Features. Cysticercosis is endemic in Mexico, Latin America, Asia, and the Southern United States. The disease accounts for about 30 percent of intracranial mass lesions in Mexico and Latin America. Cysticercosis usually occurs in childrn and young adults. The patient may present with muscle pain, severe headache, nausea and vomiting, partial or generalized seizures or confusion, delusions, and clouding of consciousness. Physical examination may reveal subcutaneous nodules and muscle tenderness. There may be papilledema or retinal detachment with visual deterioration or visual field abnormalities, cranial nerve involvement, and focal neurologic deficits. However, neurologic abnormalities may not appear for many months or years after the parasite has disseminated and matured. The course of the illness may be complicated by death of the parasite and exacerbation of symptoms as fluid is drawn into the dead organism. It may also be complicated by rupture of a cyst and dissemination of its contents.

Diagnostic Procedures.

1. Examination of the stool may reveal the presence of ova.
2. Lumbar puncture. The cerebrospinal fluid may reveal a mild eosinophilic pleocytosis with increased protein, increased gamma globulin, decreased glucose, and a positive complement fixation test (dilutions > 1:16).
3. Magnetic resonance or CT scans may reveal hydrocephalus or calcified cysts.
4. X-ray of the muscle often shows the presence of calcified cysts. The skull x-ray may show scattered calcific cysts with increased intracranial pressure, erosion of the sella, and spreading of sutures.
5. Biopsy. The organism can be demonstrated by biopsy of a subcutaneous nodule or involved muscle.
6. Indirect hemagglutination tests may be positive in blood and cerebrospinal fluid, but negative or nondiagnostic serologic studies can occur in the presence of neurocysticercosis.

Treatment. Praziquantel 50 mg/kg daily for two weeks with dexamethasone coverage will kill the parasites, the steroids limiting the inflammatory response to the foreign substance (42). Small single cysts may resolve completely following use of praziquantel (43). Albendazole 15 mg/kg daily may be useful in cases who show partial response to praziquantel therapy (44). Single cysts should be excised when they are causing hydrocephalus or acting as a mass lesion. Steroid therapy will reduce cerebral edema in the early stages of the disease, but decompression craniotomy may be necessary when elevated intracranial pressure and cerebral edema are refractory to treatment. Hydrocephalus may be treated by a shunting procedure, but the shunt is often blocked by debris (45). Seizures should be controlled with adequate doses of anticonvulsants (46).

Prognosis. The mortality is 50 percent in patients with hydrocephalus, most dying within two years after shunting. Bacterial meningitis and shunt obstruction are not uncommon. Many cases require multiple surgical procedures (47).

Hydatid Disease (Echinococcosis)

Echinococcosis is the presence of the larvae of the sheep tapeworm *Echinococcus granulosus* in the body tissues. The ova of the tapeworm are transmitted to man by petting or handling infected dogs. The ova are then ingested in contaminated food, and the larvae hatch in the intestinal tract, penetrate the mucosa, and disseminate throughout the body. Children are frequently affected. Rupture of a hydatid cyst in muscle produces an intense focal myositis. Hydatid cysts in the brain often present as slowly developing mass lesions. Rupture of the cyst and liberation of toxic contents results in a severe meningitis. There is a peripheral eosinophilia, and the diagnosis is suggested by a positive response to intradermal injection of hydatid antigen. Magnetic resonance or CT scanning will demonstrate the number and positions of the cysts and allow planning for surgical excision. Cysts should be removed unruptured to prevent spillage of fertile daughter cysts and the high risk of recurrence should this occur (48).

Viral Infections

Many different viruses have the capacity to invade the central nervous system. The type of infection depends on the degree of involvement of the central nervous system. A viral infection that is confined to the meninges results in an aseptic meningitis, while invasion of the brain parenchyma produces an encephalitis.

In general, a particular family of viruses tends to produce the same type of response. Thus the enteroviruses are usually associated with aseptic meningitis, while arthropodborne viruses often cause encephalitis (see Table 16–15).

Viral (Aseptic) Meningitis

Definition. Viral meningitis is a syndrome of headache, meningeal irritation, and monocytic pleocytosis and is most commonly caused by the enteroviruses or the mumps virus.

Etiology and Pathology. Viruses frequently associated with viral meningitis are enterovirus (*Coxsackie A*, types 7 and 9; *Cox-*

TABLE 16–15. Classification of Viruses Producing CNS Disease

Family	Genus Species	Clinical Picture
Arenavirus	Lymphocytic choriomeningitis	Meningitis, encephalitis
Bunyavirus	California encephalitis	Encephalitis
Herpesvirus	Group A HSVI, herpes B	Encephalitis
	Group A HSVII	Meningitis, encephalitis
	Group V varicella-zoster	Postinfectious encephalomyelitis, encephalitis (?), herpes zoster, Reye's syndrome
	Group B cytomegalovirus	Congenital CMV, encephalitis
	Epstein-Barr	Encephalitis
Orthomyxovirus	Influenza B	Reye's syndrome, encephalitis
Papovavirus	BK virus, JC virus	Progressive multifocal leukoencephalopathy, Jacob Creutzfeldt disease
Paramyxovirus	Paramyxovirus mumps	Meningitis, encephalitis
	Pseudomyxovirus measles	Postinfectious encephalomyelitis, encephalitis (?), subacute sclerosing panencephalitis
Picornavirus	Enterovirus—polio, echo, coxsackie A-B, encephalomyocarditis virus	Meningitis, encephalitis (paralytic disease)
Poxvirus	Orthopoxvirus variola major	Postinfectious encephalomyelitis
	Orthopoxvirus vaccinia	Postvaccine encephalomyelitis
Reovirus	Orbivirus colorado tick	Encephalitis
Rhabdovirus	Rabies	Encephalitis, postvaccine encephalomyelitis
Togavirus	Alphavirus eastern, western, Venezuelan equine	Encephalitis
	Flavivirus St. Louis, Japanese, Murray-Valley, yellow fever, dengue, West Nile	Encephalitis
	Tickborne—central European, Louping ill, Powassan	Encephalitis
	Tickborne—Russian spring-summer	Encephalitis, Russian spring-summer panencephalitis
	Rubella	Postinfectious encephalomyelitis, congenital rubella, progressive rubella panencephalitis

sackie B, types 1–6; echovirus, types 2–6, 9, 11, 14, 16, 18, and 30; poliovirus, types 1–3), paramyxovirus (mumps), and herpes virus (*Herpes simplex*, type 2). However, the majority of viruses with neurotropic properties are capable of producing the syndrome.

The leptomeninges appear grossly normal in viral meningitis but show the presence of a mild inflammatory reaction. There is a predominantly polymorphonuclear response in the early stages followed by plasma cell and lymphocytic infiltration within 8 to 12 hours. The blood vessels show perivascular cuffing.

Clinical Features. Viral meningitis is more common in children and often occurs in epidemics. Enterovirus infections are usually encountered in the summer and fall, while mumps-induced viral meningitis is more apt to occur in the winter and spring.

The condition is characterized by headache, fever, vomiting, and meningeal irritation producing a stiff neck and positive Kernig and Brudzinski signs. There may be signs of systemic involvement indicating infection by a particular virus such as parotitis in mumps or muscle paralysis in patients with poliovirus infection. However, in general complications are rare and the patient recovers completely.

Diagnostic Procedures.

1. Lumbar puncture usually reveals an elevated opening pressure and a mild pleocytosis (10–1000/cu mm) consisting of polymorphonuclear cells in the early stages with

early replacement by lymphocytes. The protein content is normal or slightly elevated, and there is a slightly decreased or normal glucose content. If the diagnosis is in doubt, the lumbar puncture should be repeated in 8 to 12 hours when there will be a change from polymorphonuclear cells to lymphocytes and/or an increase in the glucose content.

2. The demonstration of a rising antibody titer for a specific virus can be determined in serum samples drawn in the early stages of the illness and after two weeks.

3. A positive viral culture can be obtained from the cerebrospinal fluid in some cases. Counter-immunoelectrophoresis may be of value in identifying the type of virus involved.

Differential Diagnosis. See Table 16–16.

1. Early bacterial meningitis: The diagnosis may be difficult in the early stages because of the presence of polymorphonuclear cells in the cerebrospinal fluid in both conditions. However, a second lumbar puncture will demonstrate an early change to a lymphocytic pleocytosis in viral meningitis.

2. Subarachnoid hemorrhage: The presence of red cells in the cerebrospinal fluid will confirm the presence of subarachnoid hemorrhage.

Treatment. The treatment of viral meningitis is symptomatic. The prognosis is excellent.

Viral Encephalitis

Definition. Viral encephalitis is an acute, febrile illness with evidence of damage to the parenchymal tissues of the central nervous system producing seizures, alteration of consciousness, or focal neurologic signs.

Etiology and Pathology. The etiology cannot be identified in almost two-thirds of the cases of viral encephalitis. The arthropod-borne viruses (see Table 16–17) compose the largest category of identified agents in viral encephalitis. Herpes viruses and enteroviruses are also frequently reported.

Acute viral encephalitis is characterized by inflammation of and damage to the gray matter of the central nervous system. Neuronal inclusion bodies are seen in some encephalitides such as rabies and *Herpes simplex* encephalitis. There is prominent perivascular cuffing by lymphocytes and plasma cells, and the leptomeninges are inflamed. Certain viruses have a predilection for particular areas of the central nervous system. *Herpes simplex* produces an intense inflammatory response in the temporal lobes, while poliovirus infection is mainly confined to the anterior horn cells.

Clinical Features. Table 16–17 outlines the epidemiologic characteristics of the arthropod-borne encephalitides. These conditions, which constitute the most frequent forms of encephalitides, are transmitted by a blood-sucking vector. The insect, usually a mosquito or tick, acquires the virus from an animal that is unaffected by a chronic viremia.

The signs and symptoms of viral encephalitis show some variation depending on the etiologic agent. In most cases there is an acute febrile course with signs of meningeal irritation, headache, nausea and vomiting, alteration of consciousness, and focal neurologic deficits. The mortality varies from high in eastern equine encephalitis to low in Venezuelan equine encephalitis. Residual abnormalities including seizures, changes in personality, extrapyramidal signs, dementia, and motor or sensory impairment may complicate most viral encephalitides. A young age at presentation, presence of semicoma or coma, abnormal oculocephalic responses, and labora-

TABLE 16–16. **Differential Diagnosis of Aseptic Meningitis**

1. Infectious
   A. Viral
      Enterovirus (Coxsackie ECHO, polio); Paramyxovirus (mumps, measles) Herpes virus (*Herpes simplex* II, *Herpes zoster*); Arbovirus (equine, Jap. B, Russian tick, Louping ill, Colorado tick); Arenavirus (Lymphocytic choriomeningitis)
   B. Partially treated bacterial meningitis
   C. Postvaccinal, postinfectious (rabies, vaccinia, mumps, etc.), encephalomyelitis
   D. Adjacent area of infection (abscess)
   E. Spirochetal, tuberculosis, fungal, protozoan, rickettsial infections
   F. Other: sarcoid, brucellosis, listeria, mycoplasma, chlamydial, psittacosis, infectious mononucleosis, Behçet's
2. Noninfectious
   A. Irritative: any procedure involving dural puncture
   B. Neoplastic disease
   C. Toxic: lead, arsenic, systemic infection
   D. Vascular: subarachnoid hemorrhage, cerebral thrombosis, collagen disease
   E. Demyelinating disease

TABLE 16–17. Arthropod-Borne Encephalitis

Virus	Epidemiology	Reservoir	Vector	Clinical Features
Eastern equine	Eastern North America Caribbean very young or old summer-fall	Birds	Mosquito	Fulminating course, convulsions, prominent CSF pleocytosis (>1000 cells/mm 3), high mortality (50–70%), severe sequelae— especially children
Venezuelan equine	South and Central America all ages summer-fall	Small mammals, birds, rodents	Mosquito	Low mortality (<1%), moderate sequelae
Western equine	North and South America very young or old summer-fall	Birds	Mosquito	Convulsions Low mortality (<5%), severe sequelae—especially children
Japanese B	Asia, Japan, Pacific summer-fall	Birds, pigs	Mosquito	High temperature High mortality, especially in elderly, severe sequelae
St. Louis	West Hemisphere, especially central U.S. most common, adults summer-fall	Birds	Mosquito	High mortality, especially in elderly, severe sequelae
California	Midwest, south U.S. male children summer-fall	Small mammals (squirrels and rabbits)	Mosquito	Convulsions Low mortality (<5%), few sequelae
Murray-Valley	Australia, New Guinea children February-March	Birds	Mosquito	High temperature, convulsions High mortality
Russian spring-summer	Russia May–September	Birds, mammals	Tick	Bulbospinal paralysis Moderate mortality
Central European	Europe May–September	Birds, mammals	Tick	Resembles Russian spring-summer Low mortality
Colorado tick	Western U.S. May–September	Small rodents	Tick	Extreme myalgia Low mortality
Louping ill	Britain March–May	Birds, mammals	Tick	Bloody CSF Prominent cerebellar signs and symptoms, no reported mortality

tory demonstration of virus infection within the central nervous system are associated with a poor outcome (49).

Differential Diagnosis. See Table 16–17.

Diagnostic Procedures.

1. The cerebrospinal fluid is clear, and the pressure may or may not be elevated. There is an early increase in polymorphonuclear cells followed by a lymphocytic pleocytosis. The glucose content is normal, and the protein content normal or mildly elevated.

2. The virus is occasionally cultured from the cerebrospinal fluid, stool, urine, nasopharynx, or blood.

3. The most reliable method in establishing a diagnosis of viral encephalitis is the demonstration of a rise in antibody titers to a particular virus in acute and convalescent sera. Titers are quantitated by hemagglu-

tination-inhibition, complement fixation, or neutralization methods.

4. Viral antigen may be demonstrated by immunofluorescence of cells in the cerebrospinal fluid.

Treatment. The treatment of the viral encephalitides is symptomatic.

Herpes Simplex I Encephalitis

Definition. *Herpes simplex* type I encephalitis (HSVI) is an acute, frequently fatal, necrotizing encephalitis with a predilection for the temporal and orbitofrontal areas of the brain.

Etiology and Pathology. *Herpes simplex* type I virus is a large, enveloped DNA virus that may possibly spread to the brain from the trigeminal ganglion, where the virus exists in a latent stage.

Pathologic examination of the brain reveals areas of necrosis and hemorrhage, diffuse mononuclear infiltration, nerve cell loss, and eosinophilic intranuclear inclusions in surviving neurons. There is usually marked cerebral edema.

Clinical Features. The virus is the major cause of herpes labialis (cold sores), and many people have serologic evidence of prior exposure to HSVI by the second decade of life.

Herpes simplex encephalitis affects children and adults, with no sex preference. The disease begins with flulike symptoms including fever, headache, and malaise followed by the development of meningeal irritation and disorientation. There may be a prominent psychosis with hallucinations, disorientation, and disturbance of memory, followed by the appearance of focal neurologic signs such as aphasia or monoparesis. This is often followed by rapid deterioration with stupor and progression to coma.

Diagnostic Procedures.

1. The cerebrospinal fluid is under increased pressure with a monocytic pleocytosis and the presence of red blood cells in some cases. There is an elevated protein (60–150 mg%) and normal glucose content. The antibody titers to HSVI may be elevated.

2. Serology. There is a rise in anti-HSV complement-fixing antibody titers.

3. The electroencephalogram often shows periodic, high-voltage 2 to 3 Hz sharp and slow wave complexes in the temporal leads.

4. A radioactive brain scan shows a marked increased uptake in areas of severe in-

volvement and is a valuable test before selection of a potential brain biopsy site.

5. Magnetic resonance or CT scanning shows the presence of swelling and edema often more marked in one lobe or one hemisphere (50).

6. Brain biopsy is the definitive procedure in establishing the diagnosis of *H. simplex* encephalitis. Viral particles can be seen by electron microscopy and by immunofluorescence. The virus may be cultured from the biopsy material.

Differential Diagnosis. The differential diagnosis includes brain abscess, bacterial or fungal meningitis, toxoplasmosis, other viral encephalitides, septic embolization, postinfectious encephalomyelitis, acute necrotic hemorrhagic encephalitis, and toxic encephalopathy.

Treatment.

1. Acyclovir is the antiviral agent of choice for *H. simplex* encephalitis. The drug should be administered as early as possible before the onset of coma. Doses of 30 mg/kg/day should be given IV q8h and infused in one hour for a period of 14 days (51). Nephrotoxicity due to precipitation of acyclovir crystals in renal tubules can be avoided by adequate hydration to maintain a good urinary output. Toxicity with tremors, hallucinations, agitation or lethargy are rare.

2. Adenine arabinoside (Ara-A) is not as effective as acyclovir. Ara-A should be administered as early as possible before the onset of coma in doses of 10 mg/kg/day IV for 10 days. Toxic effects include nausea, vomiting, weakness, tremors, thrombophlebitis at the infusion site, and megaloblastosis of the erythroid series.

3. Dexamethasone 4 mg q6h may result in clinical improvement by decreasing cerebral edema. There is some disagreement over the use of dexamethasone because of potential suppression of interferon and antibody production. Surgical decompression may be necessary to avoid herniation in cases with rapidly increasing intracranial pressure.

Prognosis. Overall, early mortality is approximately 50 percent. In one series, 93.3 prcent of patients died or survived with severe neurologic deficits. Coma is associated with a 70 percent mortality.

Rhabdovirus—Rabies

Definition. Rabies is an acute, almost invariably fatal infectious illness caused by a neurotropic virus of the rhabdovirus family.

Etiology and Pathology. The rabies virus is a bullet-shaped, enveloped, RNA-containing virus that usually gains access to the body by a bite from a rabid animal. The virus then replicates locally in muscle cells, penetrates nerve endings, and travels in retrograde fashion up the nerve axons to the central nervous system. The virus replicates, spreads throughout the central nervous system and eventually travels out nerve trunks to all parts of the body. The virus is thought to act directly on specific membrane receptor functions.

The brain and spinal cord show perivascular and perineuronal mononuclear infiltration, and there is a mild inflammation of the leptomeninges. The disease is characterized by the presence of intracellular, intracytoplasmic, eosinophilic inclusion bodies (Negri bodies).

Clinical Features. There are approximately one to three cases of human rabies and 3,000 laboratory-confirmed animal cases reported annually in the United States. Some 30,000 courses of postexposure rabies prophylaxis are administered annually. Skunks account for more than one-half of all reported cases, bats 20 percent, and raccoons 9 percent. It has now been recognized that rabies can be transmitted by means other than an animal bite. The disease has been acquired from an infected aerosol, transmitted from an infected mother to her nursing baby, and from a rabid donor to a corneal transplant recipient.

The key to the early diagnosis of rabies is the history of exposure to a rabid or potentially rabid animal. There is an incubation period of one to two months followed by complaints of pain and paresthesias at the bite site accompanied by fever, chills, headache, and myalgia. The majority of patients develop "furious" rabies, which is characterized by periods of cyclic arousal and pharyngeal and inspiratory muscle spasm on attempted swallowing. Eventually an intense terror develops at the mere thought of water, giving rise to the synonym "hydrophobia" for rabies. Autonomic disturbances are common, and the patient may develop hypersalivation, hypotension, hyperpyrexia, and tachycardia. There may be signs of meningeal irritation and cranial and peripheral nerve palsies. The patient eventually loses consciousness and dies from respiratory arrest or circulatory failure.

Course. Some patients, particularly those bitten by bats or those who were given antirabies vaccination, may develop a clinical form of rabies termed "dumb" or "paralytic" rabies. This form of rabies is characterized by an acute ascending symmetric or asymmetric paralysis leading to respiratory and bulbar paralysis.

Diagnostic Procedures.

1. The presence of any rabies antibody in a nonimmunized patient or the presence of high serum neutralizing antibody titers or significant antibody levels in the cerebrospinal fluid of an immunized patient are evidence of rabies infection.
2. It may be possible to demonstrate rabies antigen by specific immunofluorescence of cutaneous nerve fibers in corneal smears or around hair follicles.
3. Brain biopsy may reveal the presence of rabies antigen by immunofluorescence or the presence of Negri bodies.
4. The cerebrospinal fluid is usually under increased pressure with a lymphocytic pleocytosis.

Differential Diagnosis.

1. Tetanus. Tetanus may be distinguished from furious rabies by the presence of rigidity between muscle spasms and a shorter incubation period between the bite or wound and onset of symptoms in tetanus. The cerebrospinal fluid is normal, and there is lack of hydrophobia in the tetanus patient.
2. Postinfectious encephalomyelitis. This syndrome typically appears two weeks after the first dose of vaccine administration.

Treatment.

1. All animal bites should be thoroughly treated. The wound should be vigorously flushed and scrubbed with a 20 percent soap solution. Tetanus prophylaxis and measures to control bacterial infection may be necessary.

2. Human diploid cell rabies vaccine (HDCV) is currently the treatment of choice.

a. Preexposure dosage. Individuals such as veterinarians who have a high risk of exposure to rabies virus should receive three 1 ml IM injections of HDCV, the second dose one week after the first and the third two or three weeks after the second. Serum antibody levels should be determined two to three weeks after the last dose of vaccine to be sure of a satisfactory response. A booster dose of 1 ml IM every two years is recommended when there is a continuing risk of exposure to rabies (52, 53).

b. Postexposure dosage. Human rabies immune globulin (HRIG) should be administered in a dose of 20 μ/kg, with half the dose infiltrated at the site of the wound, and the rest given IM. At the same time a 1-ml dose of HDCV should be given IM and repeated on days 3, 7, 14 and 28 after the first dose. A previously immunized person with demonstrated rabies antibody who is exposed to rabies should receive two doses of 1 ml of HDCV, one immediately and one three days after. Human rabies immune globulin is not indicated for such patients.

3. Those involved in patient care should be vaccinated and wear face masks, gloves, and gowns when in contact with the patient.

4. Rabies should be treated in an intensive care unit. Patients require careful monitoring of cardiovascular and pulmonary function, electrolytes, and parenteral fluids. The intense distress caused by hydrophobia can be reduced by adequate doses of a phenothiazine.

Prognosis. There are case reports of patients who have survived rabies. Unfortunately, the vast majority succumb to the disease.

Infection with Human Immunodeficiency Virus (HIV or HTLV-III)

The acquired immunodeficiency syndrome (AIDS) is frequently accompanied by infection of the nervous system and the human immune deficiency virus clearly possesses neurotropic properties.

Etiology and Pathology. The syndrome is transmitted by contact with infected body fluids and is more common among homosexual males and intravenous drug users. The virus enters the central nervous system at an early stage and neurologic infection may occur prior to the development of immunodeficiency.

Four distinct neurologic disorders have been recognized (54, 55):

1. Aseptic meningitis.
2. Subacute encephalitis (AIDS dementia complex) (56).
3. Peripheral neuropathy (57).
   a. Chronic symmetrical distal neuropathy.
   b. Chronic inflammatory neuropathy.
4. Vacuolar myelopathy.
5. Other neurologic conditions such as polymyositis, acute leukoencephalitis, and granulomatous angiitis are rare.

In addition, neurologic complications including opportunistic infections and primary lymphoma are frequently seen among patients with AIDS (see Figure 16–4).

The histopathology of subacute encephalitis consists of gliosis demyelination, focal tissue necrosis, microglial nodules, multinucleated giant cells, and perivascular inflammation. The axonal neuropathy is characterized by axonal loss, secondary demyelination, and mild inflammation. The chronic inflammatory neuropathy shows marked inflammation, demyelination, and secondary axonal loss. There is vacuolar degeneration of posterior and lateral columns in the vacuolar myelopathy.

Clinical Features. Aseptic meningitis presents with headache, fever, nuchal rigidity, and cranial nerve palsies.

Subacute encephalitis is characterized by progressive intellectual and cognitive deterioration with memory loss, depression, psychomotor slowing, corticospinal tract signs, ataxia, incontinence, myoclonus, and seizures. Survival time varies from several months to one year.

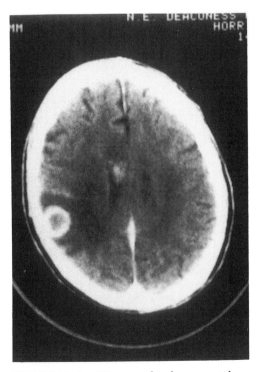

FIGURE 16–4. CT scan with enhancement showing a peripheral and a periventricular lymphoma in a case of AIDS.

The axonal type of peripheral neuropathy is associated with painful dysesthesias, numbness and paresthesias of all four limbs and autonomic dysfunction.

Chronic inflammatory neuropathy is a more diffuse disease with muscle weakness, polymononeuropathies, cranial nerve palsies, hyporeflexia, or areflexia. Occasionally a more acute form occurs and resembles postinfectious polyneuritis (Guillain Barré syndrome).

The vacuolar myelopathy is usually associated with subacute encephalitis and 90 percent of cases have dementia. The myelopathy results in lower limb weakness and ataxia, corticospinal tract and posterior column deficits and incontinence.

Diagnostic Procedures.

1. Magnetic resonance and CT scans show the presence of atrophy in subacute encephalitis with scattered areas of white matter involvement best demonstrated by MR scanning (58).
2. Lumbar puncture. The cerebrospinal fluid is abnormal in aseptic meningitis and subacute encephalitis with the presence of a mononuclear pleocytosis and an elevated protein content.
3. Serological tests for HIV infection are positive. The virus may be cultured from the cerebrospinal fluid.
4. Infection of the brain and spinal cord by opportunistic organisms must be excluded.

Treatment. There is no effective treatment at this time. Zidovudine (AZT) may delay the development and slow the progression of the disease (59).

Reye Syndrome

Definition. Reye syndrome is an acute encephalopathy that occurs predominantly in children and follows an antecedent viral illness.

Etiology and Pathology. Reye syndrome usually follows infections by influenza A or B, varicella, *H. simplex*, and paramyxovirus. Other possible causes include the combined effect of a virus infection and use of salicylates. There are characteristic pathologic changes including cerebral edema, proliferation of smooth endoplasmic reticulum, and morphologically abnormal mitochondria, which are most marked in the neurons (60). The abdominal viscera and liver are heavily infiltrated with fat, and there is mitochondrial damage in the liver cells. It is probable that the mitochondrial abnormalities affecting the brain and liver cells are the crucial pathologic changes in Reye syndrome. There is reduced activity of two of the mitochondrial urea cycle enzymes, carbamyl phosphate synthetase and ornithine transcarbamylase (61).

Clinical Features. The onset is acute. The syndrome usually presents in a child who is apparently recovering from influenza, varicella, or an upper respiratory infection. There are five stages:

1. Onset with lethargy and protracted vomiting.
2. Progressive impairment of consciousness with hallucinations, combative behavior and hyperventilation; seizures may occur.
3. Coma with intermittent decerebrate rigidity occurring spontaneously or on mimnimal stimulation; brain stem reflexes intact.
4. Coma with decerebrate rigidity, hyperventilation, and absence of brain stem reflexes.
5. Coma, respiratory failure, death.

Diagnostic Procedures.

1. Liver function tests are abnormal. Serum glutamic-oxaloacetic transaminase (SGOT) and serum glutamate pyruvate transaminase (SGPT) levels are elevated.
2. Serum glucose levels are low, and hypoglycemia occurs in some cases.
3. The plasma prothrombin time is prolonged.
4. Serum ammonia levels are elevated above 50 mg/100 ml.
5. The electroencephalogram shows symmetric slowing. Serial records are useful in assessing the course of the illness.
6. Either MR or CT scanning shows evidence of cerebral edema with decreased density in the white matter in both hemispheres.
7. There are no abnormalities in the CSF, but the glucose content may be low in the presence of hypoglycemia. Lumbar puncture should not be performed in cases with suspected increased intracranial pressure.
8. The diagnosis can be confirmed by liver biopsy, but this is not usually necessary.

Treatment. When a child is not arousable to verbal or painful stimuli, the following measures should be taken:

1. The child should be intubated with a low-pressure nasotracheal tube and placed on a mechanical respirator.

2. The mechanical respirator should be regulated to produce controlled hyperventilation, maintaining a carbon dioxide tension of 25 mmHg.
3. The prothrombin time or partial thromboplastin time should be determined. If these times are prolonged, fresh frozen plasma should be given to reduce risk of bleeding when an intracranial monitor device is inserted.
4. A ventricular or subdural pressure monitoring device should be inserted, and intracranial pressure should be continuously recorded.
5. If intracranial pressure exceeds 20 mmHg, mannitol 0.25 gm/kg should be given IV.
6. The serum osmolality should be maintained below 320 mOsm/L and should be measured every two hours.
7. A neuromuscular blocking agent such as pancuronium should be administered under the supervision of an anesthesiologist if the intracranial pressure remains elevated or the patient cannot tolerate the respirator. A neurologic examination is performed immediately before the use of the neuromuscular blocking agent, which can be discontinued briefly when further neurologic assessment is required.
8. The body temperature should be maintained below 37°C using a refrigerated blanket.
9. A Foley catheter should be inserted and the intake and output monitored.
10. Fluid and electrolyte balance should be maintained.
11. The central venous pressure and arterial pressure should be monitored.
12. Hypertonic glucose 15 to 20 percent should be given intravenously to maintain the serum glucose level between 150 and 200 mg/dl.
13. Insulin 1 unit per 10-gram glucose should be infused every four hours. The dose of insulin should be regulated to maintain glucose levels between 150 and 200 mg/dl. Glucose levels should be measured every four hours.
14. Neomycin enemas should be given to reduce serum ammonia levels.
15. The lungs should be checked frequently. Postural drainage and suctioning should be performed every two hours, or more frequently if necessary.
16. Barbiturate coma should be considered in those rare cases where intracranial pressure cannot be controlled (see p. 54).

Prognosis. Children recovering from clinical stages 1, 2, or 3 are usually neurologically normal. Recovery from stages 4 and 5 may be followed by permanent neurologic deficits, including spasticity, hemiparesis, dystonia, involuntary movements and seizures. Recurrence of Reye syndrome is rare.

SLOW VIRAL INFECTIONS

A slow viral infection is a disease process with a long latent period lasting months to years, followed by a protracted clinical course that invariably culminates in death.

There are several slow viral infections of the central nervous system; the three most important are subacute sclerosing panencephalitis, progressive multifocal leukoencephalopathy, and Jakob-Creutzfeldt disease.

Subacute Sclerosing Panencephalitis (SSPE)

Definition. The condition is a chronic progressive panencephalitis believed to be caused by measles or a measles-like virus.

Etiology and Pathology. It is believed to result from an infection by an abnormal or mutated measles virus (62), an abnormal host response to measles virus, or activation of a latent measles virus by unknown factors. The disease primarily involves white matter; inclusion bodies are prominent in the early stages, while demyelination and sclerosis are later features of the disease.

Clinical Features. The incidence of SSPE is one per million. It is three times more likely to occur in men than women, and more than 50 percent of those affected had an overt attack of measles before the age of two years.

The onset of SSPE usually occurs between 5 and 15 years of age. There are four stages in the progression of the disease:

1. Deterioration in school performance, personality change, speech difficulty, seizures, papilledema
2. Myoclonus, ataxia, spasticity, choreoathetosis, and ocular signs including cortical blindness, optic atrophy, and chorioretinitis
3. Marked mental deterioration, coma, decorticate posturing, decerebrate rigidity
4. A terminal phase of hypotonia with an exaggerated startle response to noise.

Course. The course is characterized by progressive deterioration, with death occurring three months to three years after the initial symptoms. Remissions lasting for a few weeks and occasionally for a few years have been reported. The younger the patient, the most likely remissions will occur.

Diagnostic Procedures.

1. High antibody titers to measles virus are found in both serum and cerebrospinal fluid. There is a marked increase in IgG in the CSF and measles virus particles have been demonstrated in the CSF by scanning electron microscopy.
2. The electroencephalogram shows a characteristic pattern of burst-suppression consisting of bursts of high amplitude theta activity occurring on a background of low-voltage activity.
3. Brain biopsy. Brain biopsy reveals involvement of white matter and inclusion bodies.

Treatment. There are reports that isoprinosine (Inosiplex) or amantidine has produced remissions, but the disease is invariably fatal.

Progressive Rubella Panencephalitis (PRP) and Russian Spring-Summer Panencephalitis (RSSP)

Progressive rubella panencephalitis and Russian spring-summer panencephalitis are similar to SSPE in that the clinical signs of the disease appear after a long latent period following congenital rubella encephalitis and Russian spring-summer encephalitis, respectively. The PRP commonly occurs in the 8-to-12-year age group, while signs of RSSP appear approximately 13 years after the initial infection. Both show pathologic evidence of encephalitis. The course is similar to SSPE.

Progressive Multifocal Leukoencephalopathy

Progressive multifocal leukoencephalopathy is a multifocal demyelinating disease that has been reported as a nonmetastatic complication of neoplasia. It also occurs in immunosuppressed patients with leukemia, lymphoma, tuberculosis, sarcoidosis or AIDS, and following renal transplant. The disease is thought to result from a depressed cell-mediated immune response to papoviruses.

The pathologic changes consist of areas containing numerous atypical cells showing enlarged nuclei with smudged or coarse clumped chromatin. There are numerous areas of demyelination with preservation of axons. Clinical features include progressive dementia, visual loss, and spastic quadriparesis. Death occurs less than a year after the onset of symptoms. The electroencephalo-

gram shows progressive slowing of activity over both hemispheres. The virus has been isolated from the cerebrospinal fluid.

Magnetic resonance scanning shows extensive white matter lesions bilaterally. The diagnosis is established by brain biopsy. Treatment with cytosine arabinoside or IT B interferon may delay or arrest progression of the disease (63).

Jakob-Creutzfeldt Disease

Definition. Jakob-Creutzfeldt disease (J-C disease) is a rapidly progressive spongiform encephalopathy of the central nervous system.

Etiology and Pathology. J-C disease has been transmitted to primates and man. A corneal transplant recipient and a neurosurgeon are reported to have acquired the disease from known cases. The infectious agent is thought to be a slow virus (prion) (64). Pathologic changes consist of severe generalized neuronal degeneration and astrocytic proliferation, which produces a spongy appearance in the brain.

Clinical Features. J-C disease is a rare condition that occurs sporadically in the 35-to-63-year-old group and has a worldwide distribution. The earliest symptoms include progressive loss of recent memory, dysphasia, and hallucinations. There is rapid deterioration to severe dementia, cortical blindness, and ataxia. Myoclonus is a feature of the later stages of the disease. The duration varies from six months to three years, but 80 percent die within the first year (65).

Diagnostic Procedures.

1. Magnetic resonance and CT scanning shows moderate symmetric cortical atrophy.
2. The electroencephalogram shows bursts of high voltage spike and slow wave activity.
3. The cerebrospinal fluid is usually normal, but the protein content may be elevated in some cases.
4. Brain biopsy. Brain biopsy reveals spongioform changes.

Treatment. There is no effective treatment for J-C disease.

Postinfectious Encephalomyelitis

Definition. Postinfectious encephalomyelitis (PIE) is a demyelinating disease believed to be an autoimmune response to a systemic viral disease, particularly exanthematous infections.

Etiology and Pathology.

The condition occurs most frequently after infection with measles virus and is estimated to complicate one in a thousand cases of measles. It can also occur after rubella varicella and mumps. The virus does not invade the central nervous system but infects lymphoid cells, causing abnormalities in the immune system that are directed against myelin in the brain and spinal cord (52).

The brain and spinal cord show the presence of perivascular cuffing with lymphocytes and plasma cells and scattered areas of perivascular demyelination. The primary lesion is believed to be a vasculopathy, and discrete areas of hemorrhage are seen in some cases. The condition has a similar pathologic appearance to experimental allergic encephalomyelitis.

Clinical Features. The majority of cases of PIE follow infection with the mumps virus. There has been a decrease in the incidence of PIE, which can be attributed to increased vaccination and immunization against infectious diseases. The onset usually occurs within a week of clinical evidence of infection, but the first symptoms have been reported before any signs of infection and as long as two to three months after infection. The onset is abrupt with headache, fever, anorexia, and lethargy. The subsequent course shows considerable variation. The illness may resemble a mild encephalitis with complete recovery, or there may be rapid progression to stupor and coma. Psychiatric symptoms consisting of personality changes, hallucinations, or acute paranoia are not uncommon. Seizures, sensory or motor disturbances, or dysfunction of bladder or bowel may occur.

Differential Diagnosis. Multiple sclerosis. The disseminated involvement of the central nervous system in PIE produces a clinical picture that mimics multiple sclerosis. The development of symptoms following a documented infection suggests the diagnosis of PIE.

Diagnostic Procedures.

1. Lumbar puncture. The cerebrospinal fluid is clear with normal or slightly elevated pressure. There is a lymphocytic pleocytosis, and red blood cells are present in some cases. The protein and gamma globulin contents are elevated; the glucose content is normal.
2. Electroencephalography. The EEG is abnormal in severe cerebral involvement

with diffuse slowing in the theta and delta range.

Treatment. Poly ICLC (polyinosinic–polycytidylic acid—polylysine stabilized with carboxymethylcellulose) has been suggested to be beneficial in treatment. High doses of steroids are beneficial in the early stages of the illness.

Prognosis. The mortality may be as high as 20 percent in PIE following measles. Permanent neurologic deficits occur in 30 to 50 percent of patients.

Acute Hemorrhagic Encephalomyelitis

Definition. Acute hemorrhagic encephalomyelitis is an acute, rapidly progressive demyelinating disease probably resulting from an allergic or hyperimmune process in the central nervous system.

Etiology and Pathology. Acute hemorrhagic encephalomyelitis usually follows a viral or bacterial infection and may be a manifestation of a Shwartzman reaction. The brain is swollen and shows the presence of numerous petechial hemorrhages, or hematoma formation may occur. Microscopic changes consist of necrosis of blood vessel walls and the passage of a fibrinous exudate into the perivascular spaces. There are marked white matter edema and infiltration of abnormal areas with inflammatory cells. The affected blood vessels may be surrounded by areas of necrosis and demyelination or ball or ringlike hemorrhage.

Clinical Features. The disease occurs at any age. Most cases are preceded by an upper respiratory infection, but other prodromal illnesses including the xanthemata, septicemia, pneumonia, and *H. simplex* have been reported. The prodromal symptoms often subside to be followed by clouding of consciousness, hemiplegia, dysphasia, seizures, cranial nerve palsies, and urinary incontinence. There is a high fever, and papilledema may be present.

Diagnostic Procedures.

1. The blood count shows a polymorphonuclear leukocytosis, and the sedimentation rate is elevated.
2. Cerebrospinal fluid findings vary from normal to highly abnormal. There are usually a polymorphonuclear pleocytosis, a normal glucose level, and an elevated protein content, which may be as high as 1,000 mg per 100 ml.
3. The diagnosis may be established by brain biopsy.

Differential Diagnosis. Acute purulent meningitis, acute viral encephalitis, brain abscess, epidural empyema, and lead encephalopathy should be considered.

Treatment. Large doses of corticosteroids have been advocated. Surgical decompression may be necessary when there is a dramatic rise in intracranial pressure.

Prognosis. This is a rapidly fatal disease in the majority of cases, but complete recovery has been reported following the use of corticosteroids.

Behçet's Disease

Definition. Behçet's disease is a clinical syndrome characterized by recurrent aphthous ulceration of the mouth and genitalia, posterior uveitis, cutaneous vasculitis, synovitis, and meningoencephalitis (66).

Etiology and Pathology. The etiology is unknown, but the condition is believed to be related to a viral infection.

The brain shows the presence of perivascular infiltration with neuronal loss and demyelination.

Clinical Features. Behçet's disease usually occurs in young adults. It is characterized by recurrent aphthous ulceration affecting the mouth and genitalia, and at least one of the following: posterior uveitis, cutaneous vasculitis, and synovitis. Colitis, thrombophlebitis, and large artery aneurysms have been reported.

Involvement of the nervous system is an early feature of disease and there is no characteristic clinical presentation. Any portion of the neuraxis may be involved. It may present as an aseptic meningitis or a severe, frequently fatal meningoencephalomyelitis. Intracranial hypertension, papilledema, intracerebral hemorrhage, or cerebral venous thrombosis may occur, and peripheral neuropathy has been reported (67). Relapses are frequent.

Diagnostic Procedures. There is no specific diagnostic test for Behçet's disease. The cerebrospinal fluid is frequently under increased pressure, with a lymphocytic pleocytosis and elevated protein content. Skin biopsy shows the presence of a leukocytoblastic vasculitis or a neutrophilic vascular reaction.

Differential Diagnosis.

1. Mollaret's meningitis. There is a history of recurrent meningitis but no history of recurrent aphthous ulceration.
2. Vogt-Koyanagi's syndrome. This syndrome consists of uveitis, retinal edema,

and meningoencephalitis. Alopecia and vitiligo are often present, and there is ulceration of the mouth or genitalia.
3. Inflammatory, granulomatous infections including tuberculosis, syphilis, and sarcoidosis.
4. *Herpes simplex.* This condition can be distinguished by elevated serum antibody titers to *H. simplex* and isolation of the virus by brain biopsy.

Treatment.

1. Corticosteroids, prednisone 100 mg q.d., are effective if given early.
2. Immunosuppression using azothiaprine, cyclophosphamide, chlorambusil, or cyclosporin A have been effective in cases with severe ocular and meningoencephalitic involvement.

Uveomeningoencephalic Syndrome (Vogt-Koyanagi's Syndrome)

The uveomeningoencephalic syndrome is a rare disorder characterized by progressive uveitis, meningoencephalitis, pigmentary loss of the skin and hair, and impaired hearing. The etiology is unknown. The arachnoid over the base of the brain is thickened and infiltrated with lymphocytes and histiocytes. The temporal lobes are frequently affected and show the presence of necrosis and secondary gliosis. Steroid therapy has been reported to be effective in controlling the condition. Eye involvement should be vigorously treated in an effort to avoid glaucoma and blindness.

Benign Recurrent Aseptic Meningitis (Mollaret's Meningitis)

Definition. Mollaret's meningitis is a rare, recurrent meningitis of uncertain etiology in which the patient shows complete recovery between attacks.

Etiology and Pathology. The etiology of Mollaret's is uncertain. It may be a recurrent meningeal reaction to Epstein-Barr virus (68). Pathologic changes have not been reported.

Clinical Features. The reported cases of the disorder have occurred in all ages and both sexes. The disorder consists of brief (2- to 7-day) recurrent attacks of headache and meningeal irritation. The attacks may be accompanied by fever, myalgias, nausea, and vomiting. Change in mentation, focal neurologic deficits, seizure, and coma can occur. The attacks are of variable intensity, and the patient is symptom-free between attacks. The condition resolves completely after a prolonged period of recurrent attacks (1–11 years).

Diagnostic Procedures.

1. Lumbar puncture. The cerebrospinal fluid is clear with a pleocytosis composed initially of large endothelial-like cells, which have irregular borders and lyse rapidly. These cells are eventually replaced by lymphocytes. There are a mild elevation in protein content, elevated gamma globulin, and a decrease in glucose content.

2. There may be a peripheral eosinophilia.

Differential Diagnosis. The differential diagnosis includes posttraumatic relapsing meningitis, meningitis secondary to chronic otitis or sinusitis, Behçet's disease, sarcoidosis, granulomatous meningitis, and meningitis secondary to parasitic infection and neoplasm.

Treatment. The treatment is symptomatic, and there is a rapid and complete recovery. The prognosis is excellent.

Arachnoiditis

Definition. Arachnoiditis is a chronic inflammation and fibrosis of the leptomeninges, usually occurring in the spinal canal and occasionally in the cranial cavity.

Etiology and Pathology. Arachnoiditis has been described following myelography using both water-soluble and oil contrast media. Chronic inflammation of the leptomeninges is more likely to occur following repeated myelographic studies, and it is possible that the injection of a mixture of contrast media and blood during a traumatic lumbar puncture increases the risk of arachnoiditis. There are also occasional reports of arachnoiditis following injection of antibiotics into the subarachnoid space and following spinal anesthesia. Arachnoiditis has been reported following trauma to the spinal column and spinal canal, and local arachnoiditis is not unusual at the site of a ruptured intervertebral disk. Chronic inflammatory change in the leptomeninges may follow an acute purulent meningitis or may be related to chronic infections including syphilis, tuberculosis, sarcoidosis, and fungal meningitis. Localized arachnoiditis may occur at the site of tuberculosis of a vertebral body (Pott's disease). Arachnoiditis has also been reported following subarachnoid hemorrhage, and three are rare reports of arachnoiditis in patients suffering from ankylostomiasis and ascariasis. The relationship between these conditions and arachnoiditis is not clear.

Pathologic changes consist of thickening of the leptomeninges and monocytic infiltration or granulomatous inflammation with vascular proliferation. The blood vessels are involved by an arteritis or phlebitis. The presence of thickened leptomeninges may produce constriction of nerve roots or pressure on the spinal cord. This may be compounded by ischemia of the spinal cord with circumscribed areas of necrosis and fibrosis.

Clinical Features. The chief complaint is usually weakness of the lower limbs, which may progress to severe paraparesis or paraplegia. The appearance of weakness is followed by complaints of pain, which may be of two types, a burning pain in the distribution of affected nerve roots, or a more ill-defined pain below the level of the compression. In addition, patients may complain of numbness, "deadness," and coldness in the lower limbs and trunk below the level of the arachnoiditis. Disturbances of micturition are early symptoms, and many patients develop complete incontinence. Examination shows the presence of spastic paraparesis with increased reflexes and extensor plantar responses. Sensation to pain and temperature is impaired below the level of the spinal cord compression, and posterior column involvement produces impairment of vibration and position sense.

Diagnostic Procedures.

1. X-rays of the spine may show the presence of destruction of the vertebral bodies in cases of tuberculosis.

2. Lumbar puncture reveals a spinal fluid of reduced pressure with a positive Queckenstedt test in cases of complete spinal block. The fluid is often xanthochromic, and the protein content is markedly elevated.

3. The study of choice is MR scanning. It is nontraumatic and is as effective as plain film myelography or CT myelography in the demonstration of lumbar arachnoiditis (69).

Treatment. Suspected infection should be effectively treated with antibiotics. Compression of the spinal cord should be relieved surgically in cases of localized arachnoiditis. Patients with diffuse arachnoiditis may benefit from a course of corticosteroids, which may reduce the inflammatory response. Chronic cases are difficult to treat and may require prolonged use of analgesic drugs. Transcutaneous stimulation may be useful in some cases.

Prognosis. Localized arachnoiditis treated by surgical removal of the leptomeninges usually shows good response to treatment. Patients with severe spinal cord damage can only hope to avoid further deterioration and obtain relief from pain.

REFERENCES

1. Addy, D. P. When not to do a lumbar puncture. Arch. Dis. Child. 62:873–875; 1987.
2. Gowers, D. J.; Baker, A. L.; *et al.* Contraindications to lumbar puncture as defined by computed cranial tomography. J. Neurol. Neurosurg. Psychiatry 50:1071–1074; 1987.
3. Keroack, M. The patient with suspected meningitis. Emerg. Med. Clin. North Am. 5:807–826; 1987.
4. Cann, K. J.; Rogers, T. R.; *et al.* Neisseria meningitidis in a primary school Arch. Dis. Child. 62:1113–1117; 1987.
5. Overturf, G. D.; Cable, D.; *et al.* Ampicillin-Chloramphenoical-resistant haemophilus influenzae: plasmid-mediated resistance in bacterial meningitis. Pediatr. Res. 22:438–441; 1987.
6. Smith, A. L. Pathogenesis of hemophilus influenzae meningitis. Pediatr. Infect. Dis. 6:783–786; 1987.
7. Long, J. G.; Preblud, S. R.; *et al.* Clostridium perfringens meningitis in an infant: case report and literature review. Pediatr. Infect. Dis. 6:752–754; 1987.
8. Rac, A. N. Brain abscess a complication of cocaine inhalation. NY State J. Med. 88:548–550; 1988.
9. Mempalam, T. J.; Rosenblum, M. L. Trends in the management of bacterial brain abscesses: A review of 192 cases over 17 years. Neurosurgery 23:451–458; 1988.
10. Harns, L. F.; Haws, F. P. Subdural empyema and epidural abscess: recent experience in a community hospital. South. Med. J. 80:1254–1258; 1987.
11. Weingarten, K.; Zimmerman, R. D.; *et al.* Subdural and epidural empyemas: Magnetic resonance imaging. AJNR 10:81–87; 1989.
12. Miller, E. S.; Dices, P. S.; *et al.* Management of subdural empyema. A series of 24 cases. J. Neurol. Neurosurg. Psychiatry 50:1415–1418; 1987.
13. Angtuoco, E. J. C.; McConnell, J. R.; *et al.* MR imaging of spinal epidural sepsis. AJR 149:1249–1253; 1987.
14. Mooney, R. P.; Hochberger, R. S. Spinal epidural abscess: a rapidly progressive disease. Ann. Emerg. Med. 16:1168–1170; 1987.
15. Lipman, J.; James, M. E. M.; *et al.* Autonomic dysfunction in severe tetanus: magnesium sulphate as an adjunct to deep sedation. Cont. Care Med. 15:987–988; 1987.
16. Kudrow, D. B.; Henry, D. A.; *et al.* Botulism associated with clostridium botulinum sinusitis

17. St. Louis, M. E.; Peck, S. H. S.; *et al.* Botulism from chopped garlic: delayed recognition of a major outbreak. Ann. Intern. Med. 108:363–368; 1988.
18. Mousa, A. R. M.; Kosky, T. S.; *et al.* Brucella meningitis: Presentation, diagnosis and treatment—a prospective study of ten cases. Q. J. Med. 60:873–885; 1986.
19. Shakir, R. A. Neurobrucellosis. Postgrad. Med. J. 62:1077–1079; 1987.
20. Halperin, J. J.; Little, B. W.; *et al.* Lyme disease: cause of a treatable peripheral neuropathy. Neurology 37:1700–1706; 1987.
21. Barbour, A. G. The diagnosis of lyme disease: Rewards and perils. Ann. Intern. Med. 110:501–502; 1989.
22. Diringer, M.; Halperin, J. J.; *et al.* Lyme meningoencephalitis: report of a severe penicillin resistant case. Arthritis Rheum. 30:705–708; 1987.
23. Van Eijk, R. V. W.; Wolters, E. Ch.; *et al.* Effect of early and late syphilis on central nervous system: cerebrospinal fluid changes and neurological deficit. Genitourin. Med. 63:77–82; 1987.
24. Rosenfall, U.; Lowhagen, G-B.; *et al.* Oculomotor dysfunction in patients with syphilis. Genitourin. Med. 63:83–86; 1987.
25. Musher, D. M. How much penicillin cures early syphilis? Ann. Intern. Med. 109:849–851; 1988.
26. Adendorff, J. J.; Boeke, E. J.; *et al.* Tuberculosis of the spine: results of management of 300 patients. J. R. Coll. Surg. Edinb. 32:152–155; 1987.
27. Shaw, R. H.; Holt, P. A.; *et al.* Heel pain in sarcoidosis. Ann. Intern. Med. 109:675–677; 1988.
28. Hayes, W. S.; Sherman, J. L.; *et al.* MR and CT evaluation of intracranial sarcoidosis. AJR 149:1043–1049; 1987.
29. Zaki, M. H.; Lyons, H. A.; *et al.* Corticosteroid therapy in sarcoidosis. A five year controlled follow up study. NY State J. Med. 87:496–499; 1987.
30. English, C. K.; Wear, D. J.; *et al.* Cat-scratch disease. Isolation and culture of the bacterial agent. JAMA 259:1347–1352; 1988.
31. Macdonell, R. A. L.; Donnan, G. A.; *et al.* Otocerebral mucormycosis—a case report. Clin. Exp. Neurol. 23:225–232; 1987.
32. Bradley, S. F.; McGuire, N. M.; *et al.* Sino-orbital and cerebral aspergillosis: cure with medical therapy. Mykosen 30:379–385; 1987.
33. Kasantikul, V.; Shuangshoti, S.; *et al.* Primary phycomycosis of the brain in heroin addicts. Surg. Neurol. 28:468–472; 1987.
34. Body, B. A.; Oneson, R. H.; *et al.* Use of cerebrospinal fluid lactic acid concentration in the diagnosis of fungal meningitis. Ann. Clin. Lab. Sci. 17:429–434; 1987.
35. Waterson, J. A.; Gilligan, B. S. Cryptococcal

infections of the central nervous system: a ten

36. Scott, E. N.; Kaufman, L.; *et al.* Serologic studies in the diagnosis and management of meningitis due to Sporothrix schenkeii. New Engl. J. Med. 317:935–940; 1987.
37. Dismukes, W. E.; *et al.* Treatment of cryptococcal meningitis with combination amphoreicin B and flucytosine for four as compared to six weeks. New Engl. J. Med. 317:334–341; 1987.
38. Smego, R. A. Actinomycosis of the central nervous system. Rev. Infect. Dis. 9:855–865; 1987.
39. Hall, W. A.; Martinez, A. J.; *et al.* Nocardial brain abscess: diagnostic and therapeutic use of stereotactic aspiration. Surg. Neurol. 28:114–118; 1987.
40. Danneman, B. R.; Israelski, D.; *et al.* Treatment of toxoplasmic encephalitis with intravenous Clindomycin. Arch. Intern. Med. 148:2477–2482; 1988.
41. Philpott, J.; Keystone, J. S. Severe falciparum malaria. Can. Med. Assoc. J., 137:135–136; 1987.
42. Leblanc, R.; Knowles, K. F. Neurocysticercosis: surgical and medical treatment with Praziquantel. Neurosurgery 18:419–427; 1986.
43. Rawlings, D.; Ferriero, D. M.; *et al.* Early CT re-evaluation after emperic praziquantel therapy in neurocysticercosis. Neurology 34:739–741; 1989.
44. Escobedo, F.; Penagos, P.; *et al.* Albendazole therapy for neurocysticercosis. Arch. Intern. Med. 147:738–741; 1987.
45. Sotelo, J.; Marin, C. Hydrocephalus secondary to cysticercosis arachnoiditis. A long term follow up of 92 cases. J. Neurosurg. 66:686–689; 1987.
46. Earnest, M. P.; Reller, L. B.; *et al.* Neurocysticercosis in the United States: 35 cases and a review. Rev. Infect. Dis. 9:961–979; 1987.
47. Colli, B. O.; Mortelli, N.; *et al.* Results of surgical treatment of neurocysticercosis in 69 cases. J. Neurosurg. 65:309–315; 1986.
48. Pau, A.; Brambilla, M.; *et al.* Long term follow up of the surgical treatment of the intracranial hydrated disease. Acta. Neurochir. (Wien) 88:116–118; 1987.
49. Kennedy, C. R.; Duffy, S. W.; *et al.* Clinical predictors of outcome in encephalitis. Arch. Dis. Child. 62:1156–1162; 1987.
50. Neils, E. W.; Lukin, R.; *et al.* Magnetic resonance imaging and computerized tomography scanning of herpes simplex encephalitis. J. Neurosurg. 67:592–594; 1987.
51. Vanlandigham, K. E.; Marsteller, M. B.; *et al.* Relapse of herpes simplex encephalitis after conventional acyclovir therapy. JAMA 259:1051–1053; 1988.
52. Fishbein, D. B.; Arcangeli, S. Rabies prevention in primary care. A four-step approach. Postgrad. Med. 82:83–90; 1987.

53. Fishbein, D. B.; Pacer, R. E.; *et al.* Rabies preexposure prophylaxis with human diploid cell rabies vaccine—a dose response study. J. Infect. Dis. 156:50–55; 1987.
54. Retroviruses in the nervous system. Proceedings of a symposium sponsored by the National Institutes of Health, Bethesda, Maryland. Ann. Neurol. Suppl 23:1–217; 1988.
55. Gabudza, D. H.; Hirsh, M. S. Neurologic manifestation of infection with human immunodeficiency virus. Clinical features and pathogenesis. Ann. Intern. Med. 107:383–391; 1987.
56. Ho, D. D.; Bredesen, D. E.; *et al.* The acquired immunodeficiency syndrome (AIDS) dementia complex. Ann. Intern. Med. 111:400–410; 1989.
57. Mah, V.; Vartavarian, L. M.; *et al.* Abnormalities on peripheral nerve in patients with human immunodeficiency virus infection. Ann. Neurol. 24:713–717; 1988.
58. Olsen, W. L. White matter disease in AIDS. Findings at MR imaging. Radiology 169:445–448; 1988.
59. Lane, H. C.; Faloon, J.; *et al.* Zidovudine in patients with human immunodeficiency virus (HIV) infection and Kaposi sarcoma. A Phase II randomized, placebo controlled trial. Ann. Intern. Med. 111:41–50; 1989.
60. Daugherty, C. C.; Gartside, P. S.; *et al.* A morphometric study of Reye's Syndrome. Am. J. Pathol. 129:313–326; 1987.
61. Gill, R. A.; Anderson, D. C.; *et al.* Adult Reye's Syndrome: Discordance in hepatic subcellular function testing. Minn. Med. 70:347–354; 1987.
62. Anderson, J.; Ehrnst, A.; *et al.* Visualization of defective measles virus particles in cerebrospinal fluid in subacute sclerosing panencephalitis. J. Infec. Dis. 156:928–933; 1987.
63. Tashiro, K.; Doi, S.; *et al.* Progressive multifocal leukoencephalopathy with magnetic resonance imaging verification and therapeutic trials with interferon. J. Neurol. 234:427–429; 1987.
64. Prusiner, S. B.; DeArmond, S. J. Prions causing nervous system degeneration. Lab. Invest. 56:349–363; 1987.
65. Swanson, T. H. The clinician's guide to Creutzfeldt-Jacob Disease. Henry Ford Hosp. Med. J. 35:76–83; 1987.
66. Jorizzo, J. L. Behçet's Disease. Neurology Clinics 5:427–440; 1987.
67. Namer, I. J.; Karabudak, R.; *et al.* Peripheral nervous system involvement in Behçet's disease. Eur. Neurol. 26:235–240; 1987.
68. Graman, P. S. Mollaret's meningitis associated with acute Epstein-Barr virus mononucleosis. Arch. Neurol. 44:1204–1205; 1987.
69. Ross, J. S.; Masoryk, T. J.; *et al.* MR imaging of lumbar arachnoiditis. AJR 149:1025–1032; 1987.

CHAPTER 17

TOXIC AND METABOLIC DISORDERS

CEREBRAL ANOXIA

Cerebral metabolism is almost totally dependent upon an adequate supply of oxygen and glucose. When glucose is unavailable, the high energy needs of the brain are met by anaerobic metabolism. This is less efficient, but neurologic impairment does not occur. However, as the oxygen content of arterial blood decreases there is a progressive decline in cerebral function. Higher cortical functions, particularly those associated with the frontal lobes of the brain, are the first to be affected. Vegetative functions are not involved until much later. The rate of onset of hypoxia is also important since slower rates, found for example in chronic progressive pulmonary disease, are better tolerated.

Etiology and Pathology. The most frequent causes of cerebral anoxia are listed in Table 17–1. The gray matter of the brain, due to its higher metabolic rate, is the first to be affected. The pathologic changes depend upon the length of time the patient survives after the anoxic episode. If the patient dies immediately, the brain shows acute congestion, dilated blood vessels, and petechial hemorrhages. Survival for two or three days produces additional changes including neuronal loss in the basal ganglia, particularly the globus pallidus and substantia nigra. Longer survival permits the development of cortical degeneration and gliosis. Delayed postanoxic encephalopathy, in which the patient appears to recover and later shows progressive neurologic deterioration, is characterized by diffuse demyelination.

Clinical Features. In acute hypoxia of rapid onset the decline in neurologic function is proportional to the decline in arterial oxygen content. A P_aO_2 of 50 mmHg is associated with decreased mental acuity, impairment of visual acuity, emotional lability, and loss of fine muscle coordination. A further decrease to 40 mmHg produces faulty judgment, analgesia, and a marked lack of coordination. A fall in the P_aO_2 below 32 mmHg produces loss of consciousness followed by decortication, decerebration, and respiratory arrest.

Patients who survive the initial anoxic episode may recover completely or partially with permanent neurologic deficits including intellectual difficulties and posthypoxic intention myoclonus. Patients who have suffered severe anoxia occasionally appear to make a complete recovery followed by a delayed progressive deterioration. The recovery is abruptly interrupted by the onset of irritability, apathy, and withdrawal 7 to 21 days after the anoxic episode. This is followed by the development of rigidity and psychomotor retardation, and there may be a steady progression to decerebration and death (1).

Diagnostic Procedures. The cause of the anoxia must be determined to permit appropriate therapy. If the cause is uncertain, carbon monoxide poisoning, barbiturate poisoning, and drug overdose should be excluded by

TABLE 17–1. Causes of Cerebral Anoxia

1. Decreased inspiration of oxygen: high altitudes, strangulation, drowning

2. Alveolar hypoventilation: anesthesia, postinfectious polyneuritis, myasthenic crisis, poliomyelitis, encephalitis, barbiturate poisoning, heroin, cocaine or other illegal drug overdose, trauma

3. Impaired ventilation perfusion relationship: pneumonia, chronic obstructive pulmonary disease, pulmonary embolism

4. Alveolocapillary block; hyaline membrane disease, interstitial infiltrates

5. Anemia

6. Impaired oxygen dissociation: carbon monoxide poisoning

7. Interference with cellular utilization of oxygen: cyanide poisoning

8. Ischemia: any condition that prevents adequate blood flow to the brain—cardiac arrest, trauma with massive blood loss

determination of carboxyhemoglobin and serum barbiturate levels, and a drug screen. A hemoglobin level, chest x-ray, and arterial blood gases may also provide useful information.

Diagnostic Procedures.

1. Electroencephalography. In patients who survive, the EEG shows generalized slowing in the low theta and delta range followed by gradual increase in theta activity and the appearance of alpha activity in the posterior head regions. Fatal cases show increased slowing of the EEG. In some cases, however, there may be preservation of diffuse theta activity in deep coma (theta coma) or the development of bifrontal or generalized alpha activity (alpha coma). A burst suppression pattern with periodic medium or high voltage 4 to 6 Hz activity interrupted by episodes of low voltage background activity is usually indicative of severe and fatal anoxic encephalopathy (2,3). Focal seizure activity is not unusual in severe hypoxia.

2. Magnetic resonance (MR) and computed tomography (CT) scans will show the presence of cerebral edema in severe anoxic encephalopathy. Diffuse white matter lesions are present in both hemispheres in post anoxic delayed encephalopathy.

Treatment.

1. Any condition contributing to hypoxia should be treated.

2. Increased intracranial pressure should be treated with hyperosmolar agents such as mannitol or glycerol (see page 55).

3. Patients suffering from carbon monoxide poisoning should be given pure oxygen by mask. If a hyperbaric oxygen chamber is available, the patient should be treated with hyperbaric oxygen at two atmospheres.

4. The role of calcium channel blocking agents such as nimodipine in the treatment of anoxia has yet to be clarified (4).

5. Posthypoxic intention myoclonus may respond to treatment with L-5-hydroxytryptophan or clonazepam (see p. 104).

BRAIN DEATH

The availability of mechanical respirators and the remarkable efficiency of these machines are leading to the increased use of mechanical respiratory assistance in the treatment of acute respiratory arrest. Although this procedure is usually lifesaving, it is inevitable that a number of patients given mechanical respiratory assistance have already suffered irreversible brain damage. Other cases suffer further brain damage or "brain death." Modern methods of treatment ensure that vital function, particularly respiratory and cardiac functions, and water and electrolyte balance are under adequate control. In essence this means that many body functions can continue for weeks or even months in a controlled situation despite the presence of brain death. This problem has lead to the establishment of criteria to diagnose irreversible brain damage or "brain death" in order to permit the withdrawal of life support systems when these criteria are met (5,6).

Criteria for Establishing Brain Death

1. There should be no history of drug ingestion or measurable levels of sedatives (barbiturates, hypnotics) in the blood. There should be no evidence of significant metabolic derangement.

2. Spontaneous movements should be absent. There should be no response to intense light, noise, or pain, and the limbs should be flaccid.

3. All brainstem reflexes, including pupillary, corneal, ciliospinal, reflex eye movements on head turning (doll's eye movements), gag, swallowing and coughing,

vestibulo-ocular, and tonic-neck reflexes, should be absent. The blood pressure may show a tendency to be low, and vasoactive compounds may be necessary to maintain it.

4. The body temperature should show a tendency to fall below 98°F when the patient is uncovered.

5. There is absence of spontaneous respiratory movements when $PaCO_2$ is 40 to 45 mmHg. The $PaCO_2$ should be obtained and the patient should receive 100 percent oxygen for 10 minutes before testing. The respirator is then disconnected for 10 minutes while 100 percent oxygen is delivered at 6 L/minute through an endotracheal cannula to prevent hypoxemia. This method produces sufficient rise in $PaCO_2$ to 40 to 45 mmHg to stimulate respirations.

6. Electroencephalography. There is absence of electrical activity greater than 2 μv in amplitude. A competent technician should perform the EEG and use ear electrodes and a minimum of ten scalp electrodes. Artifacts can be identified with the use of an electrocardiographic lead and a dorsal hand lead. The interelectrode resistance should be less than 10,000 ohms and greater than 100 ohms, and the interelectrode distance should be greater than 10 cm. The EEG should be run at standard gains 50 μv/5 mm for 10 minutes and then repeated at twice standard gain for an additional 10 minutes. It is also necessary to run the EEG at the slowest speed with maximum gain for a short time. There should be no response to intense stimuli, including pain, loud noise, and intense light.

When the above criteria are met the patient should be reexamined and the EEG repeated in 24 hours. If the repeat examination again meets the criteria, a diagnosis of irreversible brain damage or brain death has been established.

7. Other procedures including absence of intracranial perfusion by cerebral angiography or radionuclide scintigraphy are reliable but not essential indicators of brain death.

NEUROLOGIC COMPLICATIONS OF ELECTROLYTE DISORDERS

Hyponatremia
Definition. Hyponatremia is an abnormal decrease in serum sodium content.

Etiology and Pathology. Hyponatremia may be characterized by:

1. Increased extracellular fluid volume and edema
   a. Renal failure
   b. Congestive heart failure
   c. Hepatic cirrhosis
2. Normal extracellular fluid volume
   a. The syndrome of inappropriate antidiuretic hormone (SIADH) (see p. 305)
   b. Water intoxication
   c. Therapeutic use of oxytocin or carbamazepine (Tegretol)
3. Decreased extracellular fluid volume
   a. Renal origin: chronic diuretic use, salt-losing nephritis, hypoaldosteronism
   b. Extrarenal origin: burns, vomiting, diarrhea

The lowering of serum sodium content results in passage of fluid into cells and lowering of the intracellular sodium content. There are swelling of cells and some degree of cerebral edema.

Clinical Features. Patients with acute hyponatremia (less than 125 mEq/L) present with extreme fatigue, nausea, vomiting, hypotension, seizure, and coma. Chronic hyponatremia may cause extreme fatigue, weakness, muscle cramps, nausea and vomiting, seizures, and also confusion and delirium, which may be mistaken for a psychiatric illness.

Diagnostic Procedures.

1. The serum sodium level is abnormally low. The serum osmolality is usually low.
2. See page 305 for the characteristics of SIADH.
3. Pseudohyponatremia occurs in hyperlipemia and hyperproteinemia and is identified by elevated serum lipid or protein levels.
4. In acute cases electroencephalography shows diffuse slowing over both hemispheres with irregular high-amplitude activity in the theta range.

Treatment.

1. Hyponatremia with increased extracellular fluid should be managed by fluid restriction.
2. Hyponatremia with normal extracellular fluid volume usually responds to water restriction. Severe cases may require infusion of hypertonic saline solution. Only part of the calculated sodium deficit should be replaced (7).
3. Hyponatremia associated with decreased extracellular fluid volume should be managed by treating the cause of the problem and by replacement with normal saline at a rate of no more than 2 mEq/L per hour to a level of 128 to 130 mEq/L. A more

rapid correction to normal or hypernatremic levels may result in central pontine myelinolysis (8–10).

Hypernatremia

Definition. Hypernatremia is an abnormal increase in serum sodium content.

Etiology and Pathology. Hypernatremia may be caused by:

1. Decreased water intake. Severe dehydration may lead to hypernatremia. This is usually seen in children but can occur in elderly individuals who have significant reduction in maximal urinary concentration and an inadequate thirst response to dehydration (11).
2. Excess sodium intake. This may occur during the administration of parenteral fluids with high saline content postoperatively or following treatment of shock, or during administration of sodium bicarbonate following cardiac arrest, particularly in children.
3. Excess water loss in children with vomiting and diarrhea.
4. Enteral tube feeding or parental supplementation using supplements with a high sodium content.
5. Diabetes Mellitus with diabetic or nonketotic hyperosmolar coma.
6. Damage to osmoreceptors. Hypothalamic damage and consequent hypernatremia occasionally complicate intracranial tumors, including craniopharyngioma; Hand-Christian-Schüller disease; and inflammatory conditions involving the neurohypophysis.

Increased serum osmolality results in fluid shift from the intracellular to the extracellular compartment. This may cause tearing of intracranial vessels and hemorrhage.

Clinical Features. Early somnolence and apathy are followed by stupor, meningismus, and eventually decerebrate rigidity and coma. The course may be punctuated by chorea, myoclonus, or seizure activity.

Diagnostic Procedures. The serum sodium level is abnormally high. Urine volume is decreased, and serum osmolality is usually high.

Treatment. Rapid correction of hypovolemia may lead to water intoxication, shift of fluid into the intracellular space, and subsequent cerebral edema. This can be avoided by replacement of half of the calculated water deficit within the first 24 hours and the remainder over the next two days (12).

Chronic hypernatremia due to hypothalamic dysfunction may respond to the administration of cortisone acetate.

Prognosis. Severe acute hypernatremia has a 40 percent mortality. Approximately 50 percent of the survivors will show neurologic sequelae such as transient choreoathetosis, hemiparesis, mental retardation, or seizures.

Hypokalemia

Definition. Hypokalemia is an abnormal decrease in serum potassium content with a serum potassium less than 3.5 mEq/L.

Etiology and Pathology. Hypokalemia may result from:

1. Inadequate potassium intake, particularly with excessive water intake
2. Alkalosis, which causes a shift of serum potassium into cells
3. Gastrointestinal loss, which occurs with vomiting, diarrhea, and nasogastric suction
4. Renal loss: osmotic diuresis, aldosteronism, renal tubular disease, therapeutic use of diuretics or corticosteroids, and licorice ingestion may result in excessive renal loss of potassium
5. Drug induced: epinephrine, isoproterenol, salbutamol, terbutaline, barium, insulin (13).

Clinical Features. Symptoms do not usually develop until the serum potassium level falls below 3.0 mEq/L. Generalized muscle weakness may be followed by paresthesias, hyporeflexia, confusion, delirium, and tetany. Muscle weakness may be followed by actual paralysis in severe hypokalemia complicating renal disease or intractable vomiting, and acute quadriplegia may occur in diabetic ketoacidosis with hypokalemia. Cardiac arrhythmias such as extrasystoles are not unusual; ventricular tachycardia or fibrillation may occur with rapid onset of hypokalemia (14).

Diagnostic Procedures.

1. Serum potassium levels are abnormally low.
2. Electrocardiographic abnormalities include depression of the S-T segment, prolongation of the Q-T interval, and inverted T waves, followed by the appearance of U waves and fusion of T and U waves.
3. Primary aldosteronism is characterized by low serum potassium and elevated serum sodium levels. Urinary aldosterone exceeds 30 mg in 24 hours. There is a marked fall in urinary potassium clearance

following the administration of spironolactone, with a rise in serum potassium levels.

4. Diagnosis of secondary aldosteronism may be established by demonstrating elevated plasma renin and angiotensin levels in the presence of impaired renal function.

Treatment. The cause of hypokalemia should be corrected whenever possible. Potassium should be replaced orally in doses of 20 to 60 mEq/day. This reduces the risk of hyperkalemia. When intravenous potassium is given, the dosage should not exceed 20 mEq per hour to a total of less than 100 mEq in 24 hours. Administration should always be monitored by serial electrocardiograms and serial serum potassium levels. Primary aldosteronism will respond to resection of the adrenal adenoma.

Hyperkalemia
Definition. Hyperkalemia is an abnormally high serum level of potassium.
Etiology and Pathology. Hyperkalemia may be caused by:

1. Acidosis. Acidosis causes a shift of potassium from the intracellular to the extracellular compartment.
2. Decreased excretion. This occurs in acute renal failure and in adrenal insufficiency.
3. Endogenous and exogenous sources of potassium. Rhabdomyolysis and hemolysis serve as endogenous sources of hyperkalemia, while ingestion of foods high in potassium is an exogenous source.
4. Acute fluoride intoxication causing potassium efflux from cells (15).

Clinical Features. Hyperkalemia results in weakness and paresthesias, eventually paralysis and cardiac and respiratory arrest.
Diagnostic Procedures. The serum potassium level is abnormally high. Electrocardiography may reveal depressed S-T segments, peaked T waves, prolonged P-R intervals, and widening of the QRS complexes.
Treatment. Severe hyperkalemia may be treated with calcium gluconate, sodium bicarbonate, or cation-exchange resin therapy. Dialysis is also an effective method of treatment.

Hypomagnesemia
Definition. Hypomagnesemia is an abnormal decrease in serum magnesium content.

Etiology and Pathology. Hypomagnesemia may be caused by:

1. Inadequate intake of magnesium. This occurs with the prolonged use of intravenous fluid therapy without magnesium replacement.
2. Excess gastrointestinal loss due to prolonged diarrhea, vomiting, or continuous nasogastric suction.
3. Failure of absorption of magnesium due to intestinal obstruction, steatorrhea, or any of the malabsorptive syndromes. Bowel resection may be followed by hypomagnesemia.
4. Excess loss of magnesium through the kidney, prolonged use of mercurial diuretics, and withdrawal from alcohol in the chronic alcoholic may be followed by excessive magnesium excretion and hypomagnesemia.
5. Metabolic causes of hypomagnesemia include diabetic acidosis, porphyria, and pancreatitis. Hyperaldosteronism, hypoparathyroidism, and hyperthyroidism are often associated with hypomagnesemia.

Hypocalcemia and hypomagnesemia often occur together, in conditions such as alcoholic liver disease where hypomagnesemia induces hypoparathyroidism and hypocalcemia. Magnesium is necessary for intracellular enzymatic activity. Hypomagnesemia increases cellular membrane excitability and enhances synaptic transmission.
Clinical Features. Weakness, progressive confusion, irritability, agitation with lack of sleep, muscle twitchings, and myoclonus may be present and may be followed by seizures. Other patients show the presence of tremors, generalized hyperreflexia, personality changes, and choreoathetoid movements. There is often marked tachycardia, and Chvostek and Trousseau signs are present.
Diagnostic Procedures. Serum magnesium levels are abnormally low.
Treatment.

1. The cause of hypomagnesemia should be eliminated. If intravenous therapy is required, the patient should be treated with magnesium sulfate 2 g (16 mEq) in a 10 percent solution over a 15-minute period. Oral therapy consists of one to two, 10 grain (35 mEq) tablets per day.
2. Serial serum magnesium levels should be obtained to avoid the development of hypermagnesemia.

Hypermagnesemia

Hypermagnesemia is an abnormally high serum level of magnesium. It is most commonly the result of injudicious use of magnesium-containing pharmaceuticals (laxatives, etc.) in a patient with renal failure. The patient develops nausea and vomiting followed by muscular weakness, drowsiness, and eventually coma. Treatment, consisting of intravenous calcium gluconate, may be required in severe cases.

NEUROLOGIC COMPLICATIONS OF ORGAN DYSFUNCTION

NEUROLOGIC COMPLICATIONS OF RENAL DYSFUNCTION

The neurologic manifestations of renal disorders consist of uremic encephalopathy, uremic neuropathy, and the neurologic complications of chronic hemodialysis and renal transplantation.

Uremic Encephalopathy

Definition. Uremic encephalopathy is an encephalopathy that results from the effect of the metabolic changes accompanying kidney failure.

Etiology and Pathology. The etiology of uremic encephalopathy is unknown. The rapid resolution of signs and symptoms during dialysis suggests that small water-soluble molecules normally excreted through the kidney cross the blood-brain barrier and alter central nervous system metabolism.

There are no characteristic pathologic changes. Cerebral neuronal degeneration and necrosis of the granular cell layer of the cerebellar cortex have been described but are likely to be the result of preterminal hypoxia.

Clinical Features. The earliest signs of uremic encephalopathy are decreased alertness and awareness associated with apathy, fatigue, and poor concentration. Later in the course, perceptual disorders characterized by illusions and hallucinations may occur, and the patient may become agitated or psychotic.

Asterixis is an early feature in uremic encephalopathy and is usually accompanied by an irregular action and postural tremor. Release phenomena consisting of paratonia, sucking, rooting, and grasp reflexes appear later in the course of the disease, and meningismus may be present. Progressive visual loss with papilledema can occur in patients with uremic anemia and elevated blood pressure (16). As the disorder progresses, the patient becomes stuporous, then comatose, with myoclonus and tetany in some cases. Generalized tonic-clonic seizures are a late feature and are more characteristic of uremic encephalopathy than any other metabolic encephalopathies.

Diagnostic Procedures.

1. The standard indices of renal function, such as the blood urea nitrogen and serum creatinine, are *not* reliable predictors of the clinical course in uremic encephalopathy.
2. The electroencephalogram shows progressive, symmetric slowing of the background activity and paroxysmal bursts of slow wave activity in the anterior head regions.
3. The cerebrospinal fluid is clear and under normal pressure. There are a mild lymphocytic pleocytosis and an elevated protein content.

Differential Diagnosis.

1. Acute water intoxication. This is often coexistent and is characterized by low serum osmolality (<260 mOsm/L) and low serum sodium levels (<120 mEq/L).
2. Hypertensive encephalopathy. A history of hypertension, papilledema, and normal or minimally elevated blood urea nitrogen and serum creatinine is suggestive of hypertensive encephalopathy.

Treatment.

1. Seizures should be controlled with phenytoin (Dilantin). Serum levels of phenytoin are depressed in uremia, and seizure control may be achieved with low serum levels.
2. Slow dialysis is the definitive treatment for uremic encephalopathy. The procedure requires careful monitoring since the blood-brain barrier is slowly permeable to urea and rapid dialysis may result in water intoxication.

Uremic Neuropathy

Definition. Uremic neuropathy is characterized by distal, symmetric sensorimotor loss, which occurs predominantly in the lower limbs and affects the majority of patients with chronic renal failure.

Etiology and Pathology. The etiology of uremic neuropathy is uncertain at this time. The conditon may be due to retention of toxic metabolite or high levels of parathormone. Pathologic changes in uremic neuropathy consist of primary axonal degeneration with secondary demyelination.

Clinical Features. One of the most common symptom complexes occurring in uremic neuropathy is the "restless leg syndrome." Eventually a distal, symmetric sensorimotor neuropathy develops. Autonomic involvement may occur. The course may vary and is slowly progressive in the majority of cases. Flaccid quadriplegia is a rare complication in untreated cases.

Diagnostic Procedures. Electrophysiologic studies reveal reduced sensory and motor nerve conduction velocities and increased distal latencies. Evoked potentials show decreased amplitude, secondary peaks, and increased latency.

Differential Diagnosis. The differential diagnosis of uremic neuropathy is that of a distal symmetric sensorimotor neuropathy.

Treatment.

1. The treatment of choice is renal transplantation. Adequate dialysis may stabilize or slowly improve the clinical situation.
2. Cholestyramine, 5 mg b.i.d. or q.i.d. may reduce constant irritation in the restless leg syndrome. Carbidopa/levodopa (Sinemet) and clonidine are also effective in some cases of restless leg syndrome. Codeine 30 mg will usually abolish the abnormal sensation and movements but should be reserved for cases of a temporary nature.

Neurologic Complications of Dialysis

The neurologic complications of dialysis consist of the dysequilibrium syndrome, an increased incidence of intracranial bleeding, and dialysis encephalopathy.

Dysequilibrium Syndrome. The dysequilibrium syndrome is believed to occur as a result of shift of water into the brain during dialysis. The syndrome occurs toward the end of dialysis (17), with nausea, vomiting, headache, disorientation, convulsions and loss of consciousness indicating the presence of increased intracranial pressure. Continuous ventricular drainage and ICP monitoring will avoid uncal herniation during dialysis in these patients.

Intracranial Bleeding. There is an increased risk of intracranial bleeding during dialysis, which is probably related to systemic heparinization, hypertension, and arteriolopathy. Fifteen to 25 percent of chronic dialysis patients die of intracranial hemorrhages.

Dialysis Dementia. Dialysis dementia is a progressive, invariably fatal encephalopathy that occurs in patients undergoing chronic hemodialysis.

Etiology and Pathology. The etiology of dialysis dementia is uncertain. Current theories favor an aluminum-induced toxic encephalopathy. Pathologic findings are nonspecific.

Clinical Features. The disorder was first described in 1972 and accounts for approximately 20 percent of deaths in patients who have been on dialysis longer than three years. Initially symptoms consist of speech difficulties characterized by stammering and hesitancy. Personality changes with paranoid thinking and visual and auditory hallucinations and movement disorders such as asterixis, twitching, and motor apraxia are also seen. Eventually the patient becomes dysphasic, a global dementia develops, myoclonic jerks may be seen, and finally coma and death occur.

Early in the course of the disorder, the symptoms develop only during dialysis and clear within 24 hours. However, as the disorder progresses, the patient becomes more and more incapacitated. The typical course lasts from 6 to 12 months.

Diagnostic Procedures.

1. Electroencephalographic findings in dialysis dementia are characteristic and may precede the clinical findings by six to eight months. There are paroxysmal bursts of bilateral, synchronous delta and theta waves admixed with spike and sharp wave discharges.
2. An MR or CT scan may reveal mild to moderate hydrocephalus ex vacuo.
3. Lumbar puncture. The cerebrospinal fluid (CSF) is normal.

Treatment. Treatment of dialysis dementia is entirely symptomatic. Diazepam (Valium) is effective in decreasing symptoms and electroencephalographic abnormalities in the early stages of the disease. There is one reported case in which interruption of aluminum intake resulted in recovery.

Wernicke's Encephalopathy

This condition is a rare complication of dialysis (18) (see page 319).

Neurologic Complications of Renal Transplantation

There is an increased incidence of central nervous system infections; neoplasia, especially reticulum cell sarcoma; and progressive multifocal leukoencephalopathy in patients who receive chronic immunosuppressive therapy following kidney transplantation.

NEUROLOGIC MANIFESTATIONS OF HEPATIC DYSFUNCTION

Hepatic Encephalopathy

Definition. Hepatic encephalopathy is a metabolic encephalopathy associated with hepatic dysfunction. It is characterized by disturbances of mood and personality, asterixis, fetor hepaticus, hyperreflexia, and increased muscle tone and eventually by disturbance of consciousness.

Etiology and Pathology. The disorder is believed to be related to the inability of the liver to clear potentially toxic substances, including ammonia and fatty acids, from the blood or possibly by inability to synthesize or release essential products such as albumin and glucose.

Acute hepatic encephalopathy is characterized by the presence of diffuse cerebral edema. In chronic hepatic encephalopathy the brain shows Alzheimer type II astrocytes.

Clinical Features. Acute encephalopathy accompanies fulminant hepatic failure resulting from acute viral hepatitis, toxic liver damage, or acute fatty degeneration seen in pregnancy. In acute hepatic encephalopathy the patient develops increased muscle tone, hyperactive stretch reflexes, and extensor plantar responses. Fetor hepaticus, a sweet musty odor of the breath, may be present. Asterixis, a sudden loss and recovery of posture, may be present in the hands, feet, lips, and eyelids. There is evidence of increased intracranial pressure, and seizures occur in most cases. The patient becomes progressively confused, obtunded, and eventually comatose. The neurologic deficits usually resolve with adequate treatment.

Chronic encephalopathy, usually termed "portal systemic encephalopathy," is most commonly seen in patients with cirrhosis of the liver, often caused by chronic alcoholism. The systemic manifestations of liver disease such as palmar erythema, spider nevi, icterus, hepatosplenomegaly, and ascites may or may not be present, depending on the chronicity of the illness. The remainder of the course resembles that of acute encephalopathy without evidence of increased intracranial pressure. Some patients develop chronic cerebral degeneration that does not respond to treatment. This is a slowly progressive condition with dysarthria, cerebellar ataxis, involuntary movements, and spastic paraparesis (19).

Complications.

1. Electrolyte and acid-base disturbances are common, including hyponatremia, hypokalemia, respiratory alkalosis, and metabolic alkalosis. It is especially important to avoid alkalosis as it promotes diffusion of nonionized ammonia (NH_3) across the blood-brain barrier.
2. Renal failure may occur as a result of the hepatorenal syndrome or acute tubular necrosis.
3. Hypoglycemia may occur and is more common in acute hepatic failure.

Diagnostic Procedures.

1. There is evidence of hepatic dysfunction with elevated ammonia, serum glutamic-oxaloacetic transaminase (SGOT), serum glutamate pyruvate transaminase (SGPT), alkaline phosphatase in the serum, and abnormal coagulation studies. Hypoglycemia may be present.
2. In chronic encephalopathy, serum levels of aromatic amino acids and methionine are elevated, while branched chain amino acids are depressed. In acute encephalopathy all amino acids are markedly elevated except branched-chain amino acids, which are normal.
3. Electrolyte and acid-base abnormalities may be present. Blood urea nitrogen and serum creatinine may be elevated in renal dysfunction.
4. Lumbar puncture. In chronic cases, the cerebrospinal fluid (CSF) pressure and protein content are usually normal. The fluid may be xanthochromic and contain bilirubin, glutamine, or alpha-ketoglutarate. The CSF pressure is often elevated in acute encephalopathy.
5. Electroencephalography is a valuable tool in identifying early dysfunction. There is slowed activity with predominant delta and theta waves. Paroxysmal slow wave forms may be present.

Treatment.

1. Gastrointestinal bleeding, infection, and constipation are important precipitating and aggravating factors and should be controlled. Excessive diuresis should be avoided.
2. Initially dietary protein intake should be stopped and then gradually increased by 10–20 g/day every two to five days, depending upon the clinical response. Protein derived from milk, cheese, and vegetables is better tolerated than animal

protein. Adequate calories and vitamins should be provided.

3. The bowels should be kept as empty as possible. Neomycin 2 to 4 g q.d. p.o. or 1 percent solution by enema q.d. or b.i.d., and lactulose 50 to 150 ml q.d. with the dose adjusted to produce two to three soft stools per day will help to reduce ammonia levels.

4. The cerebral edema seen with acute encephalopathy shows a disappointing response to therapy.

5. The nonabsorbable disaccharide lactitol (β galactosido-sorbitol) or lactulose are both effective in the treatment of chronic hepatic encephalopathy. The mode of action of these substances is unknown but the benefit is established (20).

Prognosis. In patients with acute encephalopathy, the hepatocyte volume fraction (HVF) has proved a useful prognostic factor. An HVF less than 35 percent (nl—85 percent) indicates a poor prognosis. Patients with chronic encephalopathy usually recover when the precipitating event is removed.

NEUROLOGIC COMPLICATIONS OF THYROID DYSFUNCTION

Hyperthyroidism

Definition. Hyperthyroidism is a condition caused by overproduction of thyroid hormone.

Etiology. Hyperthyroidism is usually associated with a diffuse toxic goiter (Graves disease), an autoimmune condition. Single or multiple nodular goiters may begin to secrete thyroxine in patients with longstanding goiter, resulting in hyperthyroidism. Other causes include thyroiditis, functioning metastatic thyroid carcinoma, choriocarcinoma, testicular tumors, struma ovarii and some trophoblastic tumors.

Clinical Features. Hyperthyroidism is characterized by weight loss, excessive fatigue, nervousness, palpitations, heat intolerance, increased perspiration and diarrhea in an individual with goiter, tachycardia and a fine distal tremor. Exophthalmos with or without ophthalmoplegia and pretibial myxedema are seen in Graves disease.

Neurologic complications of hyperthyroidism include a symmetric, primarily motor peripheral neuropathy; proximal weakness due to myopathy; ophthalmoplegia; rarely, optic neuritis; corticospinal tract disease; chorea and seizures.

Diagnostic Procedures. Levels of triiodothyronine (T_3), thyroxine (T_4), thyroxine binding globulin (TBG) and thyroid stimulating hormone (TSH) should be obtained in all suspected cases of hyperthyroidism.

Treatment. Antithyroid drug therapy, radioactive iodine therapy and thyroidectomy all have a place in the treatment of hyperthyroidism (21). Propranolol (Inderal) is effective in reducing sympathetic overactivity and controlling tremor.

Hypothyroidism

Definition. Hypothyroidism is a condition caused by deficient production of thyroid hormone.

Etiology. Hypothyroidism may be due to a failure of the hypothalamus to secrete thyroid-releasing hormone, a failure of the pituitary to produce thyroid-stimulating hormone, or thyroid gland failure associated with chronic thyroiditis, surgical excision, or an iodine-deficient diet.

Clinical Features. The established case of hypothyroidism presents with dry skin, hoarseness of the voice, cold intolerance, bradycardia, constipation, and weight gain.

Neurologic complications include mental dullness, psychomotor retardation, headache, proximal muscle weakness, slowed tendon reflexes, and carpal tunnel syndrome. Mononeuropathies due to mucinous deposits which cause nerve damage or a symmetric sensory-motor peripheral neuropathy and/or cranial nerve abnormalities can also occur (22). Hypothyroid dementia may develop. A chronic cerebellar degeneration with progressive limb and truncal ataxia has been described. Myxedema coma is characterized by signs of hypothyroidism, coma, hypotension, hypothermia, and seizures and occurs in severe cases of hypothyroidism.

Diagnostic Procedures.

1. The diagnosis depends on demonstration of deficient production of thyroid hormone.

2. Electroencephalography reveals diffuse, low-voltage slowing in the theta range in severe hypothyroidism.

Treatment.

1. Neurologic complications of hypothyroidism resolve with replacement therapy.

2. Myxedema coma responds to symptomatic treatment and thyroid hormone replacement.

NEUROLOGIC COMPLICATIONS OF PARATHYROID DYSFUNCTION

Hyperparathyroidism

Definition. Hyperparathyroidism is a disorder caused by excessive excretion of parathormone.

Etiology. Hyperparathyroidism is usually caused by an adenoma of the parathyroid glands and results in hypercalcemia.

Clinical Features. The patient with hyperparathyroidism may develop osteitis fibrosa cystica, renal calculi, peptic ulceration, and arthralgias.

The neurologic complications of hyperparathyroidism include headache and proximal muscle weakness. Agitation, tremor, rigidity, and psychosis occur in severe cases, followed by coma and death unless prompt treatment is instituted (23).

Diagnostic Procedures.

1. Serum parathormone levels are increased.
2. Serum calcium levels are elevated above 11 mg%. Urinary calcium and ionized calcium levels are elevated. Hypercalcemia greater than 15 mg/dl should be regarded as a medical emergency requiring prompt treatment (24).
3. Magnetic resonance imaging with surface coils is useful and effective in preoperative localization of parathyroid tumors (25).

Treatment.

1. In hyperparathyroid crisis with calcium levels above 15 mg/dl the patient should be rehydrated with normal saline, then given a loop diuretic such as furosemide to increase calcinuria.
2. Removal of a parathyroid adenoma will correct parathormone excess with lowering of serum calcium levels.

Hypoparathyroidism

Definition. Hypoparathyroidism is a disorder caused by deficient production of parathormone.

Etiology. Hypoparathyroidism is usually the result of surgical treatment of hyperparathyroidism. Hypoparathyroidism produces hypocalcemia, which causes hyperexcitability of the central and peripheral nervous system. Transient hypoparathyroidism with hypocalcemia may be induced by magnesium deficiency in patients with alcoholic liver disease (26).

Clinical Features. The patient may present with seizures, paresthesias, muscle cramps, headache, or dementia. Chvostek and Trousseau signs are usually present. Papilledema occurs in 20 percent of patients, while optic neuritis is a rare occurrence. Calcification of the basal ganglia may be associated with parkinsonism. Progressive hearing loss due to altered calcium content in the inner ear occurs in longstanding hypoparathyroidism (27).

Diagnostic Procedures.

1. The serum parathormone level is abnormally low. Serum calcium levels are depressed.
2. Skull x-rays and computed tomography may demonstrate calcification of the choroid plexus, meninges, or basal ganglia.

Treatment. In acute cases the symptomatology responds to calcium administration. Chronic cases with evidence of dementia or parkinsonism will not improve with appropriate therapy, but signs of parkinsonism improve with L-dopa (see p. 109).

NEUROLOGIC COMPLICATIONS OF HYPOTHALAMIC-PITUITARY DYSFUNCTION

Diabetes Insipidus

Diabetes insipidus results from inadequate production of antidiuretic hormone. This may occur following trauma or neurosurgical procedures or damage to the supraoptic nucleus of the hypothalamus, the supraoptico-hypophyseal tract, or the posterior pituitary gland by an inflammatory process or tumor. The patient presents with excessive thirst associated with an increased volume of urine of low specific gravity. L-Desamino-8-d-arginine (Vasopressin) nasal spray produces 8 to 20 hours of antidiuresis. Carbamazepine (Tegretol) 400 mg q.d. may also be effective.

Acromegaly.

Acromegaly results from the excessive secretion of human growth hormone by a pituitary tumor.

Unilateral or bilateral carpal tunnel syndrome occurs in 50 percent of cases. A symmetric predominantly sensory peripheral neuropathy has been described in acromegaly (28).

Inappropriate Secretion of Antidiuretic Hormone (SIADH)

Definition. The condition is a disorder characterized by inappropriate secretion of antidiuretic hormone.

Etiology and Pathology. It has resulted from trauma, neurosurgical procedures, intracerebral and subarachnoid hemorrhage, cerebral infarction, acute meningitis, acute encephalitis, hydrocephalus, and such extracranial conditions as tuberculosis staphylococcal pneumonia, lung abscess and porphyria. Approximately 70 percent of cases of SIADH are related to malignancy and 70 percent of the malignancies are oat cell carcinoma of the lung. Other malignant conditions occasionally associated with SIADH include pancreatic carcinoma, Hodgkin's lymphoma, lymphosarcoma and thymoma. Drugs inducing SIADH include chlorpropamide, carbamazepine, cyclophosphamide, vincristine, antidepressant agents, antipsychotic agents, narcotics, barbiturates, and general anesthetics.

Clinical Features. The clinical features are those of hyponatremia (see p. 298).

Diagnostic Procedures.

1. The serum sodium and plasma osmolality are abnormally low in a person not taking diuretics.
2. The urine volume is reduced, and the urine osmolality is consistently higher than the serum osmolality, while the amount of urinary sodium is usually greater than 20 meq/L.
3. There is no evidence of renal disease or endocrine disorders.
4. The patient must not be taking diuretics.

Treatment.

1. The symptomatic patient with serum sodium < 125 meq/L should be given furosemide 1 mg/kg intravenous (IV) followed by hourly replacement of urinary sodium loss using 3 percent sodium chloride IV. Furosemide should be repeated as needed to maintain a negative fluid balance (29).
2. The asymptomatic patient usually responds to water restriction.
3. Chronic SIADH of unknown etiology often responds to declomycin 1200 mg daily, decreasing to a maintenance dose of 300 to 900 mg daily.

Panhypopituitarism

Definition. Panhypopituitarism is a condition caused by failure of the pituitary gland to secrete stimulating hormones.

Etiology and Pathology. Panhypopituitarism may result from infarction of the pituitary gland during pregnancy (Sheehan's syndrome) (30), head injury, gunshot wounds, tumors, internal carotid or anterior communicating artery aneurysm and inflammatory conditions (31).

Clinical Features. The patient usually develops signs and symptoms of hypothyroidism and hypoadrenalism. There is loss of axillary and pubic hair with impotence in the male and amenorrhea in the female. Patients are subject to hypotension and hypoglycemia.

Diagnostic Procedures.

1. Evidence of a pituitary, parapituitary, or hypothalamic tumor may be seen with skull x-rays or MR or CT scanning.
2. There is evidence of hypothyroidism and hypoadrenalism with lowered serum hormone levels and decreased urinary follicle stimulating hormone (FSH) levels.
3. Lumbar Puncture. The cerebrospinal fluid pressure is greater than 200 mmH$_2$O. There are no other abnormalities.

Treatment. Treatment consists of surgical excision of tumors and replacement hormone therapy with thyroxine and hydrocortisone.

Benign Intracranial Hypertension (Pseudotumor Cerebri)

Definition. Benign intracranial hypertension is a syndrome of suspected toxic or metabolic etiology characterized by the presence of increased intracranial pressure, which usually resolves spontaneously.

Etiology and Pathology. The disorder has been associated with otitis media; jugular venous obstruction; dural sinus thrombosis, particularly lateral sinus thrombosis; hypovitaminosis and hypervitaminosis A; carbon dioxide retention; and endocrine disorders, particularly hypoparathyroidism, adrenal insufficiency, and estrogen imbalance. Benign intracranial hypertension has also occurred following therapy with tetracyclines, nitrofurantoin, or chlordecane.

There are no characteristic pathologic changes. The brain appears edematous, and the ventricles are small in size.

Clinical Features. The patient is usually a child or young adult; typically an obese, adolescent female with menstrual abnormalities and evidence of increased intracranial pressure (i.e., headache, nausea and vomiting, visual difficulties, and papilledema). Minor symptoms of neck stiffness, tinnitus, distal extremity paresthesias, joint pains, and low back pain are not uncommon (32).

Diagnostic Procedures.

1. Skull x-rays. There may be separation of the skull sutures in children, and adults may show evidence of chronic increased intracranial pressure.
2. Visual field perimetry. Visual field perimetry may reveal constriction of the visual fields and enlargement of the blind spot.
3. Lumbar puncture. The only abnormality is elevation of the cerebrospinal fluid pressure.
4. Both MR and CT scans are normal. The ventricles are usually small in size.

Differential Diagnosis. Other causes of increased intracranial pressure must be excluded. Meningeal carcinomatosis may present as benign intracranial hypertension (33).

Treatment. Identifiable causes such as tetracycline therapy should be discontinued. Chronic cases may benefit from corticosteroid therapy using methylprednisone (Medrol) 64 mg q.o.d. with gradual tapering of dosage as improvement occurs.

Prognosis. Most cases resolve spontaneously in 6 to 18 months. Shunting procedures are occasionally required in patients with progressive visual failure.

NEUROLOGIC COMPLICATIONS OF SYSTEMIC ILLNESS

Diabetes Mellitus

Diabetes mellitus is a common condition, and neurologic complications occur in a high proportion of patients with this disease. The neurologic complications of diabetes mellitus include peripheral neuropathy, diabetic pseudotabes, diabetic amyotrophy, and diabetic coma.

Diabetic Neuropathy

Diabetic neuropathy is a disease of peripheral nerves which occurs in at least 50 percent of patients who have had diabetes for 25 years. The syndrome includes symmetric distal polyneuropathy, symmetric proximal motor neuropathy, focal asymmetric mono- or polymononeuropathies, and/or autonomic neuropathy. These conditions may coexist.

Etiology and Pathology. The etiology is uncertain. It is believed to be the result of vascular insufficiency of the vasa nervorum and hypoxia, or the product of one or more metabolic disturbances, including excess sorbitol production, reduction of myoinositol production due to hyperglycemia, or in-creased peripheral nerve myelin protein glycosalation resulting in demyelination (34, 35).

Clinical Features.

1. Symmetrical distal polyneuropathies.
   a. Predominantly small fiber type with pain and paresthesias, usually in the lower extremities.
   b. Predominantly large fiber type with decreased vibration and position sense, sensory ataxia and loss of ankle jerks. Painful or painless foot ulceration can occur.
   c. Mixed small and large fiber types plus autonomic involvement with dissociate sensory loss of pain and temperature, painless foot ulcers, development of Charcot joints in the lower extremities, painless distension of the bladder, and Argyll Robertson pupils (diabetic pseudotabes).

   An acute axonal degeneration involving fibers of all sizes has been termed diabetic neuropathic cachexia. This condition is more prevalent in males.
2. Symmetric proximal motor neuropathies (Diabetic amyotrophy)
   a. Acute ischemic mononeuropathy multiplex which is believed to result from asymmetric small infarcts of proximal motor nerve trunks results in a sudden asymmetric weakness of the pelvic musculature frequently associated with pain.
   b. Subacute proximal neuropathy results in a slowly progressive weakness of proximal lower limb girdle musculature and may suggest a myopathic rather than a neuropathy process.
3. Focal asymmetric mono or polymononeuropathies.
   a. Cranial neuropathies resulting in paralysis of extraocular muscles due to involvement of the third or sixth cranial nerves usually occurs in longstanding diabetes over the age of 50 years. The onset of the paralysis is usually preceded by retroorbital pain of several days duration. Pupillary sparing is not unusual, even when loss of third nerve function is complete. Resolution usually occurs within a three-month period.
   b. Painful diabetic thoracolumbar neuropathy presents with gradual onset of painful dysesthesias involving the

lower thoracic or abdominal wall. There may be some weakness of intercostal or abdominal muscles (36).

The condition resolves over a period of several months. The correct diagnosis is important since there is usually an immediate suspicion of intrathoracic or intraabdominal problems at the onset of the pain.

c. Peripheral mononeuropathies in the limbs tend to involve nerves at risk for compression such as the median nerve at the wrist, the ulnar nerve at the elbow, the radial nerve in the upper arm, the lateral cutaneous nerve of thigh (meralgia paresthetica), and the common peroneal nerve at the neck of the fibula.

4. Autonomic neuropathies
   a. Postural hypotension is probably the commonest manifestation of diabetic autonomic neuropathy. The patient experiences a sharp drop in both systolic and diastolic blood pressure without compensatory tachycardia on standing.
   b. Resting tachycardia and wide fluctuations in blood pressure are not unusual in diabetic.
   c. Silent myocardial infarction can occur in cardiac autonomic neuropathy with loss of pain conducting fibers in the cardiac sympathetic system.
   d. Involvement of the genitourinary autonomic system results in the development of an atonic painless distended bladder with overflow incontinence, male impotence with failure of ejaculation, and reduced vaginal lubrication and dyspareunia.
   e. Gastrointestinal autonomic neuropathy results in incoordination of esophageal peristalsis, gastric hypomotility, pylorospasm, intestinal hypomotility and constipation, intestinal incoordination and diarrhea, and anorectal dysfunction with incontinence.
   f. Pupillary autonomic disturbances result in miosis and failure of reaction to light—an "Argyll Robertson" like pupil.

Diagnostic Procedures.

1. Motor nerve conduction velocities are slowed but a normal result does not exclude a sensory diabetic neuropathy.
2. Tibial H reflex responses and sural nerve conduction velocities are the most sensitive studies of electrical conduction.

Treatment.

1. Maintain adequate control of diabetes and normal or near-normal glucose levels.
2. Maintain ideal body weight.
3. Painful neuropathy usually responds to tricyclics such as amitriptyline 25 mg h.s., increasing by 25 mg increments per week to as high as 50 mg t.i.d. if necessary.
4. Carbamazepine is also effective in painful neuropathy.
5. Intravenous lidocaine 5 mg/kg body weight over 30 minutes under continuous electrocardiographic monitoring should be reserved for cases with intractable pain.
6. Autonomic dysfunction and postural hypotension require elastic stockings, increased dietary sodium and fludrohydrocortisone 0.1 to 0.3 mg daily in some cases. Indomethacin 25 to 50 mg t.i.d. is also effective as is a combination of diphenylhydramine and cimetidine. An antigravity suit may be necessary in extreme cases.
7. Genitourinary problems require voiding every three hours and the use of self-catheterization. Bethanecol 10 to 25 mg t.i.d. will promote detrusor contraction. Imipramine 25 mg t.i.d. may prevent retrograde ejaculation. Impotence may require a penile prosthesis or self injection with papaverine.
8. Delayed esophageal emptying can be accelerated by bethanecol.
9. Delayed gastric emptying will respond to metoclopramide.
10. Diarrhea in diabetic patients often responds to tetracycline.

Neurologic Complications of Leukemia

An increasing number of patients with leukemia are surviving following treatment, and a number are developing neurologic complications. These include:

1. Cerebral involvement. The central nervous system may be infiltrated by leukemic cells, which produces a progressive encephalopathy. Patients with leukemia also have an increased risk of superior sagittal sinus thrombosis. Signs and symptoms include intellectual deterioration, personality change, and the development of dysphasia, hemiparesis, hemisensory loss, and hemianopia. Involvement of the ventromedial hypothalamus may result in a voracious appetite and weight gain. Patients with acute leukemia have an in-

creased incidence of intracerebral hemorrhage, subarachnoid hemorrhage, and subdural hematoma (37).

2. Meningeal involvement. Meningeal infiltration by leukemic cells can result in acute hydrocephalus with headache, vomiting, papilledema, and separation of sutures in children. Involvement of the meninges at the base of the brain produces progressive cranial nerve palsies. The oculomotor nerves are particularly susceptible to this complication. The cerebrospinal fluid is under increased pressure and may show the presence of leukemic cells. The glucose content is decreased, and the protein content is elevated.

3. Brain stem involvement. Invasion of the brain stem by leukemic cells results in progressive involvement of brain stem nuclei, progressive ataxia, and disturbance of respiration, including hypopnea and Cheyne-Stokes respiration.

4. Spinal cord involvement. Leukemic infiltration of the spinal epidural space produces spinal cord compression with progressive paraparesis, a sensory level, and sphincter involvement.

5. Peripheral nerve involvement. Infiltration of posterior root ganglia, proximal nerve roots or distal peripheral nerves can occur. A progressive polyneuropathy that resembles postinfectious polyneuritis (Guillain-Barré syndrome) may occur (38).

6. Infection. Patients with leukemia have an increased susceptibility to infection. There is an increased incidence of *Herpes zoster*, which may result in neuritis or encephalitis. Leukemic patients have an increased risk of acute pyogenic meningitis, subacute fungal meningitis, and brain abscess.

7. Complications from chemotherapy. Chemotherapy may result in neurologic complications, including leukoencephalopathy. Methotrexate may produce a diffuse arachnoiditis and progressive leukoencephalopathy with progressive dementia, spasticity, ataxis, and seizures.

Neurologic Complications of Hodgkin's Disease

The neurologic complications of Hodgkin's disease may be due to either the direct effect of the disease on the nervous system or the remote effects of a neoplastic condition. The complications include:

1. Cerebral involvement. A progressive encephalopathy with dementia has been described in Hodgkin's disease. Direct involvement has occasionally been reported with Hodgkin's sarcoma.

2. Meningeal involvement. Compression of cranial nerves, particularly of the optic chiasm, has been reported. Hypothalamic compression may result in diabetes insipidus. Subarachnoid hemorrhage is an occasional complication of Hodgkin's disease.

3. Spinal cord involvement. Cord compression may result from epidural deposits in Hodgkin's disease. Involvement of the cord and development of syringomyelia has been reported (39).

4. Peripheral nerve involvement. Peripheral nerve involvement is probably the commonest complication of Hodgkin's disease. Most cases show compression of the brachial plexus or individual nerves arising from the brachial or lumbosacral plexus. An acute, symmetric peripheral neuropathy resembling postinfectious polyneuritis has also been reported in Hodgkin's disease.

5. Remote effects of Hodgkin's disease. Many of the conditions described under nonmetastatic effects of carcinoma occur in Hodgkin's disease, including progressive multifocal leukoencephalopathy, cerebellar degeneration, and peripheral neuropathy (see p.314).

6. Increased incidence of CNS infection. Alteration and suppression of immune mechanisms in Hodgkin's disease lead to an increased risk of infections, including *H. zoster* and chronic fungal infection.

Treatment. Space-occupying lesions should be excised whenever possible. This is particularly important in paraparesis secondary to epidural deposits.

Neurologic Complications of Multiple Myeloma

Neoplastic transformation of plasma cells results in multiple myeloma. This condition may present as a single tumor, plasmacytoma, or as a disseminated condition with metastatic involvement of multiple sites. Multiple myeloma may produce osteolytic lesions in bone or extradural deposits or may directly involve the central nervous system. In addition, the abnormal plasma cells have the capacity to synthesize abnormal globulins, resulting in IgG or IgM monoclonal gammopathies, macroglobulinemia or cryoglobulinemia. Amyloidosis may occur in some patients. Involvement of bone produces hypercalcemia and hyperuricemia. Interference with coagulation mechanisms increases the risk of a hemorrhagic diathesis with hemorrhage into the brain or subarachnoid space.

The complications include:

1. Cerebral involvement. Compression of the brain by an extradural mass or infiltra-

tion of the parenchyma with production of focal signs and progressive encephalopathy have been described.

2. Meningeal involvement may lead to cranial nerve palsies.

3. Spinal cord involvement. Extradural plasma cell tumors may produce spinal cord compression and progressive paraparesis.

4. Peripheral neuropathy. A sensory motor neuropathy and a condition resembling postinfectious polyneuritis have been reported. Both conditions respond to chemotherapy and plasmapheresis. Median nerve involvement results in carpal tunnel syndrome.

5. Metabolic effects. Hypercalcemia due to increased bone destruction leads to mental changes, weakness, and increasing disability.

6. There is an increased risk of infection by *H. zoster*.

Amyloidosis

Definition. Amyloidosis is a syndrome characterized by the extracellular deposition of a fibrillar protein amyloid in one or more sites in the body.

Etiology and Pathology. Amyloidosis may be inherited, primary or secondary. Heredofamilial amyloidosis is characterized by the presence of fibrils consisting mainly of protein related to prealbumin in the serum. Primary amyloidosis is probably the result of a plasma cell dyscrasia in which clones of plasma cells produce the amyloid which consists of the amino acid terminal region of the variable fragment of an immunoglobulin light chain.

Secondary amyloidosis is associated with chronic disease such as tuberculosis, chronic osteomyelitis, leprosy, rheumatoid arthritis, systemic lupus erythematosus, polymyositis, scleroderma, tumors including Hodgkins disease, renal cell carcinoma, medullary carcinoma of the thyroid and familial Mediterranean fever. The amyloid is derived from proteolysis of the amino terminal fragments of serum amyloid-associated protein.

Clinical Features. Systemic amyloidosis occurs in approximately 0.6 to 0.7 percent of the hospital population.

1. Heredofamilial amyloidosis consists of a group of disorders all inherited as an autosomal dominant trait. Type I develops in the third or fourth decade with a progressive painful sensorimotor neuropathy affecting lower limbs more than upper limbs and often

associated with carpal tunnel syndrome, autonomic neuropathy and ulceration of the feet. Type II familial amyloidosis develops in the fourth or fifth decade with peripheral neuropathy affecting the upper limbs more than the lower limbs and carpal tunnel syndrome. Type III is characterized by a severe sensorimotor neuropathy affecting upper and lower limbs with severe amyloidosis. Type IV familial amyloidosis presents with cranial nerve palsies and a lattice dystrophy of the cornea.

2. Primary systemic amyloidosis. This condition is characterized by the deposition of amyloid in many organs and is usually associated with the production of monoclonal immunoglobulins and Bence-Jones proteinuria. There is an excessive number of bone marrow plasma cells and 20 percent of patients have multiple myeloma. Primary systemic amyloidosis is characterized by the development of a chronic peripheral neuropathy in 15 percent of cases. Other signs of amyloidosis include cardiac involvement with heart failure, pulmonary involvement, scleroderma-like lesions of the skin, and polyarthropathy. Liver, kidney, and tongue involvement may be found. The peripheral neuropathy is usually distal and resembles diabetic neuropathy. Autonomic symptoms include sexual impotence, decreased gastrointestinal motility, and orthostatic hypotension (40). Respiratory failure can occur if amyloidosis involves the respiratory muscles (41).

3. Secondary amyloidosis. This condition is associated with chronic disease. There is marked systemic involvement in secondary amyloidosis but usually little involvement of the nervous system.

Diagnostic Procedures.

1. Monoclonal immunoglobulins may be demonstrated in the serum or urine.

2. X-rays of the spine and long bones may demonstrate the presence of myeloma, and the diagnosis of myeloma can be confirmed by bone marrow biopsy.

3. Rectal biopsy will reveal amyloid deposits in approximately 80 percent of patients with systemic amyloidosis.

4. Peripheral nerve biopsy. Peripheral nerve involvement can usually be demonstrated by sural nerve biopsy.

Treatment and Prognosis. Most cases of systemic amyloidosis are fatal, and death usually results from renal failure or cardiac disease. Myeloma-associated amyloidosis has occasionally been reported to respond partially to treatment with cytotoxic drugs and prednisone (42). Dimethylsulfoximide, an amyloid-fibril denaturing agent, has resulted in the urinary excretion of amyloid subunits from renal deposits in experiments using human subjects. Its use is still experimental. It is possible that primary amyloidosis may respond to immunosuppressive drugs. In patients with secondary amyloidosis the prognosis is slightly better. If the underlying disease can be controlled, recovery may occur. Colchicine may be of value in preventing renal amyloid deposits in secondary amyloidosis.

Neurologic Complications of Macroglobulinemia

Etiology and Pathology. Macroglobulinemia may occur as a primary condition or as a secondary phenomenon in multiple myeloma, leukemia, and lymphosarcoma. The presence of macroglobulins leads to increased serum viscosity, aggregation of the cellular elements of the blood, and thrombosis of small blood vessels. Macroglobulinemia is usually associated with diffuse proliferation of leukocytes and plasma cells, which infiltrate the subarachnoid space of the brain and spinal cord. This infiltration is often associated with scattered areas of hemorrhage or infarction. Peripheral nerves may contain deposits of IgM in the myelin sheath.

Clinical Features. Increased viscosity produces decreased cerebral blood flow and hypoxia. This results in intellectual deterioration and diffuse headache. Focal signs of cerebrovascular insufficiency including dysphasia, hemiparesis, and brain stem signs with cranial nerve palsy can occur. Increasing tinnitus and decreased auditory acuity may be due to involvement of the acoustic division of the eighth nerve or hemorrhage into the cochlea. Subarachnoid hemorrhage is an occasional complication due to disturbed blood coagulation. Visual deterioration may result from increased intracranial pressure or retinal and vitreous hemorrhages. Extradural compression or vascular occlusive disease of the spinal cord will produce a progressive spastic paraparesis with bladder involvement. A condition similar to amyotrophic lateral sclerosis can result from infarction of the spinal cord. A progressive, predominantly sensory peripheral neuropathy occurs in about 40 percent of cases (43).

Diagnostic Procedures.

1. Abnormal macroglobulins can be demonstrated by serum protein electrophoresis.

2. The cerebrospinal fluid shows marked elevation of protein content with the presence of macroglobulins.
3. Decreased circulation and sludging in conjunctival vessels can be demonstrated by slit lamp examination.
4. Serum viscosity levels are elevated.
5. Sural nerve biopsy shows a demyelinating neuropathy with IgM deposits in the myelin sheath or bound to the endoneurium.

Treatment. Macroglobulinemia responds to plasmaphoresis, which should be repeated biweekly to keep the serum viscosity level below the threshold of symptom recurrence.

Neurological Complications of Plasma Cell Dyscrasias

Plasma cell dyscrasias with IgG or IgM monoclonal gammopathy are associated with peripheral neuropathy. Monoclonal IgG production is usually associated with a mixed sensorimotor neuropathy while a predominantly motor neuropathy occurs with monoclonal IgM reactive with myelin associated glycoprotein (44).

Diagnostic Procedures.

1. Motor and sensory nerve conduction velocities are slow (45).
2. Sural nerve biopsy may reveal a demyelinating or axonal degeneration.

Treatment. A combination of plasmapheresis and chemotherapy is recommended.

Neurologic Complications of Cryoglobulinemia

Cryoglobulinemia is a condition characterized by abnormal gamma globulins, which show increased viscosity and precipitation with lowering of temperature. Patients with cryoglobulinemia experience sludging or thrombosis of vessels on exposure to cold. Raynaud's phenomenon is marked. Thrombosis of skin vessels produces purpura and ecchymoses. Hemoptysis, abdominal pain, hematemesis, and hematochezia may occur. Involvement of the kidneys results in albuminuria and eventual development of hypertension and uremia. Neurologic complications include a sensorimotor neuropathy (46). Treatment with corticosteroids produces clinical improvement and lowering of cryoglobulin levels in the blood.

Neurologic Complications of Polycythemia

Etiology and Pathology. Polycythemia vera is a condition characterized by an elevated erythrocyte count, elevated hemoglobin content, increased circulating blood volume, increased blood viscosity, and marked reduction in cerebral blood flow. The cause is unknown.

Secondary polycythemia occurs as a phys-·iologic response to living at high altitudes, in chronic heart disease with right-left shunt, chronic pulmonary disease, chronic renal disease, and renal carcinoma with excess secretion of erythropoietin.

Clinical Features. The patient presents with headache, blurred vision, and lethargy. There is an increased incidence of transient ischemic attacks and cerebral thrombosis. Those who develop hypertension have an increased risk of intracerebral hemorrhage and spontaneous subarachnoid hemorrhage. Development of symptoms suggesting a posterior fossa tumor suggests the presence of an erythropoietin-secreting hemangioblastoma.

Diagnostic Procedures. Criteria for diagnosis of polycythemia vera are divided into two categories to facilitate diagnosis (47).

Category A

1. Increased red cell mass
2. Splenomegaly
3. Normal oxygen saturation

Category B

1. White cell count $> 12,000$ mm^3
2. Platelet count $> 650,000$ mm^3
3. Increased leukocyte alkaline phosphatase score.
4. Increased serum vitamin B$_{12}$ level and B$_{12}$ binding capacity.

Diagnosis established if three A criteria are present or A1 plus either A2 or A3 and two of Category B.

Treatment. Patients with mild polycythemia vera or secondary polycythemia respond to repeated venesection and removal of small volumes of blood. Replacement with low molecular weight dextran reduces the danger of cerebral thrombosis due to a sudden increase in platelets following venesection.

Refractory cases of polycythemia vera should be treated with hydroxyurea. Other agents such as chlorambucil or phosphorus 32 are leukemogenic and should be reserved for patients over 65 years of age.

Neurologic Complications of Acute Porphyrias

Definition. Acute intermittent porphyria, hereditary coproporphyria and variegate porphyria are inherited or acquired disorders caused by specific enzymatic defects in the biosynthesis of heme.

Etiology and Pathology. The acute porphyrias are all associated with excess production of heme precursors. Increased levels of delta aminolevulinic acid (ALA) and porphobilinogen are found in acute intermittent porphyria and variegate porphyria. At the same time there is a sharp decline in the production of heme which is essential for the synthesis of cytochrome oxidase in the mitochondria. This is followed by inhibition of the mitochondrial electron transport system and impaired cellular energy production (48).

There is also some evidence that excess levels of heme precursors are neurotoxic.

Neuropathologic changes consist of degenerative changes in the anterior horn cells of the spinal cord and neurons of autonomic ganglia. Degeneration of axons with areas of demyelination are found in the cerebellum and cerebral white matter.

Clinical Features. An attack of acute intermittent porphyria may be precipitated by infection, hypoglycemia, sulfonamides, anticonvulsants, barbiturates, alcohol, griseofulvin, or exposure to industrial solvents. Most patients experience abdominal pain as the initial symptom. This is believed to result from autonomic neuropathy, which also causes tachycardia, urinary retention, sweating, and hypertension. Involvement of peripheral nerves produces a predominantly motor neuropathy, which may progress to quadriparesis and respiratory failure. Muscle weakness is believed to result from failure of release of acetylcholine at the motor end plate. Cranial nerve involvement may result in dysarthria, dysphagia, facial diplegia, and external ophthalmoplegia. Optic atrophy has been described. Many patients have a history of mental disturbances including depression, paranoia, and emotional instability. An acute attack may present with mania, restlessness, visual hallucinations, and delirium. This may be followed by seizures and coma. The attacks vary in duration, frequency, and severity. A vesicular rash occurs during acute episodes of variegate porphyria.

Diagnostic Procedures.

1. Serum ALA and urinary ALA and porphobilinogen are increased in acute intermittent porphyria and variegate porphyria.
2. The urine may be brown-red in color during an acute attack. In most cases the urine will darken when placed in sunlight.
3. A normochromic, normocytic anemia may be present.
4. Electromyography shows evidence of fi-

brillation potentials in the acute phase followed by the appearance of polyphasic motor unit potentials of re-innervation six to eight weeks later. Near normal nerve conduction velocities with low amplitude compound muscle action potentials are indicative of axonal neuropathy.

5. Hypercholesterolemia is not uncommon in adults with acute intermittent porphyria (49).

Treatment.

1. Known precipitating agents should be avoided.
2. Symptomatic treatment with analgesics, antihypertensive agents, antipsychotics, and anticonvulsants may be necessary.
3. In some cases acute attacks may be aborted by administration of IV glucose, 10 gm/hour, or hematin (4 mg/kg q12h given IV over a 10-minute period). Both glucose and hematin prevent the hepatic induction of ALA-synthetase.
4. Sudden respiratory failure can occur at any time during an acute attack. Facilities for endotracheal intubation and mechanical respiration should be available for emergency use.

Neurologic Complications of Whipple's Disease

Whipple's disease, which is believed to result from a bacterial infection, may involve the central nervous system. It is probably common in AIDS.

Pathologic changes consist of inflammation of the hypothalamus, thalamus, and mammillary bodies with the presence of PAS-positive bacillary like structures in macrophages, microglial nodules and scattered in the neuropil (50).

Electron microscopic examination reveals intracellular rod-shaped bacilli. Evidence of intestinal involvement, including malabsorption, diarrhea, and steatorrhea, are not always present in patients with cerebral involvement. The disease produces dementia, supranuclear ophthalmoplegia, facial myoclonus, nystagmus, and seizures. Hypothalamic symptoms consisting of disturbed sleep-wake cycle, polydipsia, and hyperphagia have also been reported. Examination of the cerebrospinal fluid may reveal PAS-positive bacillary structures in inflammatory cells. Brain biopsy may be necessary when systemic symptoms are absent. Treatment consists of antibiotics such as penicillin and chloramphenicol that are capable of crossing the blood-brain barrier.

Neurologic Complications of Hypoglycemia

Hypoglycemia is a potent cause of neurologic symptoms in infants, children, and adults. Under aerobic conditions, glucose and oxygen are the sole source of energy in the central nervous system. There is little storage of glycogen or glucose in the brain, and available glucose supplies are exhausted within 30 minutes when hypoglycemia occurs.

Etiology and Pathology. The main causes of hypoglycemia are outlined in Table 17-2.

Pathologic changes include neuronal loss and degeneration. This may be intense in areas with a high rate of metabolism, including the visual cortex, and in Ammon's horn in the hippocampus. The subcortical gray matter and Purkinje cells of the cerebellum are all particularly susceptible to hypoglycemia. White matter is relatively resistant.

Clinical Features. Mild cases of hypoglycemia present with ataxia, hemiparesis, dysphasia, profuse perspiration, pallor, confusion, and a feeling of faintness. These symptoms are the result of sympathetic overactivity. Repeated attacks of this type may result in persistent cerebellar ataxia in some cases. Hypoglycemia occasionally causes seizures, and all patients with recent onset of seizures should have a glucose tolerance test.

In severe hypoglycemia the symptoms of mild hypoglycemia are followed by confusion, psychosis, stupor, loss of consciousness, and coma. Comatose patients may develop ir-

TABLE 17-2. Causes of Hypoglycemia

1. Deficient glucose intake: starvation, anorexia nervosa
2. Deficient absorption of glucose: malabsorption, chronic diarrhea
3. Excessive glucose utilization: fever, hyperthyroidism, malignancy
4. Excessive insulin secretion: insulinoma, leucine sensitivity, idiopathic postprandial hypoglycemia
5. Deficient glycogen synthesis: liver disease, glycogen synthetase deficiency
6. Deficient conversion of glycogen to glucose, glycogen storage diseases, prediabetic hypoglycemia
7. Diabetes mellitus: poor control, excessive insulin dose, late onset post exercise hypoglycemia (51)
8. Drugs: alcohol, biguanides, hydrazine, propoxyphene, pyribenzamine, salicylates, sulfonylureas

reversible brain damage unless the blood glucose is restored to normal levels. The encephalopathy of hypoglycemia resembles that of anoxic encephalopathy (see p. 296).

Diagnostic Procedures.

1. The diagnosis is established by demonstration of a relationship between symptoms and low serum glucose levels. The symptoms can usually be provoked by fasting for 12 to 24 hours in most cases.
2. Elevated serum insulin levels can be demonstrated in patients with hyperplasia of the beta cells; insulinoma; leucine-sensitive hypoglycemia; and idiopathic, postprandial, or alimentary hypoglycemia.
3. Liver function tests should be performed in all obscure cases of hypoglycemia. Tests for malabsorption may be required in some cases.
4. Both MR and CT scans are usually normal in early cases but may show evidence of cerebral atrophy and ventricular dilatation in patients who have suffered severe encephalopathy.
5. Electroencephalography. The EEG shows progressive slowing during an attack of hypoglycemia with the appearance of symmetric theta activity followed by the appearance of symmetric delta activity over both hemispheres. In the early stages slowing is accentuated by hyperventilation.

Treatment. Every effort should be made to identify the cause of hypoglycemia and to administer appropriate therapy. Persistent hypoglycemia will inevitably lead to brain damage.

Nonmetastatic Effects of Carcinoma

Definition. Nonmetastatic effects of carcinoma are the result of damage or dysfunction of the nervous system that occurs without evidence of direct involvement by cancer cells.

Etiology and Pathology. The etiology is unknown. Chronic viral infection, an autoimmune disorder induced by tumor antigen, and metabolic or endocrine disturbance are all possible causes of nonmetastatic complications affecting the nervous system.

The pathologic changes consist of cell loss and gliosis and/or demyelination (see Table 17-3).

Clinical Features. Nonmetastatic effects of carcinoma may involve the brain, spinal cord, peripheral nervous system, or muscle.

Involvement of the brain may present as an encephalopathy, encephalomyelopathy or subacute cerebellar degeneration (see Figure 17-1). Involvement of the spinal cord usually results in posterolateral column degeneration, necrotizing myelopathy, or carcinomatous amyotrophic lateral sclerosis. Sensory or motor neuropathy occurs when the peripheral nerves are damaged (52). Carcinomatous myopathy is the result of involvement of muscle. Any of these conditions may affect the patient before the cancer is evident (53).

In most cases the patient presents with evidence of involvement of more than one area of the nervous system. Characteristic epidemiologic features and signs and symptoms are listed in Table 17-3.

Diagnostic Procedures.

1. There is usually elevation of cerebrospinal fluid protein when the central nervous system is involved.
2. Nerve conduction velocities are slowed when peripheral nerves are affected.
3. Electromyography is abnormal and may indicate the presence of a myopathy or the myasthenic syndrome (see p. 400).

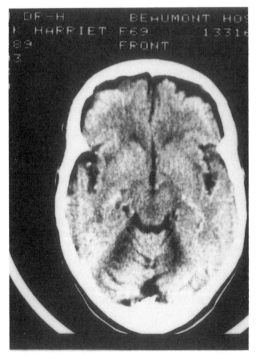

FIGURE 17-1. CT scan in a case of subacute cerebellar degeneration secondary to ovarian carcinoma.

TABLE 17–3. Nonmetastatic Effects of Carcinoma

Syndromes	Pathologic Features	Type of Carcinoma Most Frequently Associated	Characteristic Signs and Symptoms
Encephalopathy	Patchy loss of cortical neurons, microglial proliferation		Moderately rapid onset of dementia, intermittent confusion, and disorientation
Encephalomyelopathy	Loss of cortical neurons, necrosis of myelin	Oat cell carcinoma of the lung, carcinoma of the uterus	Dementia, bulbar involvement with dysphagia, dysarthria, vertigo, deafness, and/ or external ophthalmoplegia
Subacute cerebellar degeneration	Diffuse loss of Purkinje cells	Ovarian, bronchial, or breast carcinoma, see Fig. 17-1	Rapidly progressive ataxia begins in lower extremities, progresses to involve upper extremities
Posterolateral column degeneration	Demyelination of posterolateral columns		Weakness of lower extremities, hyperreflexia and extensor plantar responses, loss of vibration and proprioception
Necrotizing myelopathy	Necrosis of myelin, swollen anterior horn cells	Bronchial carcinoma	Sudden onset, pain in back, weakness of lower extremities followed by numbness and paresthesias and an ascending sensory level
Carcinomatous amyotrophic lateral sclerosis	Loss of anterior horn cells and cells of posterior root ganglia	Carcinoma of the breast, colon, thymus, prostate, and testes; basal cell carcinoma, astrocytoma, leukemia	Muscle weakness and wasting with fasciculations, loss of vibration and proprioception
Sensory neuropathy	Loss of neurons of posterior root ganglia	Bronchial carcinoma	Numbness and paresthesias of hands and feet, all sensory modalities eventually involved
Sensorimotor neuropathy	Peripheral demyelination; rarely, vasculitis	Lymphoma; carcinoma of the prostate	Symmetric distal muscle weakness and sensory impairment
Carcinomatous myopathy	May resemble polymyositis (see p. 402); atrophy of type 2 muscle fibers	Carcinoma of lung, breast, stomach, and ovary	Progressive proximal weakness, may be a rash

Treatment. The neoplasm should be removed whenever possible, although successful removal may not prevent progression of the neurologic deficits.

VITAMIN DEFICIENCIES AND INTOXICATIONS

Vitamin A

Vitamin A is a polyunsaturated, fat-soluble vitamin that can be directly absorbed or derived from carotene as it is absorbed through the intestinal wall.

Vitamin A Deficiency. Dietary vitamin A deficiency is rare in the United States, but malabsorption syndromes and biliary tract or pancreatic duct obstruction may result in a deficiency syndrome. Nightblindness is usually the presenting symptom and is due to lack of retinal, the aldehyde form of vitamin A, which is necessary for phototransduction in the retina. Prolonged deficiency may result in keratinization of epithelium with corneal necrosis and extrusion of the lens. Cranial nerve palsies, hydrocephalus, and mental retardation have also been reported.

Vitamin A Intoxication. Vitamin A intoxication is most often associated with excessive vitamin supplementation. Signs of acute vitamin A intoxication include nausea, vomiting, vertigo, drowsiness, and severe bifrontal headaches. Papilledema and mild exophthalmos are seen in cases with chronic vitamin A intoxication. Benign intracranial hypertension may be associated with hypo- and hypervitaminosis A.

Treatment. The signs and symptoms of vitamin A deficiency and intoxication resolve with replacement therapy or discontinuation of vitamin A supplementation.

Vitamin D

Altered vitamin D metabolism is thought to be the cause of the myopathy that occurs with osteomalacia. This dyscalcemic myopathy responds to the administration of 15 mg of vitamin D_2 daily.

Vitamin B$_6$ (Pyridoxine) Deficiency

Pyridoxal phosphate, the active form of pyridoxine, is a cofactor for a variety of enzymatic reactions. It is important for the conversion of tryptophan to nicotinic acid and for the conversion of glutamic acid to gamma aminobutyric acid (GABA). A deficiency of pyridoxine is associated with generalized seizures in children. Pyridoxine deficiency seizures may be related to pyridoxine's role in

the synthesis of the inhibitory neurotransmitter GABA.

Seizures develop between the ages of one month and four months. The interictal EEG is normal, and there is an excess of urinary xanthurenic acid on administration of tryptophan. Children with pyridoxine-deficiency seizures respond well to anticonvulsants or to oral doses of pyridoxine.

Chronic Pyridoxine Toxicity.

Injection of pyridoxine in megavitamin therapy has resulted in a sensory peripheral neuropathy (54).

Niacin (Nicotinic Acid) Deficiency—Pellagra

Derivatives of niacin serve as cofactors in many of the vital biologic oxidation-reduction reactions and are indispensable components of the energy transfer processes of cellular metabolism. Niacin deficiency is one of the major factors contributing to pellagra, a disease that occurs in populations who consume large quantities of corn-derived food.

Etiology and Pathology. Although niacin deficiency is a major factor in the etiology of pellagra, multiple nutritional deficiencies are usually present. Thiamine, pyridoxine, and riboflavin are also deficient, and since these compounds act as cofactors in the synthesis of niacin, the problem is compounded. The nature of the biochemical lesion in niacin deficiency is uncertain, but it probably involves impairment of respiratory chain function.

Neurons at many levels of the neuraxis are affected. Cells in the cerebral cortex, basal ganglia, brain stem, and occasionally the anterior horn cells of the spinal cord become swollen, and chromatolysis occurs.

Clinical Features. In the United States pellagra is now largely confined to chronic alcoholics. The initial symptoms of pellagra include anorexia, dizziness, insomnia, headache, muscle weakness, nervousness, and burning dysesthesias of the arms, hands, and feet.

Treatment. Patients with pellagra respond to a high-protein, low-fat diet that is high in niacinamide, thiamine, riboflavin, and pyridoxine.

Vitamin B$_1$ (Thiamine) Deficiency

See page 319.

Vitamin B$_{12}$ Deficiency

Vitamin B_{12} deficiency has a profound effect upon the nervous system due to the important role the vitamin plays in nervous system metabolism. B_{12} serves as a cofactor in the synthesis of methionine and in nucleic acid metabolism.

Etiology and Pathology. Vitamin B_{12} deficiency usually results from a deficiency of intrinsic factor which is produced in the gastric mucosa and is necessary for absorption of B_{12}. Nutritional deficiency of Vitamin B_{12} is rare but has been described in strict vegetarians, pregnancy and in infants breast fed by vegan mothers (55).

Vitamin B_{12} deficiency results in pernicious anemia and in subacute combined degeneration of the spinal cord characterized by demyelination involving the posterior columns, the pyramidal tracts, the ascending cerebellar tracts, and the anterior columns. Demyelination is followed by loss of axon cylinders and wallerian degeneration. As the disease progresses, more proximal areas of the central nervous system are affected. Demyelination and degeneration appear in the internal capsule and in the centrum semiovale and may also occur in the papillomacular bundle of the optic nerve. Cranial nerve involvement and segmental demyelination of peripheral nerves have also been reported.

Clinical Features. Patients with subacute combined degeneration usually present with numbness and tingling of the extremities. Vibration is diminished or lost, and position sense may be impaired in the toes. The lower extremities are spastic with hyperactive patellar and Achilles reflexes and bilateral extensor plantar responses. The patient becomes ataxic and may be unable to walk. Severe anemia and the resultant cerebral anoxia result in depression and other psychologic changes. A progressive dementia has been reported.

Diagnostic Procedures.

1. A complete blood count and bone marrow test will indicate the presence of anemia.
2. A Schilling test, which measures the urinary excretion of labeled B_{12} following oral administration, will be abnormal.
3. Serum B_{12} levels will be decreased.
4. Nerve conduction velocities may be slowed.
5. Somatosensory and visual evoked potentials may be abnormal.

Treatment. Treatment consists of vitamin B_{12} replacement. The vitamin is administered intramuscularly in doses of 100 μg once a day for one week and then three times weekly until the anemia disappears. Maintenance dosages of 100 μg per month for life are necessary.

Vitamin E Deficiency

Secondary Vitamin E deficiency caused by fat malabsorption disorders, abetalipoproteinemia, or long term parenteral nutrition in children and adults may lead to the development of neurologic symptoms. A few cases with idiopathic Vitamin E deficiency without fat malabsorption have been reported. Spinocerebellar degeneration and a symmetric sensorimotor peripheral neuropathy have been described (56). Spinocerebellar degeneration presents with ophthalmoplegia, proximal muscle weakness, truncal and limb ataxia, decreased vibration and position sense and hyporeflexia (57).

Treatment. Vitamin E 1000 IU supplemented by desiccated ox bile will elevate serum vitamin E levels and alleviated symptoms.

NEUROLOGIC COMPLICATIONS OF THE ALCOHOLS

NEUROLOGIC COMPLICATIONS OF ETHANOL

Fetal Alcohol Syndrome

Definition. The fetal alcohol syndrome is a congenital condition due to chronic ethanol usage during pregnancy.

Etiology and Pathology. Alcohol has a teratogenic effect on the development of the fetus, and chronic ethanol abuse affects fetal development during early embryogenesis.

Clinical Features. Affected children exhibit growth retardation and cerebellar ataxia and have an abnormal facial appearance with short palpebral fissures, micrognathia, depressed nasal bridge, long convex upper lip (fish mouth), and epicanthic folds. Attention deficit disorder, mental retardation, and epilepsy may be present (58). The neonate may show signs of acute withdrawal characterized by irritability, increased muscle tone, tremors, and tonic seizures, often accompanied by abdominal distention, and vomiting.

Treatment. Neonatal irritability should be treated with chlorpromazine (Thorazine) 2 mg per kg qd. Phenobarbital 5 mg per kg q.d. is effective in reducing symptoms and should be used to control seizures.

In adults, neurologic complications of ethanol may occur because of:

1. The direct effect of alcohol on the central nervous system
2. The effect of concomitant nutritional deficiencies

3. The indirect effect of alcohol damage to other organs
4. The increased prevalence of certain diseases in alcoholics

Acute Intoxication and Coma

Etiology and Pathology. The ingestion of large quantities of ethanol over a short period of time may lead to respiratory depression, coma, and death. In addition, there is a risk of vomiting and subsequent aspiration. Some alcoholics are prone to hypoglycemia, particularly if they ingest ethanol in association with other drugs. The combination of ethanol and depressant drugs increases the risk of coma and death.

Diagnostic Procedures and Treatment.

1. Acute intoxication with coma is a neurologic emergency. One should never assume that a patient who is in a coma and smells of ethanol is simply suffering from alcoholic intoxication. A full neurologic examination should be performed.
2. Blood should be drawn and tested for glucose level, alcohol level, and the presence of other drugs (drug screen).
3. The vital signs should be recorded every 15 minutes. The patient should be catheterized and a nasogastric tube inserted and aspirated to remove any ethanol not yet absorbed from the stomach.
4. The airway should be cleared by suction, if necessary, and the patient turned from side to side to drain secretions from the oropharynx.
5. An intravenous infusion should be started and any electrolyte imbalance corrected.
6. Upon recovery, the patient should have adequate rest, light nourishment, adequate fluid intake, and aspirin for headache.

Alcoholic Ketoacidosis.

Definition. A metabolic disturbance resulting from a prolonged intake of alcohol.

Etiology and Pathology. The condition arises from a combination of metabolic abnormalities which occur in a fasting volume depleted alcoholic following abrupt cessation of drinking (59).

Clinical Features. The condition is preceded by heavy alcohol intake of several days or weeks duration followed by abrupt cessation and starvation for 24 to 72 hours. This is followed by abdominal pain and vomiting. Examination shows tachypnea or Kussmaul breathing, tachycardia, orthostatic hypotension and signs of chronic alcoholism such as spider angiomata and an enlarged tender liver.

Diagnostic Procedures.

1. Blood alcohol levels are low or absent.
2. There is metabolic acidosis with elevated ion gap.
3. Hypokalemia, hypochloremia and bicarbonate depletion are present.
4. Serum glucose is normal or slightly elevated.
5. Urinalysis shows ketonuria without glycosuria.
6. Serum amylase and liver enzyme levels may be abnormal.

Treatment.

1. Correct volume depletion by infusion of normal saline with dextrose.
2. Give potassium supplements to correct hypokalemia.
3. Treat intercurrent processes such as pneumonia, acute pancreatitis, gastritis or gastric hemorrhage.

Delirium Tremens

Definition. Delirium tremens is a condition that occurs in chronic alcoholics 72 to 96 hours after withdrawal of alcohol. It is characterized by an acute psychosis, which may result in death.

Etiology. Delirium tremens follows the sudden withdrawal of ethanol in a chronic alcoholic and may be precipitated by infection, trauma, pancreatitis, or malnutrition.

Sudden withdrawal of alcohol produces a rebound sensitivity to carbon dioxide with hyperventilation and subsequent respiratory alkalosis. Severe dehydration and electrolyte imbalance occur. Delirium tremens probably represents the effects of respiratory alkalosis, dehydration, and electrolyte imbalance on the central nervous system.

Clinical Features. The patient presents with a prodromal phase of tremulousness, irritability, and restlessness. There is an aversion to food, sleep is disturbed, and the patient has nightmares and fragmentary illusions. The patient then passes into an acute psychotic state with hallucinations that may be visual, auditory, or rarely olfactory or tactile. During this phase there are extreme restlessness and free vocalizing, consciousness is clouded, the patient is disoriented, and speech is incoherent. Seizures may occur and are usually preceded by the delirium. Autonomic overactivity occurs with elevated temperature, tachycardia, and profuse perspiration. Severe dehydration occurs if fluids are not replaced.

On examination there is a coarse tremor involving the tongue, lips, face, limbs, and fingers. The deep tendon reflexes are hyperreflexic, and the muscles may be tender on palpation.

Treatment.

1. Alcohol should be withheld. The belief that alcohol should be given prophylactically in incipient delirium tremens is fallacious.
2. The patient should be rehydrated. The patient's water loss may be between 5,000 and 6,000 ml per day. Any electrolyte imbalance, especially magnesium and potassium, should be corrected.
3. The patient should be adequately sedated. The following are recommended:
   a. Chlorpromazine (Thorazine) up to 1 g daily in divided doses
   b. Chlordiazepoxide (Librium) 80 to 100 mg q6h
   c. Diazepam (Valium) 5 to 10 mg IM q1-4h prn
4. Supplementary thiamine hydrochloride 200 mg should be given daily intramuscularly or intravenously.
5. As improvement occurs, the patient should be given an adequate diet with a vitamin supplement.

Prognosis. Patients with delirium tremens are acutely and severely ill. Death may occur in 50 percent of cases unless treated appropriately.

Wernicke-Korsakoff Encephalopathy

Wernicke's encephalopathy is frequently associated with Korsakoff's psychosis, and the two conditions may be regarded as parts of one syndrome.

Etiology and Pathology. Wernicke's encephalopathy is due to thiamine deficiency. It occurs in approximately 12 percent of all alcoholics but it is not exclusively confined to the alcoholic population. It has been described with starvation, malnutrition, intravenous hyperalimentation, hyperemesis gravidarum, and pernicious vomiting due to high gastrointestinal obstruction. It is postulated that thiamine deficiency in a genetically predisposed individual leads to depletion of the thiamine dependent enzyme transketolase.

This results in a high concentration of pyruvate and lactate in the brain and damage to neurons (60).

The pathologic changes occur in the gray matter of the periaqueductal gray surrounding the third and fourth ventricles, the mamillary bodies, thalamus, and cerebellum. Microscopically, degeneration of neurons, demyelination, petechial hemorrhages, and capillary and astrocytic proliferation occur.

Clinical Features. The classic triad of Wernicke's encephalopathy consists of ophthalmoplegia, ataxia, and dementia. These symptoms may be followed by Korsakoff's psychosis, which presents with confabulation, loss of recent memory, and loss of retention and recall.

Diagnostic Procedures.

1. There is usually elevation of blood pyruvate levels.
2. The most sensitive test is demonstration of reduced transketolase activity in erythrocytes.

Treatment.

1. Thiamine hydrochloride 100 to 200 mg intravenously should be given, followed by 100 mg intramuscularly q12h.
2. Electrolyte imbalance should be corrected.
3. The patient should be placed on an adequate diet with vitamin supplementation and abstain from ethanol use.

Alcohol Seizures

A number of possibilities should be considered when seizures develop in an alcoholic.

1. Generalized tonic clonic seizures occur 7 to 48 hours after cessation of drinking and may be a prodromal symptom of delirium tremens in about 30 percent of cases (61).

2. Alcohol may alter the seizure threshold in a known epileptic.

3. Seizures may develop in chronic alcoholics who have had repeated head injuries. Repeated contusions lead to the development of glial scars in the cortical gray matter. Such scars may irritate neurons and create an epileptic focus. Seizures sometimes called "rum fits" are associated with hypomagnesemia, respiratory alkalosis, low arterial PCO_2, and elevated arterial pH. These patients usually have a normal neurologic examination and a normal electroencephalogram, which is abnormal only during a seizure or in the postictal period. About 50 percent of cases show

a photoconvulsive response to photic stimulation when the EEG is recorded during the period of alcohol withdrawal.

Other causes of seizures in alcoholics include the combination effect of ethanol and certain drugs. One of the commonest associations is the use of propoxyphene (Darvon) with ethanol. Propoxyphene is a commonly used analgesic; the combination of propoxyphene and ethanol in a patient who is not taking an adequate diet may produce hypoglycemia and seizures.

Alcohol Dementia

Some chronic alcoholics develop a slowly progressive dementia quite distinct from the dementia of the Wernicke-Korsakoff syndrome. The following causes of dementia should be considered:

1. Patients suffering from early Alzheimer's disease may begin to use increasing amounts of alcohol when judgment and insight become impaired.
2. In chronic alcoholics repeated head trauma produces small areas of contusion in the cerebral cortex and eventually severe neuronal loss and dementia.
3. The chronic alcoholic may suffer repeated seizures, which cause cerebral anoxia and neuronal damage.
4. The chronic alcoholic may have a chronic subdural hematoma due to frequent falls.
5. Chronic alcoholics may develop chronic hepatic encephalopathy (see p. 303).
6. Some cases are undoubtedly due to the direct effect of alcohol in susceptible individuals who suffer accelerated neuronal degeneration because of chronic alcohol abuse (62).

Clinical Features. The patient presents with symptoms of progressive dementia including loss of operational judgment, failing memory, failing insight, and an inappropriate emotional response.

Diagnostic Procedures.

1. MR or CT scanning. The scan shows diffuse cortical atrophy with relatively less enlargement of the lateral ventricles.
2. Electroencephalography. The EEG shows progressive loss of background activity with the increased presence of excess theta and eventually delta activity, particularly in the temporal leads bilaterally.
3. Neuropsychological evaluation is useful in measuring the degree of intellectual and

cognitive impairment as well as recording improvement in maintained abstinence (63).

Treatment.

1. Patients suffering from alcohol dementia should be withdrawn from ethanol, receive an adequate diet, and be given thiamine supplements.
2. All cases of dementia should be investigated for possible treatable causes. This includes a careful screening for chronic subdural hematoma.
3. Lithium therapy is reported to reduce drinking and improve chronic alcoholics who are suffering from depression. However, lithium does not have any effect on dementia.

Many chronic alcoholics who remain abstinent demonstrate a remarkable improvement in mental status (64).

Central Pontine Myelinolysis

Definition. Central pontine myelinolysis is a rare condition that occurs in chronic alcoholism and in certain nutritional deficiencies.

Etiology and Pathology. Central pontine myelinolysis has also been reported to occur in the following conditions: chronic alcohol abuse, cerebral ischemia, cerebral edema, impaired fat metabolism, neoplasia, chronic infection, liver dysfunction, impaired secretion of ADH, and electrolyte abnormalities, particularly rapid correction of hyponatremia. The common factor in the genesis of central pontine myelinolysis appears to be chronic and severe hyponatremia.

There is a symmetric demyelination of the central structures in the pons extending up into the midbrain and down into the medulla. In severe cases there may be total demyelination of the center of the pons.

Clinical Features. Central pontine myelinolysis is characterized by impairment of consciousness with progressive development of cranial nerve palsies, severe ataxia, and dysarthria.

Diagnostic Procedures. MR scanning will demonstrate the areas of demyelination in the brain stem (65).

Treatment. The patient may recover if treated in an intensive care unit with nasogastric feeding, correction of metabolic abnormalities, and immediate antibiotic therapy for intercurrent infections.

Central Demyelination of the Corpus Callosum (Marchiafava-Bignami Disease)

Definition. Marchiafava-Bignami disease seems to occur exclusively in chronic alcoholics and was first described in red wine drinkers. It also occurs following the chronic use of other alcoholic beverages.

Etiology and Pathology. The etiology appears to be similar to that of central pontine myelinolysis. Pathologic changes are confined to the corpus callosum, and there is severe central demyelination of this structure.

Treatment. There is no effective treatment. This condition has been diagnosed only at autopsy.

Alcohol Cerebellar Degeneration

Definition. Alcohol cerebellar degeneration is at present one of the most common complications of chronic ethanol abuse.

Pathology. The appearance of the cerebellum is characteristic with marked atrophy of the anterior lobes of the cerebellum and the superior vermis. The involved areas show almost complete loss of Purkinje cells and loss of the neurons in both granular and molecular layers of the cortex. Advanced cases may show some involvement of the neocerebellum, particularly the dentate nucleus.

Clinical Features. The condition is not alcohol dose dependent and occurs in alcoholics who have an unusual sensitivity to alcohol (66). The patient with alcohol cerebellar degeneration presents with severe ataxia of the lower limbs and trunk, minor cerebellar signs involving the upper limbs, and absence of nystagmus, dysarthria, and dementia.

Diagnostic Procedures. MR or CT scanning reveals atrophy of the anterior lobes of the cerebellum and the superior vermis.

Treatment. The treatment includes abstinence, adequate diet, and thiamine supplements.

Alcohol Myelopathy

Spastic paraparesis is occasionally seen in alcoholics. Most cases are probably due to cervical spondylosis aggravated by repeated falls and trauma to the neck. However, there is a rare degenerative condition involving the spinal cord due to chronic ethanol abuse and nutritional deficiencies. There are degenerative changes in the lateral and to some extent the posterior columns of the spinal cord. These patients show progressive lower limb spasticity and weakness with the presence of ankle clonus, exaggerated knee jerks and ankle jerks, and extensor plantar responses, but sparing the upper limbs and bladder function.

Alcohol Peripheral Neuropathy

Etiology and Pathology. The majority of cases of peripheral neuropathy in alcoholics are mild and appear after many years of excessive drinking. Peripheral neuropathy in alcoholics has been attributed to nutritional deficiency or to the toxic effects of alcohol on the peripheral nerve. Many chronic alcoholics have poor dietary habits, and it is reasonable to assume that both factors are involved in the development of peripheral neuropathy. The pathologic changes consist of wallerian degeneration with loss of myelin and axis cylinders.

Clinical Features. The majority of chronic alcoholics have mild symptoms of peripheral neuropathy with peripheral paresthesias and some loss of muscle bulk in the distal lower extremities. The more advanced cases show weakness involving the distal portions of all four limbs, and there may be severe pain in a majority of cases. These patients suffer extreme dysesthesias and are often unable to tolerate contact with clothing. Electromyography and nerve conduction studies are indicative of axonal degeneration (67).

Treatment. The treatment includes abstinence, adequate diet, and thiamine supplements.

Prognosis. Symptoms usually persist for many months after initial treatment despite withdrawal from alcohol, since axonal regeneration is a slow process. However, most cases will eventually recover.

Alcohol Myopathy

Alcohol myopathy occurs in three forms. It may present as acute myopathy with severe muscle pain and myoglobulinuria, acute myopathy with proximal weakness and painful spasms, or a chronic myopathy.

The acute form of alcohol myopathy with myoglobulinuria occurs after a heavy bout of drinking, and it is possible that this condition represents the effect of alcohol on a patient who is already susceptible to paroxysmal myoglobulinuria. These patients are profoundly ill and are at risk for the development of acute tubular necrosis. This should be treated in an intensive care unit with appropriate restriction of fluid, correction of electrolyte imbalance, and sedation until diuresis occurs.

The acute myopathy which follows a heavy bout of drinking is characterized by severe proximal weakness, particularly in the lower limb girdle musculature, with painful spasm of the affected muscles. Treatment consists of rest, sedation, adequate diet, and thiamine supplementation.

Chronic alcohol myopathy is a much commoner condition and is characterized by wasting of the proximal musculature, particularly in the area of the shoulder girdle. Weakness, however, is uncommon.

The treatment consists of abstinence, adequate diet, and thiamine supplements.

NEUROLOGIC COMPLICATIONS OF METHANOL

Methanol is most commonly ingested by chronic alcoholics who believe that they are drinking ethanol, but death or blindness can occur from dermal or respiratory absorption (68).

Etiology and Pathology. Methanol is found in heating agents (canned heat), solvents, cleaning agents, paints, and rubbing alcohol. Methanol itself is not toxic. It is metabolized by alcohol dehydrogenase to formaldehyde and formic acid, both of which are toxic substances.

When methanol is ingested, it is rapidly absorbed. A severe metabolic acidosis results as methanol is metabolized. Formic acid has a toxic effect on oligodendrocytes due to inhibition of cytochrome oxidase, resulting in cerebral edema and axonal compression. The optic nerve is commonly involved.

Clinical Features. Approximately 12 to 48 hours after ingestion the patient begins to complain of headache, nausea, abdominal pain, and blurred vision. The visual symptoms may progress to blindness. The patient is restless with a drunken appearance, and delirium or seizures and coma may occur.

Diagnostic Procedures.

1. Methanol and formic acid are present in the blood and urine.
2. There is evidence of a high anion-gap metabolic acidosis.
3. There may be evidence of increased intracranial pressure.

Treatment.

1. The treatment of choice is hemodialysis. It permits removal of metabolites and restoration of pH without threat of fluid overload.
2. Ethanol is a competitive inhibitor of alcohol dehydrogenase and will slow the metabolism of methanol into its toxic metabolites. It should be administered in a loading dose of 50 mg IV or 60 ml p.o. followed by 10 g% IV or 10 ml q1h.
3. Severe metabolic acidosis should be corrected with intravenous bicarbonate.

Prognosis. Ingestion of more than 100 ml of methanol is frequently fatal. Blindness is common, and parkinsonism is an occasional complication.

NEUROLOGIC COMPLICATIONS OF ETHYLENE GLYCOL

Etiology and Pathology. Ethylene glycol is found in antifreeze, detergents, and paints. It has a slightly sweet taste and may be ingested by children. Ethylene glycol is metabolized, by alcohol dehydrogenase, into toxic metabolites such as oxalic acid.

Clinical Features. The patient has a drunken appearance and develops confusion and stupor within an hour of ingestion of ethylene glycol. Seizures may occur. Between 12 and 24 hours later the patient becomes hypertensive and develops cardiopulmonary failure, acute oliguric renal failure, and coma (69).

Diagnostic Procedures.

1. Severe, high anion-gap metabolic acidosis and hypocalcemia occur.
2. Examination of the urine reveals crystalluria and the presence of oxalate or hippurate crystals.
3. Ethylene glycol is present in the blood.

Treatment. The treatment is the same as that for methanol poisoning.

NEUROLOGICAL COMPLICATIONS OF COCAINE ABUSE

A number of potentially serious neurological complications have been identified in cocaine abusers (70).

Headache, often associated with nausea, arthralgias, abdominal and chest pain, is usually benign but recurrent. Generalized tonic clonic seizures may occur within a few hours of cocaine abuse. Temporary focal neurological deficits including transient visual motor or sensory disturbances have been followed by cerebral infarction in a few cases. These latter cases are probably suffering from cerebral arteritis which can be induced by cocaine abuse. Optic atrophy has been reported.

NEUROLOGICAL MANIFESTATIONS OF POISONING AND INTOXICATION

Lead Poisoning

Etiology and Pathology. Lead and all inorganic and organic lead compounds are toxic to humans. Lead is absorbed more readily by inhalation than by ingestion, but both routes may produce toxicity. A blood lead level of more than 40 mg/100 ml is considered potentially toxic.

Absorbed lead enters all tissues but is stored preferentially in bone. Tertiary lead phosphate conversion to soluble secondary lead phosphate is enhanced by a low calcium diet, acidosis, multiple bone metastases, and excess parathormone.

The most common sources of lead poisoning are:

1. The ingestion of lead-based paint (Children may ingest lead paint flakes, which are still found in the interior of older dwellings. Lead paint is no longer available for interior decorating)
2. The ingestion of lead toys (Children may chew on lead toy soldiers)
3. The ingestion of soft water delivered through lead pipes or lead-contaminated "moonshine" whisky
4. Industrial causes: demolition workers who cut contaminated steel with oxyacetylene torches; workers exposed to dusts, fumes, or sprays containing lead

Lead enters the central nervous system as the blood concentration rises but is removed slowly when blood levels fall. Thus, intermittent exposure produces a gradual increase of lead in the central nervous system. In children, acute exposure to lead results in a sharp increase in lead concentration in the brain resulting in cerebral edema with damage to capillary endothelium, increased capillary permeability, interstitial edema, and scattered hemorrhages.

Chronic exposure to lead at any age results in neuronal damage in the central nervous system and segmental demyelination followed by axonal damage to peripheral nerves.

Clinical Features.

1. Lead encephalopathy. Affected children have a history of pica, vomiting, colic, and constipation. Cerebral edema produces drowsiness, which may proceed to coma.

Focal or generalized seizures and status epilepticus may occur. Papilledema and focal neurologic deficits are not uncommon. Increasing edema produces uncal herniation and death. Survivors may have chronic seizures, mental retardation, optic atrophy, and focal neurologic abnormalities.

2. Chronic exposure in children may lead to mental retardation, learning disabilities, behavior problems, and hyperactivity (71).

3. Adults exposed to lead show personality change, dementia, rigidity, seizures, optic atrophy, and visual failure.

4. Chronic exposure to lead may result in the development of a condition resembling amyotrophic lateral sclerosis.

5. Chronic exposure in children and adults produces peripheral neuropathy, often presenting with weakness of the hands and bilateral wrist drop (72).

Diagnostic Procedures.

1. X-rays. Skull x-rays may reveal evidence of increased intracranial pressure. The long bones may have a "lead line."
2. Examination of the peripheral blood smear vessels reveals hypochromic, microcytic anemia. Basophilic stippling of the red blood cells is usually present.
3. Nerve conduction velocities are slowed in lead neuropathy.
4. Blood lead levels are elevated above 80 μg/100 ml.
5. Urine lead levels are more than 150 g/L for every 24 hours. Coproporphyrin III levels are elevated.

Treatment.

1. In acute encephalopathy, increased intracranial pressure should be managed with mannitol, corticosteroids, and intracranial pressure monitoring.
2. Chelating agents such as calcium disodium versenate or British antilewisite should be administered. In adults penicillamine may be added.
3. The source of lead exposure should be removed.

Prognosis. The mortality of acute encephalopathy is less than 5 percent. However, severely affected children develop retardation, optic atrophy, seizure disorders, and behavior problems.

Neurologic Manifestations of Mercury Poisoning

Etiology and Pathology. Mercury is encountered in an inorganic form, as metallic mercury or a mercuric salt, or as organic mercury, usually methyl mercury. Inorganic mercury is used in the paper and pulp industry, paint manufacturing, and the electrical appliance industry. Organic mercury is used in fungicides and may be concentrated by animals and fish living in a polluted environment.

Mercury is toxic to the neurons of the occipital lobes and the granular cells of the cerebellum. The peripheral nerves show axonal degeneration and demyelination.

Clinical Features. Early mercury poisoning is characterized by a fine tremor of the fingers, eyelids, and tongue with progression to involve the arms, head, and legs. Paresthesias of the extremities followed by numbness, progressive distal weakness, and cerebellar ataxia are also seen. Tunnel vision leading to blindness, slurred speech, and impaired hearing are also frequently reported. In advanced cases seizures, mania, dementia, and hallucinations are seen.

Congenital mercury poisoning occurs at lower blood mercury levels than adult poisoning due to the ability of the fetus and placenta to concentrate the metal. Affected children are small for their age, may have a seizure disorder, and may show psychomotor retardation.

Diagnostic Procedures.

1. Hair mercury analysis. Less than 100 ppm of mercury is usually safe and asymptomatic, while levels approaching 500 ppm are always associated with symptoms. In children with congenital mercury poisoning levels greater than 100 ppm are usually associated with significant damage to the nervous system.
2. Electroencephalography. The EEG may reveal slowing of background frequency and epileptiform activity.
3. Electromyography and nerve conduction studies show delayed motor and sensory distal latencies, reduced sensory response amplitude and increased prevalence of abnormal electrical activity in muscle (73).

Treatment. Chelation with penicillamine and the use of selenium and vitamin E have been shown to be effective in reducing the neurotoxic effects of mercury poisoning.

Neurologic Manifestations of Arsenic Poisoning

Etiology and Pathology. Arsenic is found in paints, insecticides, rodenticides, and contaminated food or beer and is occasionally used in suicide attempts and homicide.

Arsenic disrupts the tricarboxylic acid cycle by interfering with pyruvate oxidase and alpha glutarate oxidase systems.

Clinical Features. A single large dose of arsenic produces vomiting followed by tachycardia, hypotension, and in some cases death. Survivors develop a peripheral neuropathy two to three weeks later (74). This is characterized by a distal numbness and intense paresthesias. Position and vibration sense are severely involved. Muscle weakness is a late development. Recovery is slow and occurs over a period of several months. Poisoning by organic arsenical insecticides may be followed by an acute, symmetrical, ascending polyneuropathy resembling postinfectious polyneuritis (Guillain-Barré syndrome).

Diagnostic Procedures.

1. Lumbar puncture. The CSF glucose and protein content is normal.
2. The blood level of arsenic is 7 ng/100 ml or greater. The urine contains greater than 1 mg/24 hr.
3. Nerve biopsy reveals demyelination and axonal degeneration.
4. Nerve conduction velocities are slowed.

Treatment. The source of arsenic should be avoided. British antilewisite (BAL) and penicillamine are effective chelating agents.

Neurologic Manifestations of Manganese Poisoning

Manganese is encountered in mining and industrial processes and enters the body by inhalation. This results in a marked neuronal loss in the basal ganglia, particularly the globus pallidus (75).

Patients with manganese intoxication present with a psychiatric disorder characterized by nervousness, irritability, and emotional lability. This is followed by generalized weakness, impotence, parkinsonism with increased muscle tone and exaggerated stretch reflexes. The blood manganese level is greater than 0.075 ppm, and the administration of 1 g of EDTA increases the urine level by 0.03 to 0.05 ppm. L-Dopa is effective in relieving some of the symptoms of parkinsonism.

Industrial Toxins

Table 17-4 lists the more common industrial toxins, where they are encountered, and

TABLE 17–4. Industrial Toxins and Neurologic Signs and Symptoms

Toxin	Exposure	Neurologic Signs and Symptoms of Toxicity
Acrylamide	Workers handling acrylamide monomer	Sensorimotor polyneuropathy Truncal ataxia
Allyl chloride	Industrial exposure	Polyneuropathy
Carbamates	Pesticides	Sensorimotor polyneuropathy
Carbon disulfide	Cellophane and textile industry Pesticides	Polyneuropathy Psychosis
Carbon tetrachloride	Fire extinguishers Cleaning agents	Polyneuropathy, optic atrophy Cerebellar ataxia, parkinsonism
Gasoline, lead-based	Gasoline sniffing Inhalant abuse	Tremor, ataxia Euphoria, visual hallucinations Irreversible encephalopathy, polyneuropathy (76)
Methyl bromide	Refrigerants, insecticides Fumigants	Sensorimotor polyneuropathy Diplopia, vertigo Ataxia, nystagmus
Methyl-n-butyl	Industrial exposure	Polyneuropathy
N-hexane	Glue sniffing Industrial exposure	Sensorimotor polyneuropathy (77)
Nitrous oxide (laughing gas)	Inhalant abuse	Polyneuropathy
Organophosphates	Insecticides, nerve gas	Early: lacrimation, twitching and convulsions, respiratory failure Delayed: sensorimotor polyneuropathy
Thallium	Rodenticides Industrial use	Motor polyneuropathy, cranial nerve palsies Convulsions, psychosis Dementia
Toluene	Spray paint Inhalant abuse	Acute: euphoria, perceptual disorders Subacute: cerebellar damage, polyneuropathy

the neurologic signs and symptoms of toxicity.

Organophosphorus and Carbamate Pesticide Poisoning

Organophosphorus compounds which are used as insecticides and carbamate pesticides have an immediate, intermediate and delayed neurotoxic effect. The immediate response following poisoning is a cholinergic crisis with respiratory failure (78). The intermediate phase consists of paralysis of motor cranial nerves, neck muscles and proximal limb muscles 24 to 96 hours after poisoning. An acute symmetrical ascending polyneuropathy resembling postinfectious polyneuritis (Guillain-Barré syndrome) can occur one to three weeks after exposure to the toxic compounds (79).

Treatment.

1. Assisted respiration with a mechanical respirator may be required at any stage.
2. The acute cholinergic phase requires large doses of atropine, beginning 2 to 4 mg IV followed by 2 mg IV every five minutes until muscarinic symptoms disappear. This should be supplemented by pralidoxime 1 to 2 g IV every five minutes, which activates cholinesterase.

Therapeutic Drug Toxicity

Table 17-5 lists common therapeutic drugs that have been reported to have toxic effects upon the nervous system. The generic drug, trade name, and toxic side effects are listed.

TABLE 17–5. Neurotoxicity of Therapeutic Drugs

Drug	Toxic Neurologic Side Effects	Drug	Toxic Neurologic Side Effects
Acetazolamide (Diamox)	Paresthesias of the hands, feet, and face Transient myopathy	Methotrexate	Intrathecal: meningismus, transverse myelitis, dementia, coma
Amiodarone	Sensorimotor polyneuropathy (80)	Metronidazole (Flagyl)	Polyneuropathy
Amphotericin B	Polyneuropathy	Nitrofurantoin (Macrodantin)	Sensorimotor neuropathy
Antidepressants/ tricyclics (Elavil, Tofranil)	Anticholinergic effects, confusion Myoclonus, choreiform movements Convulsions	Neomycin	Deafness, polyneuropathy
		Polymixin B	Polyneuropathy
		Quinidine	Progressive dementia
Bismuth (Anusol, Pepto-Bismol)	With prolonged use— encephalopathy, ataxia, tremor, myoclonus	Quinine	Optic neuritis, deafness, nystagmus
Chloramphenicol (Chloromycetin)	Painful polyneuropathy Optic neuritis	Rifampin	Encephalopathy
		Salicylates	Deafness, vertigo
Chloroquine (Aralen)	Deafness, retinopathy, myopathy	Streptomycin	Deafness, vestibular dysfunction Optic neuritis Polyneuropathy
Clioquinol	SMON syndrome (subacute myelo-optic neuropathy)	Vancomycin	Deafness
Colchicine	Proximal myopathy, polyneuropathy (81)	Vincristine (Oncovin)	Sensorimotor neuropathy Myalgia
Colistin	Polyneuropathy		
Disulfiram (Antabuse)	Polyneuropathy, cerebellar degeneration		
Ethacrynic acid (Edecrin)	Deafness		
Ethambutol (Myambutol)	Optic neuritis		
5-FU	Cerebellar ataxia, dysarthria, nystagmus		
Furosemide (Lasix)	Deafness		
Gentamicin (Garamycin)	Vestibular dysfunction		
Gold	Polyneuropathy, cranial nerve palsies Transverse myelitis, convulsions Encephalopathy		
INH	Sensory neuropathy, convulsions Euphoria, psychosis		
Kanamycin (Kantrex)	Deafness, polyneuropathy		
Lithium (Eskalith)	Twitching, tremor, ataxia, dysarthria		

REFERENCES

1. Salama, J.; Gherardi, R.; et al. Post anoxic delayed encephalopathy with leukoencephalopathy and non-hemorrhagic cerebral amyloid angiopathy. Clin. Neuropathol. 5:153–156; 1986.
2. Janate, A.; Archer, R. L.; et al. Coexistence of ectopic rhythms and periodic EEG patterns in anoxic encephalopathy. Clin. Electroenceph. 17:187–194; 1986.
3. Synek, V. M.; Synek, B. J. L. "Theta pattern coma" occurring in young adults. Clin. Electroenceph. 18:54–60; 1987.
4. Hoff, J. T. Cerebral protection. J. Neurosurg. 65:579–591; 1986.
5. Guidelines for the diagnosis of brain death. Can. J. Neurol. Sci. 14:653–656; 1987.
6. Bernat, J. L. Ethical and legal aspects of the emergency management of brain death and organ retrieval. Emerg. Med. Clin. North. Am. 5:661–676; 1987.
7. Ayus, J. C.; Krothapalli, R. K.; et al. Treatment of symptomatic hyponatremia and its relation to brain damage. A prospective study. New Engl. J. Med. 317:1190–1195; 1987.
8. Illowsky, B. P.; Laureno, R. Encephalopathy and myelinolysis after rapid correction of hyponatremia. Brain 110:855–867; 1987.

9. Nielsen, J. M. Central pontine myelinolysis complicating hyponatremia. Med. J. Aust. 146:492–494; 1987.

10. Sterns, R. H. Severe symptomatic hyponatremia treatment and outcome. A study of 64 cases. Ann. Intern. Med. 107:656–664; 1987.

11. Snyder, N. A.; Fiegal, D. W.; et al. Hypernatremia in elderly patients. A heterogenous, morbid and iatrogenic entity. Ann. Intern. Med. 107:309–319; 1987.

12. Thomas, S.; Sainsbury, C. P. Q.; et al. Treatment of hypernatremic dehydration due to diarrhea. Br. J. Clin. Pract. 40:535–536; 1987.

13. Linshaw, M. A. Potassium homeostasis and hypokalemia. Pediatr. Clin. North Am. 34:649–681; 1987.

14. Villabona, C.; Rodriguez, P.; et al. Potassium disturbances as a cause of metabolic neuromyopathy. Intensive Care Med. 13:208–210; 1987.

15. McIvor, M. E. Delayed fatal hyperkalemia in a patient with acute fluoride intoxication. Ann. Emerg. Med. 16:1165–1167; 1987.

16. Knox, D. L.; Hanneken, A. M.; et al. Uremic optic neuropathy. Arch. Ophthalmol. 106:50–54; 1988.

17. Yoshida, S.; Tajika, T. Dialysis disequilibrium syndrome in neurosurgical patients. Neurosurgery 20:716–721; 1987.

18. Jagadha, V.; Deck, J. H. N.; et al. Wernicke's encephalopathy in patients on peritoneal dialysis or hemodialysis. Ann. Neurol. 21:78–84; 1987.

19. Sherlock, S. Chronic portal system encephalopathy update 1987. Gut 28:1043–1048; 1987.

20. Morgan, M. Y.; Hawley, K. E. Lactitol vs lactulose in the treatment of acute hepatic encephalopathy in cirrhotic patients: a double blind randomized trial. Hepatology 7:1278–1284; 1987.

21. Reeve, T. S. Surgery for hyperthyroidism. Adv. Surg. 21:29–47; 1987.

22. Nemni, R.; Bottacchi, E.; et al. Polyneuropathy in hypothyroidism: clinical, electrophysiological and morphological findings in four cases. J. Neurol. Neurosurg. Psychiatry 50:1454–1460; 1987.

23. Vernava, A. M.; O'Neal, L. W.; et al. Lethal hyperparathyroid crisis: hazards of phosphate administration. Surgery 102:941–948; 1987.

24. Adams, J. E.; Burns, R. P. Hyperparathyroidism at a tertiary care facility. J. Tenn. Med. Assoc. 80:667–670; 1987.

25. Kier, R.; Blinder, R. A.; et al. MR imaging with surface cores in primary hyperparathyroidism. J. Comput. Assist. Tomogr. 11:863–868; 1987.

26. Chiba, T.; Okimura, Y.; et al. Hypocalcemic crisis in alcoholic fatty liver: transient hypoparathyroidism due to magnesium deficiency. Am. J. Gastroenterology 82:1084–1087; 1987.

27. Ikeda, K.; Kobayashi, T.; et al. Sensorineural hearing loss associated with hypoparathyroidism. Laryngoscope 97:1075–1079; 1987.

28. Jamal, G. A.; Kerr, D. J.; et al. Generalized peripheral nerve dysfunction in acromegaly: a study by conventional and novel neurophysiological techniques. J. Neurol. Neurosurg. Psychiatry 50:886–894; 1987.

29. Kinzie, B. J. Management of the syndrome of inappropriate secretion of antidiuretic hormone. Clin. Pharm. 6:625–633; 1987.

30. Lakdar, A. A.; McLaren, E. H.; et al. Pituitary failure from Sheehan's syndrome in the puerperium. Two case reports. Br. J. Obstet. Gynaecol. 94:998–999; 1987.

31. Nukta, E. M.; Taylor, H. C. Panhypopituitarism secondary to an aneurysm of the anterior communicating artery. Can. Med. Assoc. J. 137:413–415; 1987.

32. Round, R.; Keane, J. R. The minor symptoms of increased intracranial pressure: 101 patients with benign intracranial hypertension. Neurology 38:1461–1464; 1988.

33. Allen, R. S.; Sarma, P. R. Pseudotumor cerebri: meningeal carcinomatosis presenting as benign intracranial hypertension. South. Med. J. 80:1182–1183; 1987.

34. Harati, Y. Diabetic peripheral neuropathies. Ann. Intern. Med. 107:546–559; 1987.

35. Korthats, J. K.; Greron, M. A.; et al. Intima of epineurol arterioles is increased in diabetic polyneuropathy. Neurology 38:1582–1586; 1988.

36. Stewart, J. D. Diabetic truncal neuropathy: topography of the sensory deficit. Ann. Neurol. 25:233–238; 1989.

37. Peterson, B. A.; Brunning, R. D.; et al. Central nervous system involvement in acute nonlymphocytic leukemia. Am. J. Med. 83:464–470; 1987.

38. Inse, P. G.; Shaw, P. J.; et al. Demyelinating neuropathy due to primary IgM Kappa B cell lymphoma of peripheral nerve. Neurology 37:1231–1235; 1987.

39. Landan, I.; Gilroy, J.; et al. Syringomyelia affecting the entire spinal cord secondary to primary spinal intramedullary central nervous system lymphoma. J. Neurol. Neurosurg. Psychiatry 50:1533–1535; 1987.

40. Ikeda, S.; Yanegisawa, N.; et al. Vagus nerve and celiac ganglion lesions in generalized amyloidosis. J. Neurol. Sci. 79:129–139; 1987.

41. Santiago, R. M.; Scharnhorst, D.; et al. Respiratory muscle weakness and ventilatory failure in AL amyloidosis with muscular pseudohypertrophy. Am. J. Med. 83:175–178; 1987.

42. Sheehan-Dare, R. A.; Simmons, A. V. Amyloid neuropathy and myeloma: response to treatment. Postgrad. Med. J. 63:141–142; 1987.

43. Nobile-Orazio, E.; Marmiroli, P.; et al. Peripheral neuropathy in macroglobulinemia: incidence and antigen-specificity of M proteins. Neurology 37:1506–1514; 1987.

44. Smith, T.; Sherman, W. Peripheral neuropathy associated with plasma cell dyscrasia: a clinical

and electrophysiological follow-up study. Acta. Neurol. Scand. 75:244–248; 1987.

45. Smith, T.; Sherman, W.; et al. Peripheral neuropathy associated with plasma cell dyscrasia: a clinical and electrophysiological follow-up study. Acta. Neurol. Scand. 75:244–248; 1987.

46. Lippa, C. F.; Chad, D. A. Neuropathy associated with cryoglobulinemia. Muscle and Nerve 9:626–631; 1986.

47. Silverstein, M. N. Relative and absolute polycythemia. How to tell them apart. Postgrad. Med. 81:285–288; 1987.

48. Yeung-Laiwah, A. C.; Moore, M. R.; et al. Pathogenesis of acute porphyria. Q. J. Med. 63:377–392; 1987.

49. Kaplan, P. W.; Lewis, D. V. Juvenile acute intermittent porphyria with hypercholesterolemia and epilepsy: A case report and review of the literature. J. Child. Neurol. 1:38–45; 1986.

50. Adams, M.; Rhyner, P. A.; et al. Whipple's disease confined to the central nervous system. Ann. Neurol. 21:104–108; 1987.

51. Macdonald, M. J. Postexercise late onset hypoglycemia in insulin-dependent diabetic patients. Diabetic Care 10:584–588; 1987.

52. Lamarche, J.; Vital, C. Carcinomatous neuropathy—an ultrastructural study of ten cases. Ann. Pathol. 7:98–105; 1987.

53. Anderson, N. E.; Rosenbaum, M. K.; et al. Paraneoplastic cerebellar degeneration: clinical immunological correlations. Ann. Neurol. 24:559–567; 1988.

54. Waterston, J. A.; Gilligan, B. S. Pyridoxine neuropathy. Med. J. Aust. 146:640–642; 1987.

55. Ashkinazi, S.; Weitz, R.; et al. Vitamin B-12 deficiency due to strict vegetarian diet in adolescence. Clin. Pediatr. (Phila.) 26:662–663; 1987.

56. Traber, M. C.; Sokol, R. J.; et al. Lack of tocopherol in peripheral nerves of vitamin E-deficient patients with peripheral neuropathy. New Engl. J. Med. 317:262–265; 1987.

57. Yokota, T.; Wada, Y.; et al. Adult-onset spinocerebellar syndrome with idiopathic vitamin E deficiency. Ann. Neurol. 22:84–87; 1987.

58. Marcus, J. C. Neurological findings in the fetal alcohol syndrome. Neuropediatrics 18:158–160; 1987.

59. Duffens, K.; Marx, J. A. Alcoholic ketoacidosis—a review. J. Emerg. Med. 5:399–406; 1987.

60. Thompson, A. D.; Jeyasingham, M. D.; et al. Nutritional and alcoholic encephalopathies. Acta. Med. Scand. 717 (Suppl):55–65; 1987.

61. Morris, J. C.; Victor, M. Alcohol withdrawal seizures. Emerg. Med. Clin. North Am. 5:827–839; 1987.

62. Lishman, W. A.; Jacobson, R. R.; et al. Brain damage in alcoholism: Current concepts. Acta. Med. Scand. 717 (Suppl):5–17; 1987.

63. Parsons, O. A. Intellectual impairment in alcoholics: persistent issues. Acta. Med. Scand. 717 (Suppl):33–46; 1987.

64. Carlen, P. L.; Wilkinson, A. Reversibility of alcohol-related brain damage: clinical and experimental observations. Acta. Med. Scand. 717 (Suppl):19–26; 1987.

65. Rippe, D. J.; Edward, M. E.; et al. MR imaging of central pontine myelinolysis. J. Comput. Assis. Tomogr. 11:724–726; 1987.

66. Estron, W. J. Alcohol cerebellar degeneration is not a dose dependent phenomenon. Alcoholism Clin. Exp. Res. 11:372–375; 1987.

67. Shankar, K.; Thompson, C. An electrodiagnostic study in chronic alcoholic subjects. Arch. Phys. Med. Rehabil. 68:803–805; 1987.

68. Haines, J. D. Methanol Poisoning. How to recognize and treat a deadly intoxication. Postgrad. Med. 82:149–151; 1987.

69. Verrilli, M. R.; Deyling, C. L.: et al. Fatal ethylene glycol intoxication. Report of a case and a review of the literature. Cleve. Clin. J. Med. 54:289–295; 1987.

70. Lowenstein, D. H.; et al. Acute neurologic and psychiatric complications associated with cocaine abuse. Am. J. Med. 83:841–846; 1987.

71. Faust, D.; Brown, J. Moderately elevated blood lead levels. Effects on neuropsychological functioning in children. Pediatrics 80:263–269; 1987.

72. Fangsheng, H. E. Occupational toxic neuropathies—an update. Scand J. Work. Environ. Health 11:321–330; 1985.

73. Singer, R.; Valcuikos, J. A.; et al. Peripheral neurotoxicity in workers exposed to inorganic mercury compounds. Arch. Environ. Health 42:181–184; 1987.

74. Hay, R.; McCormack, J. G. Arsenic poisoning and peripheral neuropathy. Aust. Fam. Physician 16:287–289; 1987.

75. Yamada, M.; Ohno, S.; et al. Chronic manganese poisoning: a neuropathological study with determination of manganese distribution in the brain. Acta. Neuropathol. (Berl) 70:273–278; 1986.

76. Hall, D. M. B.; Ramsey, J.; et al. Neuropathy in a petrol sniffer. Arch. Dis. Child. 61:900–901; 1986.

77. King, P. J. L.; Morris, J. G. L.; et al. Glue sniffing neuropathy. Aust. Nz. J. Med. 15:293–299; 1985.

78. Senonayake, N.; Karalledde, L. Toxic effects of organophosphorus insecticides: an intermediate syndrome. New Engl. J. Med. 316:761–763; 1987.

79. Dickoff, D. J.; Gerber, O.; et al. Delayed neurotoxicity after ingestion of carbamate pesticide. Neurology 37:1229–1231; 1987.

80. Jacobs, J. M.; Costa-Lussa, F. R. The pathology of amiodarone neurotoxicity II, peripheral neuropathy in man. Brain 108:753–769; 1985.

81. Kunel, R. W.; Duncan, G.; et al. Colchicine myopathy and neuropathy. New Engl. J. Med. 316:1562–1568; 1987.

CHAPTER 18

TRAUMA

Head injury is a common neurologic and neurosurgical condition in the United States. It has been estimated that more than 1 million persons suffer head injury each year and more than one-third of accidental deaths are due to head injury. Although the majority of head injuries are trivial, a small percentage of patients suffer severe handicaps and present a major problem in terms of medical care, economic loss, and human suffering.

Most cases of severe head injury are the result of automobile and motorcycle accidents. The general acceptance of these forms of transportation as a modern "way of life" has resulted in apathetic tolerance of the increased risk of severe head injury.

Etiology and Pathology

The head and intracranial contents may be injured by forces of acceleration—the sudden linear movement of the skull; deceleration—the sudden reduction in velocity of linear movement; rotation—sudden rotary movements of the skull and contents; and lastly, missile penetration.

Forces of acceleration and deceleration produce damage to the intracranial contents because of disproportionate movement of the skull and brain. The base of the frontal lobes may be damaged by contact with the rough floor of the anterior fossa, while the tips of the temporal lobe may be injured by the edges of the sphenoid ridge. The corpus callosum may be damaged during head injury through contact with the free edge of the falx cerebri. Contact with the tentorium cerebelli may result in damage to the superior surface of the cerebellum or the brain stem.

When the head strikes a solid object, there is sudden deceleration of the head with subsequent deformity of the skull, a decrease in volume of the cranial contents, and a rise in cerebrospinal fluid pressure. A pressure wave passes from the point of impact through the cranial contents and exits at the opposite side of the brain. The initial impact and negative pressure wave produces tearing of tissue at the site of injury; the exiting pressure wave also causes tissue damage, resulting in a contrecoup injury. Rotation of the head produces shearing forces in the brain with diffuse tearing of axons in the central white matter of the hemispheres. Blood vessels and meninges may also be damaged in this manner.

Traumatic injury may result in an intracranial hemorrhage, such as epidural hematoma, subdural hematoma, subarachnoid hemorrhage, or intracerebral hematoma; a closed head injury; damage to cranial nerves; and traumatic cerebrospinal fluid (CSF) rhinorrhea and otorrhea.

TRAUMATIC INTRACRANIAL HEMORRHAGE

Epidural Hematoma

Definition. An epidural hematoma is an acute hemorrhage into the epidural space. The condition has a 20 percent mortality.

329

Etiology and Pathology. The hemorrhage usually occurs with a temporoparietal skull fracture in which the middle meningeal artery and/or vein are lacerated. In unusual cases these vessels may be torn during a severe blow to the head without the occurrence of a fracture. Because the meningeal artery is frequently involved, there is a rapid accumulation of blood in the epidural space with a rapid rise in intracranial pressure, uncal herniation, and brain stem compression.

Clinical Features. There is a history of head injury with loss of consciousness. In about 50 percent of cases the patient recovers consciousness and there is a "lucid interval" followed by a gradual decrease in level of consciousness as intracranial pressure increases and rostral-caudal deterioration occurs (see p. 50). In the remaining cases the lucid interval does not occur and loss of consciousness is followed by progressive deterioration. An epidural hematoma occasionally occurs in the posterior fossa, in which case sudden death may occur as a result of compression of the cardiorespiratory centers in the medulla. There is a poorer prognosis in patients who do not experience a lucid interval, who require early surgery and in those involved in high-speed automobile accidents (1, 2).

Diagnostic Procedures. The diagnostic procedures include:

1. Skull x-rays. X-rays of the skull typically show a linear fracture of the temporoparietal area that crosses the middle meningeal vessels. There may be displacement of the calcified pineal gland to the opposite side.

2. Either magnetic resonance (MR) or computed tomography (CT) scanning will demonstrate an acute epidural hematoma (see Figure 18–1). These hematomas cannot always be distinguished from an acute subdural hematoma, although the epidural hematoma is almost always lenticular in shape. The scan will also show shift of the midline structures and compression of the ipsilateral ventricular system with dilatation of the contralateral ventricle in about 60 percent of cases.

Treatment. Emergency neurosurgical evacuation of the hematoma is the treatment of choice. When there are signs of rapidly increasing intracranial pressure, the performance of this procedure may be based on the clinical evidence alone. Under these circumstances the surgical exploration is carried out along the site of the skull fracture.

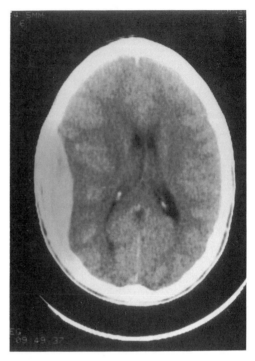

FIGURE 18–1. Epidural hematoma. CT scan showing area of increased density right epidural space. Typical lenticulate structure exerting pressure on the right cerebral hemisphere.

Acute Subdural Hematoma

Definition. An acute subdural hematoma is an acute and progressive accumulation of blood in the subdural space, which has an 80 percent mortality.

Etiology and Pathology. Acute subdural hematomas usually follow severe head injury and are associated with considerable damage to the underlying brain (3). There are a number of rarer causes of acute subdural hematoma including rupture of a berry aneurysm, bleeding from an arteriovenous malformation, lumbar puncture followed by sudden alteration in intracranial pressure and tearing of bridging veins, or as a rare complication of a bleeding diathesis or anticoagulant therapy.

Head injury causes rupture of the bridging veins that traverse the subdural space to reach the dural sinuses. The brain shows the presence of a contusion or hematoma formation and there is often considerable brain edema with displacement of the ventricular system.

Clinical Features. There is usually a history of severe head injury with rapid loss of consciousness followed by progressive deterioration with deepening coma and signs of brain stem compression. In some cases the history may suggest an epidural hematoma with the occurrence of a lucid interval. Examination may show signs of uncal herniation and rostral-caudal deterioration (see p. 50).

Diagnostic Procedures.

1. Skull x-rays. X-rays of the skull may occasionally reveal the presence of a skull fracture and displacement of a calcified pineal gland.
2. The MR or CT scanning readily reveals the presence of a subdural hematoma (see Figure 18–2). The inner edge of the hematoma may be concave or convex in relationship to the underlying surface of the brain. A convex lesion suggests the presence of an epidural hematoma or a large subdural hematoma. There are compression of the lateral ventricle on the side of the hematoma and shift of the midline structures. Cerebral edema is not unusual in acute subdural hematomas.

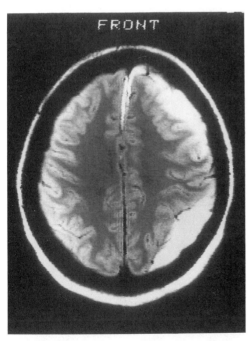

FIGURE 18–2. MR scan T1 weighted image showing an acute subdural hematoma following closed head injury.

Treatment. An acute subdural hematoma is a neurosurgical emergency, and the hematoma must be evacuated as soon as possible. Prognosis is poor where there is diffuse swelling of one hemisphere on the side of the acute hematoma (4).

Subacute Subdural Hematoma
A number of patients with acute head injury have a slow accumulation of blood in the subdural space, which occurs over a 1- to 10-day time period. These patients appear to recover from head injury, which may be quite trivial, and then develop increasing headache, drowsiness, and progressive neurologic deterioration. The diagnosis is established by MR or CT scan. The condition is treated by surgical evacuation of the hematoma.

Chronic Subdural Hematoma
Definition. A chronic subdural hematoma is an encapsulated accumulation of blood and cerebrospinal fluid in the subdural space, which requires at least 10 days to develop. The diagnosis is established by MR or CT scanning.

Etiology and Pathology. Chronic subdural hematomas often follow minor head injury. The hematoma develops as a result of tearing of bridging veins with accumulation of blood within the subdural space. The blood clots and later hemolyzes. The higher osmotic pressure of the hemolyzed blood draws cerebrospinal fluid through the arachnoid and increases the volume of the hematoma. This produces tearing of vessels at the periphery of the hematoma and bleeding into the subdural space, which further increases the osmotic pressure and attracts more fluid. Proliferation of fibroblasts occurs in the dura and arachnoid, and the collection eventually becomes surrounded by a fibroblastic membrane, which thickens over a period of several weeks. Calcification occurs in chronic cases.

Clinical Features. The condition most commonly occurs in the elderly and demented or alcoholic patients with atrophied brains. The history of head injury may not be obtained from an elderly debilitated patient or from patients with poor memory. However, younger patients often give a history of quite trivial head injury. Patients with chronic subdural hematomas are conscious but may be confused, with a characteristic waxing and waning of symptoms. When alert, the patient complains of generalized headache, and there is impairment of intellectual capacity and recent memory. Dysphasia may occur when the subdural hematoma compresses the dominant hemisphere. There is contralateral hemiparesis, with increased stretch reflexes and an extensor plantar response. The gradual increase in intracranial pressure may produce uncal herniation and progressive rostral-caudal deterioration. Papilledema is not unusual at this stage.

Diagnostic Procedures.

1. Skull x-rays. X-rays of the skull may show shift of a calcified pineal gland, evidence of skull fracture and in long-term cases calcification of the membranes of the hematoma.
2. Either MR or CT scanning is diagnostic with demonstration of a subdural collection, compression of the ipsilateral lateral ventricle, and dilatation of the contralateral ventricular system. The dilution of the blood in the subdural hematoma with the passage of time reduces the density of the hematoma, which eventually becomes isodense with the brain parenchyma when CT scanning is utilized. In such a case the displacement of the ventricular system suggests the presence of a mass lesion, and the use of intravenous contrast material increases the chances of outlining the hematoma by enhancing the surrounding membrane. Bilateral isodense hematomas

present considerable difficulty in diagnosis because of the absence of shift of the midline structures. At the same time the MR scan is abnormal (see Figure 18–3).
3. Electroencephalography. The EEG shows the presence of focal slowing and decreased voltage over the subdural collection.
4. Arteriography when MR is not available. Arteriography may be used to confirm the presence of a subdural hematoma in cases with equivocal CT scanning results.

Treatment. Small, chronic subdural hematomas that do not produce any neurologic deficit should be monitored by repeated neurologic examination and serial CT scanning. The presence of any neurologic deficit is an indication for surgical drainage. In most cases a craniotomy is necessary so that thickened membranes may be excised.

Subdural Hygroma

A subdural hygroma is an accumulation of cerebrospinal fluid in the subdural space. The most likely mechanism of formation involves tearing of the arachnoid membrane during head injury. The torn flap acts as a ball valve and allows gradual escape of cerebrospinal fluid into the subdural space during periods of temporary increase in intracranial pressure such as occurs with coughing, sneezing, or straining. Either MR or CT scanning may reveal an area of abnormality overlying the

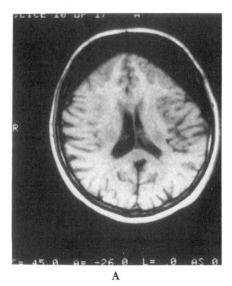
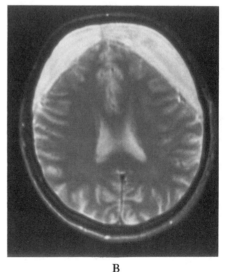

A   B

FIGURE 18–3.   Bilateral large chronic subdural hematomas over the frontal lobes extending to the mid-parietal area bilaterally. T1 (**A**) and T2 (**B**) weighted images.

brain parenchyma. The treatment of choice is surgical drainage.

Traumatic Subarachnoid Hemorrhage

See page 164.

Traumatic Intracerebral Hematoma

Definition. A traumatic intracerebral hematoma is a collection of blood in the substance of the brain following head injury.

Etiology and Pathology. Intracerebral hematomas are readily demonstrated by computed tomography and are a much commoner complication of head injury than had been believed in the past. Hemorrhage may occur at any site and result from shearing forces with subsequent rupture of blood vessels within the brain parenchyma.

Clinical Features. The level of consciousness and clinical signs and symptoms depend on the size and location of the hematoma (see p. 170). A patient who suffers a brief period of loss of consciousness may have a small hematoma in the frontal or temporal lobe, which is asymptomatic following recovery. Large or multiple areas of intracerebral hemorrhage following severe head injury may produce a rapid rise in intracranial pressure, herniation, and rostral-caudal deterioration.

Diagnostic Procedures. Intracerebral hematomas present as areas of increased density in T_2 weighted images of MR or by CT scanning. Large hematomas are associated with edema, brain swelling, ventricular displacement, and acute hydrocephalus. The hematoma may rupture into the ventricular system.

Treatment. Patients with rapidly increasing intracranial pressure require emergency treatment to reduce brain edema and swelling (5). Evacuation of the hematoma or reduction of the hydrocephalus by ventricular drainage may be necessary.

Closed Head Injury

Definition. A closed head injury is a cranial injury in which the meninges remain intact.

Etiology, Pathology, and Clinical Features. A patient with a closed head injury may experience no loss of consciousness or a temporary loss of consciousness, or may become comatose.

Closed Head Injury Without Loss of Consciousness. The majority of cases of head injury are mild and do not produce loss of consciousness. Skull fractures and intracerebral hemorrhage can occur without loss of consciousness. In general, head injury is considered mild when there is no loss of consciousness and recovery occurs in a short period of time. In most cases patients report a blow to the head followed by a feeling of confusion, headache, unsteadiness of gait, and a rapid recovery. A few patients complain of persistent headaches of a vascular nature. These are believed to result from dysfunction of autonomic control of the blood vessels of the scalp.

The juvenile head trauma syndrome is a syndrome occasionally seen in children following trivial head injury. There is a history of a mild head injury followed by apparent recovery. A few hours later the child complains of headache, becomes somnolent and irritable, and may vomit. Confusion may be a prominent symptom, and a few cases lapse into coma. Other children complain of blindness. The condition is very alarming to parents, who urgently seek medical advice. Frequently many unnecessary laboratory and radiologic procedures are performed. The syndrome usually terminates within a few minutes to a few hours. Recovery is complete. The headache resembles a severe migraine and is most likely due to severe vasoconstriction provoked by the head injury. Some children who have experienced this condition develop migraine headaches following minor head trauma later in life.

Closed Head Injury with Loss of Consciousness. A concussion is an immediate transient impairment of consciousness following head injury, believed to result from interference with the reticular activating system. There are no macroscopic changes in the brain. A contusion is an immediate, transient impairment of consciousness accompanied by neurologic deficits. The base of the frontal lobes and tips of the temporal lobes are most frequently involved. The damaged area is typically conical in shape, with the base at the surface of the brain. Layer one of the cortex is the cortical layer most frequently involved. The neurologic deficits most commonly occurring with a contusion are changes in behavior, changes in personality, loss of memory, confusion, aphasia, and the development of dementia. Many patients with brain concussion or contusion develop a "posttraumatic" syndrome. This is characterized by recurrent headaches of a vascular nature, inattention, poor memory, anxiety, irritability, lethargy, and unsteadiness of gait. Most patients make a complete and uneventful recovery.

Closed Head Injury with Coma. Moderate-to-severe head injury is associated with sudden loss of consciousness and coma with lack of response to painful stimulation. Coma may last for several hours or even several days in severe head injury and is followed by semicoma, in which the patient begins to respond to painful stimulation. This stage is followed by stupor, restlessness, and irritability. The patient attempts to avoid all stimuli and prefers to lie curled in a fetal position and sleep for many hours. The stage of stupor gradually gives way to obtundity, the restlessness increases, and the patient may require sedation. Examination reveals a disoriented patient with defective judgment and insight. There may be extreme irritability and a tendency toward combativeness even with slight frustration. Over a period of hours to days the patient gradually becomes fully conscious.

The severity of the head injury can be judged by determining the duration of post-traumatic amnesia for events following head injury. Patients with severe head injury also experience a retrograde amnesia of several hours or even days prior to the event but the duration of retrograde amnesia is less reliable in assessing the severity of brain damage. The stages of recovery from severe head injury outlined above can be arrested at any point depending upon the severity of the head injury. Some patients with very severe head injury remain comatose and die after several days, usually from increased intracranial pressure (6). Others remain comatose for days or weeks before dying from intercurrent infection. High plasma norepinephrine levels and a low Glasgow coma scale rating indicates a poor prognosis (7).

Diagnostic Procedures. Patients with severe head injury should receive diagnostic tests when they can be safely performed during the institution of emergency treatment. The procedures generally employed include:

1. X-ray of the skull, chest, and cervical spine. The high incidence of fractures of the cervical spine with severe head injury justifies the taking of cervical spine x-rays in all cases of severe head injury. Patients with upper facial fractures have a high rate of intracranial injuries (8).
2. MR scanning is extremely sensitive in detecting the presence of extracerebral or intracerebral hematoma, cerebral contusion and edema, hydrocephalus or shift of the midline structures of the brain (9, 10). Considerable white matter damage can be demonstrated in some cases who have a normal CT scan (11). Serial MR scans should be used to assess the resolution or the appearance of complications (12) (see Figures 18–4 and 18–5). CT scanning is less sensitive than MR scanning in demonstrating cerebral contusion (13).
3. Electroencephalography. In cases of mild head injury, a normal neurologic examination, and persistent subjective complaints, an EEG should be obtained. In cases with more severe injury, serial EEG's often indicate steady progression or deterioration in a patient's condition. The presence of 14 and 6 Hz positive spikes is not uncommon in children, adolescents and young adults during recovery from head injury. Persistence of this waveform is often associated with continuous symptoms of headache, nausea and vomiting, and blurred vision (14).

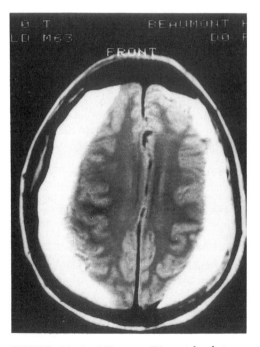

FIGURE 18–4. MR scan T2 weighted image showing increased signal in the right hemisphere due to gliosis. Scan taken more than three years after traumatic brain injury following a high speed head on collision.

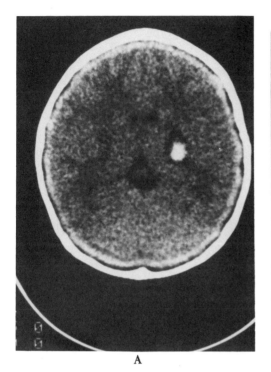 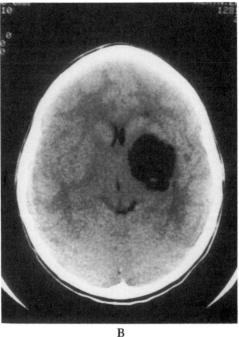

A   B

FIGURE 18–5.   CT scan showing discrete traumatic hematoma (**A**) following head injury.
Condition resolved through a cyst (**B**) containing cerebrospinal fluid indicating a connection
with the ventricular system. Treated by a shunting procedure.

4. Auditory evoked potentials (AEP). An
   AEP is valuable in providing objective evidence of damage to the brain stem in
   cases with postconcussion "dizziness"
   (15).
5. Neuropsychological testing is useful to assess the initial severity of brain damage
   and serial testing may be used not only to
   measure improvement in function but also
   to aid in the design of rehabilitative programs (16, 17).

Treatment.   Posttraumatic vascular headaches often respond to propranolol (Inderal)
20 mg t.i.d., increasing to 240 mg per day if
necessary, or amitriptyline (Elavil) 25 mg
b.i.d., slowly increasing to 150 mg daily if
necessary.
*Emergency Treatment of Severe Closed
Head Injury.*   The patient should initially be
stabilized and evaluated as described in
Chapter 2 (see p. 50).
1. Increased intracranial pressure. All patients with evidence of moderate-to-severe
head injury and increased intracranial pres-

sure should have an intracranial pressure
monitoring device inserted. The device allows more efficient and accurate titration of
the intracranial pressure using dexamethasone 12 mg q6h, Mannitol 1.5 to 2.0 G/kg
given as a 20 percent solution over 30 to 60
minutes, and controlled hyperventilation.
Decompressive craniotomy should be reserved for those cases with massive cerebral
edema or brain swelling who fail to respond
to medical treatment.
   2. Disseminated intravascular coagulation
(DIC). DIC is an occasional complication of
acute head injury due to liberation of tissue
thromboplastic following trauma. The liberated thromboplastic activates coagulation
mechanisms, and fibrin thrombi are formed in
small blood vessels throughout the body.
There is progressive reduction in platelets
and clotting factors are depleted, resulting in
a bleeding diathesis. The bleeding tendency
may increase intracranial bleeding and produce hemorrhage in other areas of the body.
Disseminated   intravascular   coagulation
should be suspected in patients with severe

head injury who show excessive or uncontrolled bleeding following venipuncture or who develop ecchymoses of the skin. DIC should be treated with intravenous heparin unless surgical procedures are contemplated. Therapy with fibrinogen, platelet concentrates, or plasma factors is also effective.

3. Patients who are restless or combative may be sedated with phenothiazines, paraldehyde, or chlordiazepoxide (Librium) (18).

4. Barbiturate coma. The induction of barbiturate coma is believed to improve the outcome in patients who suffer from severe intracranial hypertension that cannot be managed by the aforementioned means. Barbiturates reduce the cerebral metabolic rate and cerebral blood flow, which results in a fall in intracranial pressure. The induction of barbiturate coma is a major undertaking and requires careful monitoring of intracranial pressure, arterial pressure, and pulmonary gas exchange. Since the patient is "comatose," there is no way to assess the patient's neurologic status (19).

5. Limb contractures are a common complication in patients who experience prolonged coma. This debilitating complication may inhibit or delay rehabilitation. Limb position and maintenance of joint mobility are an essential part of therapy beginning in the acute stage of injury (20).

Prognosis. The majority of patients with head injury make a good recovery. A young age, good motor function and bilateral pupillary response to light usually indicate a good outcome (21). The minority, who have severe neurologic residual deficits, require a dedicated program of treatment to obtain the best results (22). The patient should enter a vocational rehabilitation program to allow maximum rehabilitation. Those with memory deficits may benefit from physostigmine 1 mg t.i.d. combined with lecithin 8 g b.i.d. (23).

Traumatic Encephalopathy

Repeated head injury may be followed by the development of traumatic encephalopathy. In the professional boxer this is known as the "punch drunk" state. The punch drunk boxer is characterized by evidence of chronic trauma (flattened nose, cauliflower ears); psychomotor retardation; poor judgment; impaired retention, recall and recent memory; and dysarthria. The mental deterioration is associated with parkinsonian-like features, titubation of the head, cerebellar ataxia of the limbs, and ataxia of gait.

Posttraumatic Seizures

When posttraumatic seizures occur, they usually follow severe head injury. Parents have a tendency to ascribe the development of seizures in children to head injury. Most children experience trivial head injuries while at play, and mild head injury rarely leads to the development of seizures.

The incidence of posttraumatic seizures following severe head injury with coma of 24 hours' duration or longer is approximately 20 percent. Thirty to 50 percent of penetrating injuries are associated with posttraumatic seizures. The early onset of seizures within 24 hours to 7 days following closed head injury has a good prognosis and rarely leads to recurrent seizure activity. Patients with a delayed onset of seizures are more likely to develop a chronic seizure disorder. High-velocity penetrating injuries, the presence of foreign bodies within the brain, and the occurrence of focal neurologic deficits are associated with a higher incidence of posttraumatic seizures. Injury to the precentral gyrus has the highest incidence of posttraumatic seizures.

Ninety percent of patients who will develop posttraumatic seizures do so within two years. The great majority of posttraumatic seizures can be totally controlled with anticonvulsant medication (see p. 75). More than 50 percent of cases cease to have seizure activity within 10 years of the head injury. When there is persistence of seizure activity despite therapeutic anticonvulsant levels, the patient should be fully investigated for the presence of a hematoma, cicatrix, or focal atrophic area. Many of these conditions are remediable by neurosurgical treatment.

Benign Positional Vertigo

Definition. Vertigo induced by rapid change in head position indicating a benign inner ear disorder.

Etiology and Pathology. Although the majority of cases are categorized as idiopathic, the commonest identifiable causes are head trauma, viral labyrinthitis, and vertebral basilar insufficiency in order of frequency. These conditions produce damage to the posterior semicircular canal.

Clinical Features. The problem is one of episodic vertigo produced by turning in bed, getting in and out of bed, sudden bending or straightening up, and extending the head to look up. The vertigo is intense, brief, lasting less than one minute, and may occur many times in one day. This may be followed by a prolonged period of lightheadedness and nausea. Bouts of vertigo are followed by periods of remission which may last for years.

Diagnostic Procedures. The diagnosis is established by demonstration of paroxysmal positional nystagmus immediately following a head hanging maneuver (24). This is a torsion nystagmus lasting about 20 seconds, the upper pole of the eye beating towards the ground.

Treatment. The condition usually resolves spontaneously but the attacks may last for more than one year. Remissions are frequent. A scopolamine patch may be helpful in some cases.

Cranial Nerve Injury

Cranial nerve injury may pass unnoticed in the comatose patient and become apparent only on recovery of consciousness. The optic nerve may be contused in the optic foramen because of sudden movement of the brain during head injury or because of fracture through the optic foramen. The patient may be blind immediately, and they may slowly recover over the next four weeks. Examination early after injury reveals a dilated pupil with absence of the direct light reflex but preservation of the consensual response. Permanent damage results in optic atrophy beginning about 1 month after the injury. Damage to the optic chiasm may result in a bitemporal or binasal, often incongruous field defect.

The third, fourth, and sixth cranial nerves are vulnerable to injury as they enter the orbit. They may be injured by sudden movement, stretching, or a fracture through the superior orbital fissure. Third nerve injury may occur during uncal herniation. Patients who recover may have a persistent third nerve palsy with a dilated pupil, an abducted eye, and ptosis. Smooth conjugate eye movements may be impaired following brain stem injury.

The fifth cranial nerve may be injured at the foramen ovale by basal skull fractures. Injuries of the face may damage branches of the trigeminal nerve. Occasionally the superior nerve is compressed at the supraorbital margin, and the inferior orbital nerve may be involved by fractures of the infraorbital foramen.

Damage to the seventh cranial nerve occurs with head injury in which the petrous portion of the temporal bone is fractured.

There is usually an associated ipsilateral hearing loss with hemorrhage into the middle ear. Facial paralysis is occasionally delayed following head injury due to the development of edema in the facial canal.

Fractures of the middle ear and petrous temporal bone are frequently accompanied by deafness due to destruction of the auditory division of the eighth nerve. This type of injury is often associated with seventh nerve paralysis. Injury to the vestibular division of the nerve results in vertigo, which may persist following the injury. The condition usually responds to treatment, but the patient may have persistent lightheadedness, ataxia, and nausea for many months after injury.

It is unusual for head injuries to involve the lower cranial nerves, although this occasionally occurs following fractures of the posterior fossa that involve the jugular foramen. This may produce damage to the ninth, tenth, and 11th nerves. Similar damage may occur with hematoma formation at the base of the skull.

Traumatic Cerebrospinal Fluid Rhinorrhea or Otorrhea

Definition. Traumatic cerebrospinal fluid rhinorrhea or otorrhea is the abnormal drainage of cerebrospinal fluid from the cranial cavity.

Etiology and Pathology. A fracture through the posterior wall of the frontal sinus may produce a tear of the dura and arachnoid, which will allow cerebrospinal fluid to leak into the frontal sinus and nasal cavity. Rupture of a congenitally weak cribriform plate or an arachnoid sleeve passing through the cribriform plate may occur with a sudden intracranial pressure wave following head injury and result in CSF rhinorrhea. Fracture of the temporal bone may tear the dura and allow CSF to drain from the ear, resulting in otorrhea.

Clinical Features. The patient usually complains of the persistent drainage of clear fluid from the nose, down the posterior pharynx, or from the ear. The drainage increases on head flexion, straining, or coughing. The condition may be complicated by the passage of air into the cranial cavity through the defect, particularly during coughing or sneezing. The air accumulates in the subarachnoid space and often enters the ventricular system causing pneumocephalus. This latter condition is associated with persistent headache and progressive intellectual deterioration.

Diagnostic Procedures.

1. Glucose and protein are present in the fluid, which distinguishes it from other nasal discharges.
2. Skull x-rays. X-rays of the skull and paranasal sinuses may show evidence of a fracture involving the cribriform plate, frontal sinus, or temporal bone. Tomography may be helpful.
3. Radioactive material may be injected into the subarachnoid space and allowed to circulate. Scintillation scanning of pledgets of cotton placed in the nose or ear canal will reveal radioactivity.
4. Metrizamide cisternography with CT scanning is the most sensitive method of demonstrating a fistula or tissue deformity at the site of leakage in a dry non-drop period (25).
5. Both MR and CT scanning will demonstrate the presence of air in the ventricular system in cases of pneumocephalus.

Treatment. Most patients respond to conservative treatment with bed rest and instructions forbidding coughing, sneezing, or straining. There is a risk of infection in all cases, and lumbar puncture should be performed if the patient develops fever and nuchal rigidity. Appropriate antibiotics should be administered if meningitis is diagnosed (see p. 259).

Surgical treatment with closure of the fistula is indicated in patients who fail to respond to two weeks of medical treatment. In order to prevent recurrence, surgical treatment should always be carried out in patients who have suffered meningitis.

Fat Metabolism

Definition. Fat metabolism is the passage of fat emboli into the circulation with consequent respiratory failure and altered levels of consciousness.

Etiology and Pathology. The majority of cases of fat embolism follow fracture of long bones. Rarer causes include concussion of long bones, bone marrow transplantation for acute leukemia (26), alcoholism, systemic lupus erythematosus, acute osteomyelitis, pancreatitis, extracorporeal circulation, steroid therapy in the presence of malignancy and injury to adipose tissue. Fat globules that break loose enter the systemic circulation and are carried to the lungs. The emboli occlude capillaries and are hydrolyzed to highly toxic and unsaturated fatty acids. This causes a leak in the pulmonary capillaries, and a hemorrhagic interstitial pneumonitis results. Occasionally fat emboli pass into the arterial circulation and enter the cerebrovascular system. In these cases the brain is characterized by numerous petechial hemorrhages and ecchymoses scattered throughout the gray and white matter with generalized edema.

Clinical Features. The fulminant form of fat embolism caused by a massive embolism may develop within hours of injury whereas the classical form of fat embolism appears within 24 to 72 hours (27). Prodromal symptoms consisting of cough, fever, dyspnea, chest pain, and wheezing are followed by agitation, confusion, disorientation, delirium, seizures, and coma. Petechiae may be seen on the upper trunk and head. Focal neurologic deficits may develop, and cerebral edema may lead to decerebrate rigidity, progressive brain stem compression, and death.

Diagnostic Procedures.

1. Blood gas analysis showing a sustained PaO_2 less than 60 mmHg.
2. A sustained $PaCO_2$ of more than 55 mmHg.
3. A pH of less than 7.3.
4. A sustained respiratory rate of 35 per minute.
5. Dyspnea with use of accessory respiratory muscles.
6. Tachycardia.
7. A chest x-ray may show pulmonary infiltration.
8. Serum free fatty acids, triglycerides, and fibrin split products are elevated.
9. Fat droplets may be demonstrated in the blood or urine.
10. The EEG shows loss of normal background activity with generalized slowing. Paroxysmal epileptic activity may occur.

Treatment.

1. Prevention is the best treatment. Long bone fractures should be promptly immobilized.
2. Oxygen should be administered. Intubation with mechanical respiration using positive end expiratory pressure (PEEP) should be initiated as soon as indicated.
3. Cerebral vasodilation may be obtained with inhalation of 5 percent carbon dioxide in 95 percent oxygen.
4. Cerebral edema may be controlled with dexamethasone (Decadron) and mannitol if necessary. Intracranial pressure monitoring is advantageous.
5. Methylprednisolone 30 mg/Kg IV re-

peated after four hours significantly reduces the incidence of symptomatic fat
embolism in patients with long bone
fractures.

Air Embolism
Definition. Air embolism is the passage
of air into the general circulation.
Etiology and Pathology. The entrance of
air into the circulation may occur following
injury, cardiac surgery, arterial catheterization, thoracic surgery, and surgical removal
of highly vascular tumors (28). Dysbaric air
embolism resulting from pulmonary over-
pressurization and lung rupture during rapid
ascent to the surface is not uncommon in
scuba divers (29). Air bubbles enter the pulmonary veins, left atrium, left ventricle and
systemic circulation causing arterial occlusion and infarction. Large volumes of air that
enter the circulation may result in acute cardiac insufficiency and death. When smaller
volumes of air enter the circulation, embolization may occur to many organs, including
the brain.
The brain shows diffuse areas of petechial
hemorrhage, generalized edema, and infarction.
Clinical Features. The passage of air
bubbles into the cerebral circulation results
in loss of consciousness, seizures, blurred vision or blindness, dysphasia or aphasia, vertigo, headache, focal weakness and paresthesias. Conscious patients may complain of
chest pain and hemoptysis.
Treatment.

1. The source of air embolism must be discontinued.
2. The patient should be placed in a steep
   Trendelenburg position and given 5 percent carbon dioxide in 95 percent oxygen
   to increase cerebral blood flow and "wash
   out" air emboli.
3. If available, treatment in a hyperbaric
   chamber is indicated. Treatment at 6 atmospheres will reduce the volume size of
   air emboli and allow their passage out of
   the cerebral circulation. Longer treatment at 3 atmospheres using 100 percent
   oxygen will improve rate of diffusion of nitrogen from emboli and reduce their volume.
4. Retrograde perfusion of the cerebral circulation through the superior vena cava to
   remove air bubbles from the cerebral circulation has been performed in massive
   air embolism following cardiac bypass
   pump failure.

Near Drowning
Definition. Near drowning is the survival
after submersion of the body in a fluid medium resulting in asphyxia secondary to submersion.
Etiology and Pathology. In the majority
of cases of near drowning, asphyxia and subsequent hypoxia are due to aspiration of fluid
into the lungs resulting in pulmonary edema.
It is believed that water destroys pulmonary
surfactant, damages pulmonary alveoli and
results in pulmonary edema with the transu-
dation of proteinaceous material into the alveolar spaces. This may be augmented by
vomiting and aspiration of gastric contents
into the lungs.
In about 10 percent of cases of near
drowning submersion is followed by persistent laryngospasm with little or no water aspiration and there is no pulmonary edema.
Treatment.

1. Clear the airway of vomitus or aspirated
   material and begin mouth to mouth resuscitation as soon as the victim is reached.
   Do not wait until the victim is ashore.
2. Once out of the water institute cardiopulmonary resuscitation (CPR) and give oxygen at highest concentration available.
3. Any near drowning victim submerged for
   more than one minute should be admitted
   to hospital or observed in an emergency
   center for 24 hours because of the risk of
   delayed pulmonary edema.
4. Obtain chest x-ray; levels of arterial blood
   gases, serum electrolytes, blood urea nitrogen (BUN), creatinine, hemoglobin;
   and a toxic screen for alcohol or drugs.
5. Any case with abnormal blood gases or
   chest x-ray should be admitted to an intensive care unit.
6. An arterial line will be required to provide
   for serial blood gas determinations.
7. Oxygen therapy can be continued by mask
   or nasal catheter if a PpO_2 of 90 mmHg
   can be maintained with an FiO_2 of 0.5 or
   less. Other cases will require intubation
   and positive pressure respiratory support
   using a mechanical respirator. This is
   also indicated in cases of apnea or impaired ventilation with $PpCO_2$ above 35
   mmHg.
8. A nasogastric tube will prevent further aspiration of stomach contents and a foley
   catheter is needed to measure urine output.
9. Cerebral edema should be anticipated in
   those who are deteriorating neurologically and can be monitored by intracranial

pressure monitoring (ICP). Measures to counter cerebral edema include hyperventilation to reduce $PpCO_2$ to 28–32 mmHg and mannitol 0.25–0.5 g/Kilo per dose to reduce ICP to less than 20 mmHg.

Prognosis. Patients with a score of 5 or less on the Glasgow Coma Scale carry a high risk of death or permanent neurologic damage. Similarly, patients who are comatosed without response or show decerebrate or decorticate state two to six hours after submersion have a poor prognosis. Those who are alert or stuporous two to six hours after submersion usually have normal or near normal recovery.

Electrical Injury to the Nervous System

Definition. Electrical injury to the nervous system may be due to electrocution or lightning.

Etiology and Pathology. In most cases damage to the nervous system following electrocution is the result of anoxia rather than the direct effect of electricity on tissue. Anoxia may result from respiratory arrest due to the electrical current passing through the brain stem and affecting the respiratory center or may be caused by cardiac arrest after lightning strike or ventricular fibrillation following high voltage electrocution (30). In some cases, however, there is direct damage to the central nervous system. The passage of electrical current through the nervous system is followed by inflammatory changes in blood vessels, leading to thrombosis and infarction; injury to neurons may result in necrosis and gliosis. These changes may occur anywhere in the brain or spinal cord depending on where the involved area lies in the path of the electrical current. The passage of an electrical current can also produce damage to peripheral nerves, particularly in the limbs.

Clinical Features. Respiratory insufficiency may result in anoxic encephalopathy and generalized seizures. Damage to the cerebrum may result in hemiplegia or homonymous hemianopia (31). The passage of an electric current through the brain stem can produce Parkinsonism, cranial nerve deficits, or corticospinal tract involvement with spasticity. Spinal cord involvement results in flaccid paralysis, which is often followed by complete recovery. In some cases damage to the anterior horn cells may present as progressive weakness and wasting of muscle associated with a progressive spasticity below the level

of the lesion. Passage of an electrical current through a limb may be followed by peripheral nerve involvement producing painful neuralgias, muscle weakness, fasciculations and atrophy, loss of reflexes, and a sensory loss corresponding to the distribution of the affected nerves. Not all neurologic sequelae are immediate and delayed complications of electrical injury may occur days or even weeks after the event and affect any part of the nervous system.

Treatment. Individuals who have been struck by lightning or electrocuted and show respiratory and/or cardiac arrest should receive immediate resuscitation. Most of the patients who are resuscitated within six minutes will survive with little or no permanent neurologic damage. Patients with electrical injury in which the current passes through the thorax should receive electrocardiographic monitoring for at least 24 hours since delayed ventricular arrhythmias may develop several hours after the injury.

Radiation Injury to the Brain and Spinal Cord

Definition. Radiation injury may occur inadvertently or during treatment of neoplastic disease. Damage to the central nervous system from ionizing radiation usually follows radiation therapy for treatment of neoplastic disease. In many cases the blood vessels of the brain and spinal cord show signs of inflammation with endothelial proliferation and obliteration of the vessel lumen or thrombosis. This suggests that the effects of radiation on the brain and spinal cord are often secondary to ischemia and infarction. Ionizing irradiation can also produce direct damage to neurons with neuronal loss and subsequent gliosis.

Clinical Features. Involvement of the circle of Willis by arteritis and thrombosis may produce scattered infarction in both hemispheres. Clinical signs include progressive dementia, spasticity, and rigidity. Involvement of one hemisphere will produce focal signs with hemiparesis and dysphasia if the dominant hemisphere is involved. Seizures are not uncommon. Focal necrosis in the area of an irradiated brain tumor may present as an expanding lesion, with increased intracranial pressure suggesting tumor recurrence (32). Damage to the brain stem may result in progressive hemiparesis, paraparesis, quadriparesis, parkinsonism, cranial nerve involvement, dysarthria, and ataxia. Irradiation for a nasopharyngeal carcinoma may be followed by damage to the hypothalamus and symptoms of hypopituitarism. Radiation myelopathy may present with

1. Acute transient radiation myelopathy. This is a transient shock like dysesthesia induced by neck flexion known as the L'hermitte sign. The neurologic examination is normal and full recovery occurs.
2. Acute paraplegia occurring within hours or days of irradiation is rare and is presumably due to cord infarction secondary to acute radiation vasculitis.
3. Lower motor neuron disease with muscle atrophy, fasciculations, and loss of stretch reflexes is also rare.
4. Chronic progressive radiation myelitis occurs 9 to 15 months after radiotherapy and presents with progressive paraplegia or quadriplegia, hyperreflexia, extensor plantar responses, sensory loss below the level of the lesion and progressive impairment of bladder function. The condition may present occasionally as a Brown-Sequard syndrome (33).

The occurrence of pain, sensory disturbance and weakness in an upper limb in a patient who has previously received radiotherapy for the treatment of carcinoma of breast may be due to metastatic involvement or radiation neuritis (34). The diagnosis is usually obtained by biopsy since radiation neuritis can be delayed for several years and breast carcinoma metastases can also present many years after treatment of the primary tumor.

Treatment. The treatment is symptomatic. Surgical decompression is indicated for cord compression following vertebral collapse after irradiation for metastatic disease.

Decompression Damage of the Central Nervous System

Definition. Decompression damage of the central nervous system is a condition in which rapid decompression from a high atmospheric pressure to a lower atmospheric pressure produces damage to the central nervous system.

Etiology and Pathology. Sudden reduction of atmospheric pressure releases gaseous nitrogen into the circulation. The bubbles of nitrogen alter the rheology of the blood, increasing the viscosity and hematocrit and encouraging erythrocyte aggregation. This results in thrombosis of the smaller vessels and infarction within the central nervous system, involving white matter more than gray matter. There are often multiple areas of infarction in the white matter of the spinal cord and

the cerebral hemispheres, particularly in the areas of marginal supply between the territories of two major cerebral vessels.

Clinical Features. Decompression sickness often presents with joint pains which increase in severity. This is associated with generalized pruritus due to bubbles of nitrogen in the skin capillaries. Involvement of the intercostal muscles and pleura produces dyspnea (the chokes) while impairment of the circulation to the abdominal viscera results in abdominal pain (the bends). When the cerebral hemispheres are involved, there may be a sudden onset of seizures, hemiparesis, aphasia, and visual field defects. Brain stem involvement may cause cranial nerve signs such as acute onset of vertigo, impairment of hearing, facial paralysis, or oculomotor palsies. In the spinal cord the thoracic cord is the commonest site of involvement with acute paraplegia, sensory loss below the level of the lesion, and sphincter paralysis.

Treatment.
1. Prevention. Deep water divers should be familiar with the regulations governing decompression when diving to depths of more than 40 feet. In general, decompression should never exceed intervals of 1.25 atmospheres (35).
2. Treatment of decompression sickness. The effective treatment is recompression in a recompression chamber. The affected individual should be placed in the chamber with pressure equal to the previous working depth or 10 to 15 lb higher than the previous working depth. Slow decompression coupled with administration of oxygen and oxygen-helium mixtures is effective in the treatment of decompression sickness.

Injury to the Spinal Canal and Spinal Cord

Etiology and Pathology. There are approximately 30 new cases of spinal cord injuries per million persons in the United States each year. The prevalence rate is approximately 906 per million. The majority of injuries occur in young adults. About 50 percent result from motor vehicle crashes, 20 percent from falls, and 15 percent from gunshot wounds and stabbings. Injury to the spinal cord may be direct, with concussion, laceration, or intramedullary hemorrhage, or indirect, due to extramedullary pressure of loss of blood supply and infarction. The mechanisms of spinal cord injury include:
1. Fracture of the vertebrae. Fracture of the vertebrae can occur with or without fracture dislocation and may involve the verte-

bral body, the pedicles, laminae, transverse processes, or spinous processes. There may be damage to the spinal cord from the concussive effect of the injury due to displaced bony fragments. Fractures may also damage blood vessels such as the vertebral arteries in the neck or the anastomotic vessels to the anterior spinal artery or result in contusion of emerging nerve roots.

2. Dislocation. Dislocation of vertebrae usually occurs at predictable sites in the spinal column. These are the areas between C_1 and C_2, C_5 and C_6, and T_{11} and T_{12}. Dislocation may be reversible or persistent with marked narrowing of the spinal canal. The results may vary from a mild concussion of the spinal cord to complete severance of the spinal cord. Dislocation may produce additional narrowing in a spinal canal already affected by cervical spondylosis, and the narrowing may be augmented by disruption and swelling of the anterior and posterior longitudinal ligaments. Dislocation can also interrupt blood supply to the spinal cord and may produce damage to emerging nerve roots. Acute dislocation is frequently associated with acute rupture of an intervertebral disk (see p. 345).

3. Penetrating wounds. The spinal cord may be injured by a high velocity missile such as a bullet, or by knife wounds with severance or partial severance of the cord.

4. Epidural hemorrhage. There is a well-defined epidural space in the spinal canal that is often the site of bleeding following trauma. The hemorrhage exerts pressure on emerging nerve roots, causing radicular pain, and results in progressive paraparesis due to pressure on the cord. This condition is a surgical emergency (36).

5. Spinal subdural hematoma. Spinal subdural hematoma is rarer than spinal epidural hematoma. The symptoms are identical and the condition is a surgical emergency that must be relieved as soon as possible to avoid permanent neurologic deficits.

6. Indirect injury to the spinal cord. The spinal cord may be injured by a pressure wave generated by a blow on the head, a fall on the buttocks, or a fall on the feet or when the individual is involved in an explosion. The degree of injury varies from minor concussion to severe cord damage with hemorrhage.

7. Intramedullary injury. This can be the result of direct pressure on the cord; passage of a pressure wave through the cord; laceration of the cord by bone, stabbing, or gunshot wound, or rupture of a blood vessel during the passage of a pressure wave through the cord with hemorrhage into the cord. Intramedullary bleeding and hematoma formation (hematomyelia) is also occasionally caused by rupture of a weakened blood vessel or a small angiomatous malformation after lifting a heavy object. The hemorrhage may extend over several segments by dissecting through the substance of the cord.

8. Ischemic damage to the spinal cord. Interruption of the blood supply to the spinal cord can result from compression of the anterior spinal artery; pressure on the anastomotic arteries; damage to major vessels, such as the vertebral arteries in the neck or the abdominal aorta, which gives rise to the anastomotic arteries to the anterior spinal artery.

Clinical Features. Injury to the spinal canal and spinal cord produces:

1. Injury to the nerve roots. This varies from minor concussion of nerve roots with pain and paresthesias in the appropriate dermatome to complete severance of a nerve root with wasting and fasciculations in the muscles supplied by the affected root and complete sensory loss in the appropriate dermatome.

2. Compression of the spinal cord. Acute compression of the spinal cord produces complete flaccid paralysis and loss of sensation below the level of the lesion. This stage of "spinal shock" resolves after several days or weeks and is followed by the development of radicular pain at the site of the lesion and the gradual development of spastic paraparesis below the level of the lesion. There is retention of urine initially with bladder distention and loss of sensation. This is followed by increasing irritability of the bladder and the eventual development, after several weeks, of a small spastic bladder with reflex emptying. In less severe degrees of spinal cord compression the patient presents with a slowly progressive spastic paraparesis, urgency and occasionally incontinence of urine, and minimal or absence of sensory loss.

3. Complete transection of the spinal cord. In a complete transection there is complete paralysis below the level of the lesion immediately after the injury with flaccidity, which changes to progressive spasticity after a period of several weeks. There is initial reflex spasm of bladder sphincters with painless distention of the bladder. With the gradual return of tone to the paralyzed limbs, the patient develops clonus, increased stretch reflexes, and extensor plantar responses. In some cases there are involuntary flexor with-

drawal spasms of the lower limbs, which may be associated with a "mass reflex" involving piloerection, sweating, and evacuation of bowel and bladder. Every effort should be made to avoid flexor spasms by adequate physical therapy and to maintain a state of paraplegia in extension, because paraplegia in flexion encourages the development of decubiti and complicates nursing of paralyzed patients.

4. Hemisection of the cord (the Brown-Sequard syndrome). Hemisection of the cord following gunshot wounds or knife wounds produces a classical picture of ipsilateral spastic monoparesis or hemiparesis with increased stretch reflexes and an extensor plantar response due to involvement of the corticospinal tracts. There is loss of pain and temperature sensation on the side opposite to the lesion because of the involvement of the lateral spinothalamic tracts and loss of vibration and position sense on the side of the lesion due to involvement of the ipsilateral posterior columns.

5. Hematomyelia. Acute hemorrhage into the central gray matter of the spinal cord may follow direct or indirect trauma to the cord. The patient experiences sudden pain at the site of the lesion followed by paralysis. There is usually rapid but partial recovery followed by the development of atrophy of muscles supplied by anterior horn cells at the site of the hematomyelia and spastic paraparesis below the level of the lesion. Sensory examination shows loss of pain and temperature sensation in the dermatomes affected by the hematomyelia, which interrupts the dissecting fibers of the lateral spinothalamic tracts (see p. 217). Sensation is preserved below the level of the hematomyelia, and posterior column function is normal.

6. Injury to the upper cervical cord is a complication of the rather unusual fracture dislocation of the atlanto-occipital joint. This occurs with violent hyperextension of the upper cervical spine. There are signs of cord injury and injury to the lower cranial nerves because of acute downward traction on these structures. A fracture or dislocation of the odontoid process may follow relatively minor trauma. The symptoms are usually mild with persistent neck pain and pain in the distribution of the greater occipital nerves. This fracture usually occurs after traffic accidents, and there is a high incidence of nonunion. This imposes a risk of severe damage to the cord if the patient is involved in further trauma. Fracture dislocation of the second and third

cervical vertebrae occurs in acute hyperextension of the neck in automobile accidents. There is bilateral fracture of the pedicles of C_2 with avulsion of the laminar arch of C_2 and forward dislocation of C_2 on C_3. The condition can be fatal and is the cause of death in judicial hanging. The fracture is termed "hangman's fracture," and there are relatively few symptoms in survivors, who usually complain of stiffness and pain in the neck accompanied by spasm of the cervical muscles.

7. Lesions of the mid- and lower cervical cord produce two distinct syndromes:
a. In the centromedullary syndrome there are contusion, edema, and hemorrhage in the central portion of the cervical cord resulting in tetraparesis; greater involvement of the upper extremities than the lower; impairment of temperature and pain sensation below the level of the lesion; and impaired sphincter control. The condition tends to show progressive improvement in survivors.
b. Anterior spinal artery occlusion with infarction of the spinal cord is a more severe syndrome producing quadriplegia, loss of sphincter control, and loss of pain and temperature sensation below the level of the lesion. Extension of the infarction into the upper cervical cord is associated with loss of sensation over the face due to involvement of the spinal tract of the trigeminal nerve and Horner's syndrome on one or both sides. This condition is often due to an acute protrusion of a cervical disk. Persistent bradycardia is common in severe injuries to the cervical cord due to disruption of the sympathetic pathway located in the cord at this level. Arrhythmias and postural hypotension may also occur during the first 14 days after injury and may be life threatening (37).

8. Lesions of the thoracic cord. Injury to the thoracic cord produces flaccid paraparesis or paraplegia with loss of bladder function and impaired or complete loss of sensation below the level of the lesion. There may be an associated and temporary paralytic ileus.

9. Injury to the conus medullaris. A compression fracture at the level of the first lumbar vertebra can injure the conus medullaris and damage the sacral segments of the spinal cord. This may produce little or no motor deficit, sensory loss in the sacral dermatomes over the buttocks and perineum, destruction of sensory and motor innervation of the bladder resulting in retention with overflow and impotence in the male.

10. Injury to the cauda equina. Lower spinal injuries involving the cauda equina are

associated with flaccid paralysis and wasting of involved muscles; sensory loss in the dermatome supplied by the involved nerves; retention of urine with distention of the bladder if there is involvement of nerve roots S_2, S_3, and S_4; and impotence in the male.

Diagnostic Procedures.

1. X-rays of the spine should be taken in anteroposterior, lateral, and oblique views. If there is any doubt about the presence of a fracture or fracture dislocation, multidirectional tomography should be obtained. X-rays of the cervical spine should be obtained in all cases of closed head injury seen in the emergency room. X-rays of the whole spine are recommended in cases of multiple injury or closed head injury and coma.
2. MR scanning produces a clear image of the spinal cord and surrounding tissues permitting precise localization of cord compression and information concerning damage to surrounding tissues (38, 39). MR is as sensitive as intrathecal contrast myelography in localizing spinal canal blockage.
3. Myelography or CT scanning following injection of contrast material into the subarachnoid space is indicated if MR scanning is not available and if there is residual function below the level of the lesion and the neurosurgeon wishes to delineate the site of compression before surgery.
4. Urodynamic studies are indicated in patients who have impaired bladder control following spinal cord injury.

Treatment. Acute Treatment of Fractures of the Cervical and Upper Thoracic Spine. There is a risk of increasing damage to the spinal cord when transporting patients who have suffered fracture or fracture dislocation of the spine. There should be as little movement as possible, and all movement should be carried out with great care. Lifting should be performed by three people, one who exerts slight traction and extension on the head by grasping the chin and the occiput, the second individual applies traction to the ankles; and the third lifts the shoulders and hips to maintain the spine in slight hyperextension. The patient should be rolled rather than lifted onto a stretcher and transported in a supine position with a roll behind the shoulders to maintain hyperextension. A cervical brace (Philadelphia collar) should be fitted as soon as the patient arrives at the emergency room, and any further movement

performed with the brace supporting the neck (40). It is usually necessary to give an analgesic to control pain. This should be given in adequate dosage to produce relief. All patients should be examined for bladder distention, and a Foley catheter should be inserted if necessary.

Fracture Dislocation of the Lower Thoracic and Lumbar Spine. The lower dorsal and lumbar spine should be maintained in extension with a rolled towel or cushion under the lumbar area. The patient should be transported to the hospital in a prone position that maintains slight extension of the spine.

Management of Cord Injuries in the Emergency Room. The immediate objective of emergency treatment is control of pain and prevention of further cord damage. Once this is achieved, further investigations should be carried out as outlined above. Neurosurgical consultation should be obtained as soon as possible. Cases who do not receive surgical decompression should receive dexamethasone (Decadron) 12 mg q6h for three days followed by 4 mg q6h daily to reduce cord edema.

Medical Management of Spinal Cord Injuries.

1. Treatment should be carried out on a unit where acute neurologic and neurosurgical nursing care is available.
2. Decubiti can be prevented by using an air mattress, frequent turning, and padding of pressure areas.
3. High cord injuries are associated with diaphragmatic paresis and paralysis of the intercostal muscles. Every effort should be made to avoid atelectasis and pneumonia by frequent turning, postural drainage, deep-breathing exercises, and percussion to the chest. Antibiotics should be given if there is any suspicion of pulmonary infection.
4. Frequent determination of arterial blood gases and vital capacity should be made when there is risk of respiratory insufficiency. An endotracheal tube and assisted respiration by mechanical respirator will be required in all C_3 level quadriplegics and may be necessary in patients with C_4 level injury.
5. Paralytic ileus is an occasional complication of cervical and thoracic spine injuries and should be treated with bowel rest and maintenance of adequate fluid and electrolyte balance with intravenous fluids.
6. An indwelling Foley catheter should be used for bladder drainage. Clamping and releasing at two-hour intervals will prevent the development of a small contracted bladder.

Urinary tract infections should be treated with appropriate antibiotics. When signs of motor recovery are observed in the lower limbs, the bladder catheter should be removed in an attempt to reestablish bladder control. Persistent bladder paralysis can be treated by the development of reflex bladder emptying or by instructing patients with intact upper limbs the technique of self catheterization.

7. The development of reflex flexor spasms in the lower limbs is an expected complication of severe paraparesis or paraplegia. This condition often precedes the development of paraplegia in flexion. Flexor spasms may respond to baclofen (Lioresal) or diazepam (Valium). These two drugs may be combined if necessary. Patients with flexor spasms benefit from the use of foam rubber or light aluminum splints, which help to preserve extension in the lower limbs. Severe adductor spasm may be treated with obturator neurectomy, and intractable flexor spasms will respond to blocking of the anterior nerve roots in the lumbosacral area with intrathecal phenol. This procedure should not be used in patients who have residual voluntary bladder function.

8. Low dose heparin or external pneumatic compression will prevent deep venous thrombosis.

9. All patients with spinal cord injury should be placed in a program of physical therapy as soon as possible after admission to the hospital. The program should be simple at first, consisting of no more than passive movements of limbs, but can be gradually developed depending upon the degree of recovery of the patient. The planned program of rehabilitation should include physical therapy and occupational therapy and should develop into a complete program of vocational rehabilitation at a later date.

Surgical Treatment. All patients with spinal cord injury and evidence of cord compression by MR who have signs of neurological function below the level of the lesion should have a decompression operation once the neurologic condition has stabilized (41).

Herniated Intervertebral Disk

Definition. A herniated intervertebral disk is characterized by protrusion of a portion of the nucleus pulposus into the spinal canal.

Etiology and Pathology. A herniated disk is one of the commoner neurologic conditions causing signs and symptoms related to the cervical and lumbar areas. The condition can occur at any age but is more frequent in middle-age and older individuals. Damage to a disk with herniation is a frequent complication of severe injury to the spinal column but may be precipitated by unaccustomed lifting or trivial trauma.

The intervertebral disks are fibrocartilaginous joints of the symphysis type situated between the vertebral bodies. There are two parts to the disk. The annulus fibrosus is an outer rim of densely fibrous tissue, while the inner nucleus pulposus consists of gelatinous material. The annulus fibrosus is firmly attached to the periosteum of the vertebral bodies and the anterior and posterior longitudinal ligaments. The nucleus pulposus has a high water content, which decreases with age. This loss is accelerated during middle age with a resulting decrease in volume of the disk. At the same time there is loss of elasticity of the annulus fibrosus, which facilitates splitting of the annulus under sudden unexpected pressure.

The initial splitting is usually a tear parallel to the circumferential fibers of the annulus fibrosus. This may or may not be associated with some bulging of the disk indicating an area of weakness. After repeated trauma the annulus tends to rupture posteriorly or posterolaterally, and herniation occurs into the spinal canal with consequent pressure on the spinal cord or spinal nerves as they exit through the intervertebral foramina (see Figure 18–6). Occasionally, fragments of the nucleus pulposus are extruded into the spinal canal as isolated cartilaginous bodies and may cause compression of the spinal cord or the

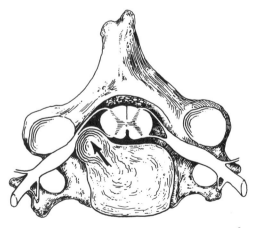

FIGURE 18–6. Diagrammatic representation of a herniated intervertebral disc.

spinal nerves. The blood supply to the annulus fibrosus is poor, and healing occurs slowly after herniation and is often incomplete. This enhances the tendency toward recurrence of symptoms of herniated disk in susceptible individuals.

Clinical Features. Herniated disks most commonly occur in the lumbosacral area, most frequently between L_4 and L_5 or L_5 and S_1. Cervical ruptures are one-tenth as common and most commonly involve the disk between C_5 and C_6. Rupture of thoracic disks is rare (42).

Fifty percent of patients have a clear-cut history of previous injury. In early cases with splitting of the annulus fibrosus rather than herniation the patient presents with pain in the lumbar area or in the neck. In more advanced cases with disk herniation numbness and weakness are present, while prolonged compression results in wasting and fasciculations of the involved muscles. The localizing signs of herniated disk are summarized in Table 18–1. In disk rupture involving the L_4, L_5, or S_1 nerve roots, straight leg-raising results in low back pain (Lasegue sign). In both cervical and lumbar ruptures examination reveals muscle spasm and tenderness in the back or neck and decreased flexion toward the side of the rupture.

The majority of disks rupture in a postero-lateral direction. In the cervical and thoracic areas midline herniation produces pressure on the spinal cord and results in progressive spastic paraparesis and urgency of micturition. A large midline rupture in the lumbar area may compress multiple nerve roots.

Diagnostic Procedures.

1. Spine x-rays. X-rays of the spine may show narrowing of the intervertebral space at the level of the suspected disk herniation.
2. Electromyography. EMG will confirm the presence of nerve root involvement in most cases with herniated disk in the cervical or lumbar areas. Fibrillations may not appear until two to three weeks after the onset of nerve compression.
3. MR scanning has replaced myelography as the study of choice to demonstrate the presence of a herniated disk. The combination of CT scan and iodide contrast myelography should be used when MR scanning is not available.

Treatment.

1. Cervical disk disease.
a. Mild pain without muscle wasting. The affected limb should be supported by a sling and the pain controlled by adequate oral analgesics. The patient should be instructed to apply heat to the neck by lying

TABLE 18–1.   Localized Signs of Herniated Disk

Level of Herniated Disk/ Nerve Root Involved	Location of Pain	Location of Numbness	Muscular Weakness and Wasting	Reflex Changes
C_4–C_5 C_5	Neck Shoulder	C_5 dermatome	Deltoid Supraspinatus	Depressed biceps reflex
C_5–C_6 C_6	Neck Lateral forearm	C_6 dermatome	Biceps	Depressed biceps brachii reflex
C_6–C_7 C_7	Neck Middle finger	C_7 dermatome	Triceps	Depressed triceps reflex
L_3–L_4 L_4	Low back, hip Posterolateral thigh Anterior leg	L_4 dermatome	Quadriceps	Depressed patellar reflex
L_4–L_5 L_5	Sacroiliac joint Posterior thigh Lateral leg to heel	L_5 dermatome	Extensors of the great toe Difficulty walking on the heels	Depressed biceps femoris reflex
L_5–S_1 S_1	Sacroiliac joint Posterior thigh Lateral foot to toes	S_1 dermatome	Plantar flexors of the toes Difficulty walking on the toes	Depressed Achilles reflex

on an electric heating pad for half an hour in the morning and half an hour in the evening.

b. Severe pain without muscle weakness. The patient should be placed on bed rest and given sufficient analgesics to abolish pain within 48 hours. Ice packs should be applied for 30 minutes twice a day. An attempt should be made to reduce swelling in an affected nerve root using dexamethasone (Decadron) in a single dose each day beginning with 30 mg and reducing the dose by 4 mg each day. Since dexamethasone tends to induce insomnia, the patient should receive adequate sedation to induce sleep at night.

c. Persistent pain, weakness, and wasting. Patients with these symptoms should be considered surgical candidates and evaluated and an MR scan should be obtained in an attempt to accurately delineate the herniated disk. Neurosurgical consultation should be obtained.

2. Lumbar disk disease.

a. Mild pain with absence of muscle weakness or wasting. The patient should be treated with bed rest on a firm mattress and restricted to one pillow. Once free from pain the patient should be fitted with a lumbosacral belt with posterior steel bars, which should be worn whenever the patient is out of bed, for at least three months. This serves to prevent sudden flexion movements on ambulation.

b. Moderately severe pain without muscle weakness or wasting. Treatment consists of bed rest on a firm mattress with ice pack to the lumbar area for 30 minutes twice a day. Adequate analgesics should be given to render the patient pain-free within 48 hours. A short course of corticosteroids should be given using dexamethasone in a single daily dose of 30 mg, reducing by 4 mg daily. The patient should be fitted with a lumbosacral belt before attempting ambulation.

c. Severe pain, muscle weakness, and wasting. These cases should be considered as surgical candidates, and if a herniated disk is demonstrated, the patient should be advised to undergo surgical treatment, and a graded program of physical therapy should be started as soon as possible after surgery. Patients are usually able to ambulate within five to seven days and should be fitted with a lumbosacral belt

and instructed to refrain from lifting heavy objects for at least six months.

Patients who fail to respond to surgical treatment or patients who do not have a herniated disk demonstrated by MR scan should receive full medical treatment, including corticosteroid treatment as outlined above.

Hyperextension-Flexion Injury to the Cervical Spine and Cervical Cord (Whiplash Injury)

Definition. A whiplash injury is an injury that results in forced hyperextension-flexion of the neck.

Etiology and Pathology. This type of injury may result from a rear-end collision which produces a sudden and violent hyperextension movement followed by an equally sudden flexion movement of the head on the neck. This may produce damage to the bony and ligamentous structures in the neck, the nerve roots as they emerge through the intervertebral foramina, the vertebral arteries as they course through the foramina in the transverse processes of the cervical vertebrae, or the cervical cord. Concussion and occasionally contusion of the brain stem may also occur.

Clinical Features. Injury to the bony and ligamentous structures of the neck is often a cause of severe pain for many months following this type of injury. There may be damage to nerve roots with pain in the distribution of the dermatome supplied by the affected nerve root. Pain in the distribution of the greater occipital nerves is not unusual following hyperextension-flexion injury and this may be associated with a persistent dull headache in the occipital area, which radiates forward bitemporally. The headache probably has a vascular component and is usually episodic and unpredictable in onset.

Injury to the vertebral arteries may result in ischemia to the brain stem. In most cases recovery occurs without neurologic sequelae, but a minority of cases show evidence of brain stem involvement with ataxia and asymmetry of stretch reflexes. Extensor plantar responses are occasionally demonstrated. This tends to occur in older patients with some degree of atherosclerosis but it can occasionally be demonstrated in younger patients. Concussion effects of injury to the brain stem can also result in permanent neurologic deficits.

The spinal cord may be damaged by the excessive movement of the vertebral column or may suffer damage from an acute herniated disk. There may be hypalgesia to pinprick over one side of the face due to involvement of the spinal tract of the trigeminal nerve. Horner's syndrome may be present on one side in some cases. Damage to the vestibulospinal tract may result in vertigo. Involvement of the spinal cord produces a mild degree of spastic paraparesis with inequality of reflexes, which also tend to be increased bilaterally.

Diagnostic Procedures.

1. Spine x-rays. X-rays of the cervical spine in the anteroposterior, lateral, and oblique views may demonstrate unexpected compression fracture of the vertebral body.
2. Electromyography. EMG is indicated in patients who have persistent pain in dermatomal distribution with some degree of appropriate muscle weakness.
3. MR scanning will demonstrate a herniated disk in cases with consistent pain due to nerve root or spinal cord compression.

Treatment.　Most patients will respond to bed rest, adequate analgesics, and the application of heat to the neck. There is a tendency to underrate the damage caused by this type of injury and to send the patients back to their occupations while acute symptoms are still present. This often prolongs the discomfort and disability. It is better to allow adequate time for recuperation. Patients with persistent neck pain and persistent headache often respond to amitriptyline (Elavil) beginning 25 mg twice a day and increasing to 150 mg daily.

Cervical Spondylosis

Definition.　Cervical spondylosis is a degenerative, arthritic disease involving the cervical spine that may result in compression of the cervical cord, cervical nerve roots, and/or vertebral arteries.

Etiology and Pathology.　The basic cause of cervical spondylosis is degeneration of the intervertebral disks in the cervical spine. There is normally a loss of water content in the intervertebral disks with aging, but the narrowing is occasionally associated with posterior herniation of the disk into the spinal canal. Herniation leads to stimulation of osteoblasts at the margins of the vertebral bodies with new bone formation, which protrudes into the spinal canal. This combination of disk protrusion and new bone formation forms a bar of tissue, which narrows the di-

ameter of the spinal canal. The normal diameter of the spinal canal (17 mm) is reduced; cord compression usually occurs when the diameter is less than 12 mm.

Spinal cord damage is enhanced by other degenerative factors, including thickening of the dentate ligaments, which normally anchor the spinal cord in the spinal canal, and thickening of the ligamentum flavum, which protrudes into the posterior aspect of the spinal canal. The spinal cord is thus anchored by the thickened dentate ligaments, making it more susceptible to compression by other spondylitic bars. Narrowing of the disk spaces produces shortening of the cervical spine and imposes additional stresses on the interpeduncular joint. These joints become the site of osteoarthritic change with formation of osteophytes, which encroach upon the intervertebral foramina and compress the cervical nerve roots. The lateral extension of the osteophytes around the interpeduncular joints will also encroach upon the vertebral arteries as these arteries ascend vertically through the neck in close relationship to the cervical spine. There is also reduction of blood supply to the nerve roots due to compression by osteophytes of segmental arteries. Osteophytic compression of the vertebral arteries, segmental arteries, and nerve roots can be enhanced by head turning, which may increase compression by the osteophytes.

The cervical cord is usually flattened in the anteroposterior diameter in cervical spondylosis, and there are loss of myelin in the posterolateral columns and loss of neurons in the anterior horns, occurring in patchy fashion throughout the cervical cord. Such changes are partially due to compression of the cord and also may result from ischemia due to compression of the anterior spinal artery and its branches.

Compression of the cervical nerve root results in wallerian degeneration.

The kinking and obstruction of the vertebral arteries that result from osteophyte formation may be enhanced by arteriosclerotic change in these arteries in the elderly. Symptoms of vertebral basilar insufficiency may occur, and there is an increased risk of infarction of the brain stem and spinal cord.

Clinical Features.　These is an increased prevalence of diabetes mellitus in patients with cervical spondylosis. Many patients with cervical spondylosis complain of intermittent pain in the neck and occipital headache. However, it is not unusual to see patients with severe x-ray changes of cervical spondylosis who have not experienced any pain or discomfort in the neck.

Patients with cervical spondylosis may experience sudden onset of nerve root pain due to an increase in disk protrusion at the level of the emergent nerve root. This is often precipitated by trauma. The pain is experienced in the distribution of the dermatome supplied by the compressed nerve root. The onset of pain is often followed by some evidence of weakness and wasting in the muscles supplied by the affected nerve root. Fasciculations are occasionally present, and the stretch reflexes innervated through the compressed nerve root are absent or depressed. Subacute or chronic compression of nerve roots produces less pain of dermatomal distribution, but there may be an insidious onset of muscle weakness and wasting with occasional fasciculations and depression of stretch reflexes.

Compression of the cervical cord rarely occurs without evidence of nerve root compression. Compression of the cord is indicated by weakness and wasting of muscles with fasciculations due to compression of anterior horn cells. There may be slow development of spastic paraparesis in the lower limbs characterized by spasticity, ankle clonus, increased stretch reflexes, and bilateral extensor plantar responses due to bilateral involvement of the corticospinal tracts. The patient may develop a spastic or spastic-ataxic gait due to involvement of the corticospinal and spinocerebellar tracts. Increased urgency and frequency of micturition may result with involvement of the descending inhibitory fibers to the bladder control centers in the sacral cord. Occasionally there is sensory impairment in the lower limbs, usually below the knees, due to involvement of the lateral spinothalamic tracts. There may be sensory loss in the lower limbs with impairment of vibration and position sense due to involvement of the posterior columns of the cord.

Compression of the vertebral arteries associated with arteriosclerotic change in these vessels may lead to the appearance of vertebral basilar insufficiency (see p. 137). These symptoms can often be precipitated by head-turning, which increases osteophytic compression of the vertebral arteries. Patients with vertebral basilar insufficiency run an increased risk of infarction of the brain stem.

Diagnostic Procedures.

1. X-rays. X-rays of the neck with anteroposterior, lateral, and oblique views and extension and flexion should be taken to evaluate fully the extent of the cervical spondylosis.
2. Electromyography. The EMG will demonstrate the extent of nerve root involvement.
3. Somatosensory evoked potentials (SEPs). The potentials will show delay in the cervical area of the cervical cord.
4. MR scanning will demonstrate compression of the spinal cord and nerve roots with exquisite clarity (43). MR has superceded myelography and CT as the procedure of choice in cervical spondylosis.

Differential Diagnosis.

1. All causes of spinal cord compression should be considered.
2. Amyotrophic lateral sclerosis can be excluded by the presence of sensory change in cervical spondylosis.
3. Patients with prominent signs of posterior column involvement should receive investigation for subacute combined degeneration of the cord.

Treatment

1. Acute radicular pain can be treated with bed rest, the application of heat to the neck, the adequate use of analgesics, and the use of an antiinflammatory agent such as naproxen 375–500 mg b.i.d. A short course of dexamethasone 30 mg initially, decreasing by 4 mg a day, is valuable in cases with severe pain and disability.
2. The patient should be placed in a program of physical therapy, combined with heat and massage, once the pain is under control.
3. The surgical treatment of cervical spondylosis should always be considered in the presence of:

   a. Persistent severe nerve root pain

   b. Progressive muscle weakness, wasting

   c. Evidence of spinal cord compression

   d. In some cases, vertebral basilar insufficiency purely related to cervical spondylosis

Surgical treatment consists of either laminectomy with decompression of the spinal cord or anterior fusion of the vertebral bodies at the affected level. If available, somatosensory evoked potentials should be monitored to evaluate spinal cord function during operative procedures (44).

Prognosis.
Many patients respond well to conservative measures as outlined here, and this can be repeated when indicated. The re-

sults of surgical treatment in selected cases are also excellent, but patients with definite myelopathy should be warned that surgery is indicated to prevent further deterioration in symptoms rather than to produce improvement.

REFERENCES

1. Rives, J. J.; Lobato, R. D.; *et al.* Extradural hematomas: Analysis of factors influencing the course of 161 patients. Neurosurgery 23:44–51; 1988.
2. Loboto, R. D.; Rioas J. J.; *et al.* Acute epidural hematoma: An analysis of factors influencing the outcome of patients undergoing surgery in coma. J. Neurosurg. 68:48–57; 1988.
3. Sahuquillo-Barris, J.; Lamorea-Cuiro, J.; *et al.* Acute subdural hematoma and diffuse axonal injury after severe head trauma. J. Neurosurg. 68:894–900; 1988.
4. Lobot, R. D.; Sarabia, R.; *et al.* Posttraumatic cerebral hemisphere swelling: Analysis of 55 cases studied with computerized tomography. J. Neurosurg. 68:417–423; 1988.
5. Dagi, T. F. Emergency management of missile injuries to the brain. Resuscitative, triage, and preoperative stabilization. Am. S. Emer. Med. 5:140–148; 1987.
6. Marmarou, A.; Maset, A. L.; *et al.* Contribution of CSF and vascular factors to elevation of ICP in severely head injured patients. J. Neurosurg. 66:883–890; 1987.
7. Hamill, R. W.; Woolf, P. D.; *et al.* Catecholamines predict outcome in traumatic brain injury. Ann. Neurol. 21:438–443; 1987.
8. Lee, K. F.; Wagner, L. K.; *et al.* The impact-absorbing effects of facial fractures and closed head injuries. J. Neurosurg. 66:542–547; 1987.
9. Levin, H. S.; Amparo, E. *et al.* Magnetic resonance imaging and computerized tomography in relation to the neurobehavioral sequelae of mild and moderate head injuries. J. Neurosurg. 66:706–713; 1987.
10. Wilberger, J. R., Jr.; Deeb, Z.; *et al.* Magnetic resonance imaging in cases of severe head injury. Neurosurgery 20:571–576; 1987.
11. Wilberger, J. E.; Deeb, Z.; *et al.* Magnetic resonance imaging in cases of severe head injury. Neurosurgery 20:571–576; 1987.
12. Levin, H. S.; Amparo, E. G.; *et al.* Magnetic resonance imaging after closed head injury in children. Neurosurgery 24:223–227; 1989.
13. Levin, H. S.; Amparo, E.; *et al.* Magnetic resonance imaging and computerized tomography in relation to the neurobehavioral sequelae of mild and moderate head injuries. J. Neurosurg. 66:706–713; 1987.
14. Gibb, F. A.; Gibb, E. L. Electroencephalographic study of head injury in childhood. Clin. Electroenceph. 18:10–11; 1987.
15. Schoenhuber, R.; Gentilini, M.; *et al.* Longitudinal study of auditory brain stem responses in patients with minor head injuries. Arch. Neurol. 44:1181–1182; 1987.
16. Heinrichs, R. W.; Celinski, M. J. Frequency occurrence of a WAIS dementia profile in male head trauma patients. J. Clin. Exp. Neuropsychology 9:187–190; 1987.
17. Freedman, P. E.; Bleiberg, J.; *et al.* Anticipatory behavior deficits in closed head injury. J. Neurol. Neurosurg. Psychiatry 50:398–401; 1987.
18. Tate, R. L. Issues in the management of behavior disturbances as a consequence of severe head injury. Scand. J. Rehab. Med. 19:13–18; 1987.
19. Eisenberg, H. M.; Frankowski, R. F.; *et al.* High dose barbiturate control of elevated intracranial pressure in patients with severe head injury. J. Neurosurg. 69:15–23; 1988.
20. Yarkomy, G. M.; Sahgal, V. Contractures: A major complication of craniocerebral trauma. Clin. Orthop. 219:93–96; 1987.
21. Choi, S. C.; Narayan, R. K.; *et al.* Enhanced specificity of prognosis in severe head injury. J. Neurosurg. 69:381–385; 1988.
22. Kern, T. F. Cognitive rehabilitation aims to improve or replace memory functions in survivors of head injury. J.A.M.A. 257:2400–2402; 1987.
23. Levin, H. S.; Peters, B. H.; *et al.* Effects of oral physostigmine and lecithin on memory and attention in closed head injury patients. Cent. Nerv. Syst. Trauma 3:333–342; 1986.
24. Baloh, R. W.; Honrubia, V.; *et al.* Benign positional vertigo: Clinical and oculographic features in 240 cases. Neurology 37:371–378; 1987.
25. Fagerlund, M.; Liliequest, B. Intermittent cerebrospinal fluid liquorrhea cerebral computed tomography in the non-drop period. Acta. Radiologica 28(2):189–192; 1987.
26. Lipton, J. H.; Russell, J. A.; *et al.* Fat embolization and pulmonary infiltrates after bone marrow transplantation. Med. Ped. Oncol. 15:24–27; 1987.
27. Lindeque, B. G. P.; Schoeman, H. S.; *et al.* Fat embolism and the fat embolism syndrome. J. Bone Joint Surg. (Br.) 69:128–131; 1987.
28. Robiesek, F.; Duncan, G. D. Retrograde air embolization in coronary operations. J. Thorac. Cardiovasc. Surg. 94:110–114; 1987.
29. Kizer, K. W. Dysbaric cerebral air embolism in Hawaii. Ann. Emerg. Med. 16:535–541; 1987.
30. Jenson, P. J.; Thomsen, P. E. B. Electrical injury causing ventricular arrhythmias. Br. Heart J. 57:279–283; 1987.
31. Gans, M.; Glaser, J. S. Homonymous hemianopia following electrical injury. J. Clin. Neuro. Oph. 6:218–221; 1986.
32. Doyle, W. K.; Budinger, T. F.; *et al.* Differentiation of cerebral radiation necrosis from tumor recurrence by [^{18}F] FD6 and ^{82}Rb positron emission tomography. J. Comput. Assist. Tomography 11:563–570; 1987.

33. Goldwein, J. W. Radiation myelopathy: A review. Med. Pediatr. Oncol. 15:89–95; 1987.

34. Hoang, P.; Ford, D. J.; *et al.* Postmastectomy pain after brachial plexus palsy: metastases or radiation neuritis? J. Hand Surg. (Br.) 11:441–443; 1986.

35. Arthur, D. C.; Margulies, R. A. A short course in diving medicine. Ann. Emerg. Med. 16:689–701; 1987.

36. Garza-Mercado, R. Traumatic extradural hematoma of the cervical spine. Neurosurgery 24:410–414; 1989.

37. Lehmann, K. G.; Lane, J. G. Cardiovascular abnormalities accompanying acute spinal cord injury in humans: incidence, time course, and severity. J. Am. Coll. Cardiol. 10:46–52; 1987.

38. Breedveld, F. C.; Algra, P. R.; *et al.* Magnetic resonance imaging in the evaluation of patients with rheumatoid arthritis and subluxations of the cervical spine. Arthritis Rheum. 30:624–629; 1987.

39. Kulkani, M. V.; McArdle, C. B.; *et al.* Acute spinal cord injury: MR imaging at last. Radiology 164:837–843; 1987.

40. Little, N. E. In case of a broken neck. Emergency Med. 21:22–30; 1989.

41. Benzel, E. C.; Larson, S. J. Functional recovery after decompression operation for thoracic and lumbar spine fractures. Neurosurgery 19:772–778; 1986.

42. Blumenkopf, B. Thoracic intervertebral disc herniations: diagnostic value of magnetic resonance imaging. Neurosurgery 23:36–40; 1988.

43. Masaryk, T. J.; Modic, J. M.; *et al.* Cervical myelopathy: A comparison of magnetic resonance and myelography. J. Comput. Assist. Tomogr. 10:184–194; 1986.

44. Veilleux, M. Monitoring of cortical evoked potentials during surgical procedures on the cervical spine. Mayo Clin. Proc. 62:256–264; 1987.

CHAPTER 19

THE PERIPHERAL NEUROPATHIES

ANATOMY OF THE PERIPHERAL NERVES

Motor nerve fibers originate from the anterior horn cells of the spinal cord and leave the cord through the anterior nerve root. The sensory fibers originate from neurons in the posterior root ganglia and enter the spinal cord through the posterior nerve root. The anterior and posterior nerve roots unite distal to the cord to form a mixed spinal nerve (see Figure 19–1). Both anterior and posterior nerve roots are covered by dura as they leave the spinal cord up to the point of exit from the spinal canal where the dura becomes continuous with the epineurium covering the mixed spinal nerve. The mixed spinal nerves unite in the cervical and lumbar areas to form the cervical, brachial, and lumbosacral plexuses. Each plexus gives rise to a number of individual mixed nerves, which are distributed to the periphery to supply muscle, skin, and blood vessels.

Each nerve contains numerous nerve fibers. The central portion of each nerve fiber consists of an axon that contains axoplasm. Axoplasm is a complex structure containing mitochondria, endoplasmic reticulum, Golgi apparatus, neurotubules, and neurofilaments, which are individual nonanastomotic fibrils that extend the entire length of the axon. The surface of the axon is covered by a limiting membrane called the axolemma and by the myelin sheath external to the axolemma. The myelin sheath is derived from the cytoplasm

of the Schwann cell and surrounds the axon in concentric layers. Large myelinated axons are either motor axons or sensory axons subserving the modalities of touch, vibration, and proprioception. Small myelinated axons serve pain and temperature, while so-called unmyelinated axons, which are invested by the Schwann cell membrane without sheath formation, carry pain and deeper ill-defined sensation. The myelin sheath is not a continuous structure but consists of sections, each derived from a single Schwann cell, which are separated by small gaps known as nodes of Ranvier. Electrical impulses are conducted by a series of "jumps" from node to node, a method known as saltatory conduction. This means that the speed of conduction is related to the distance between the nodes. Rapidly conducting axons have relatively few nodes, which are far apart. Axons that conduct more slowly have many nodes, which are close together along the extent of the axon. The so-called unmyelinated nerve fibers are very slow-conducting fibers. Axons are also capable of conducting proteins from the perineurium or cell body to the periphery, and it is known that this conduction is two-directional. There is a functional relationship between the Schwann cells and axons. Schwann cells will not survive without the presence of axons, although axons will survive in the absence of Schwann cells, but their function is markedly altered. Mixed peripheral nerves consist of many thousands of axons, each sep-

352

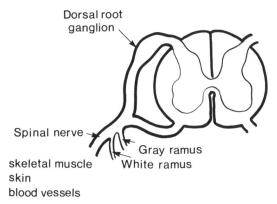

Dorsal root
ganglion

Spinal nerve

skeletal muscle
skin
blood vessels

Gray ramus
White ramus

FIGURE 19–1.   Schematic representation of the relationship of a spinal nerve to the spinal cord.

arated by a fine connective tissue called the endoneurium. Axons are collected in bundles or fascicles surrounded by perineurium, and fascicles are separated by a thicker connective tissue known as the epineurium.

Diseases of the peripheral nerves may produce changes in axons or in the myelin sheath. Axonal changes are of two types, axonal (wallerian) degeneration and axonal dystrophy. Axonal degeneration occurs following severance or infarction of a peripheral nerve. The axon dies up to the level of the first internode above the site of trauma, which may be followed by chromatolysis in the perikaryon or cell body of the neuron. The myelin distal to the site of trauma disintegrates and is digested and removed. If the cell body does not die, axonal regeneration occurs by the regrowth of nerve fibrils, which attempt to make contact with the peripheral axolemma and reestablish the previous peripheral connections. If the axolemma is destroyed, degeneration is haphazard and may result in the development of a painful, traumatic neuroma. Once the neurofibrils have regenerated, the Schwann cells reinvest the axon with myelin. A number of nutritional and metabolic disorders are associated with a second type of axonal damage called axonal dystrophy in which there is a gradual dying back of the axons from the periphery. This is commonly seen in diabetic neuropathy but also occurs in alcoholism and in many toxic conditions (1).

Segmental demyelination occurs when there is primary involvement and death of the Schwann cell. The neuron, including the perikaryon and axon, remains normal, and axonal continuity is maintained. In some cases Schwann cell regeneration occurs, but the

nodes of Ranvier are situated closer together than before demyelination. Remyelination is occasionally followed by hypertrophy of the Schwann cells, which surround axons in an "onion ring" fashion. Hypertrophic change occurs in interstitial hypertrophic neuropathy, chronic inflammatory neuropathy, and occasionally in acromegaly. Demyelination is a feature of some hereditary neuropathies and postinfectious polyneuritis. Mixed types of peripheral neuropathy with both axonal degeneration and demyelination can occur.

Several clinical patterns of peripheral neuropathy are recognized. These include:

1. Mononeuropathy. Mononeuropathy implies involvement of one peripheral nerve. This is commonly the result of trauma but also occurs in diabetes mellitus and in infarction of peripheral nerves (e.g., in polyarteritis nodosa).
2. Mononeuritis multiplex. Mononeuritis multiplex is a term used to describe involvement of several individual nerves in a haphazard fashion. The etiology is the same as for mononeuropathy.
3. Radiculoneuropathy. A radiculoneuropathy is involvement of the nerve root as it emerges from the spinal cord. This is commonly seen with herniated disks or with epidural masses (e.g. tumor).
4. Polyradiculitis. Polyradiculitis or radiculopathy is characterized by involvement of several nerve roots and is commonly seen in postinfectious polyneuritis or post-vaccinal polyneuritis.
5. Plexitis. A plexitis is an inflammation of a plexus such as the brachial plexus (brachial plexitis).
6. Polyneuritis. In polyneuritis or polyneu-

ropathy there is a symmetric involvement of peripheral nerves. The commonest causes are diabetes mellitus and alcoholism. There are, however, numerous causes of peripheral neuropathy and the identification of the etiologic agent may be difficult in unusual cases.

Neuropathies, no matter what their cause and type, present with specific signs and symptoms. Involvement of motor axons produces muscle wasting and weakness followed by atrophy and the appearance of fasciculations. The tendon reflexes supplied by the affected nerve are depressed or absent. Involvement of sensory axons produces impairment of sensation with dysethesias or paresthesias. Involvement of axons supplying autonomic function produces loss of sweating, alteration in bladder function, constipation, and impotence in the male. Causalgia, a very painful peripheral dysesthesia, is probably related to disturbance of autonomic axons in peripheral nerves.

NEUROPATHIES OF THE CRANIAL NERVES

THE THIRD, FOURTH, AND SIXTH CRANIAL NERVES

Lesions of the third, fourth, and sixth cranial nerves are conveniently considered together because of the proximity of origin of these nerves in the brain stem and the close relationship in their course through the cranial cavity to supply the extraocular muscles and intrinsic muscles of the eye. Involvement of the third, fourth, and sixth nerve nuclei or the proximal portion of these nerves in the brain stem is usually associated with other signs of brain stem dysfunction. One example is Mobius syndrome, an hereditary condition in which there is dysplasia of the nuclei of the oculomotor and seventh cranial nerves. Other causes of oculomotor palsies include brain stem trauma, encephalitis, syphilis, Wernicke's encephalopathy, tumor, infarction, multiple sclerosis, and the spinocerebellar degenerations (2). Involvement of the oculomotor nerves in the posterior fossa is common with increased intracranial pressure associated with herniation of the uncus of the temporal lobe over the free edge of the tentorium. This produces pressure on the third nerve as it crosses the tentorial edge resulting in unilateral dilatation of the pupil, followed by paralysis of the extraocular movements supplied by the third nerve. Other causes of third, fourth, and sixth nerve involvement in

the posterior fossa include meningitis, syphilis, polyneuritis, diabetes mellitus, and extraaxial tumors. Diabetic mononeuropathy involving the third nerve usually produces paralysis of the extraocular movements supplied by the third nerve with sparing of the pupil. This condition is believed to be due to infarction of the outer layer of the third nerve, which contains the motor fibers supplying extraocular muscles, while the inner core of fibers supplying the constriction of the pupil is preserved.

The third, fourth, and sixth nerves are vulnerable to pressure in the lateral wall of the cavernous sinus. The commoner causes include aneurysms of the internal carotid artery and pituitary or parapituitary tumors. Compression of the third nerve has been reported from a persistent trigeminal artery and is occasionally seen as a reversible condition in ophthalmoplegic migraine (see p. 84).

The nerves may be involved at the level of the superior orbital fissure, which may be narrowed by inflammation, by Paget's disease, or by growth of a nearby tumor, usually a meningioma. Orbital involvement of the third, fourth, and sixth nerves may follow trauma with fracture of the orbital bones. Other causes include orbital cellulitis, abscess, and temporal arteritis. Transient paralysis of the sixth nerve is sometimes seen in infants and children and is a benign condition of unknown etiology. A similar condition is sometimes induced by the use of prochlorperazine (Compazine) in children. Cyclic oculomotor paralysis is a rare condition encountered in children in which there is paralysis of extraocular movements supplied by the third nerve associated with ptosis lasting for a period varying from several seconds to several minutes.

THE FIFTH CRANIAL NERVE (TRIGEMINAL NERVE)

Trigeminal Neuralgia (Tic Douloureux)
Definition. Trigeminal neuralgia is a condition characterized by sudden, severe, lancinating pain occurring in the distribution of the trigeminal nerve.
Etiology and Pathology. Trigeminal neuralgia is probably syndromic and may be due to:

1. Degenerative changes in the trigeminal (gasserian) ganglion, producing paroxysmal discharge of neurons.
2. Pressure on the trigeminal nerve root by aberrant or arteriosclerotic vessels, by

tumor, or by displacement of the brain stem by a contralateral tumor with compression of the trigeminal nerve against a bony structure.

3. Increased angulation of the nerve root over the petrous bone caused by demineralization at the base of the skull in the elderly with upward movement of the petrous pyramid.

4. Demyelination of the most proximal portion of the trigeminal nerve root or demyelination affecting the spinal tract in the brain stem in patients with multiple sclerosis. (A similar condition occurs in patients with tabes dorsalis).

5. Paroxysmal discharges of the neurons of the spinal nucleus of the trigeminal nerve. (This concept suggests that trigeminal neuralgia is a form of seizure activity occurring at the brain stem level secondary to degenerative or vascular changes affecting the neurons of the spinal nucleus.)

Clinical Features. The disease predominantly occurs in middle-aged and elderly patients. The occurrence of trigeminal neuralgia in the younger individual suggests the diagnosis of multiple sclerosis, tumor, or aneurysm. The disorder is somewhat commoner in females. The condition is characterized by paroxysms of pain occurring in the maxillary and mandibular division of the trigeminal nerve with later spread from one division to involve the other division. Involvement of the ophthalmic division is rare and occurs in less than 5 percent of cases. Trigeminal neuralgia may involve both sides of the face, but paroxysms never occur simultaneously on the two sides. In established cases the pain may be provoked by touching the face, chewing, talking, drinking, brushing the teeth, shaving, or the movement of air across the affected side of the face. Patients recognize certain "trigger points," which will produce a typical paroxysm of pain if stimulated. Established cases exhibit sudden, severe paroxysms of pain with cessation of speech and contortion of the face often accompanied by a cry of distress. The attacks are short-lived with long periods of freedom in the early stages, but the paroxysms gradually become longer and closer together in time. This leads to constant dread of the next attack with depression, suicidal thoughts, and weight loss.

The neurologic examination is normal.

Diagnostic Procedures.

1. X-rays. The patient should have x-rays of the base of the skull with visualization of

the foramen ovale. Enlargement of the foramen ovale suggests the possibility of intracranial or extracranial tumor.

2. If there is a suspicion of the presence of tumor or aneurysm, a scan of the base of the skull should be performed.

Treatment. Medical treatment using carbamazepine (Tegretol) is successful in most cases. It should be given in small doses initially and gradually increased to effect, beginning with 100 mg at night and increasing by 100 mg every three days until the patient is receiving 800 to 1,600 mg in three divided doses daily. The slow introduction of carbamazepine will permit the establishment of therapeutic levels of the drug without the development of unpleasant side effects. See page 77 for further information on the use of carbamazepine. Oxycarbazepine is equally effective (3).

Phenytoin (Dilantin) is less effective than carbamazepine in the control of trigeminal neuralgia but should be used to treat patients who are unable to tolerate carbamazepine. Phenytoin is also useful as an adjunct when carbamazepine produces significant but incomplete control of pain. The dosage of phenytoin should always be sufficient to produce therapeutic plasma concentrations of the drug (see p. 76).

A number of surgical procedures are currently advocated for the treatment of trigeminal neuralgia. These include alcohol injection of individual nerves or the trigeminal ganglion. This form of treatment relieves pain, but the patient must clearly understand that alcohol injection produces anesthesia, and pain loss is associated with loss of sensation in the affected area of the face. Nerve regeneration often occurs after six months with return of the pain in some cases. Other surgical procedures include percutaneous radiofrequency or glycerol trigeminal gangliolysis and suboccipital craniotomy with decompression of the trigeminal nerve. This latter procedure has the advantage of relieving pain without producing anesthesia. Trigeminal tractotomy with severance of the descending spinal tract of the trigeminal nerve at the cervicomedullary junction should be reserved for intractable cases that have failed to respond to other forms of treatment.

Prognosis. The majority of cases of trigeminal neuralgia can be controlled medically with carbamazepine but many have to continue taking the drug for a prolonged period. An attempt at withdrawal should be made when the patient has been pain-free for six months. This is successful in some cases.

THE SEVENTH CRANIAL NERVE

Bell's Palsy

Definition. Bell's palsy is the acute onset of an isolated facial paralysis of the peripheral type.

Etiology and Pathology. The etiology of Bell's palsy is unknown, but the disease is believed to be the result of a viral infection involving the geniculate ganglion. It is possible that some cases are due to activation of a latent *Herpes simplex* infection.

Pathologic changes consist of inflammation and edema of the facial nerve in the facial canal. This produces increasing pressure on the nerve with paralysis of function followed by Wallerian degeneration of axons.

Clinical Features. Bell's palsy usually occurs in middle-aged and elderly individuals. There is frequently a history of exposure to cold temperatures or drafts preceding the onset of facial paralysis. Most patients give a history of pain or ache in the region of the stylomastoid foramen immediately behind the angle of the mandible some 24 to 48 hours before the appearance of the facial paralysis. The paralysis is usually appreciated for the first time on awakening in the morning, and there is a steady progression to severe weakness or total loss of function involving one side of the face. The affected side of the face sags and the eye cannot be closed because of paralysis of the orbicularis occuli. Weakness of the cheek allows food to accumulate between the teeth and the side of the mouth. There is often excess watering of the eye because of inability to move secretions across the cornea to the lacrimal duct. When the edema on the facial nerve extends proximally with involvement of the chorda tympani, there may be loss of taste. Further proximal extension produces hyperacusis because of paralysis of the nerve to the stapedius, and involvement of the geniculate ganglion results in loss of lacrimation and a dry eye. Complaints of numbness or sensory change over the face and the presence of nystagmus suggest involvement of both the trigeminal nerve and the vestibular division of the eighth nerve in some cases of Bell's palsy (4). The characteristics of seventh nerve paralysis due to lesions at particular sites and common etiologies are listed in Table 19–1.

Diagnostic Procedures. Some determination of prognosis can be obtained by obser-vation of evoked responses on stimulating the facial nerve as it emerges from the stylomastoid foramen. The demonstration of a good evoked response on stimulating the facial nerve indicates a good prognosis. Complete loss of excitability on stimulation indicates a poorer prognosis.

Treatment. The initial discomfort can be relieved with aspirin or aspirin and codeine compounds. The use of oral corticosteroids in the treatment of Bell's palsy is controversial. However, some studies indicate improvement with corticosteroids, which can be given in a single dose of methyprednisolone (Medrol) 80 mg initially with a gradual reduction of dosage over the seven-day period. Patients who are unable to close the eyelids should be treated with methylcellulose eyedrops q4h, and the eye should be protected by a patch until there is return of eyelid function.

Prognosis. The majority of patients with Bell's palsy make a complete recovery over a period of two to three weeks. The remaining 15 percent show some loss of function, including persistent facial weakness, facial spasm, ectropion, and excess lacrimation sometimes called "crocodile tears" caused by regeneration and passage of axons destined for the salivary glands to the lacrimal gland. In the older age group, hyperacusis, and a very dense paralysis are associated with a poorer prognosis.

Geniculate Neuralgia

Definition. Geniculate neuralgia is characterized by episodes of severe lancinating pain occurring in the region of the pinna and external auditory canal.

Etiology and Pathology. The etiology of this condition is unknown and is believed to be due to a neuralgia affecting the nervus intermedius. The bipolar neurons of the nervus intermedius are located in the geniculate ganglion and the afferent axons enter the spinal tract of the trigeminal nerve. The peripheral fibers are distributed to the external auditory canal and the pinna. There may also be some distribution to deeper structures of the face and hard palate.

Clinical Features. Patients experience spasmodic attacks of severe pain in the region of the pinna and external auditory canal. The pain is occasionally felt in the throat, deep in the face, and in the orbit.

Treatment. Same as for trigeminal neuralgia (see p. 354). Surgical excision of the

TABLE 19–1. Seventh Nerve Paralysis

Site	Characteristics	Etiology
Supranuclear lesions	Weakness of contralateral, lower face	Lesion involving corticobulbar tract above pons
Nuclear or pontine lesion	Total facial paralysis on side of lesion Impaired salivary secretion Taste intact Impaired lacrimation same side Associated paralysis of sixth or fifth nerve on same side Eyes may be conjugately deviated toward side of lesion Possible internuclear ophthalmoplegia Possible contralateral hemiparesis	Congenital: Mobius syndrome Infectious: encephalitis, rabies, meningitis Nutritional: Wernicke's encephalopathy Neoplastic: pontine glioma Vascular: infarction, hemorrhage Degenerative: multiple sclerosis, syringobulbia, amyotrophic lateral sclerosis
Extracranial in cerebellopontine angle	Total facial paralysis on side of lesion Hearing loss on side of lesion Episodic vertigo Corneal reflex depressed on side of lesion Impaired salivary secretion Impaired lacrimation on side of lesion	Inflammation: meningitis, tuberculosis, syphilis, fungi Neoplastic: neurilemoma, meningioma dermoid, chordoma, meningeal carcinomatosis Vascular: aneurysm of basilar artery Degenerative: multiple sclerosis
Extracranial in facial canal		Traumatic: fractures involving petrous temporal bone
a. Between internal auditory meatus and geniculate ganglion	Total facial paralysis same side Hearing loss same side Impaired lacrimation same side Impaired salivary secretion Taste lost anterior two-thirds tongue same side	Infectious: otitis media, mastoiditis, Bell's palsy (see below), *Herpes zoster* of geniculate ganglion (Ramsey Hunt syndrome) (see below), sarcoidosis, postinfectious polyneuritis (bilateral)
b. Between geniculate ganglion and origin of nerve to stapedius	Total facial paralysis same side Impaired salivary secretion Taste lost anterior two-thirds tongue same side Hyperacusis	Metabolic: diabetes mellitus Neoplastic: cholesteatoma, epidermoid temporal bone tumors, parotid gland tumors, leukemic deposits in facial canal
c. Between origin of nerve to stapedius and origin of chorda tympani	Total facial paralysis same side Impaired salivary secretion Taste lost anterior two-thirds tongue same side	
d. Distal to origin of chorda tympani	Total facial paralysis same side only	

geniculate ganglion has been performed in refractory cases.

Facial Myokymia
See page 403.

Hemifacial Spasm
Definition. Hemifacial spasm is an irregular contraction of the muscles supplied by the facial nerve on one side.
Etiology and Pathology. Hemifacial spasm is due to an irritative lesion of the facial nerve and is comparable to trigeminal neuralgia in many ways. The commonest cause is believed to be compression of the facial nerve as it emerges from the brain stem by an arteriosclerotic vessel. Other causes include multiple sclerosis, an aneurysm of the basilar artery, and tumor or arachnoiditis in the cerebellopontine angle.
Clinical Features. Hemifacial spasm usually begins with irregular contractions affect-

ing the orbicularis oculi and gradually spreads to involve all of the muscles supplied by the facial nerve on one side. The condition is always unilateral, and the movements are irregular, lasting for a few seconds to a few minutes with periods of freedom. Hemifacial spasm is increased by tension and emotional upset. Atypical facial pain may occur in some cases and suggests the presence of neoplasm (5). There are no other neurologic abnormalities on neurologic examination.

Treatment. Carbamazepine (Tegretol) and phenytoin (Dilantin) are rarely successful in controlling hemifacial spasm. Surgical treatment is indicated when hemifacial spasm becomes unacceptable to the patient. This consists of exposure of the facial nerve in the posterior fossa with identification of the compressive lesion, usually a tortuous arteriosclerotic artery.

Loss of Taste

Loss of taste has been described in some cases of Bell's palsy and also occurs in other conditions. Ageusia or dysgeusia, loss or disorder of taste, has been described after an upper respiratory tract infection and is presumably due to a viral neuritis. Other causes include exposure to certain drugs including D-penicillamine, griseofulvin, phenylbutazone, oxyphedrine, and carbamazepine. Loss of taste causes considerable distress to patients and should always be differentiated from loss of smell since most patients confuse these two senses. There is no specific treatment for loss of taste, although the use of oral zinc preparations has been suggested.

THE EIGHTH CRANIAL NERVE

The majority of eighth nerve neuropathies are due to the toxic effect of drugs. A number of antibiotics, particularly the aminoglycosides, are reported to cause eighth nerve degeneration. Streptomycin and gentamicin affect the vestibular division of the nerve, while neomycin, vancomycin, streptomycin, and kanamycin affect the auditory divisions of the nerve. Most cases follow parenteral administration of the antibiotic, but toxic neuropathy has been reported following topical application of creams containing kanamycin.

There is a rare, familial degenerative neuropathy affecting the cochlear division of the eighth nerve, which is characterized by progressive deafness. This may be associated with myoclonus and sensory peripheral neuropathy in some cases.

THE NINTH CRANIAL NERVE

Glossopharyngeal Neuralgia

Definition. Glossopharyngeal neuralgia is the occurrence of spasms of pain in the sensory distribution of the ninth and tenth cranial nerves.

Etiology and Pathology. The cause is unknown but is presumed to be pressure on or entrapment of the ninth and/or 10th cranial nerves. Glossopharyngeal neuralgia has occurred following acute infection of the pharynx but has also been related to compression at many sites, including the cerebellopontine angle, jugular foramen, base of the skull, pharynx, and tonsils.

Clinical Features. The patient experiences spasms of pain in the pharynx, often radiating into the ear. The attacks may be precipitated by swallowing, coughing, chewing, talking, sneezing, turning the head to one side, or touching the tragus of the ear. The attacks are usually brief but may last for several minutes in severe cases. Remissions are common. The neurologic examination is normal.

Attacks are occasionally associated with bradycardia, cardiac arrhythmias, hypertension, and syncope due to associated vagal stimulation. Hypersecretion of the parotid gland has been reported.

Diagnostic Procedures. A diligent search should be made for a compressive lesion in the area of the cerebellopontine angle or at the base of the skull using MR or CT scanning and x-ray views of the jugular foramen.

Treatment. Most cases respond to carbamazepine (Tegretol) as described under trigeminal neuralgia. Intracranial sectioning of the glossopharyngeal nerve has been performed in intractable cases. This procedure entails section of the upper two rootlets of the vagus nerve and may be associated with postoperative hypotension and cardiac arrhythmias.

THE TENTH CRANIAL NERVE

Superior Laryngeal Neuralgia

This rare condition is associated with episodic lancinating pain radiating over the side of the neck. The disorder may be due to entrapment of the superior laryngeal nerve as it pierces the hyothyroid membrane. Patients experience pain in the anteromedial aspect of the neck radiating up behind the angle of the mandible up to the face as high as the zygoma.

The diagnosis can be established by injection of a local anesthetic into the superior laryngeal nerve as it pierces the hyothyroid membrane. This procedure will produce temporary relief. Most patients respond to carbamazepine (Tegretol). Refractory cases require sectioning of the superior laryngeal nerve at the level of the hyothyroid membrane.

THE ELEVENTH CRANIAL NERVE

The 11th cranial nerve (accessory nerve) is subject to injury by trauma or surgical procedures or by compression due to tumors or enlarged lymph nodes in the posterior triangle of the neck. Involvement of the accessory nerve produces paralysis and wasting of the trapezius with inability to elevate the arm above the horizontal plane without external rotation. There may be pain in the neck and shoulder.

Patients may require analgesics and the use of an arm sling to relieve shoulder pain. Compression may be relieved by surgical procedures.

THE TWELFTH CRANIAL NERVE

The hypoglossal nerve is occasionally injured in surgical procedures of the neck. This produces hemiatrophy of the tongue with deviation of the tongue toward the side of the lesion on tongue protrusion.

THE CERVICAL PLEXUS

Anatomy

The cervical plexus is formed by looped connections between the anterior primary rami of C_1, C_2, C_3, C_4, and C_5 on the anterior aspect of the levator scapuli and scalenus medius muscles. Branches from C_2 supply the sternocleidomastoid, while C_3 and C_4 supply the levator scapuli. The phrenic nerve is derived from C_3, C_4, and C_5 and supplies the diaphragm. The most important sensory branch is the greater occipital nerve, which arises from C_2, and the lesser occipital nerve arises from C_2, and the greater auricular nerves from C_2 and C_3. All supply the posterior aspect of the scalp. The transverse cervical and supraclavicular nerves (C_2, C_3, and C_4) supply the neck and the anterior portion of the chest wall down to the level of the T_2 dermatome.

Occipital Neuralgia

Definition. Occipital neuralgia is a condition characterized by pain occurring in the cutaneous distribution of the greater occipital nerve.

Etiology and Pathology. The greater occipital nerve may be compressed in the neck by cervical spondylosis. It is occasionally injured during hyperextension-flexion injuries of the neck which result in contusion of the nerve root as it passes through the intervertebral foramen.

Clinical Features. The patient complains of constant pain in the distribution of the greater occipital nerve over the posterior aspect of the scalp. The nerve is tender to palpation in its course over the occipital bone.

Diagnostic Procedures. Occipital neuralgia is frequently misdiagnosed as a "headache." The diagnosis can be established by relief of symptoms with local injection of the occipital nerve as it passes over the occipital bone.

Treatment. Early cases may respond to the application of heat to the upper cervical area and the use of analgesics. Antiinflammatory agents such as naproxen 500 mg b.i.d. may help. When the pain persists, the greater occipital nerve can be injected with local anesthesia and a corticosteroid such as 40 mg of methylprednisolone (Medrol), which frequently produces permanent relief of symptoms. Treatment of cervical spondylosis is outlined on page 348.

Lesions of the Phrenic Nerve

The phrenic nerve arises from the anterior primary rami of C_3, C_4, and C_5 and passes from the neck into the thorax to supply the diaphragm. The nerve may be damaged during traumatic injury to the cervical spine with contusion or tearing of the anterior primary rami of C_3, C_4, and C_5. The nerve is occasionally involved in chronic meningitis, arachnoiditis, and cervical spondylosis. Compression by tumors of the neck, aneurysms of the major vessels, or enlarged lymph nodes in the neck may also produce phrenic paralysis. Compression in the thorax by tumors and enlarged lymph nodes or an aneurysm of the aorta is another cause of phrenic nerve involvement.

Mononeuropathy of the phrenic nerve has occasionally been reported following viral pneumonia, diptheria, and exposure to such toxins as alcohol and lead. Unilateral paralysis of the diaphragm usually produces few symptoms and the condition is often diagnosed in the evaluation of patients with tumors or enlarged lymph nodes in the neck or thorax. The sensory fibers of the phrenic nerve can be stimulated by subphrenic conditions such as subphrenic abscess, cholecystitis, pancreatitis, and carcinoma of the pancreas, or by intrathoracic inflammatory conditions producing diaphragmatic pleurisy. This produces referred pain experienced over the shoulder on the same side as the lesion. Peripheral irritation may result in persistent singultus (hiccough). This condition responds to small doses of thorazine.

THE BRACHIAL PLEXUS

Anatomy

The brachial plexus is formed by the anterior divisions of C_5, C_6, C_7, C_8, and T_1 with some variable contribution from C_4 and T_2. The plexus consists of superior, middle, and inferior trunks, which divide and reunite to form lateral, posterior, and medial cords, so named because of their relationship to the axillary artery. The trunks and cords give origin to a number of individual nerves supplying motor, sensory, and autonomic fibers to the upper thorax, shoulder, and upper limb (see Figure 19–2).

Birth Injuries to the Brachial Plexus

Etiology and Pathology. The brachial plexus may be damaged by excessive lateral traction on the head with the shoulders fixed during a difficult delivery or by excessive downward traction on the shoulders with the head fixed in a breech delivery. Both of these maneuvers produce an increase in the angle between the shoulder and the head and exert pressure on the roots of the brachial plexus.

Clinical Features. Three types of injury can occur. These include:

1. Injury to the roots of C_5 and C_6 (Erb's paralysis)
2. Injury to the roots of C_8 and T_1 (Klumpke paralysis)
3. Combined upper and lower root injury (Erb-Duchenne-Klumpke paralysis)

Erb's Paralysis. Erb's paralysis is characterized by paralysis involving the deltoid (abduction); biceps, brachialis, and supinator (elbow flexion); and supraspinatus and infraspinatus (external rotation). The infant presents with absence of movement of the affected arm. The muscles fail to develop, and the arm and shoulder assume the typical posture of adduction, inward rotation, and pronation of the forearm and hand some months after birth. There are loss of the biceps and brachioradialis reflexes and a small area of sensory loss over the upper lateral aspect of the arm.

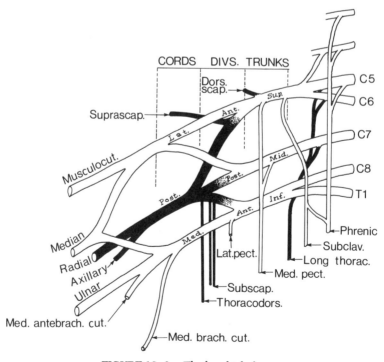

FIGURE 19–2. The brachial plexus.

Treatment.

1. All joints of the arm should be moved through a full range of motion several times a day.
2. The upper limb should be splinted in abduction with the elbow flexed to 90 degrees and the forearm in midsupination.
3. Orthopedic surgical measures, including partial section of the pectoralis major and pronator teres should be considered in cases that do not recover.

Prognosis. Recovery occurs in about 50 percent of cases.

Klumpke Paralysis. This type of paralysis is rare. Klumpke paralysis is characterized by paresis of the wrist, finger flexion, and small muscles of the hand. The fingers become extended, but the elbow is flexed. There is sensory impairment over the inner aspect of the forearm and hand. Horner's syndrome develops when there is avulsion of the cervical nerve roots.

Combined Paralysis. The combined upper (Erb) and lower (Klumpke) paralysis is extremely rare. It is characterized by paralysis of the shoulder and hand. The arm is wasted and cold, with dependent edema, and Horner's syndrome is present.

Traumatic Injury to the Brachial Plexus

Injury to the brachial plexus is not uncommon in gunshot wounds, knife wounds, competitive sports, and automotive accidents, particularly motorcycle accidents. The plexus may be stretched and damaged by carrying heavy loads on the shoulders or by prolonged backward displacement of the shoulders during coma and occasionally during general anesthesia. Traumatic injury includes:

1. A fall onto the apex of the shoulder and the side of the head. This injury abruptly increases the angle between the shoulder and the head and produces stretching or tearing of the nerve roots C_5 and C_6. This results in loss of abduction of the arm at the shoulder (deltoid, supraspinatus) and weakness of flexion at the elbow (biceps, brachialis). The biceps reflex is depressed.
2. A blow to the angle between the shoulder and the neck. This may also produce weakness of shoulder movement because of damage to the upper cord of the brachial plexus. This is associated with inability to elevate the shoulder because of damage to the accessory nerve and paralysis of the trapezius muscle.
3. A fall on the front of the shoulder. This type of injury may cause sudden extension of the shoulder with compression of the lower cord of the brachial plexus, resulting in pain and paresthesias on the medial aspect of the arm, forearm, and hand (C_8, T_1).
4. A blow to the anterior axilla. This can injure the axillary nerve producing paralysis or paresis of the deltoid muscle. A similar injury may damage the musculocutaneous nerve and result in weakness of the biceps and brachialis muscles with loss of flexion at the elbow and a sensory loss on the lateral aspect of the arm and forearm to the wrist.
5. When the force of an injury is directed upward into the axilla with the arm abducted, the entire contents of the axilla may be severely contused. The posterior cord of the brachial plexus is most vulnerable under these circumstances, resulting in loss of medial rotation of the arm (subscapularis), absence of abduction (deltoid), and paralysis of the triceps and dorsiflexors of the wrist.
6. Dislocation of the shoulder may damage the contents of the axilla, particularly the circumflex nerve, with paralysis of abduction of the arm (deltoid).
7. Gunshot wounds and knife wounds to the axilla or in the supraclavicular area often sever nerves and produce permanent damage to the brachial plexus.
8. Disability may be temporary if the plexus is contused, subjected to pressure by a hematoma, or stretched during coma or general anesthesia.
9. Traction on the brachial plexus can occur in patients with flaccid hemiplegia following a stroke. This condition can be prevented by early physical therapy and the use of a sling when the patient is walking.

Brachial Neuritis

Definition. Brachial neuritis is characterized by a sudden paralysis of muscles supplied through the brachial plexus, and is often associated with painful dysesthesia of the arm.

Etiology and Pathology. The condition occurs in known virus infections (*Herpes zoster,* Epstein Barr virus), following injection of tetanus toxoid, in putative virus infections, and as an autoimmune disorder. Pathologic changes are not well described. In *H. zoster* infections the posterior root ganglia are involved (see p. 375).

Clinical Features. There is an acute or subacute onset of pain which extends into the shoulder, upper arm, or forearm, followed by weakness, muscle wasting, and sensory loss corresponding to the involved nerves, cords, trunks, or nerve roots. Upper brachial plexus (C_5, C_6), lower brachial plexus (C_8, T_1) or whole plexus involvement can occur. The early symptoms are followed by the appearance of the typical rash within a few days in cases associated with *H. zoster*. The phrenic and recurrent laryngeal nerves are occasionally involved (6).

Diagnostic Procedures. Other causes of severe pain, such as an acute herniated cervical disk, should be excluded.

Treatment.

1. The condition is often very painful, requiring adequate doses of opioid analgesics for pain control.
2. A short course of oral corticosteroids may reduce the duration of the pain.
3. Physical therapy should be initiated once the pain is controlled to prevent joint stiffness and adhesions.

Prognosis. Most cases recover completely.

Neoplastic Involvement of the Brachial Plexus

Etiology and Pathology. Neoplastic involvement of the brachial plexus can occur due to direct extension of a bronchial carcinoma from the apex of the lung, direct extension of a breast carcinoma through the axilla, and with pressure from neoplastic lymph nodes.

Clinical Features. There is usually infiltration of or pressure on the lower trunk or medial cord of the brachial plexus. This produces severe pain in the shoulder and axilla and down the medial aspect of the upper limb with wasting of the small muscles of the hand and Horner's syndrome (Pancoast syndrome).

Treatment.

1. The condition is very painful and the patient needs adequate doses of opioid analgesics at regular intervals to reduce pain.
2. An attempt should be made to control the neoplastic process by irradiation and/or chemotherapy.

Radiation Damage to the Brachial Plexus

Radiation therapy to the axilla, as treatment for carcinoma of the breast, may be followed by fibrosis and traction on the brachial plexus. In addition, the vasa nervorum may be damaged producing an ischemic neuropathy. The symptoms are similar to neoplastic involvement of the brachial plexus, and the differential diagnosis can be very difficult.

Treatment. If metastatic recurrence can be ruled out, the patient can be treated with carbamazepine (Tegretol) 200 mg q12h, increasing slowly to 600 mg q12h. Carbamazepine can be combined with phenytoin if this drug produces additional benefit.

Surgical treatment to free the affected nerves from scar tissue may be necessary.

The Thoracic Outlet Syndrome

Definition. The thoracic outlet syndrome is due to pressure on the brachial plexus and subclavian artery.

Etiology and Pathology. The neurovascular structures of the thoracic outlet, the nerves of the brachial plexus and the subclavian artery, are compressed between the clavicle and the first rib or subjected to pressure from below by a fibrous band, cervical rib, or high first rib.

Clinical Features. Pressure on the subclavian artery produces intermittent cyanosis of the hands, which is often associated with painful paresthesias. There may be sudden, extremely painful areas at the fingertips due to emboli that originate in the subclavian artery. Numbness and tingling occur in the ulnar distribution when the medial cord of the brachial plexus is compressed. Pain in the hand may occur, particularly at night, and weakness and wasting develop in the small muscles of the hand. The patient may complain of difficulty in working with the hands elevated above the shoulders because of pain and weakness.

When pressure is exerted on the arm so that the shoulder is pulled downward and backward, the radial pulse is obliterated. A murmur may be heard over the subclavian artery on auscultation.

Diagnostic Procedures. Stenosis of the subclavian artery can be demonstrated by real time ultrasound or retrograde brachial arteriography.

Differential Diagnosis. The differential diagnosis includes wasting of the small muscles of the hand (see Table 19–2).

Treatment.

1. The shoulder should be elevated on the affected side with a full arm sling to relieve pressure on the subclavian artery and the brachial plexus.
2. Surgical excision of a fibrous band or first rib is indicated in intractable cases.

TABLE 19–2. Differential Diagnosis of Wasting of Small Muscles of the Hand

1. Anterior horn cells (acute): poliomyelitis
2. Anterior horn cells (chronic): amyotrophic lateral sclerosis, syringomyelia, peroneal muscular atrophy
3. Nerve roots: arachnoiditis, pachymeningitis, herniated cervical disk, cervical spondylosis, extramedullary tumors
4. Brachial plexus: trauma, brachial neuritis, metastasis
5. Median nerve: trauma, carpal tunnel syndrome
6. Ulnar nerve: trauma, tardy ulnar palsy, cubital tunnel syndrome
7. Muscle: polymyositis, rheumatoid arthritis, distal form of dystrophy

Prognosis. The prognosis is good. This condition has been grossly overdiagnosed in the past and is probably uncommon. Consequently, it is essential to look for other causes that can produce similar symptoms such as cervical spondylosis or the carpal tunnel syndrome.

NEUROPATHIES OF INDIVIDUAL NERVES OF THE BRACHIAL PLEXUS

Lesions of the Long Thoracic Nerve

The long thoracic nerve arises from the anterior nerve roots of C_5, C_6, and C_7 and supplies the serratus anterior muscle. The nerve may be damaged by trauma or by carrying heavy loads. It is occasionally involved by acute (probably viral) neuritis and may be severed during mastectomy. Injury to the nerve results in winging of the scapula. The scapula is medially rotated, and the acromio-clavicular joint is displaced posteriorly during pushing or lifting movements of the upper limb.

Lesions of the Suprascapular Nerve

The suprascapular nerve arises from the upper trunk of the brachial plexus (C_4, C_5, C_6) and passes through the suprascapular notch to the posterior aspect of the scapula to supply the supraspinatus and infraspinatus muscles. Entrapment of the nerve as it passes through the suprascapular notch beneath the suprascapular ligament may occur. Injury to the nerve is characterized by pain in the shoulder and wasting and weakness of the supraspinatus and infraspinatus producing weakness of abduction and external rotation of the arm. The diagnosis is confirmed by electromyography. The nerve may be infiltrated in the suprascapular notch with 2 ml of 1 percent lidocaine followed by 40 mg of methylprednisolone. If the steroid infiltration is not successful after two injections, the suprascapular ligament should be divided surgically.

Lesions of the Musculocutaneous Nerve

The musculocutaneous nerve arises from the lateral cord of the brachial plexus (C_5, C_6) and supplies the biceps, brachialis, and coracobrachialis muscles. The sensory distribution includes the anterior and posterior aspects of the lateral forearm from the elbow to the wrist. The musculocutaneous nerve may be injured in trauma to the shoulder area or following strenuous exercise such as rowing (7). Injury to the nerve is characterized by:

1. Wasting of the flexor muscles of the upper arm and weakness of elbow flexion.
2. Weakness of supination of the forearm.
3. Sensory loss of a small area on the lateral aspect of the forearm.
4. Loss of the biceps reflex.

The patient should wear a full arm sling. Physical therapy should be initiated to maintain range of motion.

Lesions of the Axillary Nerve (Circumflex Nerve)

The axillary nerve arises from the posterior cord of the brachial plexus (C_5, C_6) and supplies the deltoid and teres minor. The sensory distribution is localized to a small quadrilateral area on the upper lateral aspect of the arm.

The nerve may be injured by direct trauma to the axilla, by penetrating wounds of the axilla, and by fracture of the neck of the humerus. Isolated neuritis is not uncommon, particularly following immunizations or injection of a serum.

The patient develops weakness and wasting of the deltoid with flattening of the contour of the shoulder. There is inability to abduct the arm and weakness of external rotation. Sensory loss occurs over a small area on the upper lateral aspect of the arm.

Lesions of the Radial and Posterior Interosseus Nerves

Anatomy. The radial nerve is an extension of the posterior cord of the brachial plexus (C_5, C_6, C_7, C_8). It arises in the axilla, enters the spiral groove of the humerus, and terminates at the level of the lateral condyle of the humerus by dividing into a superficial branch and the posterior interosseus nerve. The radial nerve supplies the triceps, anconeus, brachioradialis, and extensor carpi radialis longus in the arm. The nerve also supplies forearm muscles through its posterior interosseus branch including the extensor carpi radialis brevis, supinator, extensor digitorum, extensor digiti minimi, extensor pollicis brevis, and extensor indices. The sensory distribution includes the lower dorsal forearm, dorsal and lateral aspect of the hand and thumb, and the index and lateral aspect of the middle fingers (except the distal two phalanges).

Etiology. The radial nerve is frequently injured by pressure in the axilla when falling asleep with the arm draped over the back of a chair (Saturday night paralysis), by pressure from a crutch, from penetrating injuries of the axilla, or with dislocation of the head of the humerus. A fracture of the humerus can damage the radial nerve in the spiral groove. The nerve is frequently involved in lead neuropathy.

The posterior interosseus nerve is subject to pressure as it passes through the supinator muscle just below the elbow. The nerve is subject to entrapment at the same site in the supinator muscle and may be injured in fractures of the forearm as it lies on the interosseus membrane.

Clinical Features. The clinical features depend on the location of the injury, and are as follows:

1. Radial nerve. When the radial nerve is injured, wrist drop (paralysis of extensor) associated with paralysis of extension of the elbow (triceps), weakness of elbow flexion (brachioradialis), weakness of supination (supinator), and paralysis of extension of fingers, thumb, and wrist occur.
2. Interruption of radial nerve just below the branch to the brachioradialis. Same as 1 above, except extension of the elbow remains intact.
3. Posterior interosseus nerve. Injury of the posterior interosseus nerve is characterized by progressive atrophy and weakness of the extensor muscles of the forearm. There is loss of extension of the fingers, but wrist drop does not occur because of preservation of the extensor carpi radialis. Entrapment of the nerve is associated with pain and tenderness on the lateral aspect

of the elbow and is one of the causes of "tennis elbow."
4. Sensory loss is often restricted to the dorsal surface of the thumb and the adjacent radial half of the dorsal surface of the hand.

Diagnostic Procedures. Electromyographic abnormalities of the involved muscles indicate the level of involvement of the radial nerve.

Treatment. The wrist should be splinted in extension. Physical therapy is important to prevent contractures of the fingers. Entrapment at the elbow can be treated by injection of 2 ml of 1 percent lidocaine and 40 mg methylprednisolone (Medrol) or by surgically freeing the nerve in intractable cases.

Lesions of the Ulnar Nerve

Anatomy. The ulnar nerve is the largest branch of the medial cord of the brachial plexus (C_8, T_1). The nerve passes down the medial aspect of the upper arm in close relation to the brachial artery, then inclines backward to enter the ulnar groove at the posterior aspect of the medial epicondyle of the humerus. The ulnar nerve enters the forearm between the two heads of the flexor carpi ulnaris and continues under the cover of that muscle to the wrist, where it crosses the flexor retinaculum and divides into superficial and deep branches, which terminate in the hand.

The ulnar nerve supplies the flexor carpi ulnaris and the medial half of the flexor digitorum profundus in the forearm. The deep branch of the ulnar nerve supplies the adductor pollicus, interossei, third and fourth lumbricals, palmaris brevis, abductor opponens and flexor digiti quinti, and the deep head of the flexor pollicis brevis in the hand.

The sensory distribution through the superficial branch of the ulnar nerve includes the ulnar side of the fourth finger, the whole of the fifth finger on the palmar surface, and the distal two phalanges of the fourth and fifth fingers on the dorsal surface of the hand.

Etiology. The ulnar nerve may be injured as follows:

1. At the elbow (8) by:

   a. Fracture of the medial epicondyle of the humerus.

   b. Progressive valgus deformity of the elbow following fracture of the lateral epicondyle, producing stretching of the ulnar nerve behind the medial epicondyle and paralysis occurring many years after the original injury to the elbow (tardy ulnar palsy).

    c. Pressure on the ulnar nerve in the ulnar groove behind the medial epicondyle occurring as an occupational problem (e.g., truck driving or in sedentary occupations where individuals "lean" on the elbow).

    d. Pressure on the ulnar nerve during prolonged surgical operations under general anesthesia.

    e. Entrapment of the ulnar nerve as it passes between the aponeuroses connecting the two heads of the flexor carpi ulnaris muscle just distal to the medial epicondyle (cubital tunnel syndrome).

    2. At the wrist by repeated trauma to the wrist in certain industrial occupations, by compression of the ulnar nerve in long distance bicycle (9) or motorcycle riders, or by fracture of the wrist. Rare causes of ulnar nerve involvement at the wrist include arteritis of the ulnar artery, hemorrhage secondary to hemophilia or the use of anticoagulants, and tumors of the wrist (10).

    Clinical Features. Ulnar nerve palsy is characterized by:

1. Atrophy of the hypothenar muscles.
2. Atrophy of the interossei.
3. Development of a "claw hand" with extension of the metacarpophalangeal joints and flexion of the interphalangeal joints of the second and third fingers and flexion of the metacarpophalangeal joints (paralysis third and fourth lumbosacrals) and the interphalangeal joints of the fourth and fifth digits.
4. Paralysis of the flexor carpi ulnaris, if the ulnar nerve is involved above the middle third of the forearm, producing radial deviation of the hand on flexion of the wrist and weakness of ulnar deviation of the hand.

Diagnostic Procedures.

1. Compression of the ulnar nerve at the elbow can be demonstrated by recording delayed nerve conduction in the elbow segment of the nerve.
2. Compression of the ulnar nerve at the wrist produces an increased distal latency recorded in the abductor digiti quinti and the first dorsal interosseus muscle.

    Differential Diagnosis. The differential diagnosis includes other causes of wasting of the small muscles of the hand (see Table 19–2).

Treatment.

1. Splinting is applied to prevent development of a claw hand deformity.
2. Repetitive trauma to the elbow should be prevented by transplanting the ulnar nerve from the ulnar groove to the front of the elbow.
3. Simple surgical decompression of the ulnar nerve in the cubital tunnel is required in cases of cubital tunnel syndrome.
4. Repetitive trauma to the ulnar nerve at the wrist should be avoided. Where appropriate, scar tissue should be excised and other conditions compressing the nerve should be treated.

    Prognosis. There is usually good restoration of function following adequate treatment of ulnar nerve palsy.

Lesions of the Median Nerve

    Anatomy. The median nerve arises from the lateral and medial cords of the brachial plexus. The nerve is closely related to the brachial artery as it passes down to the elbow and into the cubital fossa. It continues down the forearm connected to the deep surface of the flexor digitorum sublimis and enters the palm of the hand in close relationship to the palmaris longus tendon by passing beneath the flexor retinaculum.

    The median nerve supplies all the flexor muscles of the forearm, except the flexor carpi ulnaris and the medial half of the flexor digitorum profundus.

    The abductor pollicis brevis, flexor pollicus brevis, opponens pollicis, and the first two lumbricals are innervated by the median nerve in the hand. The sensory distribution includes the thumb, index, middle, and the radial half of the ring finger and the radial two-thirds of the palm of the hand. The "all median" hand, an anatomic variation in which most of the sensation to the hand is derived from the median nerve, is not uncommon.

    Lesions of the Anterior Interosseus Nerve. The anterior interosseus nerve arises from the median nerve in the cubital fossa, passes between the two heads of the pronator teres, and descends on the interosseus membrane to the wrist. It supplies the flexor pollicis longus, flexor digitorum profundus, and pronator quadratus.

    This nerve is occasionally involved in traumatic injury to the forearm, such as high combined fractures of the ulna and radius, or following cardiac catheterization through the antecubital fossa. Symptoms consist of pain in front of the elbow radiating down the forearm and weakness of the flexor pollicus longus and the flexor digitorum profundus in the index finger. There are no sensory changes since the anterior interosseus nerve does not carry sensory fibers from the skin. Pressure on the median nerve in the cubital fossa exaggerates the pain. This condition is frequently mistaken for "tennis elbow," particularly when there is entrapment of the anterior interosseus nerve between the two heads of pronator teres. The cubital fossa should be explored, and any constricting bands compressing the interosseus nerve should be divided.

The Carpal Tunnel Syndrome. The carpal tunnel syndrome is characterized by fluctuating numbness, paresthesia, and pain in the hand due to compression of the median nerve at the wrist. Approximately 80 percent of cases occur in women (11).

Etiology and Pathology. There are many causes of compression of the median nerve at the wrist (see Table 19–3).

The median nerve is confined in a relatively limited space as it passes beneath the transverse carpal ligament (flexor retinaculum) to enter the hand. Pressure on the nerve

TABLE 19–3. **The Carpal Tunnel Syndrome**

1. Hereditary: chronic interstitial hypertrophic neuropathy

2. Traumatic: dislocation, fracture, hematoma formation at the wrist, occupational complication of repetitive percussion to the wrist or repetitive flexion and extension of the wrist

3. Infectious: tenosynovitis, tuberculosis, sarcoidosis

4. Metabolic: amyloidosis, gout

5. Endocrine: acromegaly, diabetes mellitus, pregnancy, hypothyroidism

6. Neoplastic: lipoma, metastatic infiltration, myeloma

7. Vascular: scleroderma, systemic lupus erythematosus

8. Degenerative: rheumatoid arthritis, osteoarthritis

9. Iatrogenic: radial artery puncture, insertion of a vascular shunt for dialysis, hematoma, complicating anticoagulant therapy

leads to obstruction of the venous circulation and edema. This in turn produces ischemia, increasing pressure on the nerve, and ischemic atrophy of nerve fibers.

Clinical Features. The earliest symptoms consist of numbness and paresthesias in the sensory distribution of the median nerve in the hand (thumb, index, middle, and lateral half of the ring fingers). Later pain develops and is often ill-defined, involving the hand and wrist but also extending up into the forearm and often as high as the shoulder. The pain is worse at night, and the patient may hang the hand over the side of the bed or massage the hand in an effort to obtain relief. Complaint of weakness is a late event and is characterized by the inability to unscrew bottle caps or grip properly. Examination may show some wasting of the thenar eminence. Sensory loss is confined to the cutaneous distribution of the median nerve. This area occasionally includes the ring and little fingers if the patient has an anomaly known as the "all median hand," where the cutaneous distribution of the median nerve involves all of the fingers.

Diagnostic Procedures.

1. Electromyography. EMG may reveal fibrillations in the muscles of the thenar eminence. Lumbrical sparing can occur in some cases (12).

2. The distal latency of the median nerve is prolonged, indicating interference with conduction at the wrist.

3. Sensory nerve conduction velocities and the sensory distal latency are prolonged on stimulating the digital nerves of the index finger.

Treatment.

1. Identified causes should be removed or treated.

2. Most cases respond to injection around the median nerve in the carpal tunnel. The area around the nerve is infiltrated with 2 to 3 ml of 1 percent lidocaine followed by an injection of 40 mg methylprednisolone.

3. Cases that fail to respond to injection of corticosteroids performed on two occasions can obtain relief by surgical division of the transverse carpal ligament.

Prognosis. The prognosis is excellent if the cause is removed or treated and the affected carpal tunnel is injected wtih corticosteroids or the transverse carpal ligament is divided.

Causalgia. Causalgia is a fluctuating pain with burning and stabbing components that occurs in, and often spreads beyond, the sensory distribution of a cutaneous nerve.

Etiology and Pathology. The sympathetic system has an important but poorly defined role in the generation of the painful response. Damaged sensory axons create abnormal activity in the long tracts of the spinal cord, which is augmented by other sensory neurons along the ascending pathways to the thalamus and possibly to the cerebral cortex. Lesions close to the spinal ganglia tend to produce a more severe, painful response.

Clinical Features. The median and sciatic nerves are commonly involved, while ulnar nerve involvement is rare. The pain begins within a few days of injury or surgical repair of the wound and is incapacitating. The patient protects the affected area from unexpected contact. In severe cases the pain interferes with sleep, and the patient appears depressed and chronically ill. Many cases resolve spontaneously within two or three months.

Differential Diagnosis.

1. Entrapment conditions may mimic causalgia. Interdigital nerve entrapment following traumatic injury to the hand may mimic median nerve causalgia.
2. Neoplastic infiltration of nerves or injury from accidental injection of nerves may produce causalgia-like pain.

Diagnostic Procedures.

1. Nerve conduction velocities may be significantly slowed in the damaged nerve. Measurement of distal latencies will detect nerve entrapment syndromes.
2. A sympathetic block with local anesthesia should abolish the pain. This should always be performed before surgical sympathectomy.

Treatment. Sympathectomy produces permanent relief from pain.

Prognosis. The majority of cases resolve spontaneously or respond to sympathectomy.

THE LUMBAR PLEXUS

The lumbar plexus is a relatively simple plexus formed by the union of the anterior primary rami of L_1, L_2, L_3, and L_4 within the substance of the psoas muscle (see Figure 19–3). Lesions of the lumbar plexus are relatively rare since the nerves are well protected within the substance of the psoas mus-

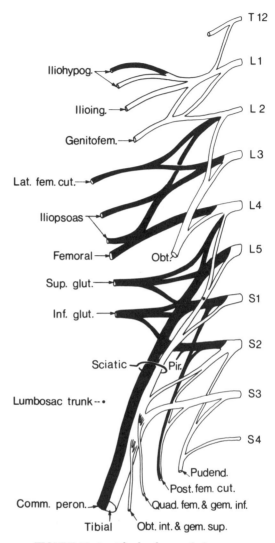

FIGURE 19–3. The lumbosacral plexus.

cle. However, the plexus may be injured by penetrating wounds or by pressure from a psoas abscess or metastatic neoplasm. Irritation of the rami gives rise to pain in the corresponding dermatome. Destruction of rami leads to muscle weakness and wasting in the appropriate myotome.

Lesions of the Iliohypogastric Nerve

The iliohypogastric nerve arises from the anterior primary ramus of L_1. The nerve may be injured as it pierces the internal oblique muscle just above the anterior iliac spine. Entrapment has also been described at this site. The patient presents with pain, paresthesias, and a small area of sensory deficit on the abdominal wall just above the pubic symphysis. Entrapment may be treated by injecting the nerve with a local anesthetic and a corticosteroid at the point where the nerve penetrates the internal oblique muscle.

Lesions of the Ilioinguinal Nerve

The ilioinguinal nerve arises from the anterior primary ramus of L_1 and traverses the abdominal wall between the transverse and internal oblique muscles to emerge through the superficial inguinal ring. The nerve supplies muscular branches to the abdominal muscles and cutaneous branches to the skin over the canal, the abdominal wall immediately above the pubic symphysis, the root of the penis, the upper part of the scrotum, and a small area on the adjacent medial aspect of the thigh.

The nerve may be compressed by enlarged lymph nodes in the inguinal area and is occasionally cut during herniorrhaphy. *Herpes zoster* involvement is not uncommon. The patient develops pain and/or sensory loss in the anatomic distribution of the nerve. Vesicles occur in the same distribution in cases of *H. zoster*. Paralysis of the internal oblique muscle may predispose to an indirect inguinal hernia.

Lesions of the Genitofemoral Nerve

The genitofemoral nerve is formed within the psoas muscle by the junction of two branches arising from the anterior primary rami of L_1 and L_2. It accompanies the iliac vessels to the level of the inguinal ligament and divides into a genital branch and a femoral branch. The genital branch enters the deep inguinal ring, traverses the inguinal canal, and supplies the cremasteric muscle, the scrotum, and the skin of the adjacent part of the thigh. The femoral branch enters the thigh beneath the middle of the inguinal ligament and supplies sensation over the femoral triangle. This nerve may also be compressed by enlarged lymph nodes or cut during herniorrhaphy. Pain and/or sensory loss occur in the anatomic distribution of the genitofemoral nerve.

Lesions of the Lateral Cutaneous Nerve of the Thigh

The lateral cutaneous nerve of the thigh arises from the anterior primary rami of L_2 and L_3, penetrates the psoas muscle, and crosses the iliacus to the anterior superior iliac spine. It enters the thigh between the two attachments of the inguinal ligament, penetrates the fascia lata, and divides into two branches about 10 mm below the inguinal ligament. The anterior branch supplies sensation to the lateral part of the anterior aspect of the thigh as far as the knee. The posterior branch supplies the upper two-thirds of the lateral aspect of the thigh and the lateral aspect of the buttock.

Etiology and Pathology. The nerve is prone to compression (entrapment) as it passes between the two attachments of the inguinal ligament or where it pierces the fascia lata. This condition seems to occur more frequently in diabetics or in individuals who suddenly gain or lose weight.

Clinical Features. Compression of the lateral cutaneous nerve of the thigh results in what is referred to as meralgia paresthetica. The patient complains of pain, paresthesias, and numbness in the distribution of the nerve.

Treatment.

1. Infiltration of the area of entrapment with 1 percent lidocaine and 40 mg of methylprednisolone (Medrol) produces permanent cure in the great majority of cases.
2. Refractory cases require incision of the fascia lata around the entrapped nerve.

Lesions of the Obturator Nerve

The obturator nerve is formed by the union of branches from L_2, L_3, and L_4. The nerve emerges from the medial border of the psoas muscle and descends through the obturator foramen to enter the thigh, where it divides into anterior and posterior branches. The obturator nerve supplies muscular branches to the adductor longus, gracilis, adductor brevis, obturator externus, adductor magnus, and (occasionally) pectineus. The cutaneous distribution is to the medial aspect of the thigh.

The obturator nerve may be injured by trauma, including fractures of the femur and gunshot wounds, and following difficult labor. A carcinoma of the cervix, rectum, or bladder may also involve the obturator nerve. The patient presents with weakness of adduction of the thigh with a tendency to abduction of the thigh when walking. Sensory loss occurs in the anatomic distribution of the nerve.

Lesions of the Femoral Nerve

The femoral nerve arises within the substance of the psoas muscle from the anterior primary rami of L_2, L_3, and L_4. It passes downward and beneath the inguinal ligament to enter the thigh lateral to the femoral artery where it divides into a number of branches. One of these branches, the saphenous nerve, accompanies the femoral vessels in the femoral canal and continues down the leg on the medial aspect of the knee joint to terminate over the medial malleolus and the medial aspect of the foot.

The femoral nerve supplies muscular branches to the iliacus, pectineus, sartorius, quadriceps femoris, and adductor longus. The cutaneous branches supply the anterior thigh (intermediate and medial cutaneous nerves of thigh) and the medial aspect of the leg and foot (saphenous nerve).

Etiology and Pathology

1. Trauma: Fracture of the femur and pelvis, gunshot wounds, hematoma of the psoas muscle from injury or manipulation.
2. Infection: Psoas abscess, sarcoidosis, diphtheria, *H. zoster.*
3. Neoplasia: Compression by pelvic tumor or metastases.
4. Vascular damage: Compression by an aortic aneurysm, polyarteritis nodosa.
5. Hemorrhage: Spontaneous bleeding with hematoma formation in leukemia, hemophilia, or other bleeding diathesis.
6. Iatrogenic damage: Hematoma of the psoas muscle or femoral canal during anticoagulant therapy.

THE SACRAL PLEXUS

The sacral plexus is formed by the union of the nerve roots L_4, L_5, S_1, S_2, S_3 and S_4 anterior to the piriformis muscle, which separates it from the lateral part of the sacrum. The most important branches include the superior gluteal nerve (L_4, L_5 and S_1), the inferior gluteal nerve (L_5, S_1, and S_2), the posterior cutaneous nerve of the thigh (S_1, S_2, and S_3), the sciatic nerve (L_4, L_5, S_1, S_2, and S_3), and the pudendal nerve (S_2, S_3, and S_4).

Lesions of the Superior Gluteal Nerve

The superior gluteal nerve leaves the pelvis through the greater sciatic foramen and supplies the gluteus medius and gluteus minimus. These two muscles act as abductors and medial rotators of the thigh. The nerve may be injured by wounds of the buttocks and is occasionally involved in fractures of the pelvis and by metastatic tumors within the pelvis. Involvement produces paralysis of the gluteus medius and minimus resulting in lat-

eral rotation of the lower limb at rest and flexion of the trunk toward the affected side when walking.

Lesions of the Inferior Gluteal Nerve

The inferior gluteal nerve enters the buttocks below the piriformis muscle and supplies the gluteus maximus. This muscle is responsible for extension of the hip, and paralysis produces difficulty in rising from a sitting position and difficulty in climbing stairs. There is marked atrophy of the affected buttock.

Lesions of the Posterior Cutaneous Nerve of the Thigh

The posterior cutaneous nerve of the thigh leaves the pelvis through the sciatic foramen and passes down the buttock and thigh on the medial aspect of the sciatic nerve. The posterior cutaneous nerve of the thigh supplies sensation to the posterior aspect of the thigh as far as the popliteal fossa. The nerve is often injured in gunshot wounds and penetrating wounds of the thigh and is occasionally injured by injections of irritating material. Damage to the nerve gives rise to a sensory deficit in the back of the thigh, the lateral part of the perineum, and the lower portion of the buttock.

Lesions of the Pudendal Nerve

The pudendal nerve leaves the pelvis through the greater sciatic foramen below the piriformis muscle and passes forward into the ischiorectal fossa. The nerve is occasionally injured in fractures of the pelvis. Damage produces sensory loss in the perineum and scrotum on the side of the lesion. Bilateral lesions produce bladder disturbances with urinary incontinence and overflow.

Lesions of the Sciatic Nerve

The sciatic nerve is the main branch of the sacral plexus and leaves the pelvis through the greater sciatic foramen to enter the buttock. The nerve then passes down the posterior aspect of the thigh to the popliteal fossa, where it divides into the tibial and common peroneal nerves. Compressive lesions of the sciatic nerve produce sciatic pain, which is distributed down the posterior aspect of the thigh, often radiating into the calf and the foot. The commonest cause is herniation of a lumbar disk between L_4 and L_5, or L_5 and S_1. Other causes of sciatic nerve compression are listed in Table 19–4. The sciatic nerve may be injured by penetrating wounds of the but-

TABLE 19–4. Causes of Sciatic Nerve Lesions
(Other than Lumbar Disk Herniation)

1. Nerve Root Involvement
   a. Cauda equina: *Herpes zoster*, arachnoiditis,
      tumors of the cauda equina, subarachnoid
      hemorrhage
   b. Vertebrae and intervertebral foramina:
      compression fractures or fracture
      dislocation, spondylosis, lumbosacral
      stenosis, tuberculosis, Paget's disease,
      metastatic tumors

2. Sacral Plexus
   Trauma with fracture of the pelvis, psoas
   abscess, pelvic abscess, direct extension of
   pelvic carcinoma, retroperitoneal metastasis,
   aneurysm of iliac vessels or branches,
   pregnancy

3. Gluteal Area
   Trauma from penetrating wounds, fracture of
   the pelvis, fracture of the femur, dislocation of
   the femoral head, traumatic hematoma,
   traumatic aneurysm of the inferior gluteal
   artery

4. Thigh
   Penetrating wounds, injection of drugs into
   sciatic nerve, sciatic nerve entrapment

5. General Involvement
   Diabetes mellitus, polyarteritis nodosa

tocks, thigh, or popliteal fossa. Sciatic nerve paralysis has also been described in association with a fracture of the femur or posterior dislocation of the femoral head. Complete interruption of the sciatic nerve produces a useless lower limb with loss of ability to flex and extend the foot at the ankle, loss of flexion and extension of the toes, and loss of inversion and eversion of the foot. Movement of the lower limb produces a flail-like movement of the foot at the ankle. In addition, there is impairment of flexion at the knee due to paralysis of the biceps femoris, semitendinosus, and semimembranous, although some movement is still possible by contraction of the sartorius and gracilis muscles supplied by the femoral and obturator nerves, respectively. Extension of the knee is preserved. There is marked sensory loss below the knee with the exception of the medial aspect of the leg and ankle, which is innervated by the saphenous nerve. Wounds of the middle portion of the posterior aspect of the thigh produce loss of function confined to the common peroneal and tibial nerve with preservation of the nerve to the hamstrings. In these cases, flexion of the knee is preserved.

Lesions of the Common Peroneal Nerve

The common peroneal nerve arises in the posterior aspect of the thigh as one of the two terminal branches of the sciatic nerve. The common peroneal nerve is injured by penetrating wounds of the lower portion of the posterior aspect of thigh or popliteal fossa. It is occasionally involved in fractures of the lower portion of the femur or the head of the fibula. Symptoms consist of foot drop with a tendency to invert the foot due to unopposed action of the tibialis posterior. There are a high-steppage gait, wasting of the muscles of the anterior compartment of the leg, and a sensory loss extending over the lateral aspect of the leg and dorsum of the foot.

Lesions of the Superficial Peroneal Nerve

This nerve arises at the level of the bifurcation of the common peroneal nerve just below the neck of the fibula. The nerve passes down the leg anterior to the fibula between the peroneal and extensor digitorum longus muscles. Lesions of the superficial peroneal nerve produce paralysis of the peroneal muscles with loss of eversion of the foot and a tendency to invert the foot on dorsiflexion. There is a variable sensory loss over the lower lateral aspect of the leg and dorsum of the foot.

Lesions of the Deep Peroneal Nerve

The deep peroneal nerve arises just below the head of the fibula as one of the two terminal branches of the common peroneal nerve. The deep peroneal nerve passes onto the interosseus membrane between the tibia and fibula and then courses downward to the ankle supplying the muscles of the anterior compartment of the leg with the exception of the peroneal group. This nerve is commonly affected by pressure over the head of the fibula, often by sitting with the legs crossed for a prolonged period of time. Deep peroneal nerve paralysis produces weakness of the dorsiflexors of the foot and extensors of the toes resulting in foot drop, steppage gait, weakness of the muscles of the anterior compartment of the leg, and a sensory deficit confined to the contiguous surfaces of the first and second toes.

Lesions of the Tibial Nerve

Tibial nerve lesions are infrequent, but the nerve is occasionally injured or compressed by cysts or hematomas of the popliteal fossa. There are weakness of plantar flexion and adduction of the foot with a sensory loss involving the sole of the foot.

The Posterior Tibial Nerve (Tarsal Tunnel Syndrome). The posterior tibial nerve is subject to compression as it passes beneath the flexor retinaculum, which forms the roof of the tarsal tunnel at the ankle. The nerve usually divides into medial and lateral plantar nerves in the tarsal tunnel, and symptoms of compression depend upon the degree of involvement of these two nerves. Symptoms consist of pain and paresthesias of the sole of the foot, which are aggravated by walking or prolonged standing. There is no weakness, but there may be some wasting of the adductor hallucis. The pain may be aggravated by pressure over the posterior tibial nerve just below the medial malleolus.

Treatment consists of infiltration of the tarsal tunnel with 1 percent xylocaine followed by 40 mg of methylprednisolone (Medrol). Surgical division of the flexor retinaculum is indicated in intractable cases.

Plantar Nerves and Interdigital Nerves. The plantar nerves are occasionally involved by inflammatory conditions such as tenosynovitis. The interdigital nerves are subject to compression as they cross the heads of the metatarsal bones. The interdigital nerve to the third and fourth toes is most commonly involved with the development of a traumatic neuroma. Symptoms consist of severe episodic pain radiating to the contiguous surfaces of the third and fourth toes (Morton's metatarsalgia). The condition may improve following infiltration with local anesthesia and methylprednisolone, but excision of the traumatic neuroma is required in most cases.

HEREDITARY NEUROPATHIES

The hereditary neuropathies are rare or uncommon conditions in which the peripheral neuropathy is the predominant, although not necessarily the sole, abnormality. The neuropathy is genetically determined and is presumably due to a metabolic disorder. Some of the metabolic abnormalities have been identified; others are as yet unknown. The essential features of this group of peripheral neuropathies are outlined in Table 19–5.

Peroneal Muscular Atrophy (Charcot-Marie-Tooth)

Definition. Peroneal muscular atrophy is a genetically determined, chronic, symmetric polyneuropathy.

Etiology and Pathology. Peroneal mus-

cular atrophy is inherited as an autosomal dominant or an autosomal recessive trait. The genetically determined metabolic abnormality producing the degenerative changes in this disease has not yet been determined.

The pathologic changes are of three types. These are:

1. Demyelination of the peripheral nerve with axonal loss and some hypertrophy of the Schwann cells, producing hypertrophic neuropathic changes.
2. Neuronal loss of anterior horn cells and posterior nerve root ganglion neurons in the lumbar and sacral segments (hereditary motor and sensory neuropathy, Type II) (13).
3. Anterior horn cell involvement with secondary axonal loss and demyelination of motor fibers.

Clinical Features. The peripheral nerve demyelinating type presents in childhood with difficulty in gait, high-arched feet, and weak ankles progressing slowly to foot drop. Marked loss of proprioception in the feet and ankles occurs in some cases. Weakness and wasting of the small muscles of the hand are seen at an early stage. The peripheral nerves are palpably enlarged in about one-third of the cases.

The hereditary, motor and sensory type begins in the second decade with foot deformity and difficulty walking. The progression is slow with muscle weakness and wasting confined to the feet and sometimes involving the leg muscles. The involvement may be asymmetric. Sensory loss involves all four modalities and is confined to the feet and lower legs. Tendon reflexes are absent in the lower limbs but normal in the arms. The anterior horn cell type presents with distal and symmetric muscle weakness and wasting beginning in the lower limbs and later involvement of the hands and forearms. Sensory loss is minimal or absent, and the nerves are not palpably enlarged.

Diagnostic Procedures.

1. Lumbar puncture. The cerebrospinal fluid protein content is normal in all types.
2. Nerve conduction velocities. Motor and sensory nerve velocities are very slow in the peripheral nerve demyelinating type but are normal or only slightly delayed in the other two types.
3. Nerve biopsy. Nerve biopsy is abnormal and should differentiate the three types of the disease.

TABLE 19–5. Hereditary Neuropathies

Name	Eponym/ Synonym	Etiology/ Inheritance	Pathology	Clinical Features	Diagnosis	Treatment	Prognosis	Remarks
Heredopathia atactica polyneuritiformis	Refsum disease	Autosomal recessive trait Failure to metabolize 3, 7, 11, 15 tetramethyl hexadecanoic acid (phytanic acid)	Loss neurons brainstem Demyelination posterior columns and cerebellar peduncles Atrophy retina Peripheral nerve hypertrophy Proliferation of Schwann cells	Night blindness Hearing loss of nerve type Peripheral neuropathy Cerebellar ataxia Ichthyosis Cardiac dysrhythmias	Retinitis pigmentosa Nerve deafness Abnormal ECG CSF protein elevated Phytanic acid in serum Slowed motor and sensory nerve conduction velocities	Diet low in phytol- and chlorophyl- containing substances	Slowly progressive unless arrested by diet	Rare condition
Alpha-lipoprotein deficiency	Tangier disease	Autosomal recessive trait Absence of high density lipoproteins in serum	Storage cholesterol esters in tissue Hepatomegaly Splenomegaly Enlarged lymph nodes	Mild peripheral neuropathy Enlarged liver, spleen, lymph nodes, tonsils	No high density lipoprotein in serum Low serum cholesterol Foam cells in bone marrow biopsy	None	Good Little disability	
Hereditary sensory neuropathy, Type 1	None	Autosomal dominant trait, etiology unknown	Progressive loss neurons in posterior root ganglia	Age 20 yr + Lightning pains Hyperkeratosis feet Painless ulcers Severe distal sensory loss and muscle wasting		Special shoes to reduce trauma Control infection, ulcers	High risk for damage to bone and deformity of feet, upper extremities occasionally involved later	Rare condition

Hereditary sensory neuropathy, Type 2	None	Autosomal recessive trait		Slowly progressive symmetric sensory loss affecting extremities beginning at second decade		None		See peroneal muscular atrophy
Hereditary motor and sensory neuropathy	None	Sex linked recessive	Axonal loss Onion bulb formation Demyelination	Severe symmetric weakness, muscle wasting begins distally, symmetric sensory loss pes cavus	Family pedigree Nerve biopsy	None	Severe disability	Rare Heterozygotes affected to lesser degree
Familial amyloid neuropathy, Type I	Portuguese type	Autosomal dominant trait	Amyloid deposits in peripheral nerves with axonal degeneration	Peripheral neuropathy of lower limbs with gastrointestinal symptoms, orthostatic hypotension, scleroderma, loss of libido and sphincter disturbance	Macroglossia Cardiopathy Charcot joints Nephropathy	None	Death Generalized amyloidosis 10 years	Rare condition
Familial amyloid neuropathy, Type II	Indiana type	Autosomal dominant trait		Carpal tunnel syndrome, followed by signs of peripheral neuropathy	Cardiomegaly Vitrous opacities Elevated CSF protein Rectal biopsy confirms diagnosis	None	Death Generalized amyloidosis 20 years +	Rare condition

373

TABLE 19–5. *Continued* **Hereditary Neuropathies**

Name	Eponym/ Synonym	Etiology/ Inheritance	Pathology	Clinical Features	Diagnosis	Treatment	Prognosis	Remarks
Familial amyloid neuropathy Type III	Iowa type	Autosomal dominant trait	Axonal loss Onion bulb formation Demyelination	Severe upper and lower limb sensorimotor neuropathy Severe renal involvement	Amyloid deposits kidneys Nerve biopsy	None	Death from uremia	Rare condition
Familial amyloid Type IV	Meretoga type	Autosomal dominant trait	Axonal loss Onion bulb formation Demyelination	Peripheral neuropathy with lattice dystrophy of cornea and cranial nerve palsies	Family pedigree Nerve biopsy	None		Rare condition
Acute intermittent porphyria								

Treatment. There is no specific treatment for peroneal muscular atrophy. Foot drop and hand deformities can be helped by splinting and orthopedic procedures.

Chronic Interstitial Hypertrophic Neuropathy (Déjérine-Sottas)

Definition. Chronic interstitial hypertrophic neuropathy is a slowly progressive, familial, peripheral neuropathy characterized by hypertrophy of peripheral nerves.

Etiology and Pathology. The condition is inherited as an autosomal recessive trait. An abnormality of pyruvate metabolism with poor conversion of lactate to pyruvate has been described. This may be due to an enzymatic abnormality with failure to utilize thiamine.

There is marked hypertrophy of peripheral nerves with proliferation of Schwann cells producing concentric rings around the axon, each ring separated by mucus-like material (onion bulb formation). The axons degenerate slowly over a period of many years.

Clinical Features. Symptoms first occur in childhood with intermittent attacks of ataxia, numbness, and weakness of the extremities accompanied by pain in the limbs. There is a gradual deterioration, leading to inability to walk by the age of 30 to 40 years. Exacerbations seem to be precipitated by infection, pregnancy, poor nutrition, and high alcohol intake. Established cases show weakness and wasting of the distal muscles in the upper and lower limbs with ataxia of gait followed by development of a wide based steppage gait due to bilateral foot drop. There is a distal sensory loss in all four extremities and absence of stretch reflexes. The peripheral nerves in the limbs and often in the neck are enlarged, nodular, and tender.

Diagnostic Procedures.

1. Nerve conduction velocities (NCV). Motor and sensory NCV are markedly slowed. Electromyography shows evidence of denervation of muscle.
2. Nerve biopsy. Nerve biopsy shows the typical "onion bulb" changes of chronic interstitial hypertrophic neuropathy.
3. Lumbar puncture. The cerebrospinal fluid protein level is elevated.

Treatment.

1. Some patients appear to benefit from daily injections of 100 mg thiamine IM during exacerbations of the disease.
2. A short course of corticosteroids, methylprednisolone (Medrol) 80 mg daily for one week followed by 80 mg on alternate days for three more weeks may help.

Prognosis. Chronic interstitial hypertrophic neuropathy is a slowly progressive disease that may lead to marked disability. Exacerbations may be reduced by a good diet and by avoiding infections and excessive use of alcohol.

Other Hereditary Neuropathies

The main features of a number of other hereditary neuropathies are described in Table 19–5.

THE INFLAMMATORY NEUROPATHIES

The inflammatory neuropathies are a group of peripheral neuropathies of various etiologies characterized by an inflammatory response involving the peripheral nerve. The most important inflammatory neuropathies are *H. zoster*, diphtheritic, infectious mononucleosis, human immunodeficiency virus (HIV) infection (14), postinfectious polyneuritis (Guillain-Barré syndrome, acute inflammatory polyradiculoneuropathy), and chronic inflammatory polyradiculoneuropathy.

Herpes Zoster (Shingles)

Definition. *Herpes zoster* is an acute, painful mononeuropathy associated with a vesicular eruption in the distribution of the affected nerve.

Etiology and Pathology. The infective agent is the varicella virus. *Herpes zoster* may represent an infection by recently acquired varicella virus in an individual who has a declining immunity to the virus or a recrudescence of activity by latent varicella virus in the presence of declining immunity.

The viral activity is predominantly located in the dorsal root ganglia or sensory ganglia of the cranial nerves. The ganglia are swollen and show areas of necrosis. There is a marked inflammatory response with necrosis of neurons. The ventral (motor) nerve root is occasionally involved, and inflammatory changes may spread to the spinal cord or brain stem. The vesicles in the skin contain *Herpes* virus, and the surrounding area shows a polymorphonuclear infiltration due to secondary bacterial infection.

Clinical Features. *Herpes zoster* is a disease of adults and rarely affects children. There is an increased incidence in patients with altered immunity due to such conditions as malignancy, Hodgkin's disease, and leukemia. The condition presents with fever followed by pain in the distribution of the involved nerve. Vesicles appear in the affected area within 24 hours and are soon involved by secondary bacterial infection, which results in severe regional lymphodermatitis. The pain usually begins to subside after a few days but may persist for months (postherpetic neuralgia). The pustules heal, and crusts separate after about three weeks, leaving pigmented scars.

Herpes zoster is not confined to sensory symptoms. Motor weakness from ventral root involvement occurs in 5 to 10 percent of cases.

Complications.

1. Involvement of the ophthalmic division of the fifth cranial nerve is frequently associated with corneal ulceration *(Herpes zoster ophthalmicus)* and may result in severe damage to the cornea. This condition is occasionally followed by retinal and intracranial arteritis, producing additional visual loss and contralateral hemiparesis.
2. *Herpes zoster* involvement of the geniculate ganglion produces a painful vesicular rash involving the pinna, external auditory meatus, and eardrum followed by ipsilateral facial paralysis (Ramsay-Hunt syndrome).
3. Sacral nerve involvement may be associated with loss of bladder and anal sphincter control.
4. *Herpes zoster* encephalitis is probably commoner than has been thought in the past (15). Careful neurological examination may reveal subtle signs of intention tremor or gait ataxia which should be regarded as encephalitic in origin. However, it is not unusual to find a cerebrospinal fluid pleocytosis in the early stages of *H. zoster* mononeuropathy.
5. Retrograde spread of the virus from the posterior root ganglion into the spinal cord occasionally produces an acute transverse myelitis. This may result in permanent cord damage with major neurologic deficits.

Differential Diagnosis. It is extremely difficult to diagnose *H. zoster* before the characteristic vesicles appear. The pain may mimic many acutely painful conditions such as pleurisy, pericarditis, perforated peptic ulcer, appendicitis, renal colic, and herniated lumbar disk.

Diagnostic Procedures.

1. The white blood count is often elevated in the presence of secondary infection.
2. Lumbar puncture will reveal a lymphocytic pleocytosis in many cases. If there is clinical evidence of central nerve system involvement, the cerebrospinal fluid abnormality is indicative of encephalitis.

Treatment

1. Herpes zoster is a systemic illness and patients should be treated with bed rest.
2. Adequate analgesia is mandatory. Narcotics are often required in the early stages.
3. A course of corticosteroids such as prednisone 80 mg daily for 7 days will produce rapid relief from pain in many cases.
4. Local applications of calamine lotion or colloidon, or application of a cream containing acyclovir, and avoidance of contact with clothing or bed clothes help to relieve pain and itching.
5. *Herpes zoster* encephalitis should be treated with acyclovir (page 285).
6. The rare occurrence of transverse myelitis may respond to intravenous acyclovir.
7. Postherpetic neuralgia is a most debilitating condition, particularly in elderly patients. The condition may persist for many months but the patient should be informed that it will eventually subside. There is no single effective remedy for this condition, but some patients obtain relief with carbamazepine (Tegretol) or phenytoin (Dilantin). These drugs may be used in combination if necessary. Alternatives include amitriptyline (Elavil) beginning 50 mg h.s. and increasing to 50 mg three times a day or to tolerance, a combination of amitriptyline and fluphenazine 1 mg q8h, or a combination of propoxyphene 65 to 100 mg q6h and fluphenazine 1 mg q8h.

Diphtheria

Approximately 10 percent of patients develop signs of neuropathy during diphtheria epidemics. Nerve involvement is the result of the neurotropic properties of the diphtheria toxin.

There are three types of involvement. These include:

1. Early involvement with paralysis of the palate and failure of accommodation occurring within a few days of the onset of the illness.
2. Delayed mononeuropathy or polymono-

neuropathy in which palatal involvement is followed by paralysis of muscles in any part of the body. (This may occur in a series with recovery of function in one area followed by paralysis of a different muscle group.)

3. A condition resembling postinfectious polyneuritis (see below).

Infectious Mononucleosis

This condition is occasionally complicated by mononeuropathy or by peripheral neuropathy resembling postinfectious polyneuritis (see below).

Postinfectious Polyneuritis (Guillain-Barré Syndrome)

Definition. The Guillain-Barré syndrome is an acute, symmetric, ascending polyneuropathy frequently occurring one to three weeks and occasionally up to eight weeks after an acute infection.

Etiology and Pathology. The Guillain-Barré syndrome often follows a non-specific respiratory or gastrointestinal illness but has also been described after a number of specific infections such as cytomegalovirus, Epstein-Barr virus, enterovirus, campylobacter jejuni or mycoplasma, and after immunization (16–18). The disease is believed to be due to lymphocytic sensitization to peripheral nerve antigen. There is diffuse, patchy, segmental demyelination of peripheral nerves. Light microscopy reveals an intense lymphocytic, inflammatory infiltrate at the sites of demyelination.

Clinical Features. There is a worldwide incidence of 1.6 to 1.9 cases per 100,000 population per year. More than 50 percent of cases have a clear history of an upper respiratory infection one to three weeks prior to the onset of neuropathy. Other antecedent conditions include immunizations, pneumonia, influenza, tonsillitis, gastroenteritis, exanthema of childhood, and organophosphate poisoning.

The syndrome often begins with myalgia or paresthesias of the lower limbs followed by weakness. About one-third of those affected develop lower limb weakness, which ascends to involve pelvic girdle, abdominal, thoracic, and upper limb muscles. Examination shows symmetric weakness of muscles with loss of tone and flaccidity. Stretch reflexes are absent. The seventh cranial nerve is frequently involved, and bilateral facial weakess is common. Involvement of the other cranial nerves may result in ptosis or facial myokymia. Dysarthria, dysphagia, and diplopia develop in severe cases. The degree of sensory involvement varies, but this is disproportionately less than the muscle involvement.

The paralysis may progress for about 10 days and then remain relatively unchanged for about two weeks. The recovery phase is much slower and may take from six months to two years for completion.

Complications. Respiratory failure occurs in about 33 percent of cases. Retention of urine occurs in the early stages in some patients due to autonomic nerve involvement. Other autonomic disturbances include orthostatic hypotension and, rarely, a persistent hypertension. Papilledema is a rare complication and the cause is unknown. Relapses and recurrences are unusual but have been reported after subsequent infections or immunizations. Death can occur from respiratory insufficiency or intercurrent infection.

Variants. Guillain-Barré syndrome may occasionally present with a descending paralysis of pharyngeal cervical brachial muscles rather than the typical ascending paralysis. Other variants include paraparesis with normal strength and reflexes in the upper limbs and an initial severe midline back pain. The Miller-Fisher syndrome of ophthalmoplegia, bilateral facial weakness, severe ataxia, absence of tendon reflexes but only mild limb weakness is believed to be another variant of Guillain-Barré syndrome although optic neuropathy may also occur in this condition (19).

Diagnostic Procedures.

1. The CSF protein content begins to rise after the first week of the illness and continues to rise for several weeks. The severity of the illness is not related to the elevation of protein in the CSF. The cell count is usually below 10 mononuclear leukocytes per cubic mm, although counts as high as 50 mononuclears per cubic mm are occasionally seen.

2. Nerve conduction velocities are less than 60 percent of normal in most cases. Evoked muscle action potentials are often absent or prolonged in latency with a marked reduction in amplitude within 48 hours of onset of weakness while sensory nerve studies are normal, indicating abnormalities in distal motor axons at an early stage. At the same time, F-wave responses are slowed, indicating proximal involvement of nerve roots (20).

About 10 percent of patients show incomplete recovery. A prolonged period (more than three weeks) from maximum weakness to initial improvement, associated with reduced motor nerve conduction velocities and with denervation by electromyography are indicative of a possible incomplete recovery.

3. Daily respiratory function tests (vital capacity) will detect impending respiratory insufficiency.

Differential Diagnosis.

1. *Poliomyelitis.* Poliomyelitis is characterized by initial fever and severe myalgia followed by asymmetric flaccid paralysis of muscles. There is an initial CSF pleocytosis, and there is no sensory involvement.

2. *Botulism.* Botulism often occurs in a group situation with ingestion of home-canned food. Symptoms begin with diplopia.

3. *Heavy metal neuropathy.* The onset of weakness is much slower. There is a history of exposure to heavy metals in industry in most cases.

4. *Periodic paralysis.* Periodic paralysis is characterized by sudden onset of generalized paralysis without respiratory involvement and hypo- or hyperkalemia.

5. *Acute polymyositis.* There is an acute onset of proximal symmetric weakness. A rash is often present in dermatomyositis. The sedimentation rate and creatine phosphokinase levels are elevated.

6. *Tick paralysis.* Tick paralysis is a flaccid paralysis without respiratory involvement that usually occurs in childhood. Examination will reveal a tick attached to the skin. There is rapid recovery after removing the tick.

7. *Acute intermittent porphyria.* Acute respiratory paralysis can occur suddenly in this condition. The urine shows the presence of porphobilinogen, and serum delta aminolevulinic acid is elevated.

8. *Myasthenia gravis.* Myasthenia gravis does not present as an ascending paralysis.

9. *Human immunodeficiency virus.* An acute inflammatory demyelinating polyneuropathy may be associated with HIV zero conversion, AIDS related complex, or AIDS (21).

Treatment.

1. Good nursing care is essential to prevent the development of pressure sores.

2. Retention of urine may occur in the early stages and require bladder catheterization.

3. Respiratory insufficiency should be treated with endotracheal intubation and the use of a respirator.

4. Physical therapy should be given from the initial stages of the disease beginning with passive movements to prevent adhesions around the joints. The program should be increased with more active participation by the patient as soon as there are signs of recovery.

5. Most studies have indicated that corticosteroids are ineffective in the treatment of Guillain Barré Syndrome.

6. Plasmaphoresis has been of benefit in several reported studies, but others report no significant improvement indicating the need for caution in the use of this mode of treatment (22).

Prognosis. Most patients with postinfectious polyneuritis recover, but the process of recovery may take years. Respiratory insufficiency poses a life-threatening situation, which should be minimized with the use of a modern, efficient respirator. A few cases show partial recovery and then develop prominent signs of peripheral neuropathy. Relapse after recovery is unusual but has been reported. Such cases may represent a distinct group with recurrent polyneuritis, and some of these are reported to show a prompt response to corticosteroid therapy.

Chronic Inflammatory Polyradiculoneuropathy

Definition. Chronic inflammatory polyradiculoneuropathy is a chronic polyneuropathy in which there is steady progression, intermittent progression, or a relapsing and remitting course over a period of years.

This condition in the past has been described as idiopathic neuritis, nonfamilial hypertrophic neuritis, nonfamilial Déjèrine-Sottas disease, relapsing neuritis, and recurrent neuritis.

Etiology and Pathology. There is often a history of a preceding infectious process or an injection of a foreign protein, but some cases of chronic inflammatory polyradiculoneuropathy develop in an apparently well individual without a history of prior infection, immunization, or vaccination. Nevertheless, the condition is believed to be an autoimmune response directed against the Schwann cells of the peripheral nerve.

The affected nerves show mononuclear cell infiltration with segmental demyelination and a reactive hyperplasia of Schwann cells producing hypertrophic neuropathy. The involvement is often predominantly proximal involving both sensory and motor nerve roots.

Brain stem involvement has been described in some cases with degeneration of neurons, microglial proliferation, and perivascular lymphocytic infiltration (23).

Clinical Features. Symptoms of sensory involvement and motor weakness occur with equal frequency. Sensory symptoms usually consist of numbness and paresthesias in the hands and feet. Pain is less frequent but occurs in some cases. Motor weakness may be proximal (24) (difficulty in arising from a chair, lifting arms above the head) or distal (poor grip, tripping due to foot drop). Intercostal, diaphragmatic, and bulbar weakness occur in less than 20 percent of cases. The course may be progressive, intermittent, or relapsing and remitting.

Weakness and wasting occur in both proximal and distal muscles and are of equal extent. Sensory loss involving touch, pinprick, vibration, and position sense occurs in symmetric fashion in upper and lower limbs. Signs of brain stem involvement are not uncommon and include Argyll-Robertson pupils, Horner's syndrome, diplopia, nystagmus, depressed corneal reflexes, sensory loss over the face, bilateral facial weakness, dysarthria and dysphagia, weakness of the tongue, and intention tremor in the upper limbs. Papilledema occurs in a small number of cases. Hyporeflexia or areflexia are observed in most patients, but hyperreflexia can occur when brain stem involvement is extensive. The peripheral nerves are palpably enlarged when the demyelinating process extends more peripherally and involves the ulnar or median nerve at the elbow.

The disease may progress to severe disability with confinement to a wheelchair or bed in a minority of cases. Most patients remain ambulatory but handicapped by the disease. Death may occur from intercurrent infection after several years in severely debilitated patients.

Diagnostic Procedures.

1. The white cell count and erythrocyte sedimentation rate are normal, but there may be an elevation of gamma globulin on serum protein electrophoresis.
2. Lumbar punctures. The cerebrospinal fluid has a normal cell content or a mild pleocytosis of less than 75 cells per dl. The cell content is predominantly lymphocytic, but some polymorphonuclear cells are present on occasion. The protein content is usually elevated and may be in excess of 500 mg/dl. The gamma globulin content is elevated in some cases.
3. Nerve conduction velocities of both motor and sensory nerve fibers are usually but not invariably slowed.
4. Nerve biopsy. Sural nerve biopsy shows evidence of demyelination with mononuclear cell infiltration of the epineurium and endoneurium, edema of the endoneurium, and Schwann cell proliferation (onion bulb formation). Teased fibers show evidence of demyelination and remyelination.
5. MR scans have demonstrated evidence of demyelination in the brain in some cases of chronic inflammatory polyradiculoneuropathy suggesting that a combined syndrome of central and peripheral demyelination may exist.

Treatment. Corticosteroid therapy (25) and immunosuppressive therapy with azothiopine or cyclophosphamide have been reported to produce improvement in some cases. Corticosteroids can be given orally in doses of 80 mg methylprednisolone (Medrol) every day, converting the patient to 128 mg every second day to reduce the development of side effects once significant clinical improvement has occurred, then decreasing the dose gradually over a three- to six-month period. Several courses can be given to those patients who appear to respond to corticosteroids.

Infusion of fresh frozen plasma or gamma globulin has produced improvement in some refractory cases (26). Plasmapheresis has also been effective.

Prognosis. Spontaneous recovery has been observed in a small number of cases. Some patients respond to corticosteroids, while others show initial improvement, then apparently fail to respond to further treatment. A number of patients fail to respond to corticosteroids and die from respiratory failure or intercurrent infection several years after the onset of the disease.

PERIPHERAL NEUROPATHIES IN VASCULAR DISEASE

Although mild peripheral neuropathy is not unusual in patients with atherosclerotic cerebrovascular disease due to atherosclerosis, such cases are nearly always due to diabetic neuropathy. Peripheral neuropathy of vascular origin is relatively rare and is related almost exclusively to arteritis (27). The term "arteritis" includes polyarteritis nodosa, giant cell arteritis (28) and systemic lupus erythematosus. Neuropathy may present as a mononeuropathy or a diffuse symmetric peripheral neuropathy. Systemic lupus erythematosus may be accompanied by a diffuse arteritis, but many of the changes in lupus erythematosus, including the peripheral neuropathy, may be due to an autoimmune reaction.

TOXIC NEUROPATHIES

Toxins are usually ingested or inhaled and may cause damage to peripheral nerves by attacking neurons, resulting in nerve cell death; by damaging Schwann cells, producing demyelination; or by directly damaging axons, producing distal axonal degeneration. Axonal degeneration is by far the commonest reaction and is usually insidious in onset following steady exposure to toxic substances. The lower limbs are affected before the upper limbs, and there is gradual development of sensory loss with a stocking type of hypalgesia. This is associated with loss of the ankle jerk. Muscle wasting and weakness develop later. Recovery is slow once toxic exposure ceases, since axonal regeneration is a slow process, and many patients show residual disabilities for months or years. Examination shows slowing of motor nerve conduction, and the CSF protein is normal. Many substances produce toxic neuropathies. The commonest encountered in clinical practice include chloramphenicol, disulfiram, isoniazid, nitrofurantoin, and phenytoin. Industrial or environmental toxins include acrylimide monomer, arsenic, carbon disulfide, n-hexane, methyl n-butyl ketone, organophosphates, triorthocresyl phosphate, polychlorinated biphenyls (PCB), and thallium.

Toxic neuropathies with segmental demyelination or following neuronal death are rare. Demyelinating peripheral neuropathy has been described in buckthorn poisoning, and the neuropathy associated with mercury poisoning is believed to follow destruction of nerve cells in the dorsal root ganglia.

METABOLIC NEUROPATHIES

A considerable number of metabolic abnormalities are associated with peripheral neuropathy. In many cases the peripheral neuropathy is one of a number of neurologic abnormalities related to the metabolic defect. The majority of the metabolic conditions and their neurologic complications are discussed elsewhere in this book.

PARANEOPLASTIC NEUROPATHIES

Peripheral neuropathies are not unusual complications in patients suffering from carcinoma. The neuropathy may be directly related to the presence of the carcinoma, may be a nonmetastatic phenomenon, or may be a complication of chemotherapeutic treatment. A number of other conditions—for example, multiple myeloma, macroglobulinemia, cryoglobulinemia—may be accompanied by a progressive and often severe peripheral neuropathy.

Carcinomatous Peripheral Neuropathy

Two forms of peripheral neuropathy have been described in association with neoplasia and must be considered to be paraneoplastic effects of cancer in that there is no direct involvement of the peripheral nerve by the neoplastic process. The commonest form of carcinomatous peripheral neuropathy is a symmetric sensorimotor neuropathy that affects the extremities, producing distal weakness and symmetric sensory loss. The condition is slowly progressive. There is a rarer sensory motor neuropathy occasionally encountered in association with malignancy. This condition begins with sensory loss involving the extremities and progresses in a chronic fashion with involvement of all four limbs. The condition sometimes becomes arrested about three months after onset and does not show further progression after that time.

Critical Illness Polyneuropathy

Definition. A diffuse polyneuropathy occurring in critically ill patients with a delay in weaning the patient from ventilatory support once the critical illness is under control (29).

Etiology and Pathology. The etiology is obscure. No toxic, metabolic, vascular or nutritional factors have been identified.

Clinical Features. The salient feature is failure to withdraw mechanical respiratory aid when the systemic illness has improved. Improvement occurs first in the upper limb and proximal limb, followed by the respiratory muscles and later by the distal lower limb musculature.

Diagnostic Procedures. The diagnosis can be established by electromyography which shows widespread denervation and by nerve conduction studies.

Treatment. The patient should receive all care necessary for a respirator dependent patient until recovery returns.

NUTRITIONAL NEUROPATHIES

Nutritional peripheral neuropathies occur in patients who are subjected to chronic deprivation of essential food constituents. These neuropathies have occurred traditionally during famine or during imprisonment and starvation. Under modern conditions they are more likely to be seen in individuals who follow strict, unbalanced diets, in food faddists, in cases of deliberate starvation to lose weight, in persons who have had alimentary bypass operations, and in alcoholics who obtain the bulk of food calories from alcohol.

Beriberi (Thiamine) Neuropathy

Definition. Beriberi neuropathy is a symmetric, distal motor and sensory neuropathy due to chronic vitamin B_1 deficiency.

Etiology and Pathology. Vitamin B_1 is essential for the metabolism of carbohydrate, and both the central and peripheral nervous systems are almost entirely dependent on carbohydrate for energy requirements. Vitamin B_1 deficiency may be due to:

1. Inadequate diet: famine, starvation, food fads, anorexia nervosa, bulimia.
2. Poor diet: alcoholism, vegetarians.
3. Poor absorption: celiac disease, adult sprue, chronic diarrhea.
4. Destruction of thiamine: presence of thiaminosis in fish and certain vegetables, thiaminolytic bacilli in the gastrointestinal tract; prevention of phosphorylation by thiamine antimetabolites such as pyrithiamine.

Vitamin B_1 deficiency results in failure of formation of thiamine pyrophosphate, which acts as a cocarboxylase in the conversion of pyruvate to active acetate. Thiamine pyrophosphate also acts in the conversion of alpha ketoglutarate to succinyl-CoA. Thiamine deficiency interferes with the citric acid cycle, and energy release is severely restricted. There is a failure of breakdown of glycose-y-phosphate into the pentose-phosphate shunt due to a lack of thiamine pyrophosphate, which acts as a coenzyme of transketolase in this cycle.

There is a concomitant loss of myelin sheaths and axonal degeneration with Schwann cell proliferation beginning distally and extending proximally.

Clinical Features. Patients complain of distal paresthesias, dysesthesias (burning feet), and muscle cramps beginning two to six months after the beginning of consistent vitamin B_1 deficiency. These symptoms may be accompanied by lethargy, anorexia, nausea, and vomiting. Early symptoms are followed by development of foot drop and steppage gait leading to paraplegia. There is an ascending glove-and-stocking sensory loss. The patient is severely ataxic and reflexes are absent. Weakness may extend to proximal muscles; muscle atrophy is late. Cranial nerve involvement usually involves the vagus nerve producing tachycardia, hoarseness, and dysphagia, and the facial nerve with bilateral facial weakness.

Acute beriberi is rare and presents with acute vomiting and tachycardia followed by rapidly ascending paralysis involving the lower, then the upper limbs. There is a high risk of death from acute heart failure. "Wet" beriberi is a subacute condition with pericardial, pleural, and peritoneal effusions, severe peripheral edema, and peripheral neuropathy.

Diagnostic Procedures.

1. Red blood cell transketolase activity is decreased.
2. Serum pyruvate and lactate levels are elevated.
3. Nerve conduction velocity measurements are slowed. An EMG shows evidence of denervation.

Treatment. Thiamine 100 mg q12h should be given by intramuscular injection. The prognosis is excellent.

Neuralgia in Pregnancy

Pregnancy may be associated with a number of neuralgias, which tend to occur in the later months of pregnancy and resolve after delivery. These neuralgias include meralgia paresthetica, carpal tunnel syndrome, sciatic neuralgia, and intercostal neuralgia.

Intercostal neuralgia may produce severe pain in the chest or upper abdomen, which may lead to an erroneous diagnosis of heart disease or acute intra-abdominal disease. The pain is usually exacerbated by movements that stretch the affected nerves, and there may be an area of sensory change in the affected dermatome. Relief may be obtained by temporary nerve block following an injection of a local anesthetic. The prognosis is excellent. The neuralgias of pregnancy resolve in the immediate postpartum period.

REFERENCES

1. Claus, D.; Eggers, R.; et al. Ethanol and polyneuropathy. Acta. Neurol. Scand. 72:312–316; 1985.
2. Galetta, S. L.; Smith, J. L. Chronic isolated sixth nerve palsy. Arch. Neurol. 46:79–82; 1989.
3. Zakrzewska, J. M.; Patsalos, P. N. Oxycarbazepine: A new drug in the management of intractable trigeminal neuralgia. J. Neurol. Neurosurg. Psychiatry 52:472–476; 1989.
4. Uri, N.; Schuchman, G. Vestibular abnormalities in patients with Bell's palsy. J. Laryngol. Otol. 100:1125–1128; 1986.
5. Perkin, G. D.; Illingworth, R. D. An association of hemifacial spasm and facial pain. J. Neurol. Neurosurg. Psychiatry 52:663–665; 1989.
6. Sanders, E. A. C. M.; Van den Neste, V. M. H.; et al. Brachial plexus neuritis and recurrent laryngeal nerve palsy. J. Neurol. 235:323–325; 1988.
7. Mastaglia, E. L. Musculocutaneous neuropathy after strenuous physical activity. Med. J. Aust. 145:153–154; 1986.
8. Stewart, J. D. The variable clinical manifestations of ulnar neuropathies at the elbow. J. Neurol. Neurosurg. Psychiatry 50:252–258; 1987.
9. Hankey, G. J.; Gubbay, S. S. Compression neuropathy of the deep palmar branch of the ulnar nerve in cyclists. J. Neurol. Neurosurg. Psychiatry 51:1588–1590; 1988.
10. Ratecas, J. C.; Daube, J. R.; et al. Deep branch ulnar neuropathy due to giant cell tumor: Report of a case. Neurology 38:327–329; 1988.
11. Stevens, J. C.; Sim, S.; et al. Carpal tunnel syndrome in Rochester, Minnesota 1961–1980. Neurology 38:134–138; 1988.
12. Logigian, E. L.; Busis, N.A.; et al. Lumbrical sparing in carpal tunnel syndrome: Anatomic, physiologic and diagnostic complications. Neurology 37:1499–1505; 1987.
13. Berciano, J.; Combarros, O.; et al. Hereditary motor and sensory neuropathy Type II. Clinicopathological study of a family. Brain 109:897–914; 1986.
14. So, Y. T.; Holtzman, D. M.; et al. Peripheral neuropathy associated with acquired immunodeficiency syndrome. Arch. Neurol. 45:945–948; 1988.
15. Mayo, D. R.; Booss, J. Varicella-Zoster- Associated neurologic disease without skin lesions. Arch. Neurol. 46:313–315; 1984.
16. Sutherland, J. M. Guillain Barre Syndrome. Med. J. Australia 146:122–123; 1987.
17. De Bont, B.; Matthews, N.; et al. Guillain Barre syndrome associated with campylobacter enteritis in a child. J. Pediatr. 109:660–662; 1986.
18. Newton, N.; Janati, A. Guillain Barre syndrome after vaccination with purified tetanus toxoid. South. Med. J. 80:1053–1054; 1987.
19. Toshnuval, P. Demyelinating optic neuropathy with Miller-Fisher syndrome. The case for overlap syndromes with central and peripheral demyelination. J. Neurol. 234:353–358; 1987.
20. Kaier, U.; Chopra, J. S.; et al. Guillain Barre Syndrome. A clinical, electrophysiological and biochemical study. Acta. Neurol. Scand. 73:394–402; 1986.
21. Parry, G. J. Peripheral neuropathies associated with human immunodeficiency virus infection. Ann. Neurol. 23(suppl):549–553; 1988.
22. Mendell, J. R.; Kissell, J. T.; et al. Plasma exchange and prednisone in Guillain Barre syndrome. Neurology 35:1551–1555; 1985.
23. Mendell, J. R.; Kolkin, S.; et al. Evidence for central nervous system demyelination in chronic inflammatory demyelinating polyradiculoneuropathy. Neurology 37:1291–1294; 1987.
24. Bradley, W. G.; Bennett, R. K.; et al. Proximal chronic inflammatory polyneuropathy with multifocal conduction blocks. Ann. Neurol. 45:451–455; 1988.
25. Sladky, J. T.; Brown, M. J.; et al. Chronic inflammatory demyelinating polyneuropathy of infancy. A corticosteroid responsive disorder. Ann. Neurol. 20:76–81; 1986.
26. Albala, M.; McNamara, M. E.; et al. Improvement in neurologic function in chronic inflammatory demyelinating polyradiculoneuropathy following intravenous gamma globulin infusion. Arch. Neurol. 44:248–249; 1987.
27. Said, G.; Lacroix-Ciaudo, C.; et al. The peripheral neuropathies of necrotizing arteritis: A clinicopathological study. Ann. Neurol. 23:461–465; 1988.
28. Golbus, J.; McCune, W. J. Giant cell arteritis and peripheral neuropathy: A report of 2 cases and a review of the literature. J. Rheumatol. 14:129–134; 1987.
29. Zochodne, D. W.; Bolton, C. V.; et al. Critical illness polyneuropathy. A complication of sepsis and multiple organ failure. Brain 110(4):819–842; 1987.

CHAPTER **20**

MUSCLE DISEASES

The differential diagnosis of muscle weakness and wasting is a commonly encountered problem in clinical situations. The first step is to determine whether the weakness is episodic, as in periodic paralysis and myasthenia gravis, or nonepisodic. The examiner should then consider the distribution of weakness since this is of value in determining etiology. Proximal weakness is usually encountered in myopathies, whereas distal weakness is more likely to have a neurogenic origin. A myopathy is a disorder of skeletal muscle due to disease of the muscle fiber itself. Muscular dystrophy is a congenital myopathy. A decrease in muscle bulk due to myopathy, dystrophy, or denervation is called muscle wasting. However, the term "muscle atrophy" should be reserved for a decrease in muscle bulk due to denervation of the muscle. Certain investigative procedures, such as serum muscle enzymes, electromyography, and muscle biopsy are invaluable in their ability to differentiate myopathic from neurogenic weakness. The distinguishing characteristics of myopathic and neurogenic disorders are summarized in Table 20–1. The differential diagnosis of weakness is illustrated in Figure 20–1.

MUSCULAR DYSTROPHIES

The muscular dystrophies are genetically determined myopathies characterized by progressive muscular weakness and degenera-

tion of muscle fibers. The muscular dystrophies are classified according to clinical features (see Table 20–2).

Duchenne Muscular Dystrophy

Definition. Duchenne muscular dystrophy is the most common form of progressive muscular dystrophy and is seen almost exclusively in young males.

Etiology and Pathology. The dystrophies are believed to be due to an inborn error of metabolism that produces abnormal cell membranes. Excessive collagen formation may also have a primary role in the degeneration of muscle fibers.

Individual muscle fibers are randomly affected, and there is a marked variation in size. Degenerative changes consisting of fragmentation of cytoplasm, focal vacuolation, hyalinization, and shrinking of the sarcolemmal sheath are present. An extensive proliferation of collagen and replacement of diagnostic muscle fibers by fat are also seen.

Clinical Features. Duchenne muscle dystrophy is inherited as a sex-linked recessive trait and occurs in one in 3,000 male births. Approximately one-third of cases are due to spontaneous gene mutation in the patient or his mother.

Affected children appear normal at birth and may be reported to be extremely placid, "good" babies. There is normal achievement of early milestones but there is a delay in

TABLE 20–1. **Distinguishing Characteristics of Myopathic and Neurogenic Disorders**

Myopathic	Neurogenic
Signs and symptoms	
Proximal weakness and wasting	Distal weakness and wasting
	± Sensory signs and symptoms
	± Fasciculations, increased tone, extensorplantar responses
Serum muscle enzymes	
Increased	Normal
Nerve conduction velocities	
Normal	Slowed
Electromyography	
Low-amplitude polyphasic motor unit potentials of brief duration	Increased insertion activity
	Fibrillations, fasciculations
	Positive sharp waves
Muscle biopsy	
Variation in fiber diameter	Angular fibers, target fibers
Internal nuclei	Pyknotic clumping
Degeneration of fibers	Type grouping
Increased endomysial connective tissue	Type I fibers: small
	Type II fibers: hypertrophied

standing and walking. The child then develops a clumsy, waddling gait and pseudohypertrophy of the calf muscles, and has difficulty climbing stairs and rising from a chair. Older children have a pronounced lumbar lordosis due to weakness of the pelvic musculature. This results in forward tilting of the pelvis, protrusion of the abdomen, and a compensatory backward arching of the upper thoracic spine and shoulders. The affected child has difficulty rising to a standing position. He must first roll to a prone position, pull himself to his hands and knees, push with his arms until only his hands and feet are on the floor, and finally, "walk" up his lower extremities until he can extend his trunk and stand. This method of assuming a standing position in the presence of severe proximal weakness has been termed "Gower's sign." Eventually the child can no longer ambulate and becomes confined to a wheelchair by the age of 10. Multiple contractures, deformities, severe scoliosis, and distal weakness and wasting are prominent features in the later stages of the disease. Typically, the patient is bedridden in the teens and succumbs in the late teens or early twenties. Many develop gastrointestinal hypomotility due to involvement of smooth muscle and fatal intestinal pseudointestinal obstruction can occur (1). Progressive involvement of heart muscle results in a steady decline in cardiac reserve, but heart failure is rare, probably because the patient leads a sedentary lifestyle. There is progressive loss of respiratory reserve, and many patients die from the effects of a relatively minor respiratory infection. Despite reports to the contrary, neuropsychologic testing does not reveal any significant impairment of intellectual or cognitive functioning in children with muscular dystrophy (2).

Diagnostic Procedures.

1. Muscle enzymes. Serum creatine phosphokinase is elevated and may be abnormal before the onset of clinical signs and symptoms. There are increased serum levels of other muscle enzymes, including glutamic-oxalacetic transaminase (GOT), glutamate pyruvate transaminase (GPT), lactic dehydrogenase (LDH), and aldolase. The elevation is high in early cases and declines with progression of the disease. Creatinuria and myoglobinuria may also be present.
2. Electrocardiography. The electrocardiogram is abnormal at an early age. The initial tachycardia is followed by increased R-wave voltage and eventually right bundle branch block and deep Q-waves occur.
3. Electromyography. The EMG is myopathic (see Table 20–1).
4. Muscle biopsy. The diagnosis is established by muscle biopsy.

Differential Diagnosis.

1. Other forms of dystrophy (see Table 20–2).
2. Neurogenic muscular atrophy (see Table 20–1).
3. Polymositis and dermatomyositis, which are characterized by inflammatory changes on muscle biopsy.
4. Polyneuritis, differentiated by its more rapid onset, slowed nerve conduction velocities, and muscle biopsy.
5. Benign congenital myopathies (see p. 389).

Differential Diagnosis of Weakness

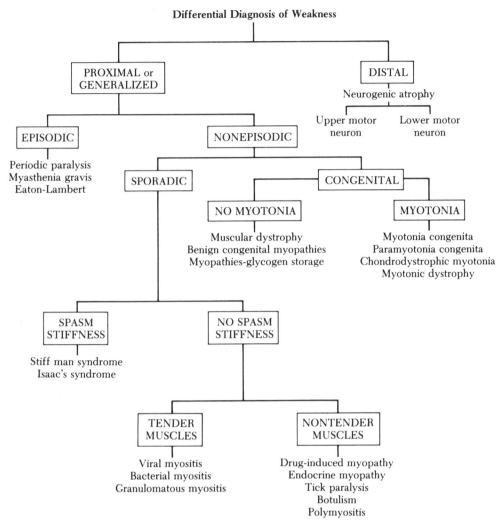

FIGURE 20–1. Differential diagnosis of muscle weakness.

Treatment.

1. There is no specific treatment for Duchenne muscular dystrophy.
2. A physical therapy program will help to delay the development of joint contractures. Obesity should be avoided.
3. Mild upper respiratory infections are potentially lethal in advanced cases and should be treated with appropriate antibiotics (3).
4. A lessening of the emotional impact of the disease on the patient and family and the development of optimal living conditions can be achieved by a combined effort of the neurologist, physiatrist, psychologist, and social worker.

5. Genetic counseling should be provided. It is important to advise the family regarding the likelihood of involvement in a subsequent pregnancy. Carriers of Duchenne dystrophy may have elevated serum creatine phosphokinase (CPK) levels (4). Carrier detection and prenatal diagnosis can be established by the use of DNA probes in both Duchenne and Becker dystrophy (5).

Prognosis. Duchenne muscular dystrophy is a steadily progressive, incapacitating disease. Death occurs in the late teens or early 20s. A better understanding of pulmonary problems and improved treatment of respiratory infections has significantly in-

TABLE 20–2. The Muscular Dystrophies

Type	Inheritance	Age of Onset	Progressive Weakness and Wasting
Duchenne	Sex-linked recessive One-third spontaneous mutation		See narrative in text
Benign sex-linked (Becker)	Sex-linked recessive	Five years or older	As for Duchenne, but slow progression
Facioscapulohumeral	Autosomal dominant	Between 10 and 20 years of age	Asymmetric involvement of lower face followed by trapezius, pectoralis major (sternal head), shoulder girdle, spinal muscles, and pelvic girdle
Scapuloperoneal	Autosomal dominant or sex-linked recessive	Early childhood	Muscles of shoulder girdle, proximal upper limb, and distal lower limb
Limb girdle type (Erb)	Autosomal recessive or dominant	Between 10 and 20 years of age	Muscles of pelvic or shoulder girdle, later both
Distal	Autosomal dominant or recessive	Adulthood	Distal muscles of upper-lower limbs
Oculopharyngeal	Autosomal dominant	Late in fourth or fifth decade	Bilateral ptosis followed by facial weakness; later onset weakness of masseters, pharynx, hands, feet

Gilchrist, J. M.; Pericak-Vance, M.; et al. Clinical and genetic investigation in autosomal dominant limb-girdle muscular dystrophy. Neurology 38:5–9; 1988.

creased the life span in Duchenne muscular dystrophy and other diseases affecting respiratory function.

Other Forms of Muscular Dystrophy

There are a number of other muscular dystrophies which are uncommon. These are outlined in Table 20–2.

MUSCLE DISEASES ASSOCIATED WITH MYOTONIA

Myotonia is a sustained contraction of muscles that may be induced by voluntary contraction, percussion, or electrical stimulation. Myotonia occurs in myotonia congenita, paramyotonia congenita, chondrodystrophic myotonia, myotonic dystrophy, and hyperkalemic periodic paralysis (see p. 394).

Myotonia Congenita

Definition. Myotonia congenita is a hereditary condition characterized by myotonia and a "herculean" appearance.

Etiology and Pathology. Myotonia is believed to be caused by an abnormality of the muscle membrane that permits excess influx of sodium ions into the muscle cell, thus prolonging depolarization. Minor pathologic changes have been described and consist of occasional atrophic fibers, increased internal nuclei, and fiber hypertrophy in surviving fibers. There is absence of type 2B fibers (6).

Clinical Features. Myotonia congenita is inherited as an autosomal dominant or autosomal recessive trait. Symptoms of myotonia first appear in infancy or childhood and consist of inability to relax muscle following con-

Heart Involvement	Diagnosis	Treatment	Prognosis
Yes—severe	See narrative in text	See narrative in text	Death in late teens or early 20s
Minimal	As for Duchenne type Enzyme elevation not as high	Nil-physical therapy to maintain activity	Still walking at 20 years Survival past 40 years
Unusual	CPK elevated 50 percent cases EMG and muscle biopsy compatible with dystrophy	Physical therapy to maintain function	Slowly progressive Many cases show minimal disability
Yes—some cases in adult life	Muscle biopsy, dystrophic and neurogenic types described	No treatment necessary	Slowly progressive, rarely disabling, not incompatible with full life span
Yes	EMG and muscle biopsy compatible with dystrophy	Physical therapy and bracing	Slowly progressive, may be wheelchair-confined after age 40 years
No	EMG and muscle biopsy compatible with dystrophy	Prosthesis, improve hand grip	Very slowly progressive Normal life span
No	EMG and muscle biopsy compatible with dystrophy Elevated IgG, IgA	Advanced forms may need tracheotomy and gastrostomy	Slowly progressive

traction. The symptoms tend to increase during childhood and adolescence but may lessen in severity in adult life. Myotonia occurs only in skeletal muscles, and the patient has difficulty initiating movement and making sudden movements. Once repetitive movements are initiated, they can be continued without difficulty. Sudden movements may initiate a sustained contraction sufficient to throw the patient off balance. Upon grasping an object, the patient is often unable to release the object for as long as 60 seconds. Patients with myotonia congenita have a well-developed musculature and have been described as "herculean" in appearance. Percussion of an affected muscle produces percussion myotonia, a dimpling of the skin and sustained contraction. Percussion may also be followed by local swelling of muscle terms "myedema."

Diagnostic Procedures. The diagnostic procedure is electromyography. There is markedly increased activity after insertion of the needle electrode. Traction or percussion of the muscle produces a series of prolonged potentials that persist when the patient is instructed to relax the contracted muscle. Contraction and relaxation of the muscle produce a typical sound on EMG examination which has been termed the "dive bomber" effect.

Treatment

1. Many cases receive some relief from myotonia with the use of phenytoin (Dilantin) beginning with 100 mg q12h and increas-

ing the dose until the serum levels are within therapeutic range.

2. A number of other drugs are known to be effective in myotonia, including procainamide HCl (Pronestyl) 50 mg/kg/day given in divided dosage four times a day and quinine 10 mg/kg/day in divided dosage. Quinine should always be followed by regular visual and audiometric tests because of the risk of optic or otic neuritis. Tricyclic antidepressants, particularly imipramine or lithium carbonate, or verapamil or nifedipine may produce improvement in some cases (7).

3. Corticosteroids are said to be effective in reducing myotonia in some cases, although long-term treatment may produce unacceptable side effects.

4. Intractable cases may respond to acetazolamine (Diamox) 8 to 30 mg/kg/day in divided dosage (8).

Paramyotonia Congenita

Paramyotonia congenita is a congenital disorder inherited as an autosomal dominant trait. It is characterized by myotonia, muscular weakness and paralysis on exertion or exposure to cold. The condition is nonprogressive, does not affect the life span, and tends to improve with age. It is probably a varient of hyperkalemic periodic paralysis (see page 394). Improvement with decreased myotonia and reduction in cold induced weakness has been reported with low doses of acetazolamide (9) or tocainide 400 to 1200 mg/day (10).

Chondrodystrophic Myotonia

Chondrodystrophic myotonia is a congenital disorder believed to be inherited as an autosomal recessive trait. It is characterized by myotonia, short stature, blepharospasm, muscle hypertrophy, and skeletal deformities.

Myotonic Dystrophy (Dystrophia Myotonia, Myotonia Atrophica)

Definition. Myotonic dystrophy is an inherited myopathy characterized by progressive muscular weakness, myotonia, cataracts, cardiac abnormalities, hypogonadism, and frontal balding.

Etiology and Pathology. Myotonic dystrophy is believed to be a systemic disorder of cellular metabolism due to a decrease of normal stimulatory effect of insulin or other trophic factors (11).

Affected muscles show evidence of fiber necrosis and degeneration with areas of phagocytosis and increased endomysial connective tissue. Surviving fibers show loss of striations and a characteristic ring fiber has been described. Histochemical studies reveal that degeneration is confined to type I muscle fibers, and that there may be some increase in the size of type II fibers.

Clinical Features. Myotonic dystrophy is inherited as an autosomal dominant trait. The signs and symptoms appear between 15 and 40 years of age. Myotonia is usually the first symptom and affects the hands, with later involvement of other muscles, particularly those of the lower limbs. Muscle wasting also affects the hands first, then spreads to the facial muscles, muscles of mastication, the sternocleidomastoids, the flexors and extensors of the forearm, the quadriceps, and the dorsiflexors of the feet. The facial appearance is characteristic with a bilateral ptosis and wating, which has been termed "hatchet face."

Patients with myotonic dystrophy usually have involvement of other organ systems. These include:

1. Cardiac abnormalities. Prolapsed mitral valve sometimes occurs in early cases, more advanced cases with severe cardiac fibrosis suffer cardiac dysrhythmias. Adams-Stokes attacks may occur (see p. 188). Subclinical cardiac involvement is not uncommon and may be responsible for sudden death in some cases.(12).

2. Ophthalmic abnormalities. Subcapsular lens opacities, which enlarge and eventually impair vision, are present in most cases.

3. Endocrine abnormalities. Primary gonadal failure and gonadal atrophy occur in both sexes. Impotence, loss of libido, and testicular atrophy occur in the male. Mild diabetes mellitus may be present in both sexes.

4. Skin and skeletal abnormalities. Frontal balding occurs at an early stage in the male. A high-arched palate may be present.

5. Smooth muscle abnormalities. There is impairment of mobility in the gastrointestinal tract with dilation of the colon in advanced cases.

6. Respiratory abnormalities. Advanced cases show evidence of respiratory insufficiency, and there is an increased risk of aspiration pneumonia.

7. Hearing loss. There is a high incidence of sensorineural hearing loss in myotonic dystrophy (13).
8. Peripheral neuropathy of axonal type is responsible for the areflexia, distal sensory impairment and fasciculations seen in some cases (14).

Children born to mothers with myotonic dystrophy may present with congenital myotonic dystrophy in the neonatal period of infancy. This condition is characterized by hypotonia, facial diplegia, dysphagia, mental retardation, a high-arched palate, and tented lips. Myotonia develops later in the course of this condition, for which the term "myotonia dysembryoplasia" has been proposed.

Diagnostic Procedures.

1. The effect of temperature change. Myotonia may be difficult to demonstrate in some cases. Submersion of the hands in cold water for several minutes may facilitate the appearance of myotonia.
2. Electromyography. The EMG is characteristic with an increase in insertional activity and typical myotonic discharges following voluntary contraction of muscle.
3. Electrocardiography. Atrial fibrillation, atrial flutter, a prolonged P-R interval, and various conduction defects may be present (15).
4. Slit lamp. Slit lamp examination may reveal the characteristic lens opacities.
5. Serum tests. There are abnormally low levels of IgG, an abnormal glucose tolerance test, and low FSH levels in most cases.
6. CT scans and skull x-rays. Thickening of the calvarium and enlargement of the frontal sinuses are often present on x-ray. There may be microcephaly and calcification of the basal ganglia in some cases (16).
7. Pure tone screening and impedence audiometry will detect sensorineural hearing loss.
8. Muscle biopsy. The diagnosis can be established by muscle biopsy.

Treatment.

1. Relief of myotonia is discussed under myotonia congenita (see pp. 386–388). The calcium channel blocking agent nifedipine, which has no effect on the cardiac conduction, decreases myotonia in doses of 10 to 20 mg t.i.d. (17).

2. In later stages, when the risk of aspiration pneumonia increases, respiratory infections should be promptly treated with appropriate antibiotics, postural drainage, and chest percussion.
3. Most anesthetic and relaxant drugs are dangerous in patients with myotonic dystrophy who require careful monitoring for cardiac and central nervous system depression during anesthesia and in the postoperative recovery period (18).

Prognosis. Myotonic dystrophy is a chronic condition with progressive deterioration in most cases. Death occurs between 40 and 60 years due to cardiac or respiratory dysfunction.

BENIGN CONGENITAL MYOPATHIES

The benign congenital myopathies are a heterogenous group of rare disorders characterized by slowly progressive or nonprogressive myopathy.

Etiology and Pathology. The etiology is unknown.

The disorders are characterized by evidence of an active myopathic process with fiber necrosis, increased internal nuclei, phagocytosis, and some replacement with connective tissue and fat. Individual fibers show abnormalities, usually detectable only by electron microscopy, which characterize the particular disorder (see Table 20–3).

Clinical Features. The congenital myopathies may become clinically apparent at any time in life. In many cases the patient presents as a hypotonic, "floppy" baby. However, signs and symptoms may not appear until childhood, adolescence, or adulthood. The common symptom is slowly progressive or nonprogressive, usually proximal muscle weakness (19). (See Table 20–3 for associated features.)

Diagnostic Procedures. The diagnosis may be established by muscle biopsy, which indicates a myopathic process (see Table 20–1). Definitive diagnosis requires electron microscopy.

Treatment. There is no specific treatment at this time.

Prognosis. In the majority of cases the congenital myopathies are slowly progressive conditions; in some cases the process appears to become arrested in adolescence or adult life. Others show a slow deterioration requiring the eventual use of a wheelchair. There is

TABLE 20–3.   **Benign Congenital Myopathies**

Type	Pathology	Clinical Features
Central	Type 1 fibers—amorphous central area (central cores) within muscle fibers which is devoid of oxidative enzymes and phosphorylase	Infancy; nonprogressive weakness, pes cavus, scoliosis
Nemaline myopathy	Rodlike muscle inclusions believed to be 10s-actin	Adolescence; progressive weakness, high-arched palate, long face, pigeon chest, kyphoscoliosis, pes cavus
Myotubular myopathy	Fetal myotube structure of muscle believed to represent arrest of development	Adolescence; progressive weakness of ocular muscles, face, and limbs
Fingerprint body myopathy	Muscle cell inclusions with concentric lamellae	Infancy; tremors, mental retardation

TABLE 20–4.   **Muscle Disorders in Glycogen Storage Diseases**

Type	Metabolic Defect	Pathology
Type 2 acid maltese deficiency	Lack of alpha 1-4 glucosidase	Excess glycogen in cells of liver, myocardium, muscle, brain, and spinal cord
Type 3 limit dextrinosis	Lack of amylo 1-6 glucosidase	Presence of limit dextrin in liver and muscle
Type 5 muscle phosphorylase deficiency (McArdle's disease)	Lack of muscle phosphorylase	Subsarcolemmal vacuoles containing glycogen in muscle
Phosphofructokinase deficiency	Lack of muscle phosphofructokinase	Similar to muscle phosphorylase deficiency
Carnitine deficiency	Defect in hepatic biosynthesis of carnitine	Severe vacuolar myopathy Vacuoles stain positive in lipid

an increased risk of respiratory infection, which may be fatal unless promptly treated.

TOXIC AND METABOLIC MYOPATHIES

Myopathies Associated with Glycogen Storage Disease

The type, metabolic defect, pathology, clinical features, and diagnostic procedures are outlined in Table 20–4.

Myopathies Associated with Thyroid Disease

Myopathy has been associated with both hyperthyroid and hypothyroid states.

Hyperthyroid Myopathy. The myopathy associated with hyperthyroidism may be acute or chronic. Acute thyrotoxic myopathy occurs during severe thyrotoxicosis or "thyroid storm." Chronic myopathy may follow thyrotoxicosis and is usually generalized; there may be marked muscle wasting in the upper limb girdle muscles. There are minimal myopathic changes on muscle biopsy.

Marked improvement occurs when the patient is restored to a euthyroid state.

Hypothyroid Myopathy. The myopathy associated with hypothyroidism may be congenital, spontaneous, or follow treatment of hyperthyroidism. It is believed to result from a disturbance of glycogen metabolism. Involved muscles show an involvement of Type 1 fibers, the presence of central "core-like" structures and hypertrophy of individual muscle fibers (20). There may be a slowness of both contraction and relaxation of muscle. Thyroid replacement hormone results in improvement.

Mitochondrial Myopathies

This heterogenous group contains many disorders which have the common feature of "ragged red fibers" indicating abnormalities of muscle mitochondria. Four groups have been recognized (21):

A. Defects of substrate utilization: pyruvate dehydrogenase deficiency; carnitine pal-

Clinical Features	Diagnostic Procedures
Autosomal recessive condition 1. Infantile: progressive cardiac enlargement, death within 1 year due to congestive heart failure 2. Childhood: progressive muscle weakness of limbs, girdle, neck, and pharynx; death before 10 years of age 3. Adult: slowly progressive muscle weakness of limbs and girdle muscles; benign course	1. Marked decrease of acid maltase in urine 2. Normal fasting blood glucose 3. Electromyography; small motor unit potentials increased short duration polyphasic potentials, occasional myotonia, fibrillations and positive waves 4. Muscle biopsy: vacuolar myopathy; lack of 1-4 glucosidase activity
Autosomal recessive condition, mild muscle weakness, mental retardation, hepatomegaly, hypoglycemic episodes	Demonstration of limit dextrin in muscle. Absence of amylo-1-6-glucosidase in muscle and liver biopsy material
Autosomal dominant or recessive condition: limitation of exercise and painful muscle cramps beginning in adolescence; myoglobinuria may occur; condition lifelong with later muscle weakness	1. Elevated serum levels of aldolase, CPK, LDH, SGOT 2. Electromyography: decreased response on repetitive nerve stimulation 3. No increase in venous lactic acid on ischemic work test 4. Muscle biopsy: absence muscle phosphorylase. Absence lactate, exaggerated IMP, low normal ATP by DNP provocation
Similar to muscle phosphorylase deficiency	As for muscle phosphorylase deficiency except for absence of phosphofructokinase in muscle biopsy specimen
1. Limb-girdle muscle weakness beginning in childhood 2. As above plus periodic episodes resembling Reyes syndrome in the systemic form of the disease°	1. Low or normal serum carnitine 2. Electromyography-myopathic pattern 3. Muscle carnitine reduced in biopsy specimens

°Rudeman, M.I.; Zito, G. Metabolic myopathies. N.J. Med. 83:36–40; 1986.

mitoyltransferase deficiency, carnitine deficiency and defects of B-oxidation enzymes.
B. Defective coupling of oxidation and phosphorylation—control of mitochondrial respiration by ADP is lost with excessive production of energy which is wasted as heat.
C. Defects of the respiratory chain.
1. Severe cytochrome c oxidase deficiency results in a profound mitochondrial myopathy, renal failure, and death before the age of one year.
2. Benign reversible muscle cytochrome c oxidase deficiency presents with severe myopathy at birth followed by spontaneous improvement and apparent normal function by the age of three years (22).
3. Subacute necrotizing encephalopathy (Leigh's syndrome). See page 210.
D. Unknown biochemical defect.

1. Kearns-Sayre Syndrome. A degenerative disorder characterized by pigmentary degeneration of the retina, progressive external ophthalmoplegia, heart block, and elevated protein in the cerebrospinal fluid. Patients are often of short stature and present with mild dementia, cerebral ataxia, hearing loss, and vestibular dysfunction. There is progressive proximal muscle weakness with demonstration of ragged red fibers on muscle biopsy. The condition develops before the age of 20 and is slowly progressive.
2. Myoclonus epilepsy with ragged red fibers (MERRF syndrome) is a familial condition characterized by myoclonus, epilepsy, generalized seizures, ataxia and muscle weakness.
3. Mitochondrial myopathy, encephalopathy, lactic acidosis and stroke-like episodes (MELAS syndrome) occurs in young children and adults who exhibit short stature, episodic vomiting, seizures and recurrent strokes causing hemiparesis, hemianopia or cortical blindness (23).

Drug-Induced Myopathy
Myopathy may occur with the use of corticosteroids; the antimalarial and amebicidal drug chloroquine; colchicine (24); meperidine (Demerol); and pentazocine (Talwin). The most common drug-induced myopathy is alcohol myopathy.
Alcohol Myopathy. Alcohol myopathy is an acute, subacute, or chronic myopathic

process related to ingestion of excessive amounts of alcohol.
Etiology and Pathology. All three forms of this condition are related to the intake of excessive amounts of alcohol. Pathologic changes in muscle are nonspecific. There are some variation in fiber size and evidence of degeneration and regeneration of muscle fibers.
Clinical Features. Alcohol myopathy may occur in an acute, subacute, or chronic form.
The acute form of alcohol myopathy, which is associated with myoglobinuria, occurs after a particularly heavy bout of drinking in the chronic alcoholic. It is possible that this condition represents the effects of alcohol in a patient who is already susceptible to paroxysmal myoglobinuria. These patients are profoundly ill with pain, tenderness, and edema in the affected muscles. There is evidence of renal damage with hyperkalemia and myoglobulinuria, and there is a risk of anuria due to blockage of renal tubules.
Subacute myopathy also occurs after heavy drinking in a chronic alcoholic. Patients develop severe proximal weakness, particularly in the lower limb-girdle musculature, with painful spasms in the affected muscles. The condition resolves over a period of several weeks.
Chronic alcohol myopathy is much more common than the acute and subacute forms. It is frequently overlooked in many hospitals with an indigent population. The condition is characterized by weakness and wasting of the proximal muscles, particularly in the area of the shoulder girdle. Pain is uncommon.
Diagnostic Procedures.

1. Serum muscle enzymes. All types of alcohol myopathy show elevation of CPK, GOT, GPT, and aldolase.
2. Myoglobinuria. Myoglobinuria is present in the acute form of alcohol myopathy. There also may be a trace of myoglobin in the urine in the subacute form.
3. In the acute form with myoglobinuria there is abnormally low elevation of serum lactate levels following ischemic exercises. Myophosphorylase activity is reported to be abnormally depressed in these cases.
4. Muscle biopsy. Muscle biopsy will reveal the nonspecific changes of variation in fiber size and evidence of degeneration and regeneration in the more chronic forms.
5. Electromyography. The EMG findings are

compatible with a myopathic process (see Table 20–1).

Treatment.

1. Patients with myoglobinuria should be treated in an intensive care unit, and appropriate treatment should be instituted if oliguria or anuria occurs.
2. Patients with other forms of alcohol myopathy should be treated with thiamine supplements and an adequate diet. Total abstinence from alcohol is essential.

Prognosis. With proper treatment all forms of myopathy improve. It may require three to six months for return of strength in the chronic form of alcohol myopathy.

DISORDERS CHARACTERIZED BY STIFFNESS AND SPASMS

Stiff-Man Syndrome

Definition. The stiff-man syndrome is a rare disorder characterized by persistent muscle stiffness, spasm, and muscle cramps, which disappear during sleep.

Etiology and Pathology. The etiology is unknown, but the condition is believed to be a dysfunction of motor neurons in the central nervous system.

Clinical Features. The patient initially experiences muscle aches and pains followed by stiffening of the muscles of the trunk, limbs, and neck. Voluntary movements are slowed. Emotional or sensory stimuli may exacerbate the stiffness and produce painful spasms. On examination the muscles are contracted and the patient is unable to relax them. The disorder is progressive and eventually results in considerable disability. A congenital form of the disorder has been reported. In these cases stiffness is present at birth and gradually resolves so that by age three the tone is almost normal. Later, in adolescence or adulthood, the stiffness reappears in a mild form.

Diagnostic Procedures.

1. Urinary neurotransmitter metabolites. There are excessive urinary metabolites of norepinephrine.
2. Electromyography reveals persistent contraction of muscle fibers and bursts of motor unit potentials during spasm.

Treatment.

1. The stiffness and spasm improve with diazepam (Valium) or clonazepam.

2. Baclofen (Lioresal) has been reported to be effective in reducing stiffness and spasm, particularly in combination with diazepam.

Isaac's Syndrome

Isaac's syndrome is a rare disorder characterized by continuous muscle twitching, generalized muscle stiffness, and hyporeflexia. The etiology is unknown, but the continuous muscle activity is believed to originate in abnormal spontaneous discharges of distal peripheral motor nerves. The diagnosis is established by demonstration of peripheral nerve origin of muscle activity. This can be accomplished with a proximal motor nerve block. Muscle biopsy reveals denervation. There is an excellent response to phenytoin (Dilantin) or carbamazepine (Tegretol).

FAMILIAL PERIODIC PARALYSIS

There are three types of familial periodic paralysis, all of which are inherited as an autosomal dominant trait. Hypokalemic periodic paralysis occur with less frequency.

Hypokalemic Periodic Paralysis

Definition. Hypokalemic periodic paralysis is a disorder characterized by episodic, flaccid muscle weakness associated with low serum potassium levels.

Etiology and Pathology. The etiology is unknown. It has been postulated that the condition might be an amplification of the normal response of muscle fibers to insulin (25).

Muscle biopsy obtained during attacks reveals large, central vacuoles in affected fibers. These are believed to represent dilated sarcoplasmic reticulum.

Clinical Features. Hypokalemic periodic paralysis is more common in males and occurs predominantly during the teens and twenties. Attacks begin at night, and the patient awakens with weakness of all skeletal muscles except those involved in respiration and speech. Involved muscles are firm and tender to palpation. The neurologic examination is normal except for weakness and hyporeflexia. The attacks last from several hours to days. Several factors have been reported to precipitate attacks. These include large meals with a high carbohydrate content; exertion; trauma; heavy alcohol ingestion; upper respiratory tract infections; cold weather; and administration of insulin, thyroid hormone, steroids, epinephrine, thiazides, or licorice.

Diagnostic Procedures.

1. Serum potassium levels are decreased below 3.5 mEq/L.
2. Electromyography shows decreased amplitude, number, and duration of motor unit potentials or electrical silence during periods of paralysis.
3. In susceptible individuals attacks may be induced by infusion of 50 g of glucose in 150 ml of water each hour to a maximum of fifteen trials.

Treatment.

1. Attacks may be terminated by oral or parenteral administration of potassium.
2. Acetazolamide (Diamox) 250 mg q4–6h or spironolactone (Aldactone) 100 mg q.d. or b.i.d. are effective in reducing the number of attacks.
3. Predisposing factors should be avoided.

Hyperkalemic Periodic Paralysis (Adynamia Episodica Hereditaria, Gamstorp Syndrome)

Definition. Hyperkalemic periodic paralysis resembles the hypokalemic forms of the disease, but the attacks are of shorter duration, occur equally in both sexes, and are associated with elevated serum potassium levels.

Etiology and Pathology. The etiology is unknown. Muscle biopsy reveals large vacuoles within the muscle fibers.

Clinical Features. Hyperkalemic periodic paralysis usually begins during childhood. The attacks are similar to those that occur in the hypokalemic form. However, the episodes are shorter, lasting one to two hours at a time. Each attack may be preceded by a sensation of heaviness or paresthesias. Mild percussion myotonia may be elicited in some cases.

Diagnostic Procedures.

1. Electromyography may reveal electrical silence during paralysis or fibrillations, positive sharp waves, and myotonic discharges during paresis. Motor unit potentials are decreased in number and duration.
2. Serum potassium levels are elevated.

Treatment.

1. Attacks can be terminated with 10 to 20 ml of IV 10 percent calcium gluconate.
2. Acetazolamide (Diamox) 250 mg q4–6h and hydrochlorthiazide (Diazide) 50 to 100 mg q.d. are effective in reducing the number of attacks.
3. Precipitating factors should be avoided.

Normokalemic Periodic Paralysis

Normokalemic periodic paralysis resembles the hyperkalemic form and is associated with normal serum potassium levels.

DISORDERS OF NEUROMUSCULAR JUNCTION

Myasthenia Gravis

Definition. Myasthenia gravis is an autoimmune condition characterized by progressive muscular weakness on exertion followed by recovery of strength after a period of rest.

Etiology and Pathology   The Normal Neuromuscular Junction. The neuromuscular junction is illustrated schematically in Figure 20–2. Acetylcholine is contained in synaptic vesicles, which fuse with the presynaptic membrane and release small quanta of acetylcholine into the synaptic cleft. The acetylcholine then diffuses across the cleft and binds to acetylcholine receptors on the postsynaptic membrane. The attachment produces a conformational change, which opens the sodium

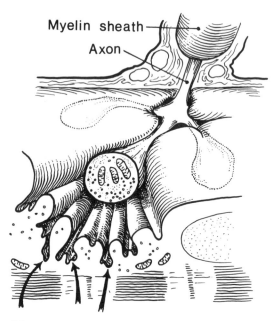

Myelin sheath

Axon

Sites of acetycholine receptors

FIGURE 20–2. The normal neuromuscular junction.

and potassium gates of the postsynaptic membrane. There is a constant and spontaneous release of acetylcholine in small quantities, which is not sufficient to depolarize the membrane but does result in what has been termed "miniature end plate potentials." Bound acetylcholine is removed by diffusion or hydrolyzed by the enzyme acetylcholinesterase, which is concentrated in the postsynaptic membrane. The receptor probably remains refractory for some time after this hydrolysis takes place.

In physiologic muscle contraction the impulse generated in the motor neuron reaches the presynaptic membrane, depolarizes it, and results in a coordinated release of acetylcholine. The acetylcholine diffuses across the cleft in sufficient quantity to produce a wave of depolarization, which is propagated down the muscle fiber. The propagated electrical discharge produces changes in the sarcoplasmic reticulum of the muscle fiber with release of calcium ions, which promotes fiber contractions. There is an ample reserve of acetylcholine receptor sites to allow repetitive depolarization of the membrane and repeated muscle fiber contraction.

Etiology and Pathology of Myasthenia Gravis. The postsynaptic membrane is abnormal in myasthenia gravis. There is a loss of secondary folds, which reduces the surface area available for binding of acetylcholine, and there is a decreased number of acetylcholine receptors. During repetitive stimulation of the nerve the available acetylcholine receptors are quickly saturated and remain refractory. This results in a state of receptor insufficiency in which there is not a sufficient number of receptors available to bind acetylcholine and produce depolarization. Therefore, repetitive stimulation will result in a decrease in the number of muscle fibers that are able to respond as each neuromuscular junction reaches a state of receptor insufficiency. Clinically, this is characterized by progressive weakness.

The reduction in functioning acetylcholine receptors in myasthenia gravis is the result of a complement mediated binding of antiacetylcholine receptor antibodies at receptor sites followed by lysis of receptors.

The antibodies which are of the IgG class are probably produced by B lymphocytes in germinal centers within the thymus in response to the presence of abnormal acetylcholine receptors. Such receptors are present on myoid or muscle like cells scattered throughout the thymus. Myoid cells are normal constituents of the thymus and the reason for their acetylcholine receptors assuming antigenic properties is not known.

However, not all myasthenics show detectable levels of antibodies to acetylcholine receptors, implying that myasthenia gravis is not a homogenous disorder and that other as yet undetected antibodies may occur in some cases.

Clinical Features. Myasthenia gravis is a rare disease with a prevalence of about 1 in 10,000. There are currently between 20,000 and 30,000 cases in the United States. The disease is more common among women than men, with a ratio of 2:1. The mean age of onset is 26 years in women and 31 years in men. The incidence in men does not show a smooth distribution. The peak incidence in the early thirties declines through middle age, but there is a second peak between 60 and 70 years of age. Why this does not occur in women is unknown. The disease can occur at any age and has been reported in the newborn. There is no significant familial occurrence.

Myasthenia gravis can be classified into four stages or types:

1. Ocular myasthenia
2. Mild generalized myasthenia
3. Severe generalized myasthenia
4. Crisis

Ocular Myasthenia. In this form of myasthenia gravis the symptoms and signs are confined to the extraocular muscles. The patient develops diplopia and ptosis usually toward the end of the day. Ocular myasthenia may develop into the second or third stage of generalized myasthenia within a period of 18 months. If generalized myasthenia does not develop within this period of time the condition usually remains localized to the extraocular muscles.

Mild Generalized Myasthenia. Mild generalized myasthenia may be preceded by ocular myasthenia or may present with symptoms of mild weakness involving the extraocular muscles and other muscle groups. There is usually some involvement of the facial muscles, muscles of mastication, and the proximal limb girdle muscles, while the extraocular muscles are frequently, but not invariably, involved. When mild generalized myasthenia develops into the severe generalized stage of the disease, the transition occurs within a period of 18 months.

Severe Generalized Myasthenia. In the severe generalized form of myasthenia gravis, there is sufficient weakness of the bulbar and limb girdle musculature to produce marked restriction in activity. The exercise tolerance is reduced, the patient has a sedentary existence, and there is a constant risk of respiratory insufficiency or respiratory failure.

Crisis. Myasthenia crisis may be defined as myasthenia gravis with respiratory failure. This is a life-threatening situation that develops in patients with severe generalized myasthenia. The onset is often sudden and crisis is usually precipitated by an infection. This usually takes the form of an upper respiratory tract infection which progresses to severe bronchitis or pneumonia.

The stages of myasthenia are not fixed and it is not unusual for progression to occur from one stage to the next within a period of 18 months. Remission can occur in any of the first three stages of myasthenia gravis. However, remission usually occurs within the first 18 months of the disease and is rare at a later stage. Some patients experience several periods of remission.

At the initial interview the patient with myasthenia gravis should receive a full general physical examination which will help to exclude a number of conditions known to be associated with myasthenia gravis, particularly thyrotoxicosis. This is followed by a full neurologic examination with careful documentation of the degree of muscle involvement. The examiner should attempt to demonstrate progressive weakness of affected muscles. In the patient with ptosis the examiner should measure the widths of the palpebral fissure and the patient should be asked to sustain upward gaze. This will produce an increasing degree of ptosis which can be observed and measured. Similarly, patients with diplopia can be asked to sustain gaze in the direction of the pull of the involved muscle, and the examiner may observe increasing deviation of the ocular axis. Patients with weakness of the masseters can be asked to bite down on a tongue blade while the examiner attempts to withdraw it. This maneuver will produce fatigue of the masseters, and biting will not be sustained after a short period of time. The patient with a generalized form of the disease may show increasing weakness on stressing any of the muscles involved in the disease process. When the hands are involved, it is possible to obtain a quantitative measure of weakness using a dynamometer.

Diagnostic Procedures.

1. Edrophonium (Tensilon) test. Edrophonium is a rapidly acting anticholinesterase which blocks the action of acetylcholinesterase. Hydrolysis of acetylcholine is prevented, thus allowing more time for attachment of acetylcholine molecules to receptor sites. The test is performed as follows:

   The examiner selects a weak muscle. For example, if the patient has ptosis, the width of the palpebral fissure can be measured. If the patient has diplopia, the degree of deviation of the ocular axis can be estimated; or if the patient has weakness of chewing, the time that the patient is able to sustain biting of the tongue blade can be recorded. The examiner then draws 10 mg (1 ml) of edrophonium into a syringe. The test begins with the intravenous injection of 2 mg (0.2 ml) of edrophonium into a vein in the forearm. The examiner then waits 30 seconds to make sure that the patient does not have any muscarinic reaction to edrophonium. This usually consists of bradycardia, hypotension, lacrimation, sweating, and/or abdominal colic. If this does not occur, the remaining 8 mg (0.8 ml) of edrophonium is injected. If the test is positive there will be a dramatic response with increasing strength of the paretic muscle within a period of 30 seconds. This increasing strength usually lasts about two minutes and then disappears. However, the patient will usually express an appreciation of the increasing strength of the weakened muscle, and the examiner will be able to observe this effect. The test is safe to perform, and side effects are unusual. If severe muscarinic side effects occur, they can be rapidly resolved by intravenous injection of atropine (0.4 mg).

2. Electromyography. The diagnosis of myasthenia gravis is usually confirmed by electromyographic (EMG) examination. This is particularly valuable when the Tensilon test is equivocal but should also be performed when it is positive. In myasthenia gravis the EMG shows variation in the amplitude of the evoked response during sustained voluntary contraction. If the patient is asked to make a maximum effort, there is gradual reduction in the amplitude of the response and finally complete loss of response. The response of an

affected muscle to repetitive nerve stimulation should also be tested. The test is carried out at supramaximal stimulation, and repetitive stimulation will produce a brief initial increase in amplitude due to increased release of acetylcholine, followed by rapid falling of amplitude, and eventually a failure to respond. When the nerve is stimulated at slow rates (e.g., two stimuli per second), the amplitude of the evoked muscle action potential declines over a period of several minutes and finally disappears.

3. Elevated levels of antibodies to acetylcholine receptors occur in most cases. Titers do not provide a measure of severity of the disease but can be used to monitor the effect of treatment on an individual basis.

Failure to detect antibody levels occur in about 10 to 15 percent of cases with the generalized form of myasthenia and about 30 percent of cases with ocular myasthenia (26).

4. Muscle biopsy. Muscle biopsy should be performed with the diagnosis is uncertain. Techniques for immunohistologic study of motor endplates and quantification of acetylcholine receptors are available.

After a diagnosis of myasthenia gravis has been established, a series of tests should be carried out to rule out associated diseases. These include:

a. A chest x-ray is taken to eliminate the possibility of a thymic tumor, which occurs in about 18 percent of patients with myasthenia gravis, particularly elderly males. If there is any doubt, laminograms of the mediastinum or computerized tomography of the thorax should be obtained.

b. Thyroid function tests should be performed to eliminate the possibility of hyperthyroidism. Antithyroid and antimuscle antibodies are available in some centers.

c. Lupus erythematosus preparation, rheumatoid factor, and antibody to nuclear antigen and anticardiolipin tests are indicated to rule out an associated lupus erythematosus.

d. Patients with the severe generalized form of the disease should have respiratory function tests performed as soon as the diagnosis is suspected and daily during the period of treatment.

Differential Diagnosis.

1. Polymyositis. The patient with polymyositis may have symmetric, proximal, limb-girdle muscle weakness. Some patients show a positive response to edrophonium, and the diagnosis can be established only by muscle biopsy.

2. Thyrotoxicosis. Thyroid myopathy presents as a proximal limb-girdle muscle weakness. The association of myasthenia gravis and thyrotoxicosis is not unusual, and the presence of myasthenia gravis in a patient with thyrotoxicosis can be suspected if improvement is seen following the edrophonium test. Patients with thyroid myopathy usually do not show improvement following the intravenous administration of edrophonium.

3. Exophthalmic ophthalmoplegia. This condition may be progressive and may resemble myasthenia gravis in the early stages. There is progressive weakness of the extraocular muscles which are replaced by fat and marked fatty infiltration of the orbit, producing exophthalmus. The response to edrophonium is absent; however, exophthalmic ophthalmoplegia and myasthenia gravis can coexist, in which case the response to edrophonium may be positive.

4. Myasthenic syndrome (Eaton-Lambert syndrome). This condition is rare and occurs in association with neoplasia. The muscle weakness involves the proximal limb-girdle muscles, and the diagnosis can be established by the characteristic findings on electromyography (see p. 400).

5. Periodic paralysis (see p. 393).

6. Botulism (see p. 265).

7. Miscellaneous. (Penicillamine, acetylcholinesterase agents—particularly organophosphorus compounds.)

Treatment. Group I and II patients may be treated as outpatients. Group III patients should be admitted to the hospital. Certain drugs may aggravate or unmask myasthenia gravis (see Table 20-5).

1. Anticholinesterase drugs. The anticholinesterase drugs were the first effective treatment for myasthenia gravis and are still widely used. There is some evidence that anticholinesterase drugs may increase damage to the postsynaptic membrane, and there is a present trend to restrict the use of anticholinesterase drugs to mild cases which show good response.

TABLE 20–5. Drugs That Aggravate or Unmask Myasthenia Gravis

1. Antibiotics (colistin, kanamycin, streptomycin, tetracyclin)
2. Cardiovascular drugs (procainamide, propranolol, quinidine)
3. Antirheumatics (chloroquine)
4. Psychotropics (chlorpromazine, lithium)
5. Anticonvulsants (phenytoin)
6. Hormonal agents (ACTH,° corticosteroids,° thyroid hormones)
7. Miscellaneous (acetylcholinesterase inhibitors,° methoxyflurane)

° Note that some of the drugs that aggravate or unmask myasthenia are those used in therapy.

Patients with mild myasthenia should be given neostigmine bromide (Prostigmin) 15 mg or the equivalent dose of pyridostigmine bromide (Mestinon) 60 mg every four hours. Pyridostigmine bromide time-span tablets (180 mg) have a longer duration of action and may be used at night. At the next outpatient visit a Tensilon test should be performed immediately before the next dose of the anticholinesterase preparation. The physician has the option of increasing the dosage or decreasing the time between administrations of the anticholinesterase drug. In this way the optimum dose of neostigmine or pyridostigmine can be calculated for each patient. The response to anticholinesterase drugs is good in about 50 percent of patients. The administration of anticholinesterase drugs may be limited by the development of cholinergic side effects, including colic, diarrhea, blurred vision, and bradycardia. Care is needed in the administration of anticholinesterase drugs to the elderly since accumulation of acetylcholine at receptor sites in the heart may result in bradycardia, nodal rhythm, atrial fibrillation or flutter. Hypotensive syncope has also been recorded (27).

Patients with group III or the severe generalized form of myasthenia should always be admitted to the hospital for treatment. Following admission an intravenous catheter should be placed; this facilitates the performance of the Tensilon test. The patient is then given 15 mg of neostigmine or 60 mg of pyridostigmine orally. The Tensilon test is performed just before the next dose is due, and the dose of medication is increased if it is positive. Again, this method allows the devel-

opment of the optimum dose for the patient.

Some patients receive additional benefit from the administration of ephedrine sulfate 25 mg three times a day or potassium chloride 0.5 g three times a day. However, when the maximum dose of the anticholinesterase drug has been achieved, the effects of ephedrine and potassium are slight.

2. Corticosteroids. Corticosteroids are widely used in the treatment of myasthenia gravis and probably act as immunosuppressants. Corticosteroids are begun in small dosages such as 20 mg of methylprednisolone (Medrol) or prednisone (Meticorten) q.d. The dosage is gradually increased to 80 mg q.d. An equivalent dose of dexamethasone (Decadron) is equally effective. At this point the patient will show improvement in strength, and the daily dosage should be maintained until maximum benefit is obtained. The patient is then converted to alternate-day therapy to reduce the development of side effects. When the patient is stabilized on an alternate-day dosage the amount is gradually decreased until the patient begins to show signs of weakness. This maintenance dosage usually varies from 16 to 32 mg of methylprednisolone. Alternate-day corticosteroid therapy can be maintained for many years but the development of side effects will eventually occur in almost all cases. Some patients with minor degrees of weakness should receive supplementary anticholinesterase medication, but the dosage requirement is often quite low.

3. Immunosuppressant Drugs. There is a good response to immunosuppression in many cases. Azothiaprine (Imuran) 2.5 mg/kg/day is usually effective but the action is slow and improvement may not occur for many months (27). Side effects including hematologic abnormalities, gastrointestinal upsets, abnormalities in liver enzymes, and infections are not uncommon (28).

4. Thymectomy. Thymectomy can be performed with very low risk and a mortality of less than 3 percent using modern surgical techniques. The therapeutic effect of the operation was first recognized in 1939 following removal of a thymoma from a patient with myasthenia gravis. The patient showed dramatic improvement, subsequently the operation was performed whether or not a thymoma was present. There is no doubt that thymomas should be removed as soon as they are detected since they are locally invasive and can spread into the lungs. However, the use of thymectomy for treatment of myasthe-

nia gravis is viewed with varying degrees of enthusiasm in different medical centers. Results of thymectomy vary from center to center, but it is apparent that the removal of a thymoma is associated with less improvement than removal of a hyperplastic thymus gland. At present it seems that thymectomy might be reserved for refractory cases who show poor or no response to anticholinesterase drugs, costeroid therapy, and immunosuppression. The risk of the operation can be reduced if efforts are made to avoid operating on patients during crisis. The postoperative patient usually requires continued support with anticholinesterase drugs and corticosteroids but the requirements are considerably reduced.

5. Plasmaphoresis. Plasmaphoresis alone or in combination with azothiaprine is effective in myasthenia. The patient will show a good response to plasmaphoresis within a short period of treatment and this response may be maintained for as long as six months. At present it seems that this form of therapy may have to be repeated at intervals varying from three weeks to six months. The treatment is limited by availability and cost.

Treatment of Myasthenic Crisis. Myasthenic crisis should be regarded as a medical emergency. The condition generally results from a gradual failure of response to anticholinesterase drugs. This failure may be precipitated by an upper respiratory tract infection, extreme fatigue, or alcoholic intoxication. The artificial division of patients into myasthenic crisis and cholinergic crisis is no longer tenable. The patient who enters in respiratory failure should simply be diagnosed as crisis and treated as follows:

1. Respiration should be assisted by whatever means necessary until intubation can be carried out. The patient should be treated in an intensive care unit where there is constant supervision.
2. All medications should be discontinued.
3. Since myasthenia crisis is often precipitated by infection, a diligent search should be made for an infectious process. Chest x-rays should be taken to rule out pneumonia or atelectasis. Infection should be promptly treated with appropriate antibiotic therapy.
4. The patient should be instructed to suction secretions from the mouth and pharynx using a soft plastic catheter. In cases of extreme weakness this must be done regularly by those in attendance.

5. The patient should be turned every two hours in bed to prevent atelectasis and encourage the flow of secretions from the lungs. This also helps to prevent the development of decubiti.
7. When the patient is free from infection, or when infection is controlled by appropriate antibiotics, corticosteroid therapy can be commenced. The patient should be given 100 mg methylprednisone IVPB daily. Corticosteroid therapy should be supplemented by antacid therapy. The corticosteroids occasionally produce increasing weakness beginning on the second or third day after the therapy is started and reaches a maximum effect on the fifth day. This is followed by rapid recovery of strength. Some patients show an increase in strength immediately following the administration of costeroids, and in other patients there may be no response for as long as three weeks. Once improvement occurs the dosage of corticosteroids can be converted to an alternate-day basis and then gradually reduced once the patient shows good response to therapy.
8. The patient should have respiratory function tests performed at the bedside at least twice a day. The determination of vital capacity is often all that is necessary and the patient can be removed from the mechanical respirator and placed on a T-bar with oxygen when the vital capacity reaches 700 ml.
9. Once the patient is extubated he should be treated as a person with a severe generalized form of myasthenia gravis.
10. An alternative form of treating patients in crisis is to perform plasmaphoresis which reduces the circulating acetylcholine receptor antibodies and often produces dramatic improvements in myasthenia crisis.

Prognosis. The prognosis in myasthenia gravis has improved dramatically in the last decade with the introduction of corticosteroids, immunosuppressants, and plasmaphoresis. The prognosis of crisis has also improved following the widespread use of reliable mechanical respirators and the wide range of drug therapy available.

Drug-Induced Myasthenia Syndrome

Drug-induced myasthenia is characterized by reversible myasthenic symptoms associated with a particular drug. Several drugs have been reported to cause a reversible myasthenic syndrome. These include antibiotics such as colistin, gentamycin, kanamycin, neomycin, polymixin B, and streptomycin; cardiovascular drugs such as oxprenolol, practolol, trimethaphan; antirheumatic drugs; D-penicillamine; anticonvulsants such as phenytoin and trimethadione; oral contraceptives; and tetanus antitoxin.

Eaton-Lambert Syndrome (Myasthenic Syndrome)

Definition. The Eaton-Lambert syndrome is characterized and believed to represent failure of release of acetylcholine at the neuromuscular junction.

Etiology. The Eaton-Lambert syndrome is an autoimmune condition associated with a number of neoplasms, particularly oat cell carcinoma of the lung. Non-cancer Eaton-Lambert syndrome occurs in about one-third of the cases in association with other autoimmune disorders. The syndrome is believed to be due to the binding of an IgG antibody to voltage dependent calcium channels in the nerve terminal (29). These channels fail to function when depolarization occurs, leading to failure of fusion of acetylcholine containing vesicles within the nerve terminal membrane and reduction in release of acetylcholine into the synaptic cleft (30).

Clinical Features. The disorder is characterized by proximal muscle weakness, which may improve on repeated effort. Hyporeflexia, peripheral paresthesias, impotence, and dry mouth are associated features.

Respiratory failure may occur spontaneously in a few cases but the usual cause is a marked increase in sensitivity to muscle relaxant drugs, particularly to those used in anesthesia (31).

Diagnostic Procedures.

1. There is little, if any, improvement in strength with anticholinesterase medications.
2. Electromyography. There is a low-amplitude response to single stimulation and further decrease occurs with low rates of stimulation. High rates of stimulation, 50 evoked potentials per second, produce marked increase in the amplitude of the evoked motor unit potential.

Treatment.

1. Improvement occurs after removal of the neoplasm.
2. Guanidine hydrochloride may improve the weakness. The drug is administered in 25-mg tablets in divided doses beginning

with one tablet t.i.d. and slowly increased until there is a satisfactory response. Doses as high as 35 mg/kg/day may be necessary but are often unattainable because of side effects including nausea, abdominal colic, and distal paresthesias.
3. 3,4.-diaminopyridine in doses of up to 100 mg per day improves muscle strength and is probably more effective than guanidine.
4. Plasmaphoresis alone or in combination with azothiaprine produces a slow but definite improvement in the Eaton-Lambert syndrome.
5. Prednisone combined with azothiaprine has also been of benefit in some cases.

Tetanus

See page 264.

Botulism

See page 265.

Tick Paralysis

Definition. Tick paralysis is an acute onset of muscle weakness proceeding to generalized paralysis associated with the attachment and injection of venom through the skin by a gravid female tick of the species dermacentor andersoni or dermacentor variabilis in North America and Ixodes holocyclus or Ixodes cornuatus in Australia (32).

Etiology and Pathology. The condition appears to be caused by the absorption of a toxic substance that prevents depolarization at the neuromuscular junction. There are no described pathologic changes.

Clinical Features. The condition has been reported in children of both sexes, and there may be a history of exposure to ticks by playing in infested grass or woods. The symptoms appear three to five days after the tick attaches itself to the skin and are often preceded by symptoms of malaise, irritability, and diarrhea. Weakness begins in the lower extremities and spreads rapidly so that the child shows complete symmetric paralysis of all voluntary muscles within 24 hours. Bulbar or respiratory muscle involvement can occur, and assisted respiration may be necessary. Examination reveals attachment of the tick, which is frequently obscured by hair on the scalp of the patient.

Diagnostic Procedures.

1. The history of possible exposure to ticks is helpful.
2. The diagnosis is established by finding the tick.

Treatment. Improvement occurs when the tick is removed. This can be accomplished by the application of petroleum jelly and removal some 20 minutes later with forceps pressed down on either side of the mouth parts to grasp the hypostome of the tick, then gentle detachment by lifting or an upward levering action.

INFLAMMATORY MUSCLE DISEASE

Myositis is an inflammation of muscle characterized pathologically by an inflammatory cell infiltrate in the muscle and clinically by weakness and occasionally tenderness of the involved muscles.

Viral Myositis

Acute viral myositis is unusual but can occasionally occur in epidemic form (epidemic pleurodynia or Bornholm disease).

Etiology and Pathology. Viral infections associated with acute myositis include Coxsackie group B, ECHO, influenza types A and B, and HIV (AIDS) (33).

Muscle biopsy shows evidence of myositis with fiber degeneration and phagocytosis, fiber regeneration, and perivascular inflammation.

Clinical Features. Acute viral myositis presents with sudden onset of severe muscular pain, which is exacerbated by movement. The pain may be confined to the intercostal and abdominal muscles (pleurodynia) or involve the neck and limb girdle muscles. The patient is febrile and often in severe distress due to myalgia and headache. Myoglobinuria can occur with the risk of renal failure. There may be an associated aseptic meningitis. The condition may be more insidious in some cases in which the patient experiences generalized muscle weakness during and following a febrile illness.

Diagnostic Procedures.

1. Serum tests. There is a polymorphonucleocytosis occasionally with eosinophilia. Serum CPK is elevated; isoenzyme study indicates a muscle origin with elevation of the M band. Levels of LDH, GOT, GPT, and aldolase are also frequently elevated.
2. The CSF shows a lymphocytic pleocytosis in cases with an associated aseptic meningitis.
3. Virus can be cultured from blood, CSF, nasopharynx, urine, or muscle. A rising titer of viral antibodies can be detected in serum over a two-week period.
4. Muscle biopsy will confirm the myositis.

Treatment. Adequate doses of a narcotic drug are needed to control pain during the first few days of acute viral myositis. The pain is often excruciating and will not respond to simple analgesics. Myoglobinuria may precipitate renal failure; oliguria and anuria should be promptly treated.

Postpoliomyelitis, Progressive Muscular Atrophy

Some individuals suffering from residual muscle weakness resulting from poliomyelitis develop new weakness and increasing atrophy years after recovery from the primary illness.

Etiology and Pathology. The condition is probably the result of excessive distal sprouting and motor unit enlargement followed by inability of the motor neuron to meet metabolic demands and atrophy of some nerve terminals (34). Muscles weakened by the original illness show areas of myopathy, recent and old neurogenic changes, while muscles originally unaffected show recent and old denervation and reinnervation.

Clinical Features. The affected muscles were previously involved by acute poliomyelitis or may have appeared to be clinically uninvolved at that time. A period of quiescence of many years duration is followed by the development of new symptoms of muscle weakness, fatigue, atrophy and fasciculations.

Diagnostic Procedures. The muscle biopsy will contain changes as described above.

Treatment. There is no effective treatment for this condition.

Bacterial Myositis

Bacterial myositis is most often the result of infection with *Clostridia*. Rare examples of infections by *Staphylococcus aureus* or *Streptococcus pyogenes* have been reported (35).

Etiology and Pathology. The organism usually involved is *Clostridium perfringens.*

Clostridial organisms proliferate under anaerobic conditions, and infection usually results from the presence of the bacteria in deep puncture wounds, compound fractures, or penetrating gunshot wounds. The clostridial exotoxin produces coagulation necrosis of muscle and breakdown of muscle glycogen with the production of carbon dioxide, which spreads through the muscle and subcutaneous tissues (gas gangrene).

Clinical Features. Patients with bacterial myositis and gas gangrene present with high fever, tachycardia, and shock due to the potent effect of the clostridial exotoxin. The affected muscles are swollen, and the presence of gas in the tissues causes crepitus on palpation.

Treatment.

1. Affected muscles should be incised, exposed, and drained.
2. Penicillin, 40 million units IV, should be administered q24h until wound cultures are sterile.
3. Hyperbaric oxygen is beneficial if available.
4. Amputation of an affect limb may be necessary in extreme cases.

Prognosis. Gas gangrene carries a high mortality unless treated immediately. All cases should be regarded as a surgical emergency.

Granulomatous Myositis

Granulomatous lesions have been seen in muscle in patients with tertiary syphilis, miliary tuberculosis, sarcoidosis, and toxoplasmosis.

The myopathy of sarcoidosis is rare and presents with chronic wasting and proximal muscle weakness. The diagnosis is established by muscle biopsy. Prolonged low dose prednisone therapy may be necessary to control the disease (36).

Trichinosis

Definition. Trichinosis is a myositis caused by the larvae of the nematode *Trichinella spiralis.*

Etiology and Pathology. Man is infected by eating raw pork products containing larvae of *Trichinella spiralis.* The larvae are liberated in the intestinal tract and develop into adult worms. After seven days the fertilized female burrows into the intestinal wall and deposits larva in the lymphatics. This process continues for about four weeks. The larvae enter the systemic circulation and are carried to all tissues but are able to survive only in skeletal muscle. The larvae grow in muscle fibers and assume a spiral form. The presence of the foreign body causes an intense inflammatory reaction, which is sufficient to kill some of the larvae. The survivors develop a connective tissue capsule in about six weeks and begin to calcify after six months. Larvae may survive for many years following an infection.

Clinical Features. Ingestion of contaminated pork products may be followed by a mild gastroenteritis. The entrance of larvae into skeletal muscles is followed by fever, severe myalgia, muscle weakness, and tenderness. Movements of the eyes, face, tongue, jaw, and neck are often painful and restricted, and there may be marked periorbital and facial edema. Intercostal muscle and diaphragmatic involvement restricts respiratory movements, which can be extremely painful. Myocardial involvement is unusual but may result in acute heart failure and death. Trichinella encephalitis is a rare but life threatening complication (37).

Diagnostic Procedures.

1. There is a polymorphonucleocytosis with a marked eosinophilia. Serum complement-fixation, precipitin, and flocculation tests are positive after three weeks.
2. The diagnosis can be confirmed by muscle biopsy, which reveals the presence of larvae.
3. A positive skin reaction can be obtained after two weeks following the intradermal injection of *Trichinella* antigen.
4. MR or CT scanning will demonstrate multifocal lesions in the brain in patients with neurotrichinosis.

Treatment.

1. The patient should be confined to strict bed rest because of the risk of heart failure. Adequate analgesia should be given to control pain.
2. Corticosteroids. Methylprednisolone 100 mg q am should be given and converted to alternate-day dosage as improvement occurs.
3. Flubendazole 40 mg/kg/day prevents larvae production and is toxic to larvae in muscle and brain (38).
4. Heart failure may be treated with fluid restriction, digitalization, low salt diet, and diuretics.

Prognosis. Recovery occurs in about six weeks in untreated cases. Treatment probably shortens this recovery period.

Cysticercosis

Myositis may occur during infection with *Taenia solium.*

Echinococcosis

Myositis may occur during infection with *Echinococcus granulosus.*

Polymyositis, Dermatomyositis

Definition. Polymyositis is an inflammatory disease of skeletal muscle of unknown etiology. When there is evidence of skin involvement the term "dermatomyositis" is used.

Etiology and Pathology. The etiology is unknown but is believed by some to be an autoimmune reaction initiated by virus infection, including the AIDS virus (39). The condition may be associated with malignancy, rheumatoid arthritis, Sjogren's syndrome, polymyalgia rheumatica, scleroderma, systemic lupus erythematosus, polyarteritis nodosa, sarcoidosis, and Wegener's granulomatosis (40).

Pathologic changes consist of inflammatory infiltration of skeletal muscle with necrosis of fibers and active phagocytosis. Central nuclei and evidence of active regeneration are seen. It is believed that the junctional sites of transverse tubules and sarcoplasmic reticulum may be the primary site of sarcoplasmic enzyme leakage. A distinct rare form of polymyositis with intranuclear and cytoplasmic inclusions: inclusion body myositis can be recognized by electron microscopy (41).

Diagnostic Procedures.

1. Polymorphonucleocytosis, lymphocytosis, hypoalbuminemia, anemia, elevated sedimentation rate, positive rheumatoid factor, antibodies to nuclear antigens (ANA), and elevated serum muscle enzymes may be present.
2. Electromyography is consistent with a myopathic process, but fibrillations, positive sharp waves, and bizarre high-frequency discharges are often present.
3. The electrocardiogram is often abnormal since there is a high prevalence of cardiac involvement in polymyositis (42).
4. A diligent search should be made for an occult neoplasm in all cases of dermatomyositis and in adult middle-aged males with polymyositis.

Treatment.

1. Treatment of any identified associated condition may reduce the symptoms.
2. Corticosteroids. Polymyositis frequently responds to prednisone 100 mg q.d. The dosage should be converted to alternate-day therapy as soon as possible to minimize side effects, then reduced to the minimum effective dose, which will control symptoms.
3. Steroid-resistant cases may repond to methotrexate, cyclophosphamide (Cytoxan), azathioprine (Imuran), or cyclosporin.
4. Immune serum globulin IV 1 g/kg/day for two consecutive days each month may produce improvement in refractory cases (43).

Prognosis. The outlook for patients with polymyositis has improved considerably since the introduction of corticosteroid therapy. However, the condition can still be fatal when progressive involvement of respiratory muscles leads to respiratory failure (44). Bedridden patients may die from pulmonary infection (44). Prolonged paralysis is a rare occurrence after anesthesia with nondepolarizing neuromuscular blocking agents. Inclusion body myositis is highly resistant to current available therapy.

MISCELLANEOUS SIGNS OF MUSCLE DISORDER

Myoglobinuria

Any disorder in which muscle cell membranes are disrupted, allowing leakage of muscle protein, may be characterized by myoglobinuria. Trauma; exercise; myositis; heat stroke; cold; diabetic acidosis; toxins such as alcohol, heroin, cocaine (45), licorice, amphotericin B, succinylcholine, epsilon aminocaproic acid, phenylpropanolamine (diet pills) (46), and IV amphetamines; ischemic insults; and certain myopathies including polymyositis, phosphorylase deficiency, phosphofructokinase deficiency, carnitine deficiency and muscle palmitoyltransferase-A deficiency may produce myoglobinuria (47). If myoglobin precipitates in renal tubules it may produce oliguric or anuric renal failure. An idiopathic form of myoglobinuria occurs and is characterized clinically by muscle weakness, pain, tenderness, cramping, and edema (48).

Myokymia

Myokymia is characterized by involuntary, fine contractions of muscle. Facial myokymia is usually a benign condition occurring in anxiety, fatigue, and ill health but has been reported in multiple sclerosis and rarely in pontine tumors. Benign myokymia is a familial disorder and consists of myokymia and painful muscle cramps, which involve the majority of the muscles of the body. There is no weakness, and electromyographic studies clearly differentiate myokymia from fasciculations.

REFERENCES

1. Barohn, R. J.; Levine, E. J.; *et al.* Gastric hypomotility in Duchenne's muscular dystrophy. N. Engl. J. Med. 319:15–18; 1988.
2. Whelan, T. B. Neuropsychological perfor-

mance of children with Duchenne muscular dystrophy and spinal muscular atrophy. Dev. Med. Child. Neurol. 29:212–220; 1987.

3. Smith, P. E. M.; Calverley, P. M. A.; *et al.* Practical problems in the respiratory care of patients with muscular dystrophy. N. Engl. J. Med. 316:1197–1205; 1987.

4. Greenberg, C. R.; Jacobs, H. K. Gene studies in newborn males with Duchenne muscular dystrophy detected by neonatal screening. Lancet 2:425–427; 1988.

5. Wood, S.; Shukin, R. J. Prenatal diagnosis in Becker muscular dystrophy. Clin. Genet. 31:45–47; 1987.

6. Heene, R.; Gabriel, R-R.; *et al.* Type 2B muscle fiber deficiency in myotonia and paramyotonia congenita. J. Neurol. Sci. 73:23–30; 1986.

7. Treatment of myotonia editorial. Lancet 1:1242–1244; 1987.

8. Trudell, R. G.; Kaise, K. K.; *et al.* Acetazolamide responsive myotonia congenita. Neurology 37:488–491; 1987.

9. Benstead, T. J.; Camfield, P. R.; *et al.* Treatment of paramyotonia congenita with acetazolamide. Can. J. Neurol. Sci. 14:156–158; 1987.

10. Streib, E. W. Paramyotonia congenita successfully treated with tocainide. Muscle Nerve 10:155–162; 1987.

11. Hudson, A. J.; Huff, M. W.; *et al.* The role of insulin resistance in the pathogenesis of myotonic muscular dystrophy. Brain 110:469–488; 1987.

12. Moorman, J. R.; Coleman, R. E.; *et al.* Cardiac involvement in myotonic muscular dystrophy. Medicine 64:371–387; 1985.

13. Wright, R. B.; Glantz, R. H.; *et al.* Hearing loss in myotonic dystrophy. Ann. Neurol. 23:202–203; 1988.

14. Cros, D.; Harden, P.; *et al.* Peripheral neuropathy in myotonic dystrophy: A nerve biopsy study. Ann. Neurol. 23:470–476; 1988.

15. Hiromasa, S.; Ikeda, T.; *et al.* Myotonic dystrophy: Ambulatory electrocardiogram, electrophysiologic study and echocardiographic evaluation. Am. Heart. J. 113:1482–1488; 1987.

16. Autahami, E.; Katz, A.; *et al.* Computed tomographic findings of brain and skull in myotonic dystrophy. J. Neurol. Neurosurg. Psychiatry 50:435–438; 1987.

17. Grant, R.; Sutton, D. L.; *et al.* Nefedipine in the treatment of myotonia in myotonic dystrophy. J. Neurol. Neurosurg. Psychiatry 50:199–206; 1987.

18. Moore, J. K.; Moore, A. P. Postoperative complications of dystrophia myotonica. Anaesthesia 42:529–533; 1987.

19. Merlini, L.; Muttutini, P.; *et al.* Non-progressive central core disease with severe congenital scoliosis: A case report. Dev. Med. Child. Neurol. 29:106–109; 1987.

20. Ono, S.; Inouye K.; *et al.* Myopathology of hypothyroid myopathy. J. Neurol. Sci. 77:237–248; 1987.

21. DiMauro, S.; Miranda, A. F.; *et al.* Metabolic myopathies. Am J. Med. Genet. 25:635–651; 1986.

22. Zeviani, M.; Peterson, P.; *et al.* Benign reversible muscle cytochrome c oxidase deficiency—a second case. Neurology 37:64–67; 1987.

23. Rudeman, M. I.; Zito, G. Metabolic myopathies. N. J. Med. 83:36–40; 1986.

24. Kungl, R. W.; Duncan, G.; *et al.* Colchicine myopathy and neuropathy. N. Engl. J. Med. 316:1562–1568; 1987.

25. DeKeyser, J.; Smitz, J.; *et al.* Rhabdomyolysis in hypokalemic periodic paralysis: A clue to the mechanism that terminates the paralytic attack. J. Neurol. 234:119–121; 1987.

26. Soliven, B. C.; Lange, D. J.; *et al.* Seronegative myasthenia gravis. Neurology 38:514–517; 1988.

27. Arsura, E. L.; Brunner, N. G.; *et al.* Adverse cardiovascular effects of anticholinesterase medications. Am. J. Med. Sci. 293:18–23; 1987.

28. Hohlfeld, R.; Michels, M.; *et al.* Azothioprine toxicity during long-term immunosuppression of generalized myasthenia gravis. Neurology 38:258–261; 1988.

29. Nagel, A.; Engel, A. G.; *et al.* Lambert-Eaton myasthenic syndrome IgG depletes presynaptic membrane active zone particles by antigenic modulation. Ann. Neurol. 24:552–558; 1988.

30. Newsom-David, J. The Lambert-Eaton syndrome. In: Johnson, R. T. (ed), *Current Therapy in Neurologic Disease.* Toronto, Decker pp. 371–375; 1985.

31. Gracey, D. R.; Southorn, P. A. Respiratory failure in Lambert-Eaton myasthenic syndrome. Chest 91:716–718; 1987.

32. Tibballs, J.; Cooper, S. J. Paralysis with ixodes cornuatus envenomation. Med. J. Aust. 145:37–38; 1986.

33. Bailey, R. O.; Turok, D. I.; *et al.* Myositis and acquired immunodeficiency syndrome. Hum. Pathol. 18:749–751; 1987.

34. Dalakas, M. C. Morphologic changes in the muscle of patients with post-poliomyelitis neuromuscular symptoms. Neurology 38:99–104; 1988.

35. Yoder, E.; Mendez, J.; *et al.* Spontaneous gangrenous myositis induced by streptococcus pyogenes: Case report and review of the literature. Rev. Infect. Dis. 9:382–385; 1987.

36. Wolfe, S. M.; Pinab, R. S.; *et al.* Myopathy in sarcoidosis: Clinical and pathologic study of four cases and review of the literature. Semin. Arthritis Rheum. 16:300–306; 1987.

37. Ryczak, M.; Sorber, W. A.; *et al.* Difficulties in diagnosing trichinella encephalitis. Am. J. Trop. Med. Hyg. 36:573–575; 1987.

38. Ellrodt, A.; Halton, P.; *et al.* Multifocal central nervous system lesions in three patients with trichinosis. Arch. Neurol. 44:432–434; 1987.

39. Dalakas, M. C.; Pezeshkpour, G. H.; *et al.* Polymyositis associated with AIDS retrovirus. JAMA 256:2381–2383; 1986.

40. Pfeiffer, J. Classification of myositis. Correlation between morphological and clinical classifications of inflammatory muscle disease. Path. Res. Pract. 182:141–156; 1987.

41. Calabrese, L. H.; Mitsumoto, H.; *et al.* Inclusion body myositis presenting as a treatment—resistant polymyositis. Arthritis Rheum. 30:397–403; 1987.

42. Behan, W. M. H.; Behan, P. O.; *et al.* Cardiac damage in polymyositis associated with antibodies to tissue ribonucleoproteins. Br. Heart J. 57:176–180; 1987.

43. Roitman, C. M.; Schaffer, F. M.; *et al.* Reversal of chronic polymyositis following intravenous immune serum globulin therapy. JAMA 258:513–515; 1987.

44. Lakhonpal, S.; Lie, J. T.; *et al.* Pulmonary disease in polymyositis/dermatomyositis: a clinicopathological analysis of 65 autopsy cases. Ann. Rheum. Dis. 46:23–29; 1987.

45. Merigian, K. S.; Roberts, J. R.; *et al.* Cocaine intoxication: Hyperpyrexia, rhabdomyolysis and acute renal failure. Clin. Tox. 25:135–148; 1987.

46. Forwell, M. A.; Hallworth, M. J. Non-traumatic rhabdomyolysis and acute renal failure. Scott. Med. J. 31:246–249; 1986.

47. Ross, N. S.; Hoppel, C. L. Partial muscle carnitine palmitoyltransferase-A deficiency. Rhabdomyolysis associated with transiently decreased muscle carnitine content after Ibuprofen therapy. JAMA 257:62–65; 1987.

48. Haverkort, P. J. E.; Joosten, E. M. G.; *et al.* Prevention of recurrent exertional rhabdomyolysis by Dantrolene sodium. Muscle Nerve 10:45–46; 1987.

INDEX